VIBRATION EFFECTS
ON THE HAND AND ARM
IN INDUSTRY

VIBRATION EFFECTS ON THE HAND AND ARM IN INDUSTRY

EDITED BY

A.J. Brammer
Division of Physics
National Research Council of Canada
Ottawa, Ontario, Canada

W. Taylor
Professor Emeritus
Department of Occupational Medicine
University of Dundee
Dundee, Scotland

A Wiley-Interscience Publication
JOHN WILEY & SONS
New York • Chichester • Brisbane • Toronto • Singapore

Library of Congress Cataloging in Publication Data:

International Symposium on Hand-Arm Vibration (3rd :
    1981 : Ottawa, Ont.)
    Vibration effects on the hand and arm in industry.

    English and French.
    Includes index.
    1. Vibration syndrome—Congresses.   2. Hand—Diseases
—Congresses.   3. Arm—Diseases—Congresses.
4. Occupational diseases—Congresses.   I. Brammer,
A. J.   II. Taylor, W. (William), 1911–
III. Title.

RC963.5.V5I58 1981   617'.57   82-24819
ISBN 0-471-88954-7

Printed in the United States of America

10 9 8 7 6 5 4 3 2 1

Preface

Exposure of the hand to vibration, leading to "white fingers" and "dead hand", is rapidly becoming recognized as an important occupational health hazard. It commonly occurs in industries that are essential to the economies of developing and industrialized countries - mining, forestry, metal-working and others in which hand-held power tools, such as pneumatic hammers, chain saws and grinders, are used. Methods for quantifying vibration exposures and their effects on man are still being developed. The mechanisms whereby vibration affects the nerves, blood vessels, and musculo-skeletal system are still being explored. As a result, there is no generally accepted limit for exposure, nor method of assessing impairment. Thus, the determination of a worker's disability is frequently a matter for litigation.

This book provides, by means of reviews and original work by acknowledged experts in the field, up-to-date information on these and related subjects. The papers have been grouped by subject to emphasize the measurement of vibration exposure, the effects of vibration on man, and the links between them in so-called dose-response relationships. These topics are complemented by papers treating the equally important subjects of objective tests for diagnosis, methods for reducing vibration exposure, and the legal ramifications for workers who become disabled.

The book is based on oral presentations at the Third International Conference on Hand-Arm Vibration, held in Ottawa (May 1981). The papers have been reviewed and edited. Matters in dispute and requiring clarification that arose during the editorial process are included in the Discussion at the end of each paper. Our introduction provides continuity and highlights major areas of concern. A subject index has also been provided to ensure ready access to treatments of similar or interrelated topics by different authors. In this way, we hope that this broadly-based collection will serve the needs of both the expert and the novice. We believe this book will be of interest to research workers and professionals concerned with occupational health, industrial hygiene, vibration acoustics, mechanical engineering, and the regulatory process.

A.J. Brammer
W. Taylor

November, 1982

Assistant Editors

Acknowledgements

We are indebted to the National Research Council of Canada, Health and Welfare Canada, and to the Acoustical Society of America for co-sponsoring the Third International Conference on Hand-Arm Vibration, on which this book is based. We also wish to express our appreciation to the Contributors, Assistant Editors, members of the Editorial Board, and to members of the Conference Organizing Committee - Dee Benwell, Hie Lee and Mike Stinson, without whose efforts this collection of papers would not have been possible.

We wish to acknowledge the many contributions to the preparation of this book, both material and professional, made by the Division of Physics, National Research Council of Canada. In particular, we would like to express our gratitude to the Head of the Acoustics Section, Dr. Edgar A.G. Shaw, for his continuing support, and to the members of the Acoustics Section for their patience and efforts in processing manuscripts, especially John Quaroni, Marina Vaillancourt and Guyane Seguin. We also wish to acknowledge the contribution of the staff of the Design Office and of Helen Cuccaro, who are responsible for the illustrations and design of the text. The layout and typing were performed by Lena Roger, to whose diligence and consummate skill this book will remain a permanent testimonial.

Contents

TOOL AND MACHINE VIBRATION

DOSE-EFFECT RELATIONS, EXPOSURE LIMITS AND STANDARDS

METHODS FOR REDUCING VIBRATION EXPOSURE

LEGAL IMPLICATIONS

Contributors

Aatola, S.A., Institute of Occupational Health, Helsinki, Finland.

Akinmayowa, N.K., Department of Psychology, University of Lagos, Lagos, Nigeria.

Ariizumi, M., Department of Public Health, School of Medicine, Kanazawa University, Kanazawa, Japan.

Asburry, W., National Institute for Occupational Safety and Health, Cincinnati, Ohio, U.S.A.

Auerbach, E.I., Sound and Vibration, Ingersoll-Rand, Easton, Pennsylvania, U.S.A.

Azuma, T., Department of Physiology, Shinshu University School of Medicine, Matsumoto, Japan.

Bakirzade, J.P., Institut National de Recherche et de Sécurité, Vandoeuvre-les-Nancy, France.

Basel, R., Westinghouse Corporation, Pittsburgh, Pennsylvania, U.S.A.

Behrens, V., National Institute for Occupational Safety and Health, Cincinnati, Ohio, U.S.A.

Bentley, S., Science & Technology Laboratories, Fisons Pharmaceuticals, Loughborough, England.

Bjerker, N., National Board of Occupational Safety and Health, Stockholm, and University of Umeå, Umeå, Sweden.

Brammer, A.J., Division of Physics, National Research Council of Canada, Ottawa, Ontario, Canada.

Chiba, M., III Department of Medicine, Kurume University School of Medicine, Kurume, Japan.

Corlett, E.N., Department of Production Engineering and Production Management, University of Nottingham, Nottingham, England.

Di Renzo, N., Institut National de Recherche et de Sécurité, Vandoeuvre-les-Nancy, France.

Doyle, T.E., National Institute for Occupational Safety and Health, Cincinnati, Ohio, U.S.A.

Edmonds, O.P., Occupational Health Service, University of Manchester, Manchester, England.

Eglin, D., Teesside Laboratories, British Steel Corporation, Middlesbrough, Cleveland, England.

Falkenberg, R.J., Alcoa Aluminum, Pittsburgh, Pennsylvania, U.S.A.

Färkkilä, M.A., Department of Neurology, University Hospital of Helsinki, Helsinki, Finland.

Fujinaga, H., Department of Public Health, School of Medicine, Kanazawa University, Kanazawa, Japan.

Fukui, T., Nagashima & Ohno, Tokyo, Japan.

Gibbs, G.W., Institute of Occupational Health and Safety, McGill University, Montreal, Quebec, Canada.

Griffin, M.J., Institute of Sound and Vibration Research, The University, Southampton, England.

Hagelthorn, G., National Board of Occupational Safety and Health, Stockholm, and University of Umeå, Umeå, Sweden.

Hanks, J.M., Department of Biological and Agricultural Engineering, North Carolina State University, Raleigh, North Carolina, U.S.A.

Harada, N., Department of Hygiene, Yamaguchi University School of Medicine, Ube, Japan.

Harrison, R.T., U.S.D.A. Forest Service, San Dimas, California, U.S.A.

Hart, W.F.D., Tanfield Associates, England.

Hoikkala, M.J., Institute of Occupational Health, Helsinki, Finland.

Holt, S., Homelite-Textron Incorporated, Charlotte, North Carolina, U.S.A.

Hursh, H.J., John Deere Medical Department, East Moline, Illinois, U.S.A.

Hyvärinen, J., Department of Physiology, University of Helsinki, Helsinki, Finland.

Itoh, N., Department of Public Health, Wakayama Medical College, Wakayama, Japan.

Iwata, H., Department of Public Health, Wakayama Medical College, Wakayama, Japan.

Kasamatsu, T., Department of Public Health, Wakayama Medical College, Wakayama, Japan.

Korhonen, O.S., Institute of Occupational Health, Helsinki, Finland.

Lidström, I-M., Health Department, Telefonaktiebolaget L.M. Ericsson, Stockholm, and University of Umeå, Umeå, Sweden.

Lindquist, B., Atlas Copco Tools AB, Stockholm, Sweden.

Lombard, R., Homelite-Textron Incorporated, Charlotte, North Carolina, U.S.A.

Lord, P., Department of Applied Acoustics, University of Salford, Salford, England.

Lukáš, E., Institute of Hygiene and Epidemiology, Centre of Industrial Hygiene and Occupational Diseases, Prague, Czechoslovakia.

Macfarlane, C.R., Institute of Sound and Vibration Research, University of Southampton, Southampton, England.

Matoba, T., III Department of Medicine, Kurume University School of Medicine, Kurume, Japan.

Matsumoto, T., Department of Public Health, Nagoya City University Medical School, Nagoya, Japan.

Mereau, P., Institut National de Recherche et de Sécurité, Vandoeuvre-les-Nancy, France.

Miwa, T., Department of Human Environmental Engineering, National Institute of Industrial Health, Kawasaki, Japan.

Miyashita, K., Department of Public Health, Wakayama Medical College, Wakayama, Japan.

Murphy, W.A., Tony Murphy Incorporated, Valyermo, California, U.S.A.

Norman, C.D., Institute of Sound and Vibration Research, University of Southampton, Southampton, England.

O'Connor, D.E., Department of Applied Acoustics, University of Salford, Salford, England.

Ohhashi, T., Department of Physiology, Shinshu University School of Medicine, Matsumoto, Japan.

Okada, A., Department of Public Health, School of Medicine, Kanazawa University, Kanazawa, Japan.

Oliver, T.P., Main Medical Centre, HM Navy Base, Portsmouth, England.

Paterson, J.C., Barrister and Solicitor, Vancouver, British Columbia, Canada.

Pathak, B.P., Institute of Occupational Health and Safety, McGill University, Montreal, Quebec, Canada.

Pelnar, P.V., Institute of Occupational and Environmental Health, Montreal, and Department of Epidemiology, McGill University, Montreal, Quebec, Canada.

Pyykkö, I., Department of Otolaryngology, University Hospital of Lund, Lund, Sweden.

Rasmussen, G., Bruel & Kjaer, Naerum, Denmark.

Reynolds, D.D., Joiner-Pelton-Rose, Incorporated, Consultants in Acoustics, Dallas, Texas, U.S.A.

Riddle, H.F.V., Civil Service Department Medical Advisory Service, Edinburgh, Scotland.

Roberson, G.T., Department of Biological and Agricultural Engineering, North Carolina State University, Raleigh, North Carolina, U.S.A.

Rodgers, L.A., Teesside Laboratories, British Steel Corporation, Middlesbrough, Cleveland, England.

Roure, L., Institut National de Recherche et de Sécurité, Vandoeuvre-les-Nancy, France.

Shiomi, S., Department of Public Health, Wakayama Medical College, Wakayama, Japan.

Sivayoganathan, K., Department of Production Engineering and Production Management, University of Nottingham, Nottingham, England.

Starck, J.P., Institute of Occupational Health, Helsinki, Finland.

Suggs, C.W., Department of Biological and Agricultural Engineering, North Carolina State University, Raleigh, North Carolina, U.S.A.

Taylor, W., Professor Emeritus, University of Dundee, Department of Occupational Medicine, Dundee, Scotland.

Tominaga, Y., Institute for Science of Labour, Kawasaki, Japan.

Toshima, H., III Department of Medicine, Kurume University School of
     Medicine, Kurume, Japan.

Wasserman, D.E., National Institute for Occupational Safety and Health,
     Cincinnati, Ohio, U.S.A.

Wilson, F.L., Garrett, Air Research Industrial Division, Torrance,
     California, U.S.A.

VIBRATION EFFECTS
ON THE HAND AND ARM
IN INDUSTRY

Vibration Effects on the Hand and Arm in Industry: An Introduction and Review

W. Taylor and A. J. Brammer

ABSTRACT: The effects of vibration on the hand and arm in industry are introduced, with emphasis on the common vascular and neurological symptoms. The
pathophysiology and differential diagnosis of these disorders is discussed,
together with schemes for classifying signs, symptoms and interference with
activities, and objective clinical tests. The factors influencing the severity
of vibration exposure and the measurement of vibration entering the hands from
power tools and machines are next considered. Finally, relations between vibration exposure and the development of some components of the Vibration Syndrome
are considered, as well as methods for limiting the consequences of occupational
exposure of the hand to vibration.

RESUME: Les effets des vibrations sur la main et le bras en industrie sont
introduits avec emphase sur les symptômes vasculaire et neurologique communs.
On discute du diagnotique pathophysiologique et différentiel de ces troubles
et des tests cliniques objectifs. On dresse aussi des plans pour classifier les
signes et symptômes de ces troubles et comment ils nuissent aux activités
quotidiens. On considère ensuite les facteurs qui influencent la gravité de
l'exposition aux vibrations et la mesure des vibrations pénétrant dans les mains
des machines et outils mécaniques. Finallement, on examine les relations entre
l'exposition aux vibrations et le développement de certains aspects du syndrome
de vibration ainsi que des méthodes pour limiter les conséquences de l'exposition
professionelle des mains aux vibrations.

INTRODUCTION

Operators of hand-held, vibrating
power tools have long complained of tingling and numbness in their hands and of
fingers blanching. These episodes of "white
fingers", "dead fingers", or "angioneurosis"
were first reported in the literature between 1911 and 1920, in the classic studies
by Loriga (1), Hamilton (2), Rothstein (3)
and Leake (4). The spasm of the arteries
in the fingers was correctly attributed to
the vibration of the rotary-percussive air
driven drills used by stonecutters and rock
miners. It was also recognized that the
vascular signs and symptoms resembled the
spontaneous vasoconstrictive phenomena
induced by exposure to cold, first described
by Raynaud in 1862, "where persons who are
ordinarily females see under the least
stimulus one or more fingers becoming white
and cold all at once, the determining cause
being the impression of cold" (5). This
clinical entity, seen to the extent of from
5 to 10% in the population, in otherwise
normal, healthy individuals, is known to
this day as *Primary Raynaud's Disease*. The

etiology of this condition is unknown and
no qualifying term can be added. With
increasing medical knowledge, however, many
causes of white fingers are now recognized,
including vibration, and these are collectively referred to as causing *Secondary
Raynaud's Phenomenon*.

With increasing technological development in the first half of this century, the
use of vibrating hand tools expanded. Out-
breaks of "white finger" arising from both
pneumatically and electrically driven tools
were reported by Seyring (6), Hunt (7),
Telford (8), Agate (9) and others. The
close association between white finger
attacks and the vibration entering the hands
led to the introduction of the descriptive
term *Vibration-Induced White Finger* (VWF).
For a time the description of traumatic
vasospastic disease was preferred by some
workers. However, it was already becoming
recognized that the vibration stimulus was
affecting components in the hand and arm
other than the vasculature, and that degenerative changes were associated with three
additional systems (10-14):
1) the peripheral nervous system;

2) tendons, muscles, bones and joints; and 3) the central nervous system. Thus, vibration-exposed persons have commonly reported paresthesia and sensory loss in the fingers, with loss of light touch, pain and temperature sensation between episodic white finger attacks. Recently, there have been reports of loss of grip strength, indicating involvement of the motor nerves and muscles (15). There is also some evidence of bone cysts in the fingers and wrists, of joint degeneration in the wrist and elbow, and of vegetative responses implying the involvement of the central nervous system. With increasing appreciation of the effects of vibration on the hand and arm, the nomenclature for this clinical entity clearly required expansion. The complex of VWF and the associated pathology occurring in other systems, in addition to the arterial system, are now termed the *Vibration Syndrome* (VS).

Acceptance of the Vibration Syndrome as an industrial disease has been hampered by several factors. Among these are:
1) the lack of recognition of the Vibration Syndrome by physicians;
2) the difficulty distinguishing between the Vibration Syndrome and other causes of similar signs and symptoms;
3) the trivial nature of the impairment in cases where there is no evidence of reduced work performance or any time lost, on or off the job; and
4) the absence of an objective test to assess impairment, much reliance having to be placed on the subject's own history of the frequency and severity of attacks, and their interference with his activities.

In this paper, the signs and symptoms commonly associated with the Vibration Syndrome are introduced, together with their underlying pathophysiology, their classification by severity, and methods for diagnosis. The factors influencing the vibration exposure of individuals and its measurement are next discussed. Finally, relations between vibration exposure and the development of some components of the Vibration Syndrome are considered, as well as methods for limiting the adverse health effects resulting from intense vibration habitually entering the hands.

I PATHOPHYSIOLOGY OF COMMON DISORDERS

When the hands are first exposed to vibration, a person will usually report tingling followed by numbness of his fingers. After regular, prolonged exposure, the fingers feel swollen, painful and inflexible, these symptoms subsiding during a weekend break from work. With further exposure (usually measured in years), the blanching of a fingertip occurs, usually in winter. This episodic blanching of fingertips, generally precipitated by cold, is often not associated with the use of vibrating tools. The time interval between the first exposure to vibration and the appearance of a white fingertip is known as the latent interval, and is related to the amplitude or level of vibration entering the hand. The shorter the latent interval, the more rapid is the rate of progression of disorders. With continuing vibration exposure, the blanching occurring during an attack extends from the fingertip to the base of the finger. Further exposure leads to the involvement of other fingers, principally those in contact with the most intense vibration. At this stage, the affected areas are often asymmetrically distributed on the hands (16). Ultimately, three or four digits bilaterally are involved, the thumb being the last to be affected.

Of equal concern as the vasospasms is the involvement of the peripheral nerves, as evidenced by complaints of numbness and paresthesia of the fingers or hands. These symptoms can cause disturbance of sleep by awakening the worker. With sufficient vibration exposure, there are measurable reductions in grip strength (15), in tactile sensitivity and in manipulative dexterity (17).

The arterial ischemia producing the blanching, the venostasis and the reactive hyperemia, all provoked by a cold stimulus, are the main phenomena of the Vibration Syndrome. At the same time, degenerative changes in the Pacinian corpuscles of the fingers give rise to tingling, numbness and paresthesia. The neurological changes run concurrently with the vasoconstrictive process, but from evidence elsewhere in this volume occur independently (18). In advanced cases, the episodes of blanching are replaced by a continuous cyanotic appearance of the fingers, the ability of the blood vessels to constrict and dilate being lost, and the lumen becoming progressively reduced. In a small number of cases (<1%), this may lead to malnutrition and atrophy of the skin at the fingertips, resulting in tissue necrosis and gangrene. Fortunately, these late manifestations of VWF are rare, since severe cases are removed (or voluntarily withdraw) from work involving vibration exposure. Regrettably, it is the loyal, dedicated worker who, unwilling to transfer to other employment and so lose his acquired skills, is most at risk.

As a person's vibration exposure increases, so the number and severity of his white finger attacks also increase, indicating that the underlying pathology is related to the cumulative energy entering the hands. The vascular tree within the fingers is the main target. Blood flow is reduced with occlusion of the digital artery, both during a VWF attack and in the basal resting state, and especially under conditions produced in a "cold" provocation test.

Raynaud assumed that the vasoconstriction was due to overactive sympathetic nerve control of the digital arteries and that the excess activity following a cold stimulus was the basis for the episodic attacks. Despite the attraction of this theory (and following 120 years of further speculation), it has never been substantiated. Also, the many treatments, directed towards minimizing sympathetic control of the vasomotor tone, including cervical sympathectomy, have been unsuccessful. On severing sympathetic nerve activity surgically, immediate dilatation of the peripheral vessels is observed; but in a matter of six to eight months, episodic attacks are again in evidence. Thus the vasomotor tone must be influenced directly by "local" factors, including chemical mediators such as serotonin and prostaglandins. The adrenergic sympathetic fibres constrict the digital arteries but the latter have no vasodilatory fibres supplying them. Reflex dilatation occurs only when the sympathetic influence is removed.

Understanding the "local" or "peripheral" factors involved in the control of the digital arteries made little progress until the discovery of the prostaglandins, and in particular thromboxane A2 (a potent vasoconstrictor), and prostacyclin (a potent vasodilator) (19). The interaction of these two compounds is thought to control the laying down (and clearance) of platelet thrombi within the vasculature. Advanced cases of Primary Raynaud's Disease and Secondary Raynaud's Phenomenon with tissue necrosis and ulceration are found to have thrombi in the small digital vessels (20-22). They are also seen in advanced VWF cases (23). In these severe cases, raised blood viscosity may also play a role (24,25).

Repeated ischemic attacks following vibration exposure produce anatomical changes in the pathology of the artery walls (26). Early cases show medial coat hypertrophy whilst still retaining the ability to constrict and to open the lumen. Late, severe cases reveal extensive intima hypertrophy, with near closure of the lumen and a permanent cyanosis of the digits. The mechanism causing these vessel wall changes is unknown. The increase in bulk of the medial coat seen in early VWF cases is said to be associated with increased sensitivity to cold. Again the mechanism is unknown. Lewis postulated that the endings of the vasoconstrictor nerves are affected and their sensitivity to cold is accentuated (27). Marshall et al. noted that the sensory loss was more proximal in the fingers than the blanching (28), again suggesting injured nerves. Magos and Okos suggested an overactive biochemical vasoconstrictor mechanism developed within the vessels when exposed to the vibration stimulus, and therefore the hypersensitivity could be due to an accumulation of vasoactive substances (29). In this context, the activity both of the prostaglandins and noradrenaline needs to be considered (30). More basic physiological research will be required to elucidate the mechanisms causing attacks in both Primary Raynaud's Disease and Secondary Raynaud's Phenomenon.

To complicate still further what was accepted as a peripheral or segmental phenomenon, Soviet investigators and others believe that the Vibration Syndrome affects the entire organism, mediated through the central nervous system (CNS). Data have been reported showing that subjects working with hand-held vibratory tools suffer from abnormal neurological and psychosomatic disorders arising from the reflex centres. These include excessive sweating of the palms of the hands, vertigo, headache, insomnia, anxiety, irritability, forgetfulness, lack of concentration and impotence - all symptomatic of a stress syndrome induced by exposure to vibration, cold and noise (31). The evidence for involving the higher centres of the autonomic nervous system in the Vibration Syndrome is strong and convincing, but requires care in interpretation. Transposing laboratory data to industrial situations and particularly to litigation cases requires consideration of two main difficulties:
a)   the adaptation of the human to stress, the initial effects tending to subside with habituation; and
b)   the difficulty of quantifying changes in the vegetative system. The role of the CNS in assessing degrees of impairment in the Vibration Syndrome (anatomical and functional) has led to confusion. Therefore, inclusion of the CNS symptomatology in a uniform classification of the Vibration Syndrome is a matter requiring immediate consideration.

II DIFFERENTIAL DIAGNOSIS

Primary Raynaud's Disease (or constitutional white finger) is distinguished by its early onset (60% of persons affected by age 30 years), its bilateral, symmetric appearance in response to cold and often to stress, its familial predisposition and the absence of any predisposing disease or trauma. Secondary Raynaud's Phenomenon is, in contrast, associated with many diseases including occlusive arterial diseases, neurovascular entrapment syndromes (costoclavicular), connective tissue diseases (scleroderma) and trauma (lacerations and fractures of the hand and forearm). A complete list of causes of Secondary Raynaud's Phenomenon is given in Table 1 (32). What these associated conditions have in common is that their pathophysiological changes all affect blood flow which, when reduced, produces white fingers through changes in pressure gradient, vessel diameter

Table 1. Causes of Secondary Raynaud's Phenomenon (Adapted from Ref. 32, with Permission of W. Taylor and P.L. Pelmear).

Connective Tissue Disease	Scleroderma Systemic lupus erythematosus Rheumatoid arthritis Dermatomyositis Polyarteritis nodosa Mixed connective tissue disease

Trauma	1. Direct to Extremities
	  (a) Following injury, fracture or operation
	  (b) Of occupational origin (vibration)
	  (c) Frostbite and Immersion Syndrome
	
	2. To Proximal Vessels by Compression
	  (a) Thoracic outlet syndrome (cervical rib, scalenus anterior muscle)
	  (b) Costoclavicular and hyperabduction syndromes

Occlusive Vascular Disease	Thromboangiitis obliterans Arteriosclerosis Embolism Thrombosis
Dysglobulinemia	Cold hemagglutination syndrome Cryoglobulinemia Macroglobulinemia
Intoxication	Acro-osteoylis Ergot Nicotine Vinyl chloride
Neurogenic	Poliomyelitis Syringomyelia Hemiplegia

or blood viscosity. Acute, abrupt changes in the vasculature of the fingers may result, however, from injuries (lacerations and fractures) or from cold (frostbite). In an epidemiological survey of a vibration-exposed population, causes of Secondary Raynaud's Phenomenon unrelated to vibration exposure may account for a substantial prevalence of the white fingers reported.

The presence of peripheral nerve degeneration requires the scope of the differential diagnosis to include neurological diseases. This has proved to be more difficult than for the circulatory diseases, in that early changes in the neurological system are more difficult to quantify, especially subjective complaints such as tingling, numbness, clumsiness and difficulty controlling fine movements of the fingers. The need for an age- and sex-matched control group of manual workers handling similar weight tools but without vibration exposure becomes imperative. Recently, median nerve compression within the carpal tunnel at the wrist (carpal tunnel syndrome), which results in sensory loss over the median nerve distribution in the fingers (thumb and index, middle and half the ring fingers, on the palmar side), has been recognized as a complication that also needs to be excluded in epidemiological studies of the Syndrome.

In the search for degenerative changes in the hand-arm system (blood vessels, nerves, bones, joints, connective tissue) due to vibration, it has proved difficult to differentiate between the effects of vibration, and those of heavy manual work involving constant, repetitive movements of the hands and arms to manipulate the tool or work piece. It is also necessary to appreciate that the neurological effects of long-term exposure may be of even greater significance than the circulatory effects, depending on the spectral content of the vibration entering the hands. However, the main complaints of vibration-exposed subjects tend to focus on the disruption to outdoor activities caused by the white finger episodic attacks. Occupational surveys using an accepted classification of signs and symptoms, together with accurate measurements of the vibration stimulus and exposure time, will ultimately enable the extent of degeneration in each system to be established.

III CLASSIFICATION OF DISORDERS, IMPAIRMENT AND OBJECTIVE TESTS

The consequences of these disorders are usually related to the extent and frequency of attacks, and the ease with which they are provoked. There is also always the possibility that the reduction in grip strength that accompanies vibration exposure (18), and so occurs daily, may be sufficient to reduce the ability to hold or control an object, particularly the work tool.

Outdoor workers exposed to low temperatures are most prone to early morning attacks, especially if they ride bicycles or motorcycles to work, or have a morning work break in unheated shelters. With increasingly frequent attacks, workers report interference with home, leisure and hobby activities, e.g. gardening, house and car maintenance, bathing, fishing, golfing, skiing, and skating. These complaints are difficult to quantify but constitute a definite reduction in the "quality of life". When attacks occur year round, subjects report interference with the performance of their work, the fingers ultimately becoming stiff and clumsy, leading to difficulty with fine work and with handling small objects. Some people whose condition becomes this severe find that they are unable to continue working outdoors during cold weather (33).

Because of the reliance on a person's history of his attacks and impairment, it is not surprising that several different schemes for classifying the symptoms and defining the extent of impairment have been developed. Only the two most commonly used classification schemes will be considered here.

The Taylor-Pelmear clinical grading of VWF into Stages has been used extensively in the United Kingdom since 1968, and more recently in the U.S.A., Canada, and elsewhere (32). A Stage 1 (early case) complains of blanching confined to one or more fingertips; there is no interference with work or leisure activities. These early cases usually suffer first from tingling sensations, on and off the job, followed by numbness which may or may not persist after the blanching is noticed. A Stage 3 (advanced case) will have bilateral finger blanching extending to the base of the fingers, and interference with activities at home and at work owing to the number and severity of attacks. These attacks will occur in summer as well as winter. There will be inability to perform fine tasks and there is likely to be paresthesia and disturbance of sleep.

In Japan, the U.S.S.R. and some countries in Eastern Europe, the classification is based on the Soviet work of Andreeva-Galanina, and consists of Levels again emphasizing the person's signs and symptoms (34). In Level I, Secondary Raynaud's Phenomenon is dormant but there may be numbness, intermittent pain of the fingers and forearm, and light sweating of the palms. In Level II, there is occasional Secondary Raynaud's Phenomenon with increasing numbness, pain, coldness, and muscle pain and joint stiffness in the fingers and forearm. A decline in muscle power of the upper arm and gripping force also appears. Dull headaches are frequent complaints, and sweating of the palm increases. In Level III, there is frequent Secondary Raynaud's Phenomenon with increased symptoms in the fingers and forearm. There is slight muscle contracture and occasional appearance of ulnar nerve paralysis. Changes in the bones of the elbow joint are frequently detected and extreme sweating of the palms occurs. Symptoms indicating neurosis, such as anxiety, state of depression and interference with sleep, also appear. In Level IV, Secondary Raynaud's Phenomenon is very frequent and prominent, and may also appear in the legs. Muscle contracture, peripheral nerve paralysis, and changes in the bones of the elbow joint become apparent. Nervous instability and symptoms indicating neurosis increase further; nausea and dizziness also occasionally appear.

Clearly, there is a substantial difference between these classification schemes and in the interpretation of the dominant effects of vibration on the hand-arm system. Some of the reported effects may be due to constant tool manipulation rather than vibration exposure. Others, such as anxiety and headache, are difficult to quantify and also may be unconnected with the vibration stimulus.

Objective tests, not dependent on the subject's history, have been devised for the three principal biological systems known to suffer damage from vibration exposure: the peripheral circulatory and sensory systems, and the motor-musculo-skeletal system. The early physicians, Hamilton, Rothstein and Leake (2-4), measured finger temperature, sensory loss, loss of pain sensation and of temperature appreciation in their clinical examinations of stone-cutters. In the 1950's and 1960's, blood flow (plethysmography) was investigated before and after provocative cooling, which was used to simulate the characteristic vasoconstriction of Secondary Raynaud's Phenomenon triggered by cold. More recently, the vibration perception threshold of the finger pulps and its temporary shift with vibration exposure (TTS) have been investigated. Although failing to relate perception thresholds directly to VWF impairment, Lidström et al. were able to detect significant differences in TTS between vibration-exposed and control populations, by using a provocative vibration dose and controlled hand grip in the laboratory (35). A recent attempt by Wasserman et al. to correlate the presence of bone cysts in the finger and wrist bones with the VWF Stage assessment was, however, inconclusive (36).

The many objective tests for the Vibration Syndrome evaluated to date include, in the peripheral vascular field, skin temperature (with provocative cooling), brachial artery compression tests, cold pressor recovery tests (CPRI), plethysmography, with and after cooling, and with measurement of recovery time, finger pulse plethysmography (after Kadlec and Pelnar), nail bed tests (Lewis-Prusik), whole blood viscosity index and brachial arteriography. Neurological changes investigated include vibro-tactile finger pulp thresholds, tactile discrimination tests (esthesiometry), electroneuromyographic (EMG) measurements of the motor and sensory conduction velocities (MCV, SCV) of the median and ulnar nerves, and conduction velocity motor fibre tests (CVSP). Changes in the musculo-skeletal system have been investigated with the following tests: grip force, pinching power (between thumb and little finger), tapping ability, tonic vibration reflex (TVR) and urinary hydroxyproline excretion tests (from collagen fibre breakdown).

Unfortunately, the neurological tests in their present form (especially the nerve conduction velocity tests) have been found to be unspecific, in that they detect a range of polyneuropathies frequently found in industrial workers not exposed to vibration (37). In the vibro-tactile threshold determinations, there exists a broad overlap in the threshold values of vibration-exposed and normal subjects, although the more severe the VS symptoms, the greater the difference between the populations (38).

Close examination of the available statistics relating any of the objective tests with impairment reveals that they succeed only in demonstrating a significant difference between vibration-exposed and control groups, and not between individuals. The tests have not been directly correlated with Levels or Stages, and thus a precise, objective measure of the severity of the Syndrome cannot be made. To date, no single objective test for assessing impairment in an individual has yet been described. It is believed that all the tests would apply to individual cases if a baseline for each subject were obtained, that is if the tests are applied prospectively.

This method of comparative measurements will apply especially to plethysmography, where it is difficult to control the variables regulating peripheral blood flow (vasomotor tone, core body temperature and emotional state). Time of day for determining blood flow is another important variable which requires standardization to permit the comparison of results. It is the experience of all investigators that VWF attacks in early (Stages 1 and 2) and late cases (Stage 3) cannot be triggered at will by cooling the extremities, or even by reducing core temperature. In neurological tests, it is essential to ensure that the subject be free from vibration exposure for at least 24 hours before testing, in order to remove TTS from vibro-tactile measurements. A further complication in objective testing is that impairment as measured by

objective tests may reverse when the subject is withdrawn from vibration exposure. There is evidence that Stage 1 and early Stage 2 cases will reverse, as measured by a reduction in the number and severity of VWF attacks. A recent report contains evidence that even Stage 3 cases may reverse to Stage 0 (no signs or symptoms) (39). Thus, the time interval between testing and the last known vibration exposure may be important. A similar situation exists when measuring noise-induced permanent threshold shift, where it is essential to ensure a noise-free interval (up to 6 months) to remove all temporary threshold shift. Since there is some evidence that noise and vibration (both stressors) may act synergistically, objective tests should be conducted in a quiet environment (40).

Finally, the clinical tests for the perception of light touch, pain and temperature favoured by early physicians are open to serious objections, namely: a) observer bias; b) poorly designed instrumentation with uncontrolled variables; and c) inadequate preparation of the subject vis-a-vis ambient temperature and vibration exposure. These and other objective tests that at present fail to reveal differences between individuals may benefit from further development. This could include the design and careful evaluation of improved apparatus in which the pertinent variables are controlled.

IV FACTORS INFLUENCING VIBRATION EXPOSURE AND ITS MEASUREMENT

A complete listing of the many factors known or believed to influence the severity of vibration exposure is given in Table 2 (41-46). Studies of groups of workers in industry who have been engaged in the same work for many years have shown that the risk of developing the Vibration Syndrome increases with the duration of exposure, and with the amount of vibration entering the hand. The former is determined by the consecutive years of employment involving vibration exposure and the duration of exposure each work day, which are combined by some investigators to form the total operating time (TOT). The latter is determined by the dominant amplitudes and frequencies of the source of vibration, be it a hand-held power tool or a work piece (such as a casting being ground), and by the coupling between the source and the hand.

Both source intensity and the source-hand coupling may vary substantially over a period of time, even for the same power tool, or industrial process, and operator. Increases in source vibration usually result from deterioration in the condition of the tool (e.g. from lack of maintenance, excessive wear, and ageing), and from a failure to control the efficiency of the work process. Examples of the latter are

Table 2. Factors Known or Believed to Influence the Severity of Occupational Exposure of the Hand to Vibration.

Physical	Dominant vibration amplitudes entering the hand
	Dominant vibration frequencies entering the hand
	Years of employment involving vibration exposure
	Total duration of exposure each work day
	Temporal pattern of exposure each work day
	Dominant vibration direction relative to the hand
	Non-occupational exposure to vibration
Biodynamic	Hand grip forces (compressive and push or pull forces)
	Surface area, location and mass of parts of the hand in contact with the source of vibration
	Posture (position of the hand and arm relative to the body)
	Other factors influencing the coupling of vibration into the hand (e.g. texture of handle - soft compliant v rigid material)
Individual	Factors influencing source intensity and exposure duration (e.g. state of tool maintenance, operator control of tool or machine work rate, skill and productivity)
	Biological susceptibility to vibration
	Vasoconstrictive agents affecting the peripheral circulation (e.g. smoking, drugs, etc.)
	Predisposing disease or prior injury to the fingers or hands (trauma, lacerations, etc.)
	Hand size and weight
	Epidemiological factors, such as age

incorrectly sharpened saw chains and eccentric grinding wheels. The worker can also strongly influence the vibration entering the hands, by the method of operating the tool or machine (e.g. speed and throttle controls), by the manner he holds or supports the tool or work piece, and by the forces he exerts to control the process. Thus, differences in work practices, skill and productivity will lead to variations in the severity of exposure for workers performing the same task with the same tool or machine, by introducing both biodynamic and motivational factors. Biological differences in the susceptibility of humans to vibration also affect the severity of exposure.

A complete specification of exposure would thus require measuring the vibration amplitudes and frequencies entering each hand, and the hand grip forces, in well-defined directions, and perhaps even the surface area and location of flesh in contact with the source, all as a function of time. To monitor daily all these parameters for each worker, including his posture and other factors, is clearly impractical. It is hence necessary to reduce the problem to manageable proportions, by identifying those parameters that may be expected to dominate and hence effectively determine the severity of vibration exposure. These form the first group listed for each category in Table 2.

Even with this simplification, it is essential to recognize that it is only possible in practice to establish a *typical* vibration exposure for a large group of

workers engaged in the same work, by performing measurements on a subset from that population. In consequence, the vibration exposure of population groups needs to be expressed statistically, as does the corresponding development of the Syndrome in industry. These considerations inevitably lead to dose-response relations that describe a typical (or average) rate of progression of disorders, and a measure of the variation in the rate between individuals (which may arise from differences in exposure time, hand grip, susceptibility, etc). Dose-response relations expressed in this form have only recently been reported (47).

There are several techniques for determining the vibration stimulus, some of which may provide an inaccurate measure of the vibration entering the hand-arm system. A common and convenient practice is to monitor the vibration of a tool handle, or work piece, close to the positions occupied by the hands. However, the coupling between the hands and a lightweight vibrating structure may alter its flexural modes of vibration, tending to introduce constraints to motion at the points of contact. Hence, the levels recorded near the hands may be greater than those entering the hand-arm system. A more satisfactory technique is to record the vibration of surfaces directly in contact with the hands. This is done by attaching a transducer to the source that is sufficiently small to fit between the hand and the vibrating surface without greatly disturbing the flesh (48). When a glove is worn, the motion of the source-glove interface is monitored. There is usually little need to adjust the levels observed at this interface to obtain those entering the hand, as the transmissibility of common gloves is close to unity at frequencies of up to 500 Hz (49).

The vibration measured at either of these sites will be strongly influenced by the hand grip employed by the operator, especially for tools with vibration-isolated handles (48). This results from the mechanical impedance of the hand-arm system depending on the grip and push forces, as well as the posture adopted by the worker. Paradoxically, a tighter (more compressive) grip will tend to reduce the vibration of the handle, or work piece, yet increase the transmission of vibration into the hand and arm (50).

Several methods for overcoming the variable coupling of vibration into the hand-arm system have been developed. Some involve attaching a transducer to the flesh of the hand or wrist, preferably as close to a protruding bone as possible. Although, intuitively, a flesh mounted detector is desirable for measuring the vibration of the hand, it is difficult to demonstrate that the motion recorded at one location is representative of the general motion of the hand. Equally importantly, it is also difficult to demonstrate that the motion is not significantly influenced by the size, weight, and rigidity of the device attached to the flesh. An elegant solution, at least to this latter problem, is to mount an extremely small and lightweight transducer on a fingernail (49). An alternative approach is to determine the vibrational energy transmitted to the hand-arm system, by measuring simultaneously the dynamic force and velocity at the surface of the hand (51).

As most transducers respond primarily to motion in one direction, it is desirable to record the vibration entering the hands in specific directions, both to relate exposures to the physiology of the hand-arm system, and to permit meaningful comparisons between measurements performed independently. For these purposes, an orthogonal system of coordinates centred on the head of, and with its primary (Z) axis along the length of, the third metacarpal has been proposed by the International Organization for Standardization (ISO) (41). In this biodynamic coordinate system, the Y axis lies in the plane of the hand and the X axis is normal to the palm. A related basicentric coordinate system, in which the Y and Z axes are rotated slightly to align the former with the axis of a cylinder gripped between the thumb and the fingers, appears more practical. However, the origin of the coordinate system will usually be determined in practice by the position of the transducer.

The vibrations commonly occurring in industry and believed responsible for the Vibration Syndrome possess frequencies of from 5 to 1000 Hz, accelerations of from 0.5 to approximately 5000 m/s^2, and transient displacements at low frequencies of up to 5 cm. This range of vibration amplitudes and frequencies, plus the requirement for extremely small size and weight, suggests that miniature accelerometers will serve as the most satisfactory type of contact transducer. However, traditional methods of attaching an accelerometer to a vibrating surface (rigid stud mounts, adhesives, double-sided adhesive tape, etc.) (52,41), while suited to measuring the low level vibration of rigid surfaces, do not provide a precise measure of the motion of flesh, other than at the source-hand interface, or of large impacts. Contrary to popular belief, a rigidly mounted (mechanically underdamped) shock accelerometer does not guarantee accurate measurement of repetitive large displacements such as occur in rotary-percussive tools. In the most extreme cases (the chisels of chipping hammers, rock drills, and road breakers), physical destruction of the transducing element often occurs, frequently within an hour of commencing measurements. More important, however, are the physical processes, little understood at present, that result in non-linear transduction at large displacements. These are responsible for grossly exaggerated accelerations being reported for many pneumatic tools at low frequencies (53). A possible solution to this problem may lie in the insertion of a low-pass mechanical filter between the source of vibration and accelerometer. This is designed to reduce excitation of the accelerometer's internal (underdamped) mechanical resonance by impacts, though whether this procedure suppresses all mechanisms responsible for non-linear transduction is unclear at present.

An attractive and convenient method of mounting an accelerometer is to employ a hand-held mount, gripped between the fingers, somewhat like a knuckle-duster, and held against the tool handle or work piece (54). This technique combines a low-pass mechanical filter (the frictional coupling between the vibrating source and mount) with a location for the transducer that is close to the origin of the biodynamic coordinate system. However, the performance of the mechanical filter is ill-defined, and may be expected to vary with hand grip. In addition, since the mount is also in contact with two fingers and the palm, its motion is influenced both by the localized elastic properties of flesh and by the motion of the hand. The consequences of these complex interactions on the performance of the mount require further study.

In summary, although the recording and analysis of vibration exposures follow

Taylor et al.: Introduction

accepted acoustical practices (41,52,54,55), the method of measuring the vibration coupled to the hands has to be carefully defined.

V DOSE-RESPONSE RELATIONS, STANDARDS, PREVENTION AND TREATMENT

In parallel with efforts to provide epidemiological and exposure data for vibration-exposed population groups in industry, there have been several attempts to develop dose-response relations. Ideally, such relations should apply to all persons and to all occupations involving hand-transmitted vibration. They should be quantitative in nature and permit both prediction of the development of the Syndrome, and identification of tolerable vibration exposures. No dose-response relations devised so far completely satisfy all these requirements, mainly because of a lack of reliable epidemiological and exposure data from a wide range of occupations. However, some recent relations provide considerable insight into the onset and progression of the vascular component of the Syndrome among full-time, vibration-exposed workers (47,56).

In view of the pressing need for occupational health guidelines for exposure to hand-transmitted vibration, it is not surprising that standards have been developed almost independently of dose-response relations. Hence, present-day standards contain vibration limits based mainly on subjective laboratory experiments, involving human response to vibration stimuli (42). In consequence, the limits currently specified in different countries vary in magnitude by approximately a factor of five and, in addition, differ as functions of frequency. The only international consensus on a tolerable vibration limit is contained in the Draft International Standard (DIS) of the ISO that is referred to repeatedly in this book, ISO/DIS 5349 (1979) (41). This DIS is currently being replaced by a second (in press), at which time the current DIS will be withdrawn. Following the recent policy of not proposing exposure limits, believing these to be the responsibility of Governments and Regulatory Agencies, the second DIS contains procedures for measuring vibration exposure, but no vibration limit. Instead, the dose-response relations reported by Brammer (Table 3 of Ref. 56) are contained in an appendix.

The specification of tolerable vibration exposures is thus open to interpretation, though, based on the dose-response data selected by the ISO, a threshold limit close to that proposed elsewhere in this volume is implied to prevent the onset of VWF (56). More precise specification of a vibration limit will require more epidemiological data, with more detailed and accurate measurement of vibration exposures, especially for groups operating pneumatic

tools. This information should provide further evidence for contours of equinoxious vibration amplitudes and frequencies, and for the effect of work breaks throughout the work day. Also, in the development of measurement procedures for testing the compliance of power tools with a vibration standard, the use of mechanical simulation of the hands, perhaps incorporated into a test machine, will overcome much of the variability arising from hand grip (57).

That many existing power tools and industrial processes transmit excess vibration to the hands is evidenced by the prevalence of the Vibration Syndrome in many occupations (44). The extent to which the vibration of existing power tools may be reduced depends on their principle of operation and design. Many current designs would benefit from the addition of vibration-isolation systems to the handles (58), and future power tools should employ operating principles that minimize vibration entering the hands. It should be noted that a significant reduction in the prevalence of VWF among chain saw operators has followed the introduction of saws with vibration-isolated handles. However, a recent prospective study of professional lumberjacks, who have only used this type of saw, reveals that a further reduction of saw vibration is needed to prevent the occurrence of the Syndrome (39). This may require the development of more sophisticated vibration-isolation systems and the re-design of some saws.

Until power tools and processes are developed that eliminate the risk of developing the Vibration Syndrome, preventive measures will have to be employed to minimize the hazard (59). These may involve:
a) pre-employment screening, to identify those persons with Primary Raynaud's Disease and diseases that may cause Secondary Raynaud's Phenomenon (see Table 1);
b) establishing previous vibration exposure; and
c) an annual medical examination to detect those susceptible to the Syndrome.
When there is a choice of power tool or process, models resulting in the least severe vibration exposure should be selected (see Table 2), and the equipment should be properly maintained. Workers should receive training and be advised to:
a) wear sufficient clothing, including gloves, to keep warm;
b) avoid continuous exposure, by introducing rest periods;
c) employ a minimum hand grip consistent with safe operation of the tool or process; and
d) rest the tool on the work piece whenever practicable.
It is also desirable that there be a medical policy to remove persons from further vibration exposure at a definite Stage or Level of the Syndrome, preferably Stage 1 or early Stage 2 in the Taylor-Pelmear classification.

Taylor et al.: Introduction

Deteriorating cases will require close supervision, in view of the strong epidemiological evidence of a direct relationship between the signs and symptoms of the Syndrome and the cumulative vibrational energy entering the hands.

For subjects with the Vibration Syndrome, no cure or treatment is presently available. Therapy is essentially palliative. Vasodilatation of the peripheral vessels by direct action through chemotherapy has been unsuccessful and is dangerous in many cases, owing to undesirable side-effects which affect balance. The failure of drugs or chemotherapy is due to the absence of a therapeutic agent which acts specifically on the digital arteries. In advanced cases, the sympathetic nerves are either blocked or severed. Vasodilatation of the digital vessels following surgery is immediate but, as in the case of Primary Raynaud's Disease, the improvement is temporary and the vasoconstrictive attacks return. Recent reports indicate some success with serial plasmapheresis, although it is difficult to understand the mechanism of this treatment, since involvement of plasma fibrinogen, cold hemagglutins or cryoglobulins has not been demonstrated conclusively in VWF. The use of ketanserin has also been reported recently for the treatment of Secondary Raynaud's Phenomenon (60). In addition, some success has been claimed for biofeedback therapy (61).

VI CONCLUSIONS

In summary, habitual exposure of the hand and arm to vibration leads to damage of the peripheral blood vessels and nerves. Other systems, including the central nervous system and the musculoskeletal system may also be involved. Diagnosis is complicated by the need to separate the effects of vibration exposure from those of heavy manual work, by the occurrence of similar vascular signs and symptoms in other diseases, and by the lack of an effective objective test for individuals.

The development of complete dose-response relations and, in turn, more precise specification of tolerable exposures, are dependent on the availability of reliable and comparable epidemiological data from occupational studies. Such information can only be obtained by the establishment and use of an internationally accepted medical classification for the Syndrome, and by the accurate measurement of vibration exposures.

REFERENCES

1. Loriga G. Il lavoro con i martelli pneumatici. Boll Inspett Lavoro 1911; 2: 35-60.

2. Hamilton A. A study of spastic anemia in the hands of stonecutters. Washington: Government Printing Office, 1918. (Bull US Bureau of Labor Statistics, no. 236: Ind Accidents and Hygiene Series, no. 19): 53-66.

3. Rothstein T. Report of the physical findings in eight stonecutters from the limestone region of Indiana. Washington: Government Printing Office, 1918. (Bull US Bureau of Labor Statistics, no. 236: Ind Accidents and Hygiene Series, no. 19): 67-96.

4. Leake JP. Health hazards from the use of the air hammer in cutting Indiana limestone. Washington: Government Printing Office, 1918. (Bull US Bureau of Labor Statistics, no. 236: Ind Accidents and Hygiene Series, no. 19): 100-113.

5. Raynaud M. On Local Asphyxia and Symmetrical Gangrene of the Extremities. London: The New Sydenham Society, 1888. (Selected Monographs).

6. Seyring M. Diseases caused by working with pneumatic tools. Arch Gewerbepath Ccworbhyg 1930; 1: 359-375. (in German).

7. Hunt JH. Raynaud's phenomenon in workmen using vibrating instruments. Proc Roy Soc Med 1936; 30: 171-178.

8. Telford ED, McCann MB, MacCormack DH. "Dead hand" in users of vibrating tools. Lancet 1945; II: 359-360.

9. Agate JN. An outbreak of cases of Raynaud's phenomenon of occupational origin. Br J Ind Med 1949; 6: 144-163.

10. Teleky L. Pneumatic tools. In: International Labour Office, ed. Occupation and Health: Encyclopedia of Hygiene, Pathology and Social Welfare. Geneva: International Labour Office, 1938. (Supplement): 1-12.

11. Hasan J. Biomedical aspects of low-frequency vibration: a selective review. Work Environ Health 1970; 6: 19-45.

12. Pyykkö I. Vibration syndrome: a review. In: Korhonen O, ed. Vibration and Work. Helsinki: Inst of Occup Health, 1976: 1-24.

13. Klimková-Deutschová E. Neurologische aspekte der vibrationskerankheit. Int Arch Gewerbepath Gewerbehyg 1966; 22: 297-305.

14. Kumlin T, Wiikeri D, Sumari P. Radiological changes in carpal and metacarpal bones and phalanges caused by chain saw vibration. Br J Ind Med 1973; 30: 71-73.

15. Färkkilä MA, Pyykkö I, Starck JP, Korhonen O. Hand grip force and muscle fatigue in the etiology of the vibration syndrome. In: Brammer AJ, Taylor W, eds. Vibration Effects on the Hand and Arm in Industry. New York: Wiley, 1982: 45-50.

16. Färkkilä M, Starck J, Hyvärinen J, Kurppa K. Vasospastic symptoms caused by asymmetrical vibration exposure of the upper extremities to a pneumatic hammer. Scand J Work Environ Health 1978; 4: 330-335.

17. Banister PA, Smith FV. Vibration-induced white fingers and manipulative dexterity. Br J Ind Med 1972; 29: 264-267.

18. Pyykkö I, Korhonen OS, Färkkilä MA, Starck JP, Aatola SA. A longitudinal study of the vibration syndrome in Finnish forestry workers. In: Brammer AJ, Taylor W, eds. Vibration

Effects on the Hand and Arm in Industry. New
York: Wiley, 1982: 157-167.

19. Moncada S, Higgs EA, Vane JR. Human arterial
and venous tissues generate prostacyclin
(prostaglandin X) - a potent inhibitor of
platelet aggregation. Lancet 1977; I: 18-20.

20. Lewis T, Pickering GW. Observations upon
maladies in which the blood supply to digits
ceases intermittently or permanently, and upon
bilateral gangrene of digits; observations
relevant to so-called "Raynaud's Disease".
Clin Sci 1934; 1: 327-366.

21. Lewis T. The pathological changes in the
arteries supplying the fingers in warm-handed
people and in cases of so-called "Raynaud's
Disease". Clin Sci 1938; 3: 287-313.

22. Pickering GW. Vascular spasm. Lancet 1951;
II: 845-850.

23. James PB, Galloway RW. Arteriography of the
hand in men exposed to vibration. In: Taylor W,
Pelmear PL, eds. Vibration White Finger in
Industry. London: Academic Press, 1975: 31-
41.

24. Pringle R, Walder DN, Weaver JPA. Blood viscosity and Raynaud's disease. Lancet 1965; I:
1086-1088.

25. Okada A, Ariizumi M, Fujinaga H. Diagnosis of
the vibration syndrome by blood viscosity. In:
Brammer AJ, Taylor W, eds. Vibration Effects
on the Hand and Arm in Industry. New York:
Wiley, 1982: 67-70.

26. Ashe WF, Cook WT, Old JW. Raynaud's phenomenon
of occupational origin. Arch Environ Health
1962; 5: 333-343.

27. Lewis T. Vascular Disorders of the limbs. 2nd
ed. London: Macmillan, 1949.

28. Marshall J, Poole EW, Reynard WA. Raynaud's
phenomenon due to vibrating tools: neurological
observations. Lancet 1954; I: 1151-1156.

29. Magos L, Okos G. Raynaud's phenomenon: the
situation in the Hungarian iron, steel and
engineering industry. Arch Environ Hlth 1963;
7: 341-345.

30. Azuma T, Ohhashi T. Pathophysiology of vibration-induced white finger: etiological considerations and proposals for prevention. In:
Brammer AJ, Taylor W, eds. Vibration Effects
on the Hand and Arm in Industry. New York:
Wiley, 1982: 31-38.

31. Matoba T, Kusumoto H, Mizuki Y, Kuwahara H,
Inanaga K, Takamatsu M. Clinical features and
laboratory findings of vibration disease: a
review of 300 cases. Tohoku J Exp Med 1977;
123: 57-65.

32. Taylor W, Pelmear PL. Introduction. In:
Taylor W, Pelmear PL, eds. Vibration White
Finger in Industry. London: Academic Press,
1975: XVII-XXII.

33. Laroche GP. Traumatic vasospastic disease in
chain saw operators. Can Med Assoc J 1976;
115: 1217-1221.

34. Matoba T, Kusumoto H, Takamatsu M. A new
criterion of the severity of the vibration
disease. Jpn J Ind Health 1975; 17: 211-214.
(in Japanese).

35. Lidström I-M, Hagelthorn G, Bjerker N. Vibration perception in persons not previously
exposed to local vibration and in vibration-

exposed workers. In: Brammer AJ, Taylor W, eds.
Vibration Effects on the Hand and Arm in
Industry. New York: Wiley, 1982: 59-65.

36. Wasserman DE, Taylor W, Behrens V, Samueloff S,
Reynolds D. Vibration White Finger Disease in
US Workers Using Pneumatic Chipping and Grinding
Hand Tools. I - Epidemiology. Cincinnati, OH:
Dept of Health and Human Services, 1982 (NIOSH
publication no. 82-118).

37. Chatterjee DS, Barwick DD, Petrie A. Explora-
tory electromyography in the study of vibration-
induced white finger in rock drillers. Br J
Ind Med 1982; 39: 89-97.

38. Pelmear PL, Taylor W, Pearson JCG. Clinical
objective tests for vibration white finger.
In: Taylor W, Pelmear PL, eds. Vibration White
Finger in Industry. London: Academic Press,
1975: 53-81.

39. Taylor W, Riddle HFV, Bardy DA. Vibration-
Induced White Finger in Chain Saw Operators in
Thetford Chase Forest, Norfolk, England. Report
to the UK Forestry Commission, 1980. (unpublished).

40. Pyykkö I, Starck JP, Korhonen OS, Färkkilä MA,
Aatola SA. Link between noise-induced hearing
loss and the vasospastic component of the
vibration syndrome. In: Brammer AJ, Taylor W,
eds. Vibration Effects on the Hand and Arm in
Industry. New York: Wiley, 1982: 51-58.

41. International Organization for Standardization.
Principles for the Measurement and the Evaluation of Human Exposure to Vibration Transmitted
to the Hand. Geneva: International Organization for Standardization, 1979. (Draft International Standard ISO/DIS 5349).

42. Griffin MJ. Vibration Injuries of the Hand and
Arm: Their Occurrence and the Evolution of
Standards and Limits. London: Her Majesty's
Stationery Office, 1980. (Health and Safety
Executive Research Paper 9).

43. Miyashita K, Shiomi S, Itoh N, Kasamatsu T,
Iwata H. Development of the vibration syndrome
among chain sawyers in relation to their total
operating time. In: Brammer AJ, Taylor W,
eds. Vibration Effects on the Hand and Arm in
Industry. New York: Wiley, 1982: 269-276.

44. Taylor W, Pelmear PL, eds. Vibration White
Finger in Industry. London: Academic Press,
1975.

45. Matsumoto T, Yamada S, Harada N. A comparative
study of vibration hazards among operators of
vibrating tools in certain industries. Arh Hig
Rada Toksikol 1979; 30: 701-717.

46. Färkkilä M, Pyykkö I, Korhonen O, Starck J.
Hand grip forces during chain saw operation
and vibration white finger in lumberjacks. Br
J Ind Med 1979; 36: 336-341.

47. Brammer AJ. Relations between vibration exposure and the development of the vibration
syndrome. In: Brammer AJ, Taylor W, eds.
Vibration Effects on the Hand and Arm in
Industry. New York: Wiley, 1982: 283-290.

48. Brammer AJ. Influence of hand grip on the
vibration amplitude of chain saw handles. In:
Wasserman DE, Taylor W, Curry MG, eds. Proc of
the Int Occup Hand-Arm Vibration Conf. Cincinnati,
OH: Dept of Health and Human Services, 1977
(NIOSH publication no. 77-170): 179-185.

49. Griffin MJ, Macfarlane CR, Norman CD. The transmission of vibration to the hand and the influence of gloves. In: Brammer AJ, Taylor W, eds. Vibration Effects on the Hand and Arm in Industry. New York: Wiley, 1982: 103-116.

50. Reynolds DD. Hand-arm vibration: a review of 3 years' research. In: Wasserman DE, Taylor W, Curry MG, eds. Proc of the Int Occup Hand-Arm Vibration Conf. Cincinnati, OH: Dept of Health and Human Services, 1977 (NIOSH publication no. 77-170): 99-128.

51. Lidström I-M. Vibration injury in rock drillers, chiselers, and grinders. In: Wasserman DE, Taylor W, Curry MG, eds. Proc of the Int Occup Hand-Arm Vibration Conf. Cincinnati, OH: Dept of Health and Human Services (NIOSH publication no. 77-170): 77-83.

52. Broch JT. Mechanical Vibration and Shock Measurements. 2nd ed. Naerum: Bruel & Kjaer, 1980.

53. O'Connor DE, Lindquist B. Method for measuring the vibration of impact pneumatic tools. In: Brammer AJ, Taylor W, eds. Vibration Effects on the Hand and Arm in Industry. New York: Wiley, 1982: 97-101.

54. Rasmussen G. Measurement of vibration coupled to the hand-arm system. In: Brammer AJ, Taylor W, eds. Vibration Effects on the Hand and Arm in Industry. New York: Wiley, 1982: 89-96.

55. International Organization for Standardization. Second Draft Proposal for Human-Response Vibration Measuring Instrumentation. Committee document ISO/TC 108/SC 3 N99, 1982. (unpublished).

56. Brammer AJ. Threshold limit for hand-arm vibration exposure throughout the workday. In: Brammer AJ, Taylor W, eds. Vibration Effects on the Hand and Arm in Industry. New York: Wiley, 1982: 291-301.

57. Reynolds DD, Falkenberg RJ. Three- and four-degrees-of-freedom models of the vibration response of the human hand. In: Brammer AJ, Taylor W, eds. Vibration Effects on the Hand and Arm in Industry. New York: Wiley, 1982: 117-132.

58. Miwa T. Vibration-isolation systems for hand-held vibrating tools. In: Brammer AJ, Taylor W, eds. Vibration Effects on the Hand and Arm in Industry. New York: Wiley, 1982: 303-310.

59. International Organization for Standardization. Guide for the Measurement and the Assessment of Human Exposure to Vibration Transmitted to the Hand. Committee document ISO/TC 108/SC 4 N95, 1980. (unpublished).

60. Stranden E, Roald OK, Krohg K. Treatment of Raynaud's phenomenon with the 5/8 HT2 receptor antagonist ketanserin. Br Med J 1982; 285: 1069-1071.

61. Sedlacek K. Bio-feedback for Raynaud's disease. Psychosomatics 1979; 20: 538-544.

PHYSIOLOGICAL EFFECTS

Studies on the Etiological Mechanism of the Vasospastic Component of the Vibration Syndrome

I. Pyykkö, J. Hyvärinen and M. Färkkilä

ABSTRACT: The etiological mechanism of the vasospastic component in the Vibration Syndrome has been studied in 99 subjects working with vibrating tools and 33 healthy controls. They were exposed to vibration, noise and body cooling. Finger-pulse plethysmography revealed strong vasospasms during simultaneous vibration exposure, particularly at frequencies from 80 to 125 Hz, and significantly more often in subjects than in the controls. Body cooling and exposure to loud noise potentiated the vasospasms produced by vibration. Contralateral muscle work generally caused vasodilatation of the finger vessels, but simultaneous vibration exposure could inhibit this dilatation or cause constriction. The occurrence of vasoconstriction was correlated with an index of the severity of vibration-induced white finger (VWF). The findings are compatible with the idea that sensory vibration receptors contribute to VWF through over-excitation of the Pacinian corpuscles, which produce reactions in vasculature by a reflex linkage with the sympathetic nervous system.

RESUME: Le mécanisme étiologique de la composante vasopasmodique du syndrome des vibrations a été étudié chez 99 sujets travaillant avec des outils vibrants et 33 témoins en santé. Les sujets furent exposés à des vibrations, à du bruit et à un refroidissement corporel. L'étude pléthysmographique du pouls dans le bout des doigts révéla des angiospasmes intenses au cours d'une exposition simultanée des vibrations, surtout aux fréquences entre 80 et 125 Hz, et beaucoup plus souvent chez les sujets que chez les témoins. Le refroidissement corporel et l'exposition à des bruits forts amplifia les angiospasmes produits par les vibrations. Des travaux musculaires contralatéraux provoquèrent en général la vasodilatation des vaisseaux sanguins des doigts, mais l'exposition simultanée à des vibrations pouvait inhiber cette dilatation ou provoquer une constriction. La présence de vasoconstriction fut corrélée avec un indice de la sévérité du doigt blanc dû aux vibrations (VWF). Les résultats sont compatibles avec la théorie selon laquelle les récepteurs sensoriels de la vibration contribuent aux doigts blancs par surexcitation des corpuscules de Pacini, qui produisent des réactions dans le système vasculaire par l'entremise d'une liaison de réflexe avec le système nerveux sympathique.

INTRODUCTION

The vascular symptoms of the Vibration Syndrome resemble the spontaneous vasoconstrictive disease first described by Raynaud (1), where paroxysmal ischemia in fingers is provoked by cold weather. The vasoconstriction of finger vessels usually lasts from 5 to 15 minutes, during which the fingers look white and pale (2,3). Recovery is achieved by massage, or local or general warming. These vasoconstrictions seldom lead to malnutrition or atrophy of the skin, even though a few such cases have been reported (4,5). These symptoms are known by a variety of names e.g. Raynaud's Phenomenon of occupational origin (6), white fingers, dead fingers (7,8), traumatic vasospastic disease (TVD) (3,9,10) and vibration-induced white finger (VWF) (11).

The etiological mechanism of VWF is still unknown. Knowledge of the patho-physiological effect of vibration on the circulation is based on sparce animal data. Folkow et al., and Hallbäck and Folkow showed that vibration is a powerful stimulator of the sympathetic nervous system in hypertensive rats (12,13). Acute exposure to vibration caused increase in heart rate and in blood pressure, while chronic exposure to vibration led to permanent hypertension within a period of three weeks. The vascular changes were induced by an increase in peripheral vascular tone. In the acute stage, this was a result of activation of the vasoconstrictor nerves, which in the chronic stage led to hypertrophy of the muscular layer of the vessel wall.

In experiments with an isolated blood vessel (the portal vein of a rat), Ljung and Sivertsson showed that longitudinal vibration caused an immediate relaxation of the vessel (14), and stimulation at 200 Hz was more effective than at 80 or 125 Hz. Thus a direct effect of vibration on smooth muscle is to cause a relaxation of the vessel, whereas chronic exposure of an intact organism to vibration causes vasoconstriction.

Some recent findings indicate that continuous stimulation of the Pacinian corpuscles, which are very sensitive to vibration at frequencies from 60 to 700 Hz (15), might lead to continuous activation of the sympathetic nervous system (16,17). Miyamoto and Alanis stimulated the hind leg of cats with low-amplitude vibration at a frequency of 175 Hz, and found synchronous activity in the ipsilateral splanchnic nerves (18). Furthermore, stimulation of the sympathetic nervous system leads to a decrease in the activation threshold of the Pacinian corpuscles (19,20), which is a result of efferent activity of a sympathetic nerve axon within the corpuscle (21). Thus, there is a reciprocal connection between the sympathetic nervous system and the Pacinian corpuscles.

The present studies were undertaken to examine whether such a vasoconstrictor mechanism triggered by vibration might operate in humans exposed occupationally to vibration, and whether Pacinian corpuscles might operate as an afferent receptor system in the reflex arc. The results of these studies have been reported earlier (16,17,22-25).

I MATERIAL AND METHODS

In the first part of this study, 99 workers with VWF and 36 healthy controls were exposed to different test stimuli. The occupations of the subjects, their ages, and the number of years of exposure to vibration are listed in Table 1.

Testing took place in laboratory rooms which varied in temperature from 21 to 25°C. Provocation tests were started only after the subjects had been in the room for at least 15 minutes. During the various provocation tests, the subject sat attached to the recording system, bare above the waist and with his arms flexed about 20 cm below the level of the heart. The palm of the hand was exposed to vibration of various frequencies and amplitudes, presented in a mixed order. When a hand was vibrated, the pulse wave from the most affected finger of the same hand was recorded by a plethysmograph. An airfilled piezoelectric pulse plethysmograph (Elema-Shönander type 510 B), with a glass cylinder covering the two distal phalanges of the finger, and a locally-constructed photoelectric plethysmograph, with the transducer placed on the nail-fingerpad region, were used. Simultaneously, as an indicator of the activation of the sympathetic skin nerves, the galvanic skin response (GSR) was recorded as a change in skin conductance by a silver chloride disc electrode cutaneously applied to two adjacent fingers. For clarification of the role of muscle receptors activated by vibration, the tonic vibration reflex (TVR) was recorded by strain gauges attached to metal rods compressed by the subjects (26).

The skin temperature of both hands was periodically measured by thermocouple electrodes and recorded by a strip chart recorder (Ellab Instruments model Z8). The amplified signals of the pulse plethysmograph, GSR and TVR were recorded on paper using a portable, 3-channel, ink-writing polygraph recorder (Watanabe type H611). The acceleration was monitored by a Bruel & Kjaer accelerometer attached to the moving parts of the vibrator (EA1250 of MB Electronics, Textron Inc.) and connected through an impedance matching preamplifier

Table 1. Occupations, Ages and Exposure Times to Vibration for Subjects with VWF and for Controls.

Subject	N	Occupation	Age range (yrs)	Vibrating tool	Exposure (yrs) Mean	Range
With VWF	43	forest worker	30 - 61	chain saw	12.8	5 - 20
	47	forest worker	20 - 58	chain saw	11.5	5 - 20
	2	metal stamper	40	Pullmax iron plate stamper	9.5	6 - 13
	2	rock driller	46 - 49	Atlas Copco pneumatic drill	13	11 - 15
	5	grinder	20 - 41	carborundum grinding wheel	3.4	1 - 8
Without VWF	13	forest worker	30 - 61	not exposed		
	23	student	21 - 33	not exposed		

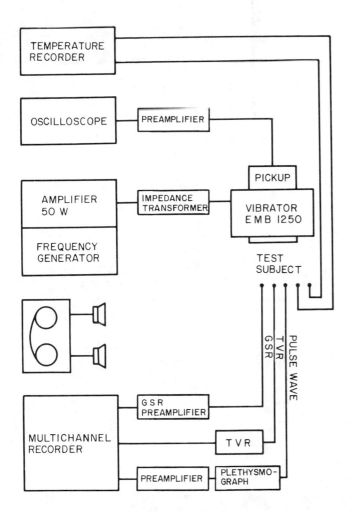

Fig. 1 Block diagram of the apparatus.
(From Ref. 16, with permission of Work
Environ Health).

to an oscilloscope. The accelerometer
readings were converted to peak-to-peak
displacement amplitudes. The apparatus is
shown schematically in Fig. 1.

Sinusoidal vibration, body cooling,
chain saw noise from loudspeakers (103-
107 dB(A)), and an arithmetic task (to
multiply 7 × 13) were the stimuli used in
the provocation tests.

Vibration frequencies of 40, 80, 125,
250, and 500 Hz were applied to the palm
of the hand most affected by VWF. These
were given in random order to each
subject at least once. At the same time
as the amplitude of the vibration was
increased, the amplitude of the pulse
volume was also being monitored, and the
lowest amplitude of vibration at which a
strong vasoconstriction could be elicited

was thereby determined. A vasoconstriction
in which the pulse wave fell below one-half
of its initial value was classified as
strong.

Psycho-physical threshold values for
vibration detection were estimated in 25
subjects with VWF and in 15 control subjects. The method used for this estimation, which involved the presentation of
vibration frequencies of 2, 10, 20, 40, 60,
100, 200, 300, and 400 Hz to the distal pad
of the third finger of the left hand, has
been reported elsewhere (16,22).

These measurements typically lasted
eight hours for each subject. Several
subjects came to the tests during two consecutive days. The measurements were
usually started early in the morning and
continued up to the afternoon.

In the second part of the study, vasodilatation was induced by muscle work and
the effect of vibration was studied in the
contralateral hand by means of plethysmography. A total of 63 lumberjacks were
examined. The mean age of the lumberjacks
was 39.7 years and they had used chain saws
an average of 10 000 hours (range 1500 to
26 800 h).

The vibration was generated by a
dynamic shaker (Ling model 403), which was
driven by a signal generator and power
amplifier (TPO 300). The handle of the
shaker consisted of two metal bars (diameter 25 mm, length 140 mm) with strain
gauges (Honeywell-Selcom) for the measurement of muscle force. Acceleration levels
of 5 G rms were used at frequencies of 30
and 60 Hz, and 10 G rms at frequencies of
100, 200, and 400 Hz. The subject sat on
a chair with his right hand resting on the
table and his left hand compressing the
handle. The pulse wave was recorded from
the right hand while the left hand was
working.

The subjects exerted maximum compression of the handle for 2.5 s, and then
relaxed the hand for another 2.5 s, and so
on, for 5 min. This test was repeated six
times, once without vibration and once with
each of the following vibration frequencies:
30, 60, 100, 200, and 400 Hz, applied in
random order. The interval between the
tests was 6 min. The pulse wave of the contralateral hand was recorded by a photoelectric plethysmograph placed on the nail-
fingerpad region of the third finger. The
amplified signals of pulse plethysmography
were recorded by an ink-writer (Watanabe
H611).

The mean pulse amplitude was estimated
at the beginning and at the end of each
minute by visually fitting a line through
approximately ten pulse waves. A change in
pulse amplitude was indicated by a difference
between the levels of these two lines that
was greater than 25%; smaller changes were
not taken into account.

Pyykkö et al.: Etiological mechanism

II   RESULTS

2.1   Vascular Reaction, GSR and TVR During Vibration Exposure of Ipsilateral Hand

2.1.1   Finger-Pulse Plethysmography

Exposure of the palm of the hand to vibration normally produced vasoconstriction in the ipsilateral finger. Exceptionally, vasodilatations were noticed, and these occurred mainly at the lowest frequencies of vibration (at 40 and 80 Hz). Vasoconstrictions in the control subjects were generally mild, but in three subjects out of 36, a vasoconstrictor response exceeding 50% of the initial value was observed.

In the 99 subjects who had been occupationally exposed to vibration, this stimulus in the laboratory produced strong vasoconstrictions in 44, small and variable responses, similar to those recorded in control subjects, in 44, and no response in 11. The difference in the occurrence of vasoconstrictions between control subjects and subjects with VWF was statistically highly significant ($\chi^2(1)$ = 15.7, p<0.001).

In subjects responding with strong vasoconstriction, the vasoconstrictions appeared immediately after the onset of vibration, whereas in others, several long exposures to vibration were needed before vasoconstrictions were observed. A gradual restoration of the pulse wave to the initial volume, even during the vibratory stimulus, was noticed in the recordings of most subjects. In spite of individual variability in those subjects in whom vasoconstrictions could be readily elicited, the response to vibration did not adapt in repeated presentations.

A representative recording of vasoconstriction triggered by vibration is displayed in Fig. 2. The subject was a lumberjack who had suffered from severe VWF for four years. He had operated a chain saw for 14 500 h. Vibration at high amplitude regularly caused a vasoconstriction, whereas vibration at lower amplitudes occasionally triggered a vasoconstriction during the initial cycles of the stimulus.

Since the vasoconstrictions adapted easily and even varied spontaneously, the vibration provocation trials were presented in random order. Each trial consisted of all frequencies, and the 64 most representative trials were selected. The frequencies at which vasoconstrictions were most often provoked were 80 and 125 Hz. These frequencies caused vasoconstrictions 41 and 46 times, respectively, out of the 64 times that they were presented. The other frequencies were less effective in provoking vasoconstrictions, as is shown in Fig. 3.

The amplitude of vibration that produced strong vasoconstrictions was determined by gradually increasing the vibration

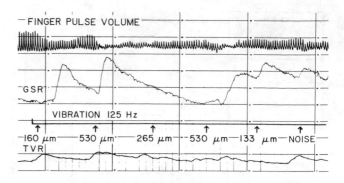

Fig. 2 Vasoconstrictions during vibration exposure (uppermost curve); the vibration frequency is 125 Hz and the subject is exposed to different amplitudes from 160 to 530 µm. The middle curve displays skin conductance (GSR) and the lowest curve muscle force (TVR). (From Ref. 16, with permission of Work Environ Health).

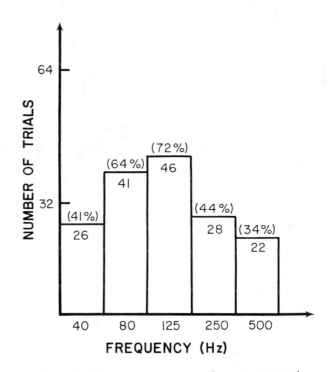

Fig. 3 The occurrence of vasoconstriction in 64 representative trials. (From Ref. 22, with permission of Work Environ Health).

amplitude until the pulse volume fell to less than half its initial value, or until the maximum amplitude possible has been reached. The means and standard errors for the threshold displacement amplitudes that

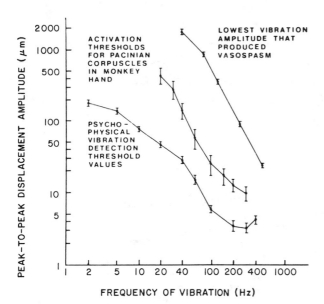

Fig. 4 The amplitude-frequency relationship of vibration provoking strong
vasoconstrictions (uppermost curve).
The middle curve displays activation
thresholds for Pacinian corpuscles in
the monkey hand (27). The lowest curve
displays psycho-physical vibration-
detection threshold values in 25 forest
workers. (From Ref. 17, with permission of Lancet).

provoked strong vasoconstrictions at different frequencies are shown in Fig. 4
(uppermost curve). This threshold curve
follows closely the psycho-physical vibration-detection thresholds for subjects
exposed to vibration (lowest curve). For
comparison, a curve displaying threshold
activation for Pacinian corpuscles when
the receptors are responding to sinusoidal
vibration with one spike for each sine wave
is also shown (middle curve). This curve
is derived from the individual threshold
values of Pacinian afferents in the monkey
hand, recorded by Mountcastle et al. (27).

Activation of the Pacinian corpuscles
is most common at frequencies from 60 to
700 Hz, where the receptors respond at the
psycho-physical vibration-detection threshold. At frequencies below 40 Hz (not
illustrated), the threshold values for the
Pacinian corpuscles are higher than those
for vibration detection (27). The vibration
detection thresholds for the monkey hand
are, furthermore, much the same as those
for man (15).

Strong vasoconstrictions were also
produced by chain saw noise at peak amplitudes of 107 dB(A) in 14 subjects, by the

cold towel test in 15, and by the arithmetic
task in 8. When testing was performed under
laboratory conditions, vibration produced
vasoconstrictions more often than the next
most powerful stimulus, the cold towel test.
In actual working conditions, however, it
is usually cold that triggers an attack.

When the vibration provocation test
was conducted in combination with noise or
cold provocation, the subsequent vasoconstrictions were often stronger than those
occurring when any one of the stimuli was
presented alone. Figure 5 illustrates how
noise potentiated the vasoconstriction produced by vibration.

The pulse volume was measured bilaterally in 25 subjects and, in most cases,
vasoconstrictions evoked by vibration were
observed in both hands. The vasoconstrictions that occurred in the hand contralateral to vibration were, however, weaker
than those in the ipsilateral hand; in only
a few subjects did the pulse volume fall to
the same extent in both hands during vibration provocation (Fig. 6).

2.1.2 Tonic Vibration Reflex (TVR)

When displacements of between 500 to
600 μ at frequencies of 60 to 250 Hz were
applied to the muscles and flexor tendons
at the palm, a gradual development (during
0.5 to 1 min) of the tonic vibration reflex
in hand flexor muscles was observed in all
patients. The same phenomenon was also
observed in normal control subjects. The
activation of TVR was not excessive in
chain-saw operators as compared with normal
subjects (Figs. 2 and 5).

When the tonic vibration reflex was
recorded simultaneously with finger-pulse
plethysmography, the increases in skeletal
muscle tone did not appear simultaneously
with the vasoconstrictions. These observations led us to the tentative conclusion
that the activation of muscle receptors, as
recorded by the development of the tonic
vibration reflex, is not associated with
vibration-induced white fingers.

2.1.3 Galvanic Skin Response (GSR)

In the lumberjacks with VWF, the galvanic skin response, which reflects the
activation of cholinergic sudomotor nerves
of the skin, was variable. Similar variability was observed in the healthy control
subjects. The GSR reacts readily to various
forms of mental activity, such as arithmetic
tasks, deep breathing, sudden noise, etc.
These reactions were seen both in controls
and in patients with VWF.

When the recordings of GSR and finger
plethysmography were done simultaneously
during exposure of the hand to vibration,
a decrease in pulse amplitude and an increase in skin conductivity often occurred
at the same time (Fig. 2). This association

Pyykkö et al.: Etiological mechanism

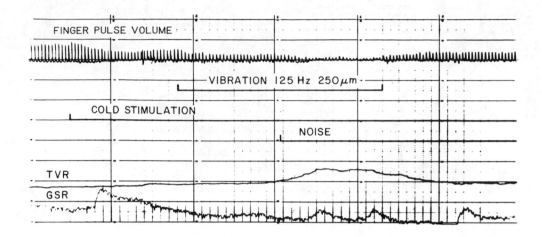

Fig. 5 Effect of cold, vibration and noise on finger pulse volume, muscle tone (TVR) and skin conductance (GSR). (From Ref. 17, with permission of Lancet).

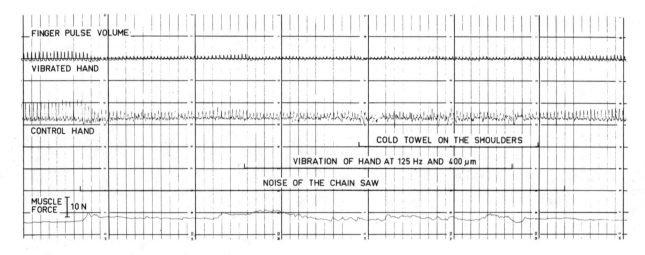

Fig. 6 Bilateral recording of finger pulse volume during simultaneous exposure to loud noise, vibration of the hand, and body cooling with a cold towel. A weak tonic vibration reflex (lowest curve) is also recorded. (From Ref. 24, with permission of Angiologia).

was loose, however, and the vasospasms could also occur without a GSR.

These observations suggest that vibration does excite the sympathetic nervous system, as recorded by the GSR, but that the association of vibration with the activation of the sympathetic sudomotor nerves is variable.

2.2 Effects of Vibration on the Heart

Disturbances in the cardiac rhythm of heart pulsation were observed in some subjects during exposure to noise, vibration, and cold. Extrasystoles were recorded in the finger plethysmograms of 13 subjects: for only two of these did electrocardiograms show extrasystoles during rest (Fig. 7). In some subjects the occurrence of extrasystoles was determined by the intensity of vibration, as illustrated in Fig. 8.

2.3 Vascular Reaction During Vibration Exposure of Contralateral Hand and Muscle Work

Vascular responses during muscle work and vibration exposure were studied in 63 lumberjacks (25). Vasodilatation of the skin vessels was the normal response to prolonged muscle work and was seen in 47

Pyykkö et al.: Etiological mechanism

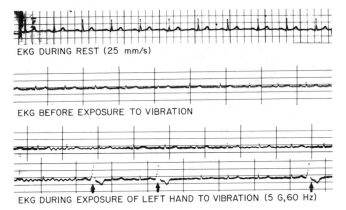

EKG DURING REST (25 mm/s)

EKG BEFORE EXPOSURE TO VIBRATION

EKG DURING EXPOSURE OF LEFT HAND TO VIBRATION (5 G,60 Hz)

Fig. 7 Electrocardiography when res-
ting and during exposure to vibration.
(From Ref. 23, with permission of Acta
Chir Scand).

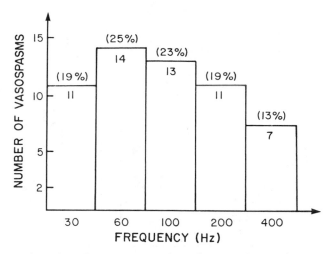

Fig. 9 The occurrence of vasoconstrictions in 56 trials. (From Ref. 25, with
permission of Scand J Work Environ
Health).

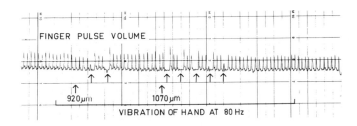

FINGER PULSE VOLUME

920μm   1070μm

VIBRATION OF HAND AT 80 Hz

Fig. 8 Reflexion of disturbances in
heart rhythm in finger pulse volume
during vibration exposure. Extrasystoles are marked with arrows.
(From Ref. 22, with permission of
Work Environ Health).

subjects; no changes to the pulse wave were
observed in the others.

During exposure to vibration, vasodilatation induced by muscle work was
inhibited in 25 subjects, who displayed a
significant vasoconstriction in their
finger-pulse recordings. In 11 subjects,
no significant change in pulse wave was
observed, and vasodilatation only occurred
in 27 subjects. However, 20 subjects who
reacted with vasoconstrictions also displayed short periods of vasodilatation
(Table 2). Vibration frequencies between

60 and 100 Hz were found most commonly to
provoke vasoconstrictions, and were observed
in 56 of the 315 tests (Fig. 9).

The subjects were classified according
to pulse-wave response and severity of VWF
(Fig. 10). The latter was based on an
index recording the extent of blanching of
the fingers during an attack of VWF, the
recovery time, the frequency of attacks,
the weather conditions provoking attacks
and the results of a cold provocation test.
The subjects with severe VWF exhibited
strong vasoconstrictions during simultaneous vibration and muscle work, whereas
subjects either with less severe VWF or
without VWF exhibited no change in pulse
wave, or vasodilatation (25).

III DISCUSSION

3.1 The Etiology of VWF

Lewis's original hypothesis for the
explanation of Raynaud's Phenomenon was
that the mechanisms operating at the endings
of the vasoconstrictor nerves were primarily
affected, and therefore their reaction to
cold was increased (28). Magos and Okos

Table 2. Vascular Reaction in Lumberjacks During Vibration Exposure and Muscle Work.

Pulse Wave Response	N	Age (yrs) Mean	SD	Sawing time (h) Mean	SD	Prevalence of VWF (%)
Vasodilatation	27	37.2	6.7	9400	4600	30
No pulse change	11	40.9	7	10 700	2900	55
Vasospasm and dilatation	20	41.5	7.9	10 000	4500	60
Vasospasm	5	43	8	13 400	6700	80

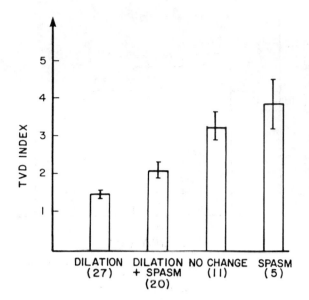

Fig. 10 The relationship of finger
pulse volume with severity of VWF as
expressed by a TVD-index. The numbers
in parentheses indicate the number
of subjects examined. (From Ref. 25,
with permission of Scand J Work Environ
Health).

suggested that an overactive biochemical
vasoconstrictor mechanism gradually develops
in the blood vessels during exposure to
vibration (29). The vessels not only
become increasingly sensitive to locally
applied cold, but also lose their capacity
for cold-induced vasodilatation. They also
proposed that hypersensitivity could be the
result of the accumulation of vasoactive
substances that cannot be destroyed in the
affected vessels.

According to a hypothesis of Stewart
and Goda (30), exposure to vibration produces "friction" in the skin of fingers and
leads to the formation of subcutaneous
callosities. The calloused finger pads
cause capillary occlusion, which decreases
the blood volume in capillaries, and hence
"weakens the buffer action to the finger
circulation" during sudden contractions of
the finger vessels and therefore leads to
an attack of TVD. Marschall et al. noticed
that in an attack of VWF the numbness was
more proximal in the fingers than the
changes in colour (31). They therefore proposed that, as in some neurological diseases
(see Burch and Philips (32)), the primary
reason for Raynaud's Phenomenon was injured
nerves.

Soviet authors have suggested that the
Vibration Syndrome is a disease of the entire
organism and that the regulatory function of
the central nervous system is disturbed (33).

The vascular reflexes are more pronounced
because of disorders in the reflex centres
(34). This hypothesis is supported by the
fact that many persons working with vibrating tools suffer from nervous disorders,
and, in many, abnormal neurological findings
have been reported in the central nervous
system (35).

Up to now, no conclusive proof for any
of these theories has been provided. In
fact, determination of the metabolites of
noradrenaline during a cold provocation
test has failed to show any breakdown of
these substances in subjects with VWF (36).
Furthermore, biopsies of fingerpads made by
other researchers have not shown excessive
accumulation of callosities (9,37), whereas
both intimal thickening and hypertrophy of
the muscle layer of the vessel wall have
been reported (37).

In laboratory conditions, exposure to
vibration produced vasoconstriction in the
fingers of healthy subjects as well as in
vibration-exposed workers. This is in good
agreement with the findings of Folkow et al.
(12,13), who showed that vibration increases
the peripheral vascular tone of rats by
activating the central vasoconstrictor mechanism. As indicated by Ljung and Sivertsson
(14), vasodilatation occurs initially in
situations where a denervated blood vessel
is exposed to vibration. Thus, vibration
acts on muscle tissue by causing a relaxation of the contraction. Therefore the
vasoconstrictions in lumberjacks were probably not caused by a direct effect of vibration on the smooth muscle tissue of the
vessel wall, but through activation of a
nervous reflex. However, if vibration
breaks down the contraction mechanism of
muscles in the vessel wall, this may lead,
in time, to compensatory reactions resulting
in hypertrophy (Folkow B, personal communication).

When a person operates a vibrating
tool many hours a day for a prolonged period
of time, its vibration continually activates
the vasoconstrictor nerves, and may be
capable of producing hypertrophy of the
vessel wall as a result of the exercise.
Such hypertrophy of the vessel walls has
been reported in subjects with VWF (37).
If the hypertrophy narrows the lumen of the
vessel sufficiently, the circulation is
somewhat reduced even during the intervals
between attacks.

When a person with hypertrophy of the
vessel walls is exposed to cold while
working, the blood flow is markedly reduced.
At the critical closing pressure of the
digital vessels (38), they collapse,
triggering an attack of VWF. Such hypertrophy of the vessel walls may well be
important in the etiology of VWF, and may
even provide the sole explanation why
exposure to cold triggers attacks of VWF.
Hypertrophy of the vessel walls is, however,
the end result of vibration exposure and

21

does not explain why vibration causes VWF. Nevertheless, it clearly indicates a role for the central nervous system in the etiology of the disease, inasmuch as the central nervous system regulates the vasoconstrictor reflexes that ultimately produce the hypertrophy. However, local factors in the vessel wall may also contribute to the hypertrophy.

3.2 The Role of the Central Nervous System

The vasoconstrictor centre in the pontine region of the brain has close connections with the thermoregulatory centre and with the emotional centres in the hypothalamus (39). Activation of the latter centres is reflected in changes in the circulation of the skin in normal subjects (40). If activation of the emotional centres is excessive, pronounced responses in the peripheral organ may ensue.

Locally applied vibration causes a strong alerting response in the central nervous system (41), and the adaption to vibration is poor (42). Because of poor adaptation, the responses to vibration may well become pronounced. Occupational exposure to vibration may therefore trigger vascular reflexes, which may operate through the spinal cord as well as through higher centres in the central nervous system. Thus, during simultaneous exposure to cold, noise and vibration, the response may be additive, as shown in laboratory experiments, and in consequence result in more pronounced vasoconstriction.

The health hazards caused by vibration seem not to be limited to upper limbs only, but more generalized changes have been reported (34,43). The reason might be that during exposure of the hand to vibration, activation of the sympathetic nervous system, both localized and systemic, occurs (18). If the stimulus is repeated, the sympathetic reflexes may become activated especially in the cardiovascular system. Whereas conditioned reflexes originate in the higher levels of the central nervous system (44), specific organization of sympathetic reflexes takes place in the spinal cord and sympathetic ganglia (45). In the stellate ganglia that are in charge of most of the sympathetic ennervation of the hands, overlap of preganglionic fibres, the subliminal fringe, occlusion, and spatial and temporal summation all participate in integrating the nervous outflow to a specific sympathetic response (46). Hence different synaptic mechanisms and the extensive divergence and convergence of sympathetic nerves make it possible for one effector to be affected by the outflow from both segmental and central nerves. Such mechanisms can explain why VWF is limited to the hands and, most notably, to that hand

most exposed to vibration. In support of this idea, we note that the vasoconstrictions elicited during the vibration provocation tests were greatest in the hand exposed to vibration, although vasoconstrictions were also recorded to a lesser degree in the contralateral hand.

3.3 The Afferent Reflex Arc in Triggering the Vasoconstrictor Reflex

When vibration is applied locally to the skin, the spreading surface waves cause a large number of receptors to respond by generating one or more impulses for each oscillation. Moreover, these impulses are phase-locked to the oscillation and thus occur in synchrony (47). Although receptors usually adapt to most stimuli and decrease their response rates, vibration is an exceptional sensory stimulus in that receptors follow it perfectly in synchrony for long periods of time without much adaptation (27, 47-49). A phase-locked response is also obtained for long periods in cells of the central nervous system (27,42). Since the signal arrives synchronously at the CNS cells from many receptors, and, on higher levels, synchronously from many higher order cells, a powerful spatial and temporal summation takes place at the synapses of the afferent pathway. Such a strong, synchronous barrage from a large number of afferent inputs may travel further and cross more synapses than responses that lack the property of synchronous discharge.

Heavy vibrating tools often generate vibration within the body at some distance from the hand, as vibrations are transmitted by the bones and tendons, particularly at low frequencies (50). The Pacinian corpuscles are very sensitive to high frequency vibrations occurring at a distance (48,49). Because of the synchrony of synaptic activation, responses to vibration may pass the successive synaptic levels in the CNS more easily than responses to other stimuli, and, finally, cause on the output side a discharge in the efferent sympathetic nerves.

The parallelism of the curves for the mean threshold values of vibration detection, and the mean amplitude of vibration producing vasoconstrictions are indications that Pacinian corpuscles might trigger the vasoconstrictor reflex. Recent studies, furthermore, point to a close connection between Pacinian corpuscles and the sympathetic nervous system (18,21).

IV CONCLUSIONS

Contrary to the effect of vibration on isolated blood vessels, vibration causes vasoconstriction in intact blood vessels. This response seems to be stronger in subjects with VWF than in controls. If subjects are simultaneously exposed to vibration and

Pyykkö et al.: Etiological mechanism

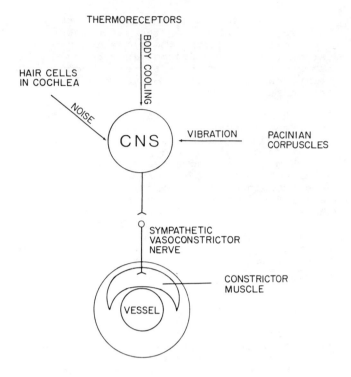

THERMORECEPTORS

HAIR CELLS
IN COCHLEA

NOISE

BODY COOLING

CNS

VIBRATION

PACINIAN
CORPUSCLES

SYMPATHETIC
VASOCONSTRICTOR
NERVE

CONSTRICTOR
MUSCLE

VESSEL

Fig. 11 The hypothetical mechanism
leading to vascular changes in VWF.

loud noise, or to vibration and cold, the
vasoconstriction is greater than when the
three stimuli are applied separately. It
seems probable that vibration causes vasoconstriction by activating the central
nervous system. The vasoconstrictions occur
in the frequency range where the Pacinian
corpuscles are most sensitive to vibration,
and the threshold curve for vasoconstriction
is parallel to the threshold curve for
Pacinian corpuscles. It is therefore plausible that the afferent reflex arc for the
vasoconstrictor reflex is triggered by
Pacinian corpuscles. When a person operates
a vibrating tool many hours a day for a prolonged period of time, continual activation
of the vasoconstrictor reflex may lead to
hypertrophy of the vessel wall.

The skin circulation is under close
control of the thermoregulatory system, and
this is why cold overcomes the other environmental stimuli in activating the sympathetic vasoconstrictor mechanisms. When a
person with VWF is exposed to stimuli like
cold, noise or vibration, the result is an
excessive vasoconstriction, in advanced
cases, because of hypertrophy of the medial
layer of the vessel wall. If the intra-
luminal flow decreases to a sufficiently low
level, the vessel wall collapses triggering
an attack of VWF. A diagram summarizing
the postulated mechanism leading to an
attack of VWF is shown in Fig. 11.

REFERENCES

1. Raynaud M. De l'asphyxie et de la gangrène
symétrique des extrémités. Thesis. Rignou,
Paris. 1862. cited by Birnstingle. The Raynaud
Syndrome. Postgrad Med J 1971; 47: 297-310.
2. Hellstrom B, Lange Andersen K. Vibration injuries in Norwegian forest workers. Br J Ind
Med 1972; 29: 255-263.
3. Pyykkö I. The prevalence and symptoms of
traumatic vasospastic disease among lumberjacks
in Finland. Work Environ Health 1974; 11:
118-131.
4. Teleky L. Pneumatic tools. Occup Health Saf
1938; 1: 1-12.
5. Blair HM, Headington JT, Lynch PJ. Occupational
trauma, Raynaud phenomenon, and sclerodactylia.
Arch Environ Health 1974; 28: 80-81.
6. Agate JN. An outbreak of cases of Raynaud's
phenomenon of occupational origin. Br J Ind
Med 1949; 6: 144-163.
7. Hamilton A. A study of spastic anemia in the
hands of stonecutters. Washington: Government
Printing Office, 1918. (Bull US Bureau of Labor
Statistics, no. 236: Ind Accidents and Hygiene
Series, no. 19). cited by Agate (Ref. 6).
8. Hamilton A. A vasomotor disturbance in the
finger of stonecutters. Int Arch Gewerbepat
Gewerbehyg 1930; 1: 348-358.
9. Gurdjian ES, Walker LW. Traumatic vasospastic
disease of the hand (white fingers). JAMA
1945; 129: 668-672.
10. Kumlin T, Wiikeri M, Sumari P. Radiological
changes in carpal and metacarpal bones and
phalanges caused by chain saw vibration. Br J
Ind Med 1973; 30: 71-73.
11. Taylor W. Introduction. In: Taylor W, ed.
The Vibration Syndrome. London: Academic Press
1974: 1-12.
12. Folkow B, Hallbäck M, Weiss L. Cardiovascular
responses to acute mental "stress" in spontaneously hypertensive rates (SHR). Acta Physiol
Scand 1972; 7-8 A.
13. Hallbäck M, Folkow B. Cardiovascular responses
to acute mental "stress" in spontaneously
hypertensive rats. Acta Physiol Scand 1974;
90: 684-698.
14. Ljung B, Sivertsson R. Inhibition of vascular
smooth muscle contraction by vibration. Acta
Physiol Scand 1973; Suppl 396: 95.
15. Mountcastle VB, La Motte RH, Carli G. Detection
thresholds for stimuli in humans and monkeys:
comparison with threshold events in mechanoreceptive afferent nerve fibers innervating
the monkey hand. J Neurophysiol 1972; 35:
122-136.
16. Pyykkö I, Hyvärinen J. The physiological basis
of the traumatic vasospastic disease (TVD): a
sympathetic vasoconstrictor reflex triggered by
high frequency vibration. Work Environ Health
1973; 10: 36-47.
17. Hyvärinen J, Pyykkö I, Sundberg S. Vibration
frequencies and amplitudes in the aetiology of
traumatic vasospastic disease. Lancet 1973;
I: 791-794.
18. Miyamoto J, Alanis J. Reflex sympathetic
response produced by activation of vibrational
receptors. Jpn J Physiol 1970; 20: 725-740.

19. Loewenstein WR, Altamirado-Orrega R. Enhancement of activity in a Pacinian corpuscle by sympathomimetic agents. Nature 1956; 178: 1292-1293.
20. Edelberg R. The relationship between the galvanic skin response, vasoconstriction, and tactile sensitivity. J Exp Psychol 1961; 62: 187 105.
21. Santini M, Ibata Y, Pappas D. The fine structure of the sympathetic axon within the Pacinian corpuscle. Brain Res 1971; 33: 279-287.
22. Pyykkö I. A physiological study of the vasoconstrictor reflex in traumatic vasospastic disease. Work Environ Health 1974; 11: 170-186.
23. Pyykkö I, Hyvärinen J. Vibration induced changes of sympathetic vasomotor tone. Acta Chir Scand 1976; Suppl 465: 23-26.
24. Hyvärinen J, Pyykkö I. On the etiological mechanisms in traumatic vasospastic disease. Angiologia 1977; 7: 241-246.
25. Färkkilä M, Pyykkö I. Blood flow in the contralateral hand during vibration and hand grip contractions of lumberjacks. Scand J Work Environ Health 1979; 5: 368-374.
26. Eklund G, Hagbarth K-E. Normal variability of tonic vibration reflexes in man. Exp Neurol 1966; 16: 80-92.
27. Mountcastle VB, Talbot WH, Darian-Smith I, Kornhuber HH. Neural basis of the sense of flutter vibration. Science 1967; 155: 597-600.
28. Lewis T. Vascular Disorders of The Limbs. 2nd ed. London: MacMillian, 1949.
29. Magos L, Okos G. Cold dilatation and Raynaud's phenomenon. Arch Environ Health 1963; 7: 402-410.
30. Stewart AM, Goda DF. Vibration syndrome. Br J Ind Med 1970; 27: 19-27.
31. Marschall J, Poole EG, Reynard WA. Raynaud's phenomenon due to vibrating tools. Lancet 1954; I: 1151-1156.
32. Burch GE, Philips J. Peripheral vascular diseases - diseases other than atherosclerosis. In: American Physiological Society, eds. Handbook of Physiology (vol II, section 2). Baltimore: Waverly Press, 1963: 1215-1249.
33. Teisinger J. Vascular disease disorders resulting from vibrating tools. JOM 1972; 14: 129-133.
34. Nalca IF. Vascular disorders and their pathogenesis in connection with vibration disease. Sov Med 1971; 34: 11-14. (English abstract).
35. Klimková-Deutschová E. Neurologische aspekte der vibrationskrankheit. Int Arch Gewerbepat Gewerbehyg 1966; 22: 297-305. (in German).
36. Okada A, Yamashita T, Nagano C, Ikeda T, Yachi A, Shibata S. Studies on the diagnosis and pathogenesis of Raynaud's phenomenon of occupational origin. Br J Ind Med 1971; 28: 353-357.
37. Ashe WF, Cook WT, Old JW. Raynaud's phenomenon of occupational origin. Arch Environ Health 1962; 5: 333-343.
38. Roddie IC, Shephard IT. Evidence for critical closure of digital resistance vessels with reduced transmural pressure and passive dilatation with increased venous pressure. J Physiol (Lond) 1957; 136: 498-506.
39. Ingram WR. Central autonomic mechanism. In: American Physiological Society eds. Handbook of Physiology (vol II, section 1). Baltimore: Waverly Press, 1960: 951-978.
40. Fox RH. Effects of cold on the extremities. Proc Roy Soc Med 1968; 61: 785-787.
41. Pyykkö I, Matsuoka I, Ito S, Hinoki M. Enhancement of eye motor response and electrical brain activity during noise and vibration exposure in rabbits. Otolaryngol Head & Neck Surg. (in press).
42. Hyvärinen J, Sakata H, Talbot WH, Mountcastle VB. Neuronal coding by cortical cells of the frequency of oscillating peripheral stimuli. Science 1968; 162: 1130-1132.
43. Pyykkö I, Starck J, Färkkilä M, Hoikkala M, Korhonen O, Nurminen M. Hand-arm vibration in the etiology of hearing loss in lumberjacks. Br J Ind Med 1981; 38: 281-9.
44. Hillarp N-A. Peripheral autonomic mechanisms. In: American Physiological Society, eds. Handbook of Physiology (vol II, section 1). Baltimore: Waverly Press, 1960; 979-1006.
45. Koizumi K, Brooks CM. The integration of autonomic system reactions: a discussion of autonomic reflexes, their control and their association with somatic reactions. In: Ergebnisse der Physiologie. Vol 67. Wurtzburg: Universitatsdruckerei H. Sturz AG, 1972: 1-68.
46. Sato A, Schmidt RF. Ganglionic transmission of somatically induced sympathetic reflexes. Pflugers Arch 1971; 326: 240-253.
47. Johnson KO. Reconstruction of population response to a vibratory stimulus in quickly adapting mechanoreceptive afferent fiber population innervating glabrous skin of the monkey. J Neurophysiol 1974; 37: 48-72.
48. Merzenich MM, Harrington T. The sense of flutter-vibration evoked by stimulation of the hairy skin of primates: comparison of human sensory capacity with the responses of mechanoreceptive afferents innervating the hairy skin of monkeys. Exp Brain Res 1969; 9: 236-260.
49. Talbot WH, Darian-Smith I, Kornhuber HH, Mountcastle VB. The sense of flutter-vibration: comparison of the human capacity with response patterns of mechanoreceptive afferents the monkey hand. J Neurophysiol 1968; 31: 301-334.
50. Pyykkö I, Färkkilä M, Toivanen J, Korhonen O, Hyvärinen J. Transmission of vibration in the hand-arm system with special reference to changes in compression force and acceleration. Scand J Work Environ Health 1976; 2: 87-95.

DISCUSSION

T. Azuma: What is the mechanism by which vasoconstriction is brought about by vibratory stimulation?

Authors' Response: The vasoconstriction observed during acute exposure to vibration presumably was induced by stimulation of the sympathetic nervous system. It is noteworthy that the subjects showed hyperreactivity to all stimuli used in all of our tests.

Did you measure the level of critical closing pressure in human digits?

Pyykkö et al.: Etiological mechanism

Authors' Response: No, we did not. The critical closing pressure in digital vessels has been documented in several reports, but the majority of the reports deal with subjects with VWF.

J.A. Rigby: Are you suggesting that noise alone can cause VWF or are you saying that noise potentiates vibration in causing VWF?

Authors' Response: I don't think that noise alone is able to induce VWF. Allegedly, noise assists the development of vascular changes in the Vibration Syndrome, as can be seen from plethysmographic recording in this work and from our noise-induced hearing loss study (see elsewhere in this volume).

Has anyone proved that there is more VWF in a noisy situation as opposed to a quiet situation?

Authors' Response: Yes, Jansen's results indicate that workers exposed to high noise levels have a higher prevalence of Raynaud's Phenomenon than workers exposed to low noise levels. However, it is difficult to draw conclusions. Where there is vibration, there is usually high level noise.

Cardiovascular Features of the Vibration Syndrome: An Adaptive Response

T. Matoba, M. Chiba and H. Toshima

ABSTRACT: The Vibration Syndrome is a systemic condition induced by the action of stressors such as vibration, noise and a cold environment. In fact, not only peripheral disorders such as Raynaud's Phenomenon in the fingers, but systemic disorders may also occur. Consequently, these disorders would include the adaptive responses to the stressors, in addition to the direct injuries caused by vibration. The prevalence of resting bradycardia, cardiomegaly, increased stroke volume, increased left ventricular ejection fraction and abnormalities of the electrocardiogram were distinctly higher in patients with vibration disease than in controls. The clinical features were similar to those found in well-trained athletes, the mechanism of which would be an adaptive response in the cardiovascular system. The adaptations usually regressed within several years after discontinuing the use of vibratory tools, according to the results of a four-year follow-up study.

RESUME: De syndrome des vibrations est une maladie systémique provoquée par des facteurs stressants comme les vibrations, le bruit et l'environnement froid. En fait, il peut se produire des désordres non seulement périphériques, comme le phénomène de Raynaud dans le bout des doigts, mais systémiques. Par conséquent, ces désordres comprendraient des réactions d'adaptation aux causes du stress, en plus des blessures directement provoquées par les vibrations. La prévalence de bradycardie au repos, de cardiomégalie, de l'augmentation du volume sanguin, de l'augmentation de la fraction éjectée du ventricule gauche et d'anomalies dans l'électrocardiogramme étaient nettement plus grande chez les patients ayant la maladie de vibration que chez les témoins. Les caractéristiques cliniques étaient analogues à celles qu'on rencontre chez les athlètes bien entraînés, chez lesquels le mécanisme constituerait une réaction d'adaptation du système cardiovasculaire. L'adaptation régressait en général au bout de plusieurs années après l'abandon de l'utilisation des outils vibratoires, d'après les résultats d'une étude de rappel de quatre ans.

INTRODUCTION

It is well known that the use of vibratory tools such as chain saws, pneumatic hammers, or electric grinders for long periods of time results in injuries of the peripheral blood vessels and nerves, and in Raynaud's Phenomenon in the fingers (1). Recently, this disease has been recognized to be systemic, in that it impairs not only the peripheral circulatory and nerve functions but also the central, especially the autonomic nervous function (2). As to pathogenesis, three major stressors usually affecting the operator of a vibratory tool are vibration, noise and a cold environment (3). Accordingly, the clinical features of vibration disease may include the adaptive responses to the stressors in addition to direct injuries caused by vibration. In these circumstances, it is appropriate to consider how the cardiovascular system responds to these stressors, and what further changes then occur if patients terminate their exposures.

The present study was undertaken to establish the cardiovascular features in patients with vibration disease, and to ascertain whether such cardiovascular responses to the stressors change after cessation of exposure.

I SUBJECTS AND METHODS

The study was in two parts: first, a study of the cardiovascular features in patients with vibration disease; and, second, changes in these features after discontinuing the use of vibratory tools.

1.1 Cardiovascular Features

The groups consisted of 35 male

patients with vibration disease and 35 healthy men. Subjects from the two groups were matched by age and were from 36 to 64 years old. Chain saws and jack hammers had been used by 20 men and 15 men respectively, for 15.9 ± 4.6 years (mean ± SD). The period of time from last using the tools to the examination was 2.9 ± 1.4 years. Physical examination and laboratory tests confirmed that the control subjects were healthy men without cardiovascular or hormonal diseases.

A standard M-mode echocardiogram was recorded in all subjects by the same doctor. The left ventricular ejection fraction was calculated by measuring the left ventricular end-diastolic and end-systolic dimensions from the echocardiogram. Intraventricular septal thickness, left ventricular posterior wall thickness, aortic diameter and left atrial diameter were also measured at end-diastole and at end-systole.

A 12 lead electrocardiogram was recorded in a supine position at a paper-speed of 25 mm/min. The following parameters were observed: the resting heart rate, from the mean of five consecutive beats; the algebraic sum of the Q, R, and S deflections in the standard leads (R_I+S_{III}) and the precordial leads ($S_{V_1}+R_{V_5}$); and the ratio of the amplitudes of T and R waves in the leads I, V_5 and V_6.

The level of autonomic nerve activity was observed by means of digital plethysmography with auditory stimuli (4,5).

In order to avoid inter-observer variation, all measurements were made by the same observer. The significance of the means was calculated by Student's t-test.

1.2 Follow-Up Study

The subjects were 51 male patients with vibration disease, ranging in age from 43 to 62 years. All the subjects had used chain saws for 10.9 ± 4.2 years on average. The first examination was 2.9 ± 2 years after discontinuing exposure to vibration. The period from the first to the last follow-up examination was 3.8 ± 1.1 years. During the follow-up period, the subjects were not exposed to vibration in their jobs and they worked half of the usual work load. They also received treatment at a clinic once a week.

The following physical and laboratory examinations were performed: physical examinations in internal medicine, orthopedic surgery and otolaryngology, blood pressure, electrocardiogram, chest X-ray, X-rays of the joints, the autonomic nervous function test, electrocardiogram, electroencephalogram, gastrointestinal series and blood analyses.

II RESULTS

2.1 Cardiovascular Features of Vibration Disease

The left ventricular ejection fraction (EF) was significantly higher in patients with vibration disease than in the controls (p<0.002). EFs of the patients and the controls were 0.787 ± 0.041 and 0.744 ± 0.062, respectively. As shown in Table 1, the increase in EF of the patients appears to result from the increased left ventricular end-diastolic dimension and possibly from the small decrease in left ventricular end-systolic dimension. The stroke volume of the patients was also larger than that of the controls. Concerning the relation between EF and the level of autonomic nerve activity, increases in EF were found to be proportional to the enhancement of autonomic nerve activity, as shown in Fig. 1. Even in the hyporeactive subgroup, the EF was apparently higher than that of the controls. However, there were no statistically significant differences among these types. Approximately 68% of the patients had abnormal levels of autonomic nerve activity. In other parameters of echocardiographic

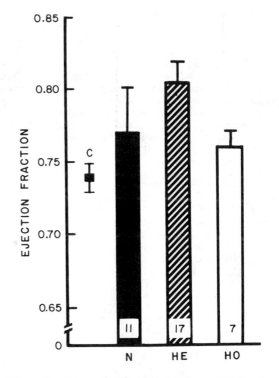

Fig. 1 Mean (and SD) left ventricular ejection fraction (EF) for each level of autonomic nerve activity: N - normoreactive; HE - hyperreactive; HO - hyporeactive; and C - controls.

Matoba et al.: Cardiovascular features

Table 1. Echocardiographic Measurements of Vibration Diseases and Controls (mean ±SD).

Measurement	Vibration Disease (N=35)	Controls (N=35)	p Values
Left ventricular end-diastolic dimension (mm)	49.1 ± 3.3	46.3 ± 5.2	<0.05
Left ventricular end-systolic dimension (mm)	29.2 ± 2.7	30 ± 5	NS
Ejection fraction (%)	78 ± 4	74 ± 6	<0.002
Intraventricular septal thickness (mm)	9.4 ± 1.1	10.2 ± 0.8	<0.01
Left ventricular posterior wall thickness (mm)	9.6 ± 1.2	9.9 ± 0.9	NS
Aortic diameter at end-diastole (mm)	29.7 ± 2.8	31.9 ± 2.7	<0.002
Left atrial diameter at end-diastole (mm)	30.2 ± 4.7	34 ± 4.3	<0.002
Heart rate (beats/min)	59 ± 1.4	67 ± 9.3	<0.001

measurements, the intraventricular septum thickness, left atrial dimension and aortic dimension were all significantly smaller in the patients with vibration disease than in the controls.

From the electrocardiographic data, the amplitude of the T waves is given in terms of the ratio of T to R waves in the limb lead I and the precordial lead V_5 and V_6. These ratios were slightly greater for the patients than for the controls. There was a statistically significant difference in the precordial lead V_6 (Table 2). The flat T waves in all leads were observed in one patient and three controls. The algebraic sum of the Q, R, and S deflections was also analyzed: the sum of $R_I + S_{III}$ was slightly smaller for the patients than in the controls, whereas the sum of $S_{V_1} + R_{V_5}$ was slightly larger in the patients.

The resting heart rate was significantly lower in the patients than in the controls (p<0.001), namely 59 ± 8.1 and 67 ± 9.3, respectively. As to blood pressure, hypertension was observed in two patients (5.7%), and the others were within the normal range. No statistically significant differences were seen between the cardiothoracic ratio of the patients and of the controls.

2.2 Follow-Up Study

A follow-up study of the cardiovascular features was performed approximately four years later on 51 male patients with vibration disease. All had ceased vibration exposure.

Figure 2 shows changes in the prevalence of normotension, borderline hypertension and hypertension between the first and last examinations (A and B, respectively). The prevalence of hypertension increased from 7.8% to 27.5% (p<0.05). The prevalence of normotension at the first examination was 82.4%: at the last follow-up examination, however, it had decreased to 58.8%. Thirteen of the 42 cases of normotension (30.9%) have changed to borderline hypertension or hypertension.

The increased prevalence of hypertension may be associated with an increase in subjective symptoms of the Vibration Syndrome. It is evident from Fig. 3 that the prevalence of subjective symptoms reported at the first examination had increased by the time of the final examination, with the exception of complaints of Raynaud's Phenomenon. The increased complaints suggest that, as well as lesions of the joints and muscles occurring in the vibration disease, which are difficult to treat, these patients are psychologically and socio-economically impaired.

Table 2. Electrocardiographic Findings in Patients With Vibration Diseases and Controls (mean ± SD).

	Vibration Disease (N=35)	Controls (N=35)	p value
T/R wave ratio: I	0.399 ± 0.218	0.363 ± 0.206	NS
V_5	0.267 ± 0.14	0.237 ± 0.075	NS
V_6	0.315 ± 0.127	0.239 ± 0.112	0.05
$R_I + S_{III}$	6.14 ± 2.34 mm	7.67 ± 4.3 mm	NS
$S_{V_1} + R_{V_5}$	29.1 ± 9.3 mm	28 ± 7.21 mm	NS

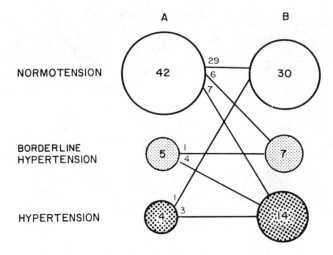

Fig. 2 Assessment of blood pressure
in 51 patients with vibration disease
at the initial (A) and final (B)
examinations. The time between
examinations was approximately four
years.

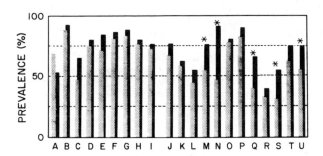

Fig. 3 The prevalence of subjective
symptoms reported at the first and
last examinations (dotted and solid
bars, respectively): A - Raynaud's
Phenomenon; B - numbness; C - pain;
D - cold sensation; E - stiffness;
F - nuchal pain; G - stiff shoulders;
H - elbow pain; I - lumbago; J - heavy
feeling in head; K - headache; L -
difficulty falling asleep; M - disturbance of sound sleep; N - early morning
awakening; O - palmar hyperhidrosis;
P - forgetfulness; Q - irritability;
R - depressive mood; S - suppressed
motivation; T - fatigue; and U - tin-
nitus. Statistically significant
changes are indicated by asterisks
(p<0.05).

By the time of the follow-up examination, the prevalence of resting bradycardia (less than 50/min) had decreased

from 15.7% to 9.8%. The electrocardiographic results at the last examination
revealed nothing unusual in nearly all
patients (94.1%), compared with the findings
of the first examination, (72.5%). At the
original examination, eleven of the 51 cases
were diagnosed as possessing left ventricular
hypertrophy from the electrocardiogram; they
had regressed to normal by the time of the
follow-up.

Figure 4 shows changes in the level of
autonomic nerve activity as recorded by
digital plethysmography with auditory
stimuli (4,5). The activity levels were
divided into four types: normoreactive type,
intermediate and delayed types (hyperreactive), and a poor response type (hyporeactive). At the first examination, the level
of autonomic nerve activity was abnormal in
approximately four-fifths of all patients.
These abnormal activity levels reverted to
normal during the follow-up period in most
patients, so that the prevalence decreased
from 82.3% to 29.4% (p<0.01).

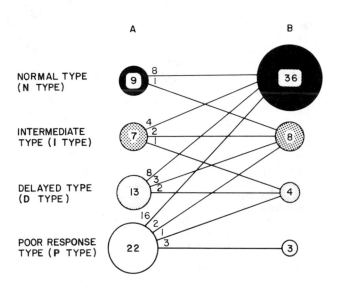

Fig. 4 Assessment of the level of
autonomic nerve activity in 51 patients
with vibration disease at the initial
(A) and final (B) examinations. The
hyperreactive types, intermediate (I)
and delayed (D) responses; and the
hyporeactive type, poor (P) response
decrease in prevalence. The normoreactive (N) type increases during this
period.

Spindle shaped fast activity in the
electroencephalogram was frequently observed
in patients with vibration disease (2,6).
The prevalence of the fast activity decreased from 19.6% to 11.7%. These findings
provide circumstantial evidence for the
regression of an adaptive response in the
cardiovascular system.

Matoba et al.: Cardiovascular features

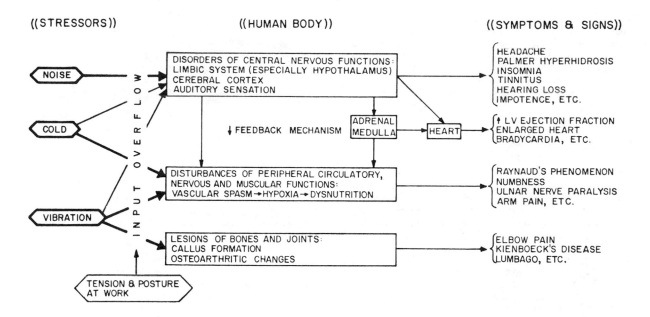

Fig. 5 Hypothetical scheme representing the pathogenesis of the vibration disease. Vibration, noise and cold act as stressors on the human body (modified from Matoba (3)).

III DISCUSSION

Vibration and noise from vibratory tools, and cold environments are stressors which affect the human body. Typical levels of tool vibration are from 90 to 140 dB (0.316 to 100 m/s^2) and of tool noise are from 80 to 120 dB(A). These stressors may excite the hypothalamus and the limbic lobe in the cortex, in which the higher centre of the autonomic nervous system exists. Consequently, the sympathetic tone could be significantly augmented, and the circulating catecholamines may be increased. In these situations, defense mechanisms to the stressors may be provided in the human body, so that an adaptive response can be produced.

Thus, habitual operation of vibratory tools could result in the production of an adaptation to the stressors. With regard to the cardiovascular features of the disease, resting sinus bradycardia, low blood pressure, cardiomegaly and abnormalities of the electrocardiogram have been observed in a study of 300 patients with vibration disease (2). In the present work, an increase in the left ventricular ejection fraction and stroke volume have been found. These findings are similar to the results of studies on endurance athletes (7-10). Well-trained athletes are adapted to physical training and possess, at rest, sinus bradycardia, cardiomegaly, comparatively lower blood pressure, increased stroke volume and left ventricular ejection fraction, increased cardiac output, and abnormalities of the electrocardiogram. Therefore, it is plausible that adaptation can be

produced in patients with vibration disease. The mechanism responsible for these adaptations is unclear, though the most frequently cited explanation involves alterations in the autonomic nervous system (11). Thus, it is emphasized that the clinical features of the vibration disease can include adaptive responses to the stressors, in addition to direct injuries induced by vibration.

It is relevant to question when the adaptation will regress after the use of vibratory tools is stopped. According to our results, the cardiovascular changes in the vibration disease may subside in six to eight years after discontinuing the use of vibratory tools. In fact, the adaptation of well-trained athletes regresses after training ceases (11).

The hypothetical pathogenesis of vibration disease is shown in Fig. 5. The chronically repeated action of stressors on the human body may overload and impair not only the peripheral systems, but also the central nervous system. If input overloading occurs, the sympathetic tone in the autonomic nervous system is elevated and increases the nerve impulses to the effectors. The increased nerve impulses result in vasoconstriction, leading to hypoxia and lack of nutrition in the tissues. Symptoms such as Raynaud's Phenomenon, numbness and others may develop in the fingers. As to the central nervous system, the excitation of the hypothalamus and the limbic system in the brain produces an increase in the circulating catecholamines from the adrenal medulla. On the other hand, if input overloading of the limbic system continues, the

Matoba et al.: Cardiovascular features

limbic system might exhaust itself and the feedback mechanism to the peripheral systems would become weak. These processes may lead to an enormous increase in vasoconstriction and an excitation of the heart. In these situations, the adaptation observed in endurance athletes may be produced in operators of vibratory tools, and various symptoms and signs would be observable.

IV   CONCLUSIONS

Cardiovascular features in patients with vibration disease are similar to those in well-trained athletes. These clinical symptoms and signs may indicate adaptation of the human body to the stressors. This adaptation is observed to regress for several years after discontinuing the use of vibratory tools. Accordingly, the clinical features of the vibration disease may include the adaptive responses to stressors as well as the direct injuries caused by vibration.

REFERENCES

1. In: Taylor W, ed. The Vibration Syndrome. London: Academic Press, 1974: 1-11.
2. Matoba T, Kusumoto H, Mizuki Y, Kuwahara H, Inanaga K, Takamatsu M. Clinical features and laboratory findings of vibration disease: A review of 300 cases. Tohoku J Exp Med 1977; 123: 57-65.
3. Matoba T. Vibration disease and the autonomic nervous system. The Autonomic Nervous System 1979; 16: 131-5.
4. Matoba T, Kusumoto H, Omura H, Kotorii T, Kuwahara H, Takamatsu M. Digital plethys-mographic responses to auditory stimuli in patients with vibration disease. Tohoku J Exp Med 1975; 115: 385-92.
5. Matoba T, Mizobuchi H, Ito T, Chiba M, Toshima H. Further observations on the digital plethysmography with auditory stimuli and its clinical applications. Angiology 1981; 32: 62-72.
6. Arikawa K, Shirakawa T, Kotorii T, Ohima M, Nakazawa Y, Inanaga K, Kuwahara H. An elec-troencephalographic study of patients with vibration disease. Folia Psychiatr Neurol Jpn 1978; 32: 211-22.
7. Ikäheimo MJ, Palatsi IJ, Takkunen JT. Non-invasive evaluation of the athletic heart: Sprinters versus endurance runners. Am J Cardiol 1979; 44: 24-30.
8. Bekaert I, Rannier JL, Van De Weghe C, Van Durme JP, Clement DL, Pannier R. Non-invasive evaluation of cardiac function in professional cyclists. Br Heart J 1981; 45: 213-8.
9. Roeske WR, O'Rourke RA, Klein A, Leopold G, Karliner JS. Non-invasive evaluation of ventricular hypertrophy in professional athletes. Circulation 1976; 53: 286-92.
10. Van Ganse W, Versee L, Eylenbosch W, Vuylsteek K. The electrocardiogram of athletes: comparison with untrained subjects. Br Heart J 1970; 32: 160-4.
11. Scheuer J, Tipton CM. Cardiovascular adapta-tions to physical training. Annu Rev Physiol 1977; 39: 221-51.

DISCUSSION

I. Pyykkö: The autonomic nervous system per-forms several functions, for example, cardiovascular and sudomotor functions, which operate independently. Hence one can increase and the other decrease (e.g. vasodilatation in skin circulation and increase in sweat production in warm temperatures). Further-more, in the cardiovascular system, the cardiac and peripheral circulation can be dissociated in function (e.g. palpitation of the heart and vaso-dilatation - see Koizumi and Brooks, Ergebniss der Physiologie 1972; 67: 1-67). In your paper, you classified subjects according to hypo-, normo- or hyperactive sympathetic tone. What were your criteria?

Authors' Response: The autonomic tone has been assessed by digital plethysmography with auditory stimuli (Ref. 4,5). It is based on a physiological method, namely stimulation of the brain and its response as measured by digital blood flow. This method reflects the activity level of the higher centres of the autonomic nervous system.

What were your criteria for assessing the severity of the Vibration Syndrome?

Authors' Response: The severity, classified by us into four Stages, has been assessed using our own criteria (Matoba et al. Jpn J Ind Health 1975; 17: 211-214). The activity of the autonomic nervous system is increasing with Stage to the hyperreactive level. At the end of Stage III, the autonomic tone is decreasing to hyporeactive. Recovery from the hyporeactive state to normoreactive is via the hyperreactive state.

H.F.V. Riddle: Have any studies been made of the personalities of affected individuals in view of the claims of generalized autonomic response to vibration and noise?

Authors' Response: We have done a study of the relationship between the Cornell Medical Index scores and the activity level of the autonomic nervous system (Ref. 5). Approximately 20% of the patients tended to be neurotic. The scores of III (near neurotic) and IV (neurotic) were comparatively higher in the hyperreactive type.

Pathophysiology of Vibration-Induced White Finger: Etiological Considerations and Proposals for Prevention

T. Azuma and T. Ohhashi

ABSTRACT: The response of arterial smooth muscle to noradrenaline was suppressed during, and enhanced soon after, vibratory stimulation. This hyperresponse was not induced by vibration frequencies less than 10 Hz and it was reduced, or eliminated, by periodic stimulation with rest intervals. Pretreatment of arterial smooth muscle with verapamil considerably inhibited the contractile responses to noradrenaline in the hyperresponsive state, as well as those before vibration exposure. The contraction of arterial smooth muscle was markedly reduced in plasma containing vitamin E. Based on the hypothesis that the vibration-induced hyperresponse of arterial smooth muscle to noradrenaline is associated with the development of VWF, four methods are suggested for counteracting the development of a local circulatory insufficiency: 1) use of a low-pass mechanical filter to reduce vibration entering the hand; 2) use of intermittent vibration exposures; 3) administration of calcium antagonists; and 4) continued use of vitamin E.

RESUME: La réaction des muscles lisses artériels à la noradrénaline fut supprimée pendant, et amplifiée peu après, une stimulation vibratoire. Cette hyper-réaction ne fut pas provoquée par des fréquences vibratoires inférieures à 10 Hz et fut réduite, ou éliminée, par une stimulation périodique avec intervalles de repos. Le pré-traitement des muscles artériels avec du vérapamil a considérablement inhibé les réactions de contraction à la noradrénaline dans l'état hyper-réactif, ainsi qu'avant l'exposition aux vibrations. La contraction du muscle lisse artériel fut nettement réduite dans du plasma contenant de la vitamine E. Partant de l'hypothèse que l'hyper-réaction, due aux vibrations, du muscle lisse artériel à la noradrénaline, est liée au développement des doigts blancs (VWF), quatre moyens sont proposés pour contrer le développement d'une insuffisance circulatoire locale: 1) l'utilisation d'un filtre mécanique passe-bas pour réduire les vibrations pénétrant dans la main; 2) utilisation d'expositions aux vibrations intermittentes; 3) administration d'antagonistes au calcium; et 4) utilisation continuelle de vitamine E.

INTRODUCTION

Vibration disease is becoming recognised as an important occupational disease, because of the large number of people affected. A characteristic feature of the disease is Raynaud's Phenomenon in the fingers. We have used a physiological approach to study the pathogenesis of vibration-induced white finger, and found that the response of arterial smooth muscle to noradrenaline was strikingly elevated after the imposition of vibratory stimulation (1,2). The human body may be in a condition of severe stress when exposed to intense vibration and loud noise in a cold environment. Furthermore, the output of catecholamines from the adrenal medulla will be enhanced and the sympathetic vasoconstrictor tone will be elevated under these conditions. A concurrent rise in the response of arterial smooth muscle to noradrenaline in fingers exposed to vibration can lead to local vasoconstriction, which impairs blood supply to the fingers. The hyperresponse may thus be a basis for the appearance of VWF. The present study was undertaken to investigate the mode of appearance of the vibration-induced hyperresponse in detail and to find ways of inhibiting its development.

I MATERIALS AND METHODS

1.1 In Vitro Experiments

Forty mongrel dogs of both sexes, weighing from 7 to 24 kg, were anesthetized with intravenous administration of sodium pentobarbital (30 mg/kg) and killed by bleeding. Segments were isolated from the femoral, popliteal, celiac, superior mesenteric and renal arteries, and the abdominal aorta.

1.1.1 Dose-Response Relationships for Noradrenaline

After removal of the connecting tissue surrounding the arterial segments, helical strips of 15 mm length and 5 mm width were dissected at an angle of 15° to the transverse axis of the vessels. Each of these strips was placed in an organ bath filled with a modified Locke's solution of the following composition (in mM): NaCl, 154; KCl, 5.6; $CaCl_2$, 2.2; $NaHCO_3$, 8; and glucose, 5.5. The solution was kept at 37°C and bubbled continuously with 95% O_2 and 5% CO_2 to give a pH of 7.4. The upper end of the strip was connected to a force-displacement transducer (Shinko Tsushin UL-20-120) and the lower end to the movable shaft of a special electromagnetic vibrator (3). Tension development in the strip was recorded isometrically by means of a strain amplifier (Shinko Tsushin DS6-RJ) and an electronic polyrecorder (Towa Denpa EPR-2TS). Before commencing experiments, each strip was elongated until its in vivo length was regained, and allowed to equilibrate for 60 min in the bathing medium.

The response of the strip to dl-noradrenaline (Sankyo) was studied at intervals of 1 h by the use of cumulative dose-response relationships. Vibratory stimulations, 1 to 70 Hz in frequency, 300 or 500 μm in amplitude, and 0.5 to 6 h in duration, were applied to the strips after the first dose-response relationships were obtained. The tension developed in the specimen was expressed relative to the maximum value induced by noradrenaline before the application of vibratory stimulation. The effects of verapamil (Eizai) and vitamin E (Eizai) on the contraction of arterial smooth muscle induced by noradrenaline were also investigated.

1.1.2 Histological Examination

After being elongated until their in vivo lengths were regained, segments of the aforementioned arteries were fixed in a 10% formalin solution. After dehydration in alcohol, the segments were embedded in paraffin and cut into transverse sections. The sections were stained with Mallory-azarin and examined by an optical microscope (Olympus FH). The wall thickness of an artery, D, and the width of its media, d, were measured by means of a micrometer attached to the microscope, and the smooth muscle content of the arterial wall, θ, calculated as:

$$\theta = (d/D) \times 100. \qquad (1)$$

1.2 In Vivo Experiments

Twenty-four mongrel dogs of both sexes, weighing from 10 to 16 kg, were anesthetized with sodium pentobarbital (30 mg/kg) and ventilated artificially by means of a respirator (Harvard 613). Both ends of a looped polyethylene catheter, equipped with an electromagnetic flow probe (Nihon Koden FF020T), were inserted into the femoral artery of a hindlimb (test limb) to measure the rate of arterial inflow. The probe was connected to an electromagnetic flowmeter (Nihon Koden MF-27). A side branch of the artery and of the ipsilateral femoral vein were cannulated with polyethylene catheters, to record arterial and venous pressures respectively, by the use of pressure transducers (Toyo Baldwin MPU-0.5-290 and LPU-0.1-350) and strain amplifiers (Sanei Sokki Type 1236 and Type 1237). These pressures, together with the rate of arterial flow, were displayed on a direct-writing oscillograph (Sanei Sokki 8S). Peripheral vascular resistance was calculated as the ratio of the mean pressure difference between the artery and vein to the rate of blood flow in the femoral artery.

A handmade vibrator was connected to the ankle of the test hindlimb. The output of the vibrator was set to 0.22 mm displacement at 60 Hz (corresponding to an acceleration of 3 G), to provide a fixed vibratory stimulation to the test limb for three hours. Administrations of 3 μg/kg dl-noradrenaline hydrochloride (Sankyo) were made via a catheter in the external jugular vein before, during, and after application of the vibratory stimulation, to observe changes in peripheral resistance. The changes were statistically evaluated by Student's t-test (unpaired), and differences in means were considered significant when values were less than 0.05.

II RESULTS

2.1 Responses of Femoral Arterial Strips to Noradrenaline

Cumulative dose-response relationships for noradrenaline were obtained with strips prepared from the femoral artery. The upper panel of Fig. 1 shows the results of a control experiment. The time elapsed after the start of incubation in the bathing medium is given at the top of each curve, which shows the change in tension caused by increasing doses of noradrenaline. No appreciable time-dependent change was observed in the threshold dose or the tension developed at each concentration of noradrenaline. As demonstrated in the lower panel, the response to noradrenaline was considerably suppressed during a vibratory stimulation of three hours' duration.

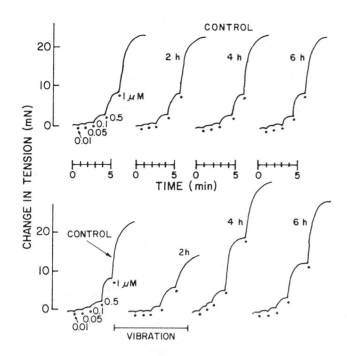

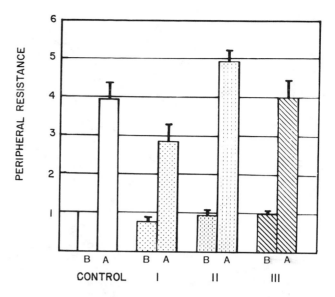

Fig. 1 Cumulative dose-response relationships, shown as tension versus
time, for noradrenaline obtained with
femoral arterial strips: upper panel-
stable responses of a strip without
vibratory stimulation; and lower panel-
suppression of the response during, and
enhancement of the response after, a
vibratory stimulation (50 Hz, 500 μm,
3 h). The time elapsed after incubation in the bathing medium is shown
at the top of each curve. The moment
at which a given concentration of noradrenaline was administered is represented by a dot, and the horizontal bar
indicates the period of vibratory stimulation.

The magnitude of the maximum response was
reduced by about 30%, and the threshold
concentration was increased by a factor of
2 or 3. On the other hand, the response
was markedly enhanced after interruption
of the stimulation. The magnitude of the
maximum contraction obtained 1 h after the
end of the stimulation was 160 to 170% of
that in the control, and the threshold concentration was reduced by a factor of 0.2.
These changes were statistically significant. The response, once elevated, gradually faded away and returned to the control
level 5 h after the end of the stimulation.

2.2 Effects of Vibratory Stimulation on Noradrenaline-Induced Changes in Peripheral Resistance in Vivo

The peripheral vascular resistance in
the hindlimbs of anesthetized dogs was

Fig. 2 Mean vibration-induced change
in the peripheral vascular resistance
of canine hindlimb (+ SEM), from ten
experiments. Each set of bars indicates
stationary resistance before (B) and a
maximum resistance after (A) administration of 3 μg/kg noradrenaline: control-
before vibration imposed upon the ipsilateral ankle; I - during vibratory
stimulation (50 Hz, 3 G, 0.22 mm, 3 h);
II - 1 h after stimulation; III - 3 h
after stimulation. All resistances are
expressed relative to the stationary
resistance (B) in the control. (From
Ref. 2, with permission of Cardiovasc Res).

increased by the intravenous administration
of 3 μg/kg noradrenaline. The maximum
resistance was calculated at the moment at
which arterial blood pressure reached a
peak. This resistance was compared with
the value observed in a stable state before
noradrenaline administration (stationary
resistance). The stationary and the maximum
resistances were calculated before, during,
and after a fixed vibratory stimulation
imposed upon the ipsilateral ankle (Fig. 2).
Each of the resistances was expressed relative to the stationary resistance recorded
before application of the vibratory stimulation.

Before the vibratory stimulation, the
administration of noradrenaline elevated
the peripheral resistance by a factor of
3.97. During the stimulation, the stationary resistance was significantly lowered,
from 1 to 0.78. Administration of noradrenaline in this period raised the resistance by only a factor of 2.89, which was
significantly less than the maximum resistance before the stimulation. The stationary and maximum resistances calculated 1 h
after the end of the vibratory stimulation

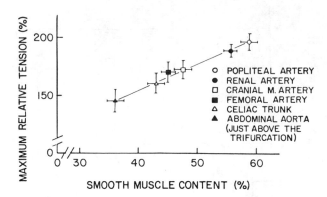

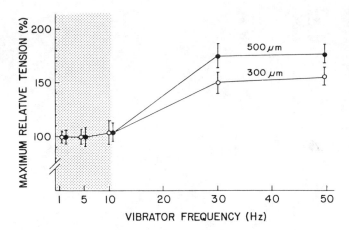

Fig. 3 The relationship between smooth muscle content and its response to noradrenaline, in vitro, after a vibratory stimulation (30 Hz, 500 μm, 1 h): mean values ± SEM (horizontal and vertical bars) from five experiments (r=0.98). The magnitude of the maximum response to noradrenaline 1 h after the end of vibratory stimulation is expressed relative to that before the stimulation (maximum relative tension), and the smooth muscle content is expressed as a ratio of the thickness of the media to the width of the arterial wall.

were 0.91 and 5.03, respectively. The latter was significantly higher than the maximum resistance before the stimulation. The increased response to noradrenaline disappeared 3 h after the end of the stimulation.

These results support the conclusion of our in vitro experiments, namely, that the response of arterial smooth muscle to noradrenaline decreases during, and increases soon after, vibratory stimulation.

2.3 Smooth Muscle Content and Noradrenaline Response

Figure 3 shows the relationship between the extent of vibration-induced hyperresponse to noradrenaline and the smooth muscle content of various arteries. The magnitude of the maximum isometric response of an artery to noradrenaline 1 h after the end of a fixed vibratory stimulation (30 Hz, 500 μm, 1 h) has been expressed relative to the corresponding control value, i.e. the maximum tension in the same artery developed by noradrenaline before the vibratory stimulation. The smooth muscle content of an artery is expressed as the ratio of the thickness of its media to the width of the wall (eqn. 1).

The maximum response after the stimulation exceeded 190% of the control value in the popliteal artery, the smooth muscle

Fig. 4 Effects of the frequency and amplitude of vibratory stimulation (for 3 h) on the vibration-induced increase in noradrenaline response of femoral arterial strips, expressed in terms of the maximum relative tension. Open and solid circles represent the mean responses ± SEM induced by stimulations of 300 and 500 μm amplitude, respectively, in ten experiments. (From Ref. 1, with permission of Cardiovasc Res).

content of which amounted to 59%. In the abdominal aorta, on the other hand, the maximum response and the smooth muscle content were 145% and 36% respectively. Values obtained from the other arteries were greater than those in the aorta and smaller than those in the popliteal artery. Generally speaking, the more the smooth muscle content, the greater the extent of the vibration-induced hyperresponse to noradrenaline.

2.4 Effects of Vibration Parameters

The maximum tension developed in femoral arterial strips by noradrenaline, 1 h after a 3 h vibratory stimulation, was expressed relative to that before the stimulation, and plotted as ordinate with the vibration frequency as abscissa (Fig. 4). The larger the vibration amplitude, the more pronounced the effect became. No hyperresponse was induced by any stimulation of less than 10 Hz. The effect increased with increasing frequency up to 30 to 40 Hz and then reached a plateau. Because of the restricted frequency range of our vibrator, no vibratory stimulation of more than 70 Hz was applied to the preparations.

Figure 5 demonstrates the time course of the hyperresponse of smooth muscle to noradrenaline in the femoral artery, induced by vibratory stimulations of different duration. Vibration frequency and amplitude were set during these experiments at 30 Hz and 500 μm, respectively. After the end

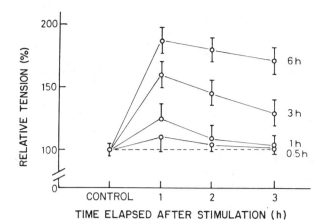

Fig. 5 Time course of vibration-induced hyperresponse to noradrenaline, in vitro, after the end of vibratory stimulation (30 Hz, 500 μm). The magnitude of the maximum response to noradrenaline at a given time is expressed relative to that before stimulation (relative tension). Results are for the mean ± SEM from 10 experiments. The duration of the stimulation is shown to the right of each curve.

of vibratory stimulation, the maximum tension developed by noradrenaline was measured every 1 h, expressed as a ratio relative to the magnitude of the maximum response in the control, and plotted as a percentage.

In general, the hyperresponse to noradrenaline became more pronounced, and the time required for its disappearance become longer, as the duration of the stimulus increased from 0.5 to 6 h. The hyperresponse induced by stimulation for 6 h was long lasting, the magnitude of the maximum response at the third hour still amounting to 170% of the control. The effect of stimulation for 3 h had largely disappeared at the third hour, whereas the response to stimulation for 1 h had almost disappeared after two hours. The response of arterial smooth muscle to stimulation for 30 min tended to increase for another hour: the increase, however, was not statistically significant. Under these experimental conditions, the threshold for the appearance of the effect seemed to involve exposures in excess of 30 minutes.

Accordingly, the total duration of the vibration exposure was set at 1 h and femoral arterial strips were then stimulated in three different ways (Fig. 6). A continuous 1 h stimulation was applied to the preparations in group A. Two 30 min stimulations were applied to those in group B, with a 30 min pause between exposures. The preparations in group C were stimulated

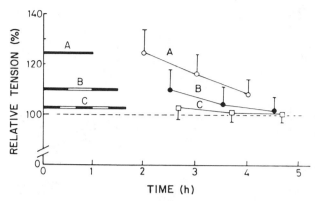

Fig. 6 Time course of vibration-induced hyperresponse to noradrenaline, in vitro, measured from the commencement of stimulation: A - continuous stimulation for 1 h (30 Hz, 500 μm); B - stimulation for two 30 min periods separated by a 30 min rest interval; and C - stimulation for three 20 min periods separated by two 20 min rest intervals. The ordinate is the same as in Fig. 5. Results are for the mean ± SEM from 10 experiments.

three times for 20 min each, at intervals of 20 min. The response of these preparations to noradrenaline was examined every hour after the end of vibration exposure. In group A, a statistically significant hyperresponse was found after the first and second hour. In group B, the response tended to increase after the first hour: the increase, however, was statistically insignificant. No hyperresponse was induced in group C.

2.5 Effects of Drugs

The hyperresponsive state may be induced not only by an increase in the sensitivity of the noradrenaline receptor in smooth muscle membranes, but also by a facilitation of the contractile mechanism which is known to be intimately associated with Ca^{2+} influx. Pretreatment of the preparations with 10^{-4} M verapamil, a calcium antagonist, inhibited contractile responses to noradrenaline in a hyperresponsive state as well as those in the control, shifting both dose-response relationships toward the lower right (Fig. 7). In this figure, the magnitude of a response is expressed relative to the maximum tension developed before vibratory stimulation, and plotted as ordinate against noradrenaline concentration as abscissa. The responses to noradrenaline at concentrations of less than 5×10^{-5} M were completely suppressed in both cases. The response to 5×10^{-4} M noradrenaline were reduced by about 50%.

Azuma et al.: Pathophysiology

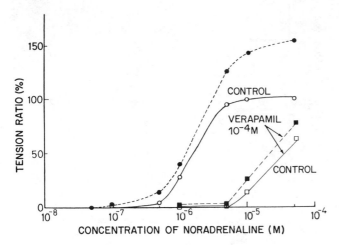

Fig. 7 Effect of verapamil on dose-response relationships for noradrenaline, obtained with femoral arterial strips. Mean ratio of the tension developed by a given concentration of noradrenaline relative to the maximum value before vibratory stimulation (tension ratio) ± SEM, from 10 experiments: solid curves - before vibratory stimulation; and dashed curves - 1 h after vibratory stimulation (30 Hz, 500 μm, 3 h). Data are shown by circles before, and squares after, the administration of verapamil.

Pretreatment of arterial preparations with 10^{-5} M phentolamine also moved the dose-response relationships after vibratory stimulation to the right, though the respective maximum tensions remained unchanged. The dose-response relationships thus appeared to be parallel.

Vitamin E (α-tocopherol) has been said to improve blood flow through peripheral tissues. At first, we studied the effect of vitamin E on the contractile response of arterial smooth muscle to noradrenaline. When the modified Locke's solution was used as a bathing medium, the presence of vitamin E at concentrations of between 10^{-5} and 10^{-3} g/ml did not affect the contraction of femoral arterial smooth muscle induced by 10^{-6} M noradrenaline. However, when we used canine plasma or whole blood as the bathing medium, the vitamin dose inhibited the contraction. The solution of vitamin E did not influence the muscle contraction in either of the bathing media.

Figure 8 shows dose-response relationships for noradrenaline obtained with arterial strips bathed in canine plasma. As shown by the data from control samples, a marked reduction in the noradrenaline threshold concentration was observed in this medium. The relationship obtained 1 h

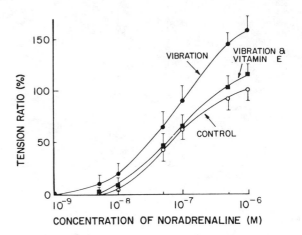

Fig. 8 Effect of vitamin E on dose-response relationships for noradrenaline, obtained with femoral arterial strips bathed in canine plasma. Mean tension ratio ± SEM, from 10 experiments: open circles - control; solid circle - 1 h after vibratory stimulation (30 Hz, 500 μm, 3 h); and squares - 1 h after vibratory stimulation in plasma containing 10^{-3} gm/ml of vitamin E. The ordinate is the same as in Fig. 7.

after a vibratory stimulation (30 Hz, 500 μm, 3 h) showed a lowering of the threshold and an increase in the tension developed at each concentration of noradrenaline. Thus, a hyperresponsive state was also induced by vibratory stimulation in this bathing medium, the maximum tension amounting to 158% of that in the control. Hyperresponsiveness after vibratory stimulation did not occur, however, in samples bathed in canine plasma containing 10^{-3} g/ml vitamin E. In this bathing medium, the maximum tension only increased by 18% 1 h after the end of the vibratory stimulation. This increase was not statistically significant.

III DISCUSSION

3.1 Possible Etiology

As shown in Figs. 1 and 2, the response of arterial smooth muscle to noradrenaline was suppressed during, and enhanced soon after, the application of vibratory stimulation (1,2). The suppression may be related to a vibration-induced reduction of the tension in portal and ureteral smooth muscles that have been in a state of contracture (4). Bhattacharya et al. reported a decrease in the total peripheral resistance of conscious dogs exposed to whole-body vibration (5).

Azuma et al.: Pathophysiology

The degree and duration of the hyper-responsiveness after a vibratory stimulation depended upon the frequency, amplitude, and duration of the stimulation (Figs. 4 and 5). A linear relationship between the extent of hyperresponsiveness and smooth muscle content in arterial walls suggests that the greatest increase in responsiveness to noradrenaline will take place in arterioles where the relative thickness of the media reaches a maximum (Fig. 3). The hyperresponsiveness seems to be a key to the development of vibration-induced white finger, since an intense, long-lasting constriction of digital arterioles will give rise to a profound impairment of local circulation.

Based on the experimental results so far obtained, we infer the mode of appearance of vibration-induced white finger as follows. An increase in output of catecholamines from the adrenal medulla and a rise of vasoconstrictor tone will take place in a human body exposed to an intense vibration accompanied by loud noises, as a reaction to these stressors. Vascular smooth muscle will thus be in readiness for vasoconstriction. Assuming that our results from acute experiments can be applied to human digital arteries, an elevated response of arteries and arterioles to noradrenaline in fingers exposed to vibration will lead to a profound local vasoconstriction, which continues for up to two hours and reduces the blood supply to the fingers. According to Johshita et al., iterative elevations in circumferential tension of the rabbit carotid artery caused intimal thickening and medial muscular hyperplasia followed by degeneration (6). Intimal thickening and medial fibrosis appeared in the rat mesenteric arteries in which a sustained, intense vasoconstriction was induced daily for two weeks by topical application of methoxamine hydrochloride (7). Repeated vibration-induced local vasoconstriction may therefore play an important role in the gradual development of the white fingers. The localized occurrence of circulatory insufficiency in vibration disease may thus be understood in terms of a vibration-induced hyperresponsiveness of arterial smooth muscle to noradrenaline.

Most of the patients suffering from vibration disease are said to complain that paresthesia in the hands was relieved during, and intensified after, operating vibrating tools (Terayama K, personal communication). This complaint seems to have been overlooked, because, as far as we are aware, no such description is to be found in clinical reports. The improvement of paresthesia during the operation of power tools can easily be understood from the viewpoint of the reduction in responsiveness to noradrenaline during vibratory stimulation.

3.2 Possible Means for Prevention

From the preceding discussion, it appears that the occurrence of the hyper-response may be a basis for the development of vibration-induced white finger. Hence any means that can restrict this hyper-response should effectively prevent the development of local circulatory insufficiency in fingers operating vibrating tools. The results of our experiments suggest the following four methods which may possibly counteract the development of vibration-induced white finger.

3.2.1 Use of Mechanical Filter

As shown in Fig. 4, no hyperresponse to noradrenaline was induced in arterial smooth muscle by vibratory stimulations at frequencies less than 10 Hz. In addition, the larger the vibration amplitude, the more pronounced the effect became. Similar frequency and amplitude dependence of the spontaneous rhythm in portal venous smooth muscle was also observed during vibratory stimulation (4). For protection against the occurrence of white finger, therefore, it seems to be important to reduce the amplitude of vibration and to inhibit the transmission to the hand of components at frequencies greater than 10 Hz. The interposition of an appropriate mechanical filter between a vibrating machine and the hand may thus be useful in protecting the fingers from circulatory impairment.

3.2.2 Division of Work Time

The vibration-induced hyperresponse of arterial smooth muscle to noradrenaline became more pronounced, and the time required for its disappearance become longer, as the duration of stimulation increased while other parameters remained unchanged (Fig. 5). A significant increase in the response to vibratory stimulation was not observed when the exposure was divided into two or three periods, and applied at intervals (Fig. 6). These findings suggest that dividing the work time into several short periods, separated by vibration-free periods of an appropriate duration, will be an effective measure in the prevention of white finger.

3.2.3 Administration of Calcium Antagonists

The dose-response relationship for noradrenaline obtained with arterial preparations in a vibration-induced hyper-responsive state was not a simple vertical shift of the relationship found in the control strips (see Figs. 7 and 8). The difference between these two relationships increased with increasing noradrenaline

concentration. Pretreatment with phentolamine did not alter the magnitude of the
maximum response in the hyperresponsive
state or in the control. Pretreatment
with verapamil, on the other hand, generally inhibited the contractile responses of
arterial smooth muscle to noradrenaline
(Fig. 7). The maximum tension developed
was decreased by about 50% in the hyperresponsive state. Administration of
calcium antagonists is thus thought to be
useful for prophylactic and therapeutic
purposes.

3.2.4 Continued Use of Vitamin E

Vitamin E did not affect the nor-
adrenaline-induced contraction of arterial
smooth muscle in a physiological saline
solution. The vitamin, however, considerably reduced the contraction in plasma or
whole blood. The magnitude of the vibration-induced hyperresponse to noradrenaline
was considerably reduced in plasma containing vitamin E (Fig. 8). An elevation in
the plasma level of vitamin E may therefore
be effective for the prophylaxis of white
finger in vibration disease.
The present discussion of the pathogenesis and prophylaxis of vibration-
induced white finger has been inferred from
the results of our acute experiments.
Chronic experiments on the vibration-induced
hyperresponse of arterial smooth muscle to
noradrenaline are needed in the future.

REFERENCES

1. Azuma T, Ohhashi T, Sakaguchi M. Vibration-
   induced hyperresponsiveness of arterial
   smooth muscle to noradrenaline: with special
   reference to Raynaud's phenomenon in vibration
   disease. Cardiovasc Res 1978; 12: 758-764.
2. Azuma T, Ohhashi T, Sakaguchi M. An approach
   to the pathogenesis of "white finger" induced
   by vibratory stimulation: acute but sustained
   changes in vascular responsiveness of canine
   hindlimb to noradrenaline. Cardiovasc Res
   1980; 14: 725-730.
3. Sakaguchi M, Ohhashi T, Azuma T. A new vibratory stimulator: with special reference to
   its physiological application. IEEE Trans-
   action on Biomedical Engineering 1978; BME-25:
   484-486.
4. Ohhashi T, Azuma T, Sakaguchi T. Effect of
   microvibration on activity of ureteral and
   portal smooth muscles. Am J Physiol 1979;
   236: C192-C201.
5. Bhattacharya A, Knapp CF, McCutcheon EP,
   Edwards RG. Parameters for assessing
   vibration-induced cardiovascular responses
   in awake dogs. J Appl Physiol 1977; 42: 682-
   689.
6. Johshita T, Sakata N, Yoshida K, Yoshida Y,
   Ooneda G. Arterial circumferential tension
   and atherosclerosis. J Jpn College Angiol
   1978; 18: 857-862.
7. Masawa N. Pathological study on the arterial
   lesions by repeated arterial contraction (spasm)
   in rats. J Jpn College Angiol 1979; 10: 863-
   876.

DISCUSSION

N. Olsen: Does exposure to vibration increase
the concentration of noradrenaline in the blood of
the animals studied?
Authors' Response: We are preparing for the
measurement of the noradrenaline concentration.
At present, however, we have no data.

M. Färkkilä: Do you think that vibration
exposure can increase the noradrenaline levels in
human beings to the concentrations used in your
experiments with dogs?
Authors' Response: I cannot answer this
question on the basis of our animal experiments.
A review of the literature indicates that cold
exposure or severe hemorrhage increases the blood
concentration of noradrenaline by several times.
(Johnson DG et al. J Appl Physiol 1977; 43: 216-
220, Johnson MD et al. Am J Physiol 1979; 236: H463-
H470.)

I. Pyykkö: Your results appear to be in good
agreement with the findings of Sjöqvist and Ljung
(Acta Physiol Scand 1980; 110: 381-384), who showed
that vibration causes immediate relaxation of an
isolated blood vessel (denervated rat portal vein).
However, when a vessel's wall is isolated from the
nerve, its sensitivity to adrenaline increases after
a certain latent period. Thus, could the effects of
adrenaline be a result of the so-called denervation
syndrome of the vessel wall?
Authors' Response: We cannot completely deny
the possibility that the observed hyperresponse of
arterial smooth muscle to noradrenaline may be
related to a rise of noradrenaline sensitivity after
denervation. As shown in Fig. 1, however, the
responses of arterial smooth muscle to noradrenaline
in the control were unchanged for several hours.
In addition, the vibration-induced hyperresponse was
not only observed to noradrenaline, but also to
serotonin and angiotensin (unpublished data). These
findings indicate that the above mentioned possibility may be invalid.

Were all the experiments performed on
anesthetized dogs, or did your controls consist of
intact, unanesthetized animals?
Authors' Response: All of our in vivo experiments were performed on anesthetized dogs.

Peripheral Nervous System and Hand–Arm Vibration Exposure

E. Lukáš

ABSTRACT: Two hundred and forty-five persons, exposed to hand-arm vibration, were examined clinically and by measuring the conduction velocities of the motor and sensory fibres of the ulnar and median nerves (N.). The results are compared with X-ray findings of the cervical vertebral column and the elbow joint. The clinical and EMG studies indicate mostly isolated damage of the N. medianus, which resembles the carpal tunnel syndrome. Isolated damage of the N. ulnaris was usually observed simultaneously with damage to the elbow-joint processes (arthropathy). Combined lesions of both nerves occurred predominantly in subjects with a diagnosis of vasoneurosis. A small group of persons with traumatic vasoneurosis, a group with industrial vasoneurosis and a control group were also examined by EMG. The results indicate that in the initial stage of vibration damage, the vessel component is an important factor leading to ischemic neuropathy.

RESUME: On a fait subir un examen clinique à 245 personnes dont le système main-bras est exposé à des vibrations et mesuré la vitesse de conduction des fibres nerveuses motrices et sensorielles des nerfs (N.) cubital et médian. On a ensuite comparé les résultats de ces examens à des radiographies de la colonne cervicale et du coude. Les examens cliniques et les électromyographies révèlent surtout une altération du N. median seul, ce qui s'apparent au syndrome du canal carpien. En général, on observait une altération du N. cubital seul lorsque l'articulation du coude était atteinte (arthropathie). Les lésions touchaient les deux nerfs à la fois surtout chez les sujets souffrant de vasoneurose. On a également étudié l'EMG d'un petit groupe de personnes atteintes de vasoneurose traumatique, d'un groupe de personnes souffrant de vasoneurose industriel et d'un groupe témoin. Les résultats révèlent qu'au premier stade de l'altération que provoquent les vibrations, les vaisseaux sanguins constituent un important facteur d'évolution vers la neuropathie ischémique.

INTRODUCTION

It is well known that exposure of the hand to vibration may cause nerve signs and symptoms indicating damage to the peripheral neurons. It is not known, however, whether such lesions are the primary damage sites, or whether they should be considered second-ary disturbances due to damage of the circulatory and/or locomotive system.

The basis for a discussion of this problem must be an objective neurological and electro-physiological diagnosis of potential lesions in the peripheral nervous system. As such lesions are also found in persons not exposed to vibration, a wide-spread differential diagnosis is essential.

In order to develop our experience in this field, we have followed a large group of patients exposed to hand-arm vibration for a period of ten years. The results of this work are presented here.

I RESULTS AND DISCUSSION

Two hundred and forty-five subjects were divided into two subgroups according to the nature of their exposure to vibration (see Table 1). In all cases a neurological

Table 1. Age, Occupation and Exposure Duration of Subjects.

	Subgroup I N=108	Subgroup II N=137
Mean Age (yrs)	45.3	44.7
Industrial Group	various and combined (tunnelers, stone-cutters, coal miners, forest workers, grinders)	homogeneous (ore miners)
Mean Exposure time (yrs)	11.8	13.9

examination was performed. Either the patients themselves had complained of some neurological symptoms, or a physician had diagnosed symptoms associated with a suspected vibration-induced nerve lesion during a periodic survey. Thus the group consisted of subjects either with a history of nerve symptoms or a positive finding of nerve injury.

Some characteristic symptoms were reported by the subjects, in particular finger paresthesia, white fingers, pain (in the neck, muscles and joints), hypoesthesia and hypodynamia. The objective examination consisted of signs mostly of hypoesthesia, hyporeflexia C5-8, acrovasal syndrome, and symptoms of amyotrophy and myohypotony. The frequency of the signs and symptoms is given in Table 2.

Table 2. Signs and Symptoms Found in Subjects.

		Subgroup I	Subgroup II
Subjective Signs and Symptoms	finger paresthesia	50%	74%
	white fingers	49%	69%
	pains-neck	28%	24%
	muscles	39%	52%
	joints	32%	65%
	hypoesthesia	23%	24%
	hypodynamia	34%	43%
Objective Signs and Symptoms	hypoesthesia	59%	71%
	hyporeflexia C5-8	33%	47%
	acrovasal syndrome	30%	37%
	amyotrophy & myohypotonia	27%	26%

For an objective diagnosis, we have standardized a procedure involving simultaneous measurement of the nerve conduction velocities in fast motor and sensory fibres. The method involves antidromic stimulation of the sensory fibres and the use of finger ring electrodes for the observation of the neurograms (see Figs. 1 and 2).

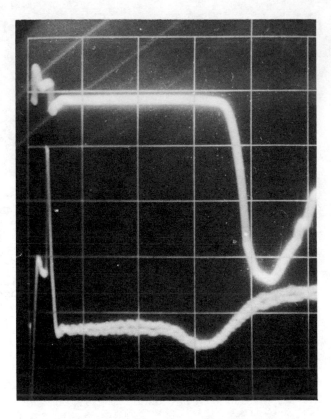

Fig. 2 Simultaneous stimulation of the sensory and motor fibres of the median nerve. Upper trace - motor fibres (vertical scale 200 μV/div; horizontal scale 1 ms/div); lower trace - sensory fibres (vertical scale 60 μV/div).

An interesting finding from our electromyographic test is that isolated pathological phenomena were found more often in only one of the nerves tested, and seldom in both nerves (see Table 3). The prevalence of mononeural lesions may indicate

Table 3. Results of Electromyographic Tests.

Site of Lesion(s)	Subgroup I	Subgroup II
N. medianus or N. ulnaris	25.9%	32.1%
N. medianus and N. ulnaris	3.7%	9.5%

that the damage is caused by something other than the direct effect of vibration. Vibration should, in fact, stimulate the whole hand and thus lesions in both nerves are to be expected. To exclude nerve trapping syndromes as a source of the

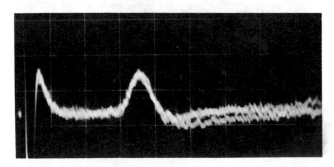

Fig. 1 Neurogram after stimulation of the sensory fibres of the ulnar nerve above the wrist (vertical scale 60 μV/div; horizontal scale 1 ms/div).

Lukáš: Peripheral nervous system

Table 4. Results of X-Ray Examination of the Cervical Spine and Elbow Joint.

		Subgroup I	Subgroup II
Megatransversus C7		16%	11%
Cervical Spine	praespondylotic changes	37%	
	osteoarthritis discopathy	47%	47%
Elbow Joint	arthrosis ossification (olecranon) epicondyl appositions	67%	70%

mononeuropathic lesions, X-ray examinations of the cervical spine and the elbow joint region were performed. The results are shown in Table 4.

The first critical region is the upper thoracic aperture. The increased prevalence of megatransversus C7 in our groups is certainly striking, and the anomalous position of the hands during work (frequently hyperabduction or hyperelevation) may explain not only the subjective symptoms, but also the pathological changes resulting from compression of the nerve bundles. The symptoms were unfortunately accompanied in practically all cases by other signs of lesions of the locomotive system, and it was not possible to evaluate the influence of the megatransversus in isolation.

In addition to the symptoms resulting from spondylotic and praespondylotic changes in the cervical spine region, signs of spinal compression from discopathy appeared in both our groups a total of 13 times (5.3%). The clinical picture is of symptoms characteristic of the development of compressive myelopathy (entrapment of the first and second neuron), a syndrome previously shown to be associated with vibration exposure. In our experience, such a syndrome is an indication for pneumoperimyelography. In five of the patients on whom this examination was performed, a prolapsed disc was detected and later verified surgically.

The excursion of the N. ulnaris in the sulcus during repeated flexion and extension of the arm, or during a prolonged static arm load when the elbow is flexed, may lead to a permanent irritation of the stem of this nerve. This anomaly was found in 29.9% of our subjects, but is only expected in approximately 12 to 18% of a control population.

The condition of the elbow region can influence the development of neurological complications, if the joint has been affected by arthrosis, epicondylar appositions, or if ossification of the olecranon occurs. Pathological findings were observed in the elbow joints of 67% and 70% of subjects in subgroups I and II, respectively. These findings may be a result of overstrain and overuse, and are associated with various occupations involving heavy work. Both

objective and subjective symptoms of a lesion of the ulnar nerve may be observed, especially when excessive excursions of the N. ulnaris occur.

During work, the holding of the tool, the force applied, and the need to maintain a given direction often require a very firm grip of the tool handle, and can subject the wrist to certain stresses. Perhaps for this reason, it is often possible to diagnose the complex of symptoms of the carpal tunnel syndrome among vibration-exposed workers. This syndrome was found in 21% of cases of the first subgroup and in 32.8% of the second subgroup.

Symptoms of compression of the median nerve may again be a consequence of overload of the wrist. Work with a pneumatic tool requires not only a given grip, which frequently leads to an unfavourable position for the wrist, but also a considerable force to be exerted on the tool. Owing to these factors, a tenosynovitis may develop, which may be responsible for the initial damage to the nerve.

As already mentioned, a minority of pathological EMG findings were bineural. All persons with such a finding also had symptoms of industrial traumatic vasoneurosis, diagnosed objectively by means of plethysmography, a cooling test, and/or by the Lewis-Prusik compression test. The association of vascular and neurological symptoms leads to the suspicion that the peripheral neuron is damaged by ischemia of the nerve.

To study the influence of ischemia on the peripheral neuron, a group of workers with occupational traumatic vasoneurosis and a group with Raynaud's Disease were examined by EMG. The minimum duration of vasoneurosis in patients from either group was five years. The results from the two groups are compared in Table 5, including data for a control group. The findings may be summarized as follows. The mean values of the conduction velocities in the terminal part of the sensory fibres of the ulnar and median nerves, and in the terminal part of the motor fibres of the median nerve are significantly less in the groups with vasoneurosis than in the control group. As other factors which are possibly responsible for nerve injuries have been excluded (as a result of X-rays on the cervical spine and

Lukás: Peripheral nervous system

Table 5. Nerve Conduction Velocities in Controls, a Group with Occupational Traumatic Vasoneurosis, and a Group with Non-Occupational Vasoneurosis.

	Control Group N=24	Occupational Traumatic Vasoneurosis N=24	Non-Occupational Vasoneurosis N=23	F-Test	Probability
N. ULNARIS					
Motor fibres					
forearm velocity	55.1 ± 5.4	56.1 ± 7.9	56.9 ± 6.5	0.8	NS
terminal velocity	28.4 ± 3.8	28.2 ± 3.5	27.7 ± 3.0	0.48	NS
Sensory fibres					
forearm velocity	55.9 ± 4.9	55.7 ± 5.2	56.6 ± 5.9	0.39	NS
distal velocity	56.8 ± 5.7	50.8 ± 7.5	52.9 ± 6.5	10.7	p<0.01
N. MEDIANUS					
Motor fibres					
terminal velocity	26.4 ± 3.0	24.0 ± 3.9	23.2 ± 3.4	10.9	p<0.01
Sensory fibres					
distal velocity	58.8 ± 6.3	51.1 ± 8.9	53.3 ± 7.1	13.1	p<0.01

Mean values are given in m/s with ±1 SD
NS = statistically not significant

on the wrist, of negative clinical findings in the wrist region, and of similar acral skin temperatures), these results suggest that the vascular component plays an important role in the development of damage to the peripheral nerves by vibration, and may be the cause of the neuropathy.

II CONCLUSIONS

Most of the neurological signs and symptoms that can be diagnosed in persons whose hands are exposed to vibration are the result of long exposure times, usually more than ten years. The present study has shown that the lesion of the peripheral nerves due to vibration appears to be a result of complex damage to the vascular, joint and muscle systems of the upper extremities. It may be secondary to excess stress in the hand-arm system, in combination with ischemia due to vasoneurosis.

REFERENCES

1. Alaranta H, Seppäläinen AM. Neuropathy and the automatic analysis of electromyographic signals from vibration exposed workers. Scand J Work Environ Health 1977; 3: 128-134.
2. Gálik L, Pelikán F. Contribution to the problem of myelopathy in vibration disease. Acta Univ Pal Olomucensis 1974; 69: 107-111.
3. Jandová D, Krofta V, Titman O. Electromyographic investigation of ulnar nerve lesion in workers under risk of vibration. Cesk Neurol 1971; 2: 64-68. (in Czech).
4. Klimková-Deutschová E. Neurologische Aspekte der Vibrationskrankheit. Int Arch Gewerbepat Gewerbehyg 1966; 22: 297-305. (in German).
5. Lukáš E. Conduction velocity in sensory fibres of N. ulnaris and N. Medianus Cesk Neurol 1970; 6: 281-287. (in Czech).
6. Lukáš E. Lesion of the peripheral nervous system due to vibration. Work Environ Health 1970; 1: 67-79.
7. Lukáš E, Kuzel V. Klinische und elektromyographische Diagnostik der Schädigung des peripheren Nervensystems durch lokale Vibration. Int Arch Arbeitsmed 1971; 239-249.
8. Sakurai T. Vibration effects on hand-arm system. Part 1. Observation of electromyogram. Ind Hyg 1977; 1-2: 47-58.
9. Seppäläinen AM. Nerve conduction in the vibration syndrome. Work Environ Health 1970; 1: 82-84.
10. Seppäläinen AM. Peripheral neuropathy in forest workers. A field study. Scand J Work Environ Health 1972; 3: 106-111.
11. Teisinger J, Louda L. Vascular disease disorders resulting from vibrating tools. J Occup Med 1972; 14: 129-137.

DISCUSSION

N. Olsen: How is the nerve conduction velocity of controls and of vibration-exposed persons, both with and without vibration-induced white finger, influenced by cooling of the arm?

Author's Response: The condition velocity must be estimated before cooling tests because a decrease in skin temperature influences the velocities measured on each person, whether for controls or for persons with damage of the peripheral nervous system. In persons with ischemic neuropathy, a relative greater decrease of conduction velocity after cooling of the arm may be expected. This was not systematically followed up in our groups.

Lukás: Peripheral nervous system

A.J. Brammer: Are the neurological disturbances you have described in vibration-exposed workers reversible if their exposure to vibration is reduced?

Author's Response: The neurological entrapment symptoms improved mostly during a period of one year after cessation of vibration exposure. The symptoms of an ischemic lesion are dependent on the development of the vasoneurosis, which proceeds at a slower rate. A simple reduction of the exposure is technically difficult to realise, and therefore cases with serious neurological symptoms should be removed from further vibration.

M. Färkkilä: Did you find any correlation between the severity of the white fingers and the motor or sensory conduction velocity?

Author's Response: An exact correlation between the severity of VWF and nerve conduction velocities is difficult. Decrease in the conduction velocity is the result of long-term damage. On the other hand, the success of the objective tests for vasoneurosis is much more dependent on the vascular damage, which, in turn, is influenced by many environmental factors.

P.V. Pelnar: This paper supports our opinion that neurological disorders are not necessarily part of the vibration disease (Kadlec K, Pelnar P. Onset, course and prognosis of the "pounder's disease".

Cas Lek Cesk 1944; 83: 1251-1259. (In Czech); and Pelnar P, Pacina V. Evaluation of the occupational traumatic vasoneurosis in miners in ore mines. Proc 8th Cong on Occup Health, Marianske Lazne, Czechoslovakia, 1964. (In Czech)). It is becoming more and more plausible that there are two streams of symptomatology caused by long-term work with vibrating tools: one vascular (Raynaud Phenomenon, cyanosis, eventually trophic changes, gangrene of fingers), and one involving the peripheral sensory and/or motor neurons. Both vascular and neurological syndromes are often present simultaneously, but they may occur separately or they may be present in varying degrees, because their respective pathogenesis is not identical. Färkkilä and Pyykkö alluded to this possibility when they observed that lumberjacks with whitening of the fingers experienced vasoconstriction in the hand not stimulated by vibration, whereas workers with numbness experienced vasodilation (Färkkilä M, Pyykö I. Blood flow in the contralateral hand during vibration and hand grip contractions of lumberjacks. Scan J Work Environ Health 1979; 5: 368-374). Disturbances to the more proximal structures (muscles, bones and joints of the arms), and neurological syndromes of amyotrophic lateral sclerosis and similar disorders appear to be more related to the consequences of heavy musculo-skeletal stress than to the pathogenesis of the peripheral vascular and neurological disturbances.

Hand Grip Force and Muscle Fatigue in the Etiology of the Vibration Syndrome

M. A. Färkkilä, I. Pyykkö, J. P. Starck and O. S. Korhonen

ABSTRACT: The role of hand grip force and muscle fatigue in the etiology of the Vibration Syndrome was studied in a series of experiments. The first study measured the hand grip forces of 51 lumberjacks and seven controls. The second study measured hand grip force in 88 lumberjacks and 31 controls during a two minute compression-relaxation task. The third study measured hand grip forces for 89 professional lumberjacks during the operation of chain saws. The hand grip forces were then compared with the symptoms caused by occupational exposure to vibration. The strength of the hand grip may play a significant role in the etiology of the Vibration Syndrome. A positive correlation exists between the occurrence of vibration-induced white finger (VWF) and the use of large hand grip forces. Chronic exposure to occupational vibration may lead to decreased muscle force.

RESUME: On a réalisé une série d'expériences pour étudier le rôle de la force de préhension et de la fatigue musculaire dans l'étiologie du syndrome de vibration. On a premièrement mesuré la force de préhension de 51 bûcherons et de sept témoins. En second lieu, on a mesuré la force de préhension de 88 bûcherons et de 31 témoins pendant un exercice de contraction et de décontraction de 2 minutes. Enfin, on a mesuré la force de préhension de 89 bûcherons professionnels pendant qu'ils utilisaient une tronçonneuse. La force de préhension a ensuite été comparée avec les symptômes d'exposition professionnelle aux vibrations. Il se peut que la force de préhension joue un rôle important dans l'étiologie du syndrome de vibration. Il existe en effet une corrélation positive entre le symptôme des doigts blancs (VWF) et l'application d'une grande force de préhension. L'exposition chronique à des vibrations peut provoquer une diminution de la force musculaire.

INTRODUCTION

The effects of vibration on the hand-arm system have been studied for decades, with most attention focused on the vascular symptoms (1,2). A few authors have described muscle weakness, atrophy and nerve changes among workers exposed to vibration (3-6). People working with vibrating tools have also reported diminished muscle force in the upper extremities (2,7-11). However, objective measurements have not confirmed excessive muscle fatigue in workers exposed to vibration (7).

The understanding of the effects of vibration varies in different countries. The vascular symptoms represent only a part of the Syndrome, which comprises symptoms related to the blood circulation (2), the peripheral nerves (12), the muscles (4) and the bones and joints (13). In our experience, the symptoms can appear together or separately (Fig. 1) (14).

In controlled studies, the prevalence of a diminished grip force has been

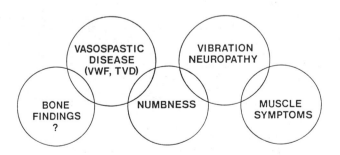

Fig. 1 Symptoms of the Vibration Syndrome and their possible relationships.

significantly more common among lumberjacks than among workers without exposure to vibration (9,10). Our studies among grinders and lumberjacks have found a common history of diminished muscle force.

This paper considers the effects of vibration on muscle force, the meaning of muscle symptoms in the Vibration Syndrome, and the effect of compression force, which increases the transmission of vibration to the extremities and hence may influence the vascular symptoms.

I SUBJECTS AND METHODS

The role of muscle force in the Vibration Syndrome was investigated in three different studies. The subjects for each study are shown in Table 1.

Table 1. Age, Vibration Exposure and Number of Subjects.

Study	Group	Age mean and (range)(yrs)	Exposure Time mean and (range) (h)	N
I	lumberjacks	40.7 (26-57)	11 500 (3900-26 800)	51
	controls	28.4 (19-44)	-	7
II	lumberjacks	35.8 (19-53)	9320 (1500-24 100)	88
	controls	37.4 (20-58)	-	31
III	lumberjacks	37.8 (18-54)	9760 (1100-18 400)	89

In the first study, we used a dynamic shaker to vibrate the hand. For the measurement of grip force, a strain-gauge dynamometer was built into the handle of the shaker (15). The selected subjects were divided into different groups according to the symptoms they reported (see Table 2). During the experiment the subject compressed the handle repeatedly with maximal force, following the pace set by a metronome. Each compression lasted 2.5 seconds and was followed by a pause for another 2.5 seconds, and so on, for five minutes. This measurement was repeated six times for each man at handle vibration frequencies of 30, 60, 80, 100, 200 and 400 Hz.

In the second study, we measured fatigue of the hand grip force in 88 lumberjacks, and in 31 controls who had not been occupationally exposed to vibration (Table 1). From the knowledge gained in the first study, we followed the fatigue for only two minutes and used only vibration at a frequency of 80 Hz. Otherwise the experimental procedure was similar to the first study (16).

In the third experiment, we measured the grip force used by 89 professional

lumberjacks (Table 1). The tests were performed using a Partner model R22 chain saw with strain-gauge dynamometers built into the front and rear handles. At the beginning of the test, the maximal voluntary compression force (MVC) exerted on the handles was measured. The subject then cut slices of pine logs four times (Fig. 2). Each subject was instructed to use his normal way of sawing with no time limits. The mean amplitude of the grip force during sawing was used to represent the hand grip force (HGF) of the subject. The ratio HGF/ MVC was used to compare the subject groups.

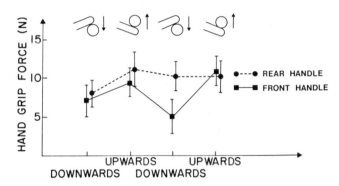

Fig. 2 Muscle forces of 89 lumberjacks during the four stages of the sawing test (mean values ± SEM). (From Ref. 26, with permission of Br J Ind Med).

The compression forces were also compared in a matched pair test with lumberjacks with VWF (N=20) and lumberjacks without VWF (N=20).

II RESULTS

Our studies of the lumberjacks in Suomussalmi, Finland, revealed cases of the Vibration Syndrome where the subject suffered only from attacks of white finger and had never experienced diminished grip force (11). We also found cases where the lumberjacks reported only numbness of the hands and/or diminished grip forces (15). The prevalence of subjectively-diminished grip force was 21% among 187 lumberjacks. Seven men experienced considerable occupational disability from the symptom (11).

Compression force diminished in every person with age. The grip forces of lumberjacks were clearly diminished in the age group of 35-44 years, as can be seen from Fig. 3. The fatigue curve of muscle force is similar to the standard curve (17). Muscle forces were equal among lumberjacks and controls when the hand was not subjected to vibration. During vibration, the force

Färkkilä et al.: Hand grip force

Table 2. Grouping of Subjects According to Symptoms Reported. (From Ref. 15, with permission of Scand J Work Environ Health).

Grip Force Reduced?	White Fingers?	Mean Age ± SD (yrs)	Mean Exposure Time and (range) (h)	N	Remarks
No	No	37.1 ± 4.7	8720 (3900-12 800)	6	
No	Yes	39.7 ± 7.6	12 100 (7500-26 800)	16	Cold provocation test positive in 75%
Yes	No	39.8 ± 6.5	11 650 (4200-22 800)	15	Reduced force history 53% bilaterally, others unilaterally (left)
Yes	Yes	44.4 ± 7.4	11 840 (3900-12 800)	14	
No	No	28.4 ± 9.4	-	7	Controls

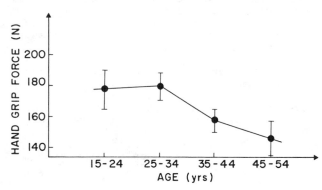

Fig. 3 The effect of age on the hand grip force of lumberjacks (mean values ± SEM).

exerted by the hands of the lumberjacks was reduced from the very beginning of the fatigue curve (Fig. 4)(16).

Muscle force was significantly diminished among workers who reported numbness of the hands, diminished muscle force or pain in the upper extremities. Exposure to vibration diminished the grip force of these workers more than for those lumberjacks who did not complain of such symptoms. The vibration frequency used in the experiment did not affect the muscle fatigue curve (Fig. 5).

In the compression-relaxation experiment, the muscle force of lumberjacks with VWF as the only symptom of their disease was significantly less than that of lumberjacks who had diminished grip force and numbness, but not white fingers (Fig. 6). In the same experiment, the muscle forces of healthy controls were the same as the muscle forces of lumberjacks with VWF. Therefore, diminished muscle force does

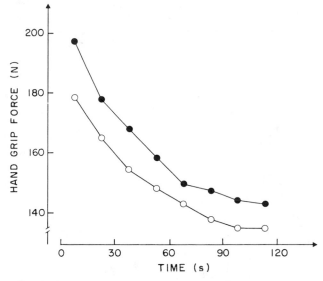

Fig. 4 Mean hand grip force of 88 lumberjacks during vibration (lower curve) and without vibration (upper curve), showing the effect of fatigue. (After Ref. 16, with permission of Eur J Appl Physiol).

not seem to be associated with white fingers.

A history of muscle weakness in the hands was associated with occupational exposure to vibration. A history of diminished grip force was not found among those who had been sawing less than 5000 hours, and both the prevalence and severity of this symptom increased with exposure time, as seen in Fig. 7. The measured muscle force was not dependent on the time of exposure to vibration.

Färkkilä et al.: Hand grip force

48

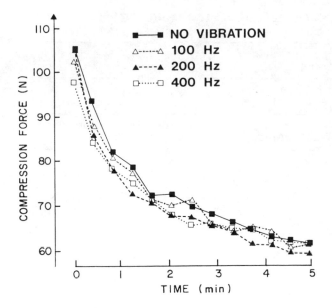

Fig. 5 Muscle fatigue occurring at
different vibration frequencies. (From
Ref. 15, with permission of Scand J
Work Environ Health).

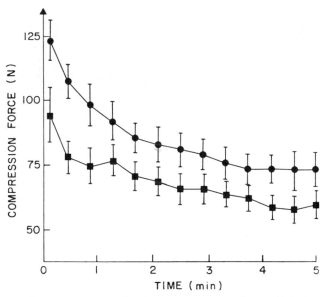

Fig. 6 Comparison between hand grip
forces of lumberjacks with VWF as the
only symptom (upper curve), and lumberjacks with diminished grip force but who
never experience attacks of VWF (lower
curve) (mean values ± SEM). (From Ref.
15, with permission of Scand J Work
Environ Health).

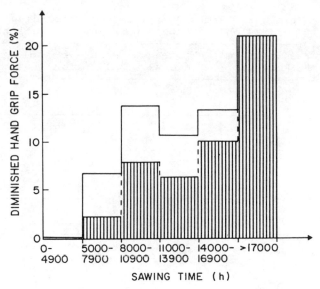

Fig. 7 The distribution of lumberjacks
suffering from diminished grip force
when classified according to occupational
vibration exposure time. The lined
columns represent those who had severe
symptoms. (From Ref. 16, with permission
of Eur J Appl Physiol).

   The measurement of compression force
during sawing showed that those lumberjacks
who have white fingers used significantly
stronger force when cutting logs than was
used by lumberjacks who had not developed
VWF (Fig. 8). Our previous measurements
show that an increase in compression force
increases the transmission of vibration to
the upper extremities (18).

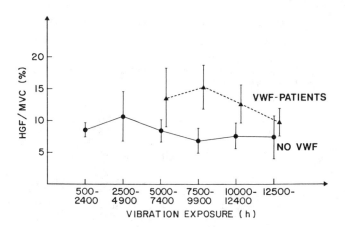

Fig. 8 Muscle forces observed at the
front handle during sawing from 20 lumberjacks with, and 69 without, VWF (mean
values ± SEM). (From Ref. 26, with
permission of Br J Ind Med).

Färkkilä et al.: Hand grip force

III DISCUSSION

In clinical studies, the weakening of hand grip force is common among lumberjacks, although Agate postulated that diminished grip force is not a symptom of the Vibration Syndrome (2). In our studies, the weakening of hand grip force was associated with vibration exposure. The symptom was not found in lumberjacks with a vibration exposure of less than 5000 hours, and the severity of the symptom increased with increasing use of a chain saw. This indicates a dose-response relationship.

In our experiments, vibration frequencies of 30, 60, 80, 100, 200 and 400 Hz were used. We were not able to find any differences in the effect of vibration frequency on muscle force during the short exposure times of our experiments. No electromyographic changes were noticed when subjects were exposed to vibration at frequencies of 30, 60, 125 or 250 Hz (19).

The muscle force fatigue followed the curve of Rohmert (17). The fatigue curves of lumberjacks closely followed those of the controls. The shape of the fatigue curve was also alike for the controls and the lumberjacks. The reason for muscle fatigue is thought to be metabolic in origin (20). It seems, therefore, that hand muscle metabolism is normal in lumberjacks, and that the measured decrease of hand grip force is caused by other factors.

In these experiments, we found a significant decrease of grip force in those lumberjacks who gave a history of diminished grip force. The finding of normal grip force among lumberjacks whose only symptom of vibration exposure is white fingers, and, at the same time, the finding of decreased grip force among a group of lumberjacks not suffering from VWF but who reported diminished grip force suggests that there are possibly two different mechanisms. The first would be a vasospastic disease caused by the central sympathetic vasoconstrictor reflex (21). The second would be vibration neuropathy caused by the local effects of vibration on the nerves and muscles. Vibration is known to affect the peripheral nerves (5,6). The present findings suggest that a clinical polyneuropathy also affects the lower extremities of many lumberjacks (Juntunen J, personal communication). Numbness of the hands, a very common symptom among workers exposed to vibration, as well as the weakened muscle force could be a sign of neuropathy. Numbness can also be a symptom of muscle or nerve ischemia. We consider numbness a very non-specific symptom.

Exposure to vibration may also directly affect the muscles, and cause the sudden decrease in muscle force that was observed in our experiments. In an isolated smooth muscle, relaxation caused by vibration has been reported (22); in this study it was thought that vibration may mechanically affect the actin and myosin filaments in muscle cells.

Vibration affects muscle tension by activating the muscle spindles. These reflexively trigger a muscle contraction known as the tonic vibration reflex (TVR). This reflex facilitates the agonistic muscles to contract while the antagonistic muscles are inhibited (23). During hand-arm exposure to vibration, the muscle spindles of both the flexor and extensor muscles are activated, and there is simultaneous inhibition and facilitation of both muscle groups; the net effect is diminution of muscle force. The activation of the tonic vibration reflex can explain the momentary decrease in muscle force in the lumberjacks at the beginning of exposure to vibration. The weakening of grip force is yet to be explained. One possibility is vibration neuropathy.

According to laboratory measurements of the transmission of vibration in the hand and arm, the compression of the handle increases the acceleration levels of vibration measured in different parts of the upper extremity (24,25,18). Our measurements during sawing showed that those lumberjacks who compressed the handles tightly had contracted VWF more often than the others (26). This can be due to the increased transmission of vibration in the upper extremities. Thus in order to avoid vascular symptoms from vibration exposure, the hand grip force needed to hold the device should be minimized.

IV CONCLUSIONS

The symptom of diminished grip force was not associated with white fingers. There was a dose-response relationship between diminished grip force and vibration exposure. These findings suggest that the observed decrease in muscle force is a symptom of the Vibration Syndrome. The exact pathophysiological mechanism remains obscure. One possibility is a neurogenic muscle dysfunction.

REFERENCES

1. Loriga G. Cited by Teleky L. Pneumatic tools. In: Occupation and Health Supplement. International Labor Office, Geneva 1938: 1-12.
2. Agate JN. An outbreak of cases of Raynaud's phenomenon of occupational origin. Br J Ind Med 1949; 6: 144-163.
3. Teleky L. Pneumatic tools. Occup Health Saf 1938; 1: 1-12.
4. Marshall J, Poole EB, Raynaud WA. Raynaud's phenomenon due to vibrating tools. Lancet 1954; I: 1154-56.
5. Andreeva-Galanina ET, Karpova NI. On the degeneration and regeneration of peripheral nerves under the effect of experimental vibration. Gig Tr Prof Zabol 1969; 13: 4-7. (English summary).

Färkkilä et al.: Hand grip force

6. Seppäläinen A-M. Peripheral neuropathy in forest workers: a field study. Work Environ Health 1972;9: 106-111.
7. Hellström B, Lange Andersen K. Vibration injuries in Norwegian forest workers. Br J Ind Med 1972; 29: 255-263.
8. Laitinen J, Puranen J, Vuorinen P. Vibration syndrome in lumbermen (working with chain saws). JOM 1974; 16: 552-556.
9. Matsumoto K, Itoh N, Kasamatsu T, Iwata H. A study on subjective symptoms based on total operating time of chain saw. Jpn J Ind Health 1977; 19: 22-28. (in Japanese).
10. Korhonen O, Nummi J, Nurminen M, Nygård K, Soininen H, Wiikeri M. Metsätyöntekijä: Osa 2. Työterveyslaitoksen tutkimuksia 126, Työterveyslaitos, Helsinki 1977, 1-100. (in Finnish).
11. Pyykkö I, Sairanen E, Korhonen O, Färkkilä M, Hyvärinen J. A decrease in the prevalence and severity of the vibration-induced white fingers among lumberjacks in Finland. Scand J Work Environ Health 1978; 4: 246-254.
12. Klimkova-Deutschova E. Neurologische Aspekte der Vibrations-krankheit. Int Arch Gewerbepat Gewerbehyg 1966; 22: 297-305. (in German).
13. Taylor W. Introduction. In: Taylor W, ed. The Vibration Syndrome. London: Academic Press, 1974: 1-12.
14. Pyykkö I. The prevalence and symptoms of traumatic vasospastic disease among lumberjacks in Finland: a field study. Work Environ Health 1974; 11: 118-131.
15. Färkkilä M. Grip force in vibration disease. Scand J Work Environ Health 1978; 4: 330-335.
16. Färkkilä M, Pyykkö I, Korhonen O, Starck J. Vibration-induced decrease in the muscle force in lumberjacks. Eur J Appl Physiol 1980; 43: 1-9.
17. Rohmert W. Ermittlung von Erholungspausen fur statische Arbeit des Menschen. Inter Z Angew Physiol 1960; 18: 123-164. (in German).
18. Pyykkö I, Färkkilä M, Toivanen J, Korhonen O, Hyvärinen J. Transmission of vibration in the hand-arm system with special reference to changes in compression force and acceleration. Scand J Work Environ Health 1976; 2: 87-95.
19. Sakurai T. Vibration effects on hand-arm system, part 1: observations of electromyogram. Ind Health (Japan) 1977; 15: 47-58.
20. Kearney JT, Stull GA, Kirkendal D. Isometric grip-flexion fatigue in females under conditions of normal and occluded circulation. Am Correct Ther J 1976; 30: 7-11.
21. Hyvärinen J, Pyykkö I, Sundberg S. Vibration frequencies and amplitudes in the etiology of traumatic vasospastic disease. Lancet 1973; I: 791-794.
22. Ljung B, Sivertsson R. Inhibition of vascular smooth muscle contraction by vibrations. Acta Physiol Scand Suppl 1973; 396: 1-95.
23. Eklund G, Hagbarth K-E. Normal variability of tonic vibration reflex in man. Exp Neurol 1966; 16: 80-92.
24. Hempstock TI, O'Connor DE. Assessment of hand transmitted vibration. Ann Occup Hyg 1978; 21: 57-67.
25. Suggs CW. Modelling of the dynamic characteristic of hand-arm system. In: Taylor W, ed. The Vibration Syndrome, London: Academic Press, 1974; 169-186.
26. Färkkilä M, Pyykkö I, Korhonen O, Starck J. Hand grip forces during chain saw operation and vibration white finger in lumberjacks. Br J Ind Med 1979; 36: 336-341.

DISCUSSION

N. Olsen: You suggested that the stronger hand grip force in subjects with VWF may have given them their white finger symptoms. Can you exclude that the hand grip force was increased to compensate for clumsy fingers in subjects with VWF?

Authors' Response: The lumberjacks in our study did not report clumsy fingers except during their attacks of VWF.

J.R. Barron: Were the environmental conditions controlled during the experiment, as the temperature at which the test was performed could affect the result?

Authors' Response: The room temperature during the tests was constant. Temperature compensation of the strain gauges was a problem, but did not affect the conclusions.

Link Between Noise-Induced Hearing Loss and the Vasospastic Component of the Vibration Syndrome

I. Pyykkö, J. P. Starck, O. S. Korhonen, M. A. Färkkilä and S. A. Aatola

ABSTRACT: The connection between noise-induced permanent threshold shift (NIPTS) and vibration-induced white finger (VWF) has been studied to examine whether vibration-induced circulatory disturbances in the fingers could provide a basis for increased hearing loss. The subjects studied, 72 lumberjacks in 1972 and 203 in 1978, were grouped according to their history of VWF, age, duration of use of chain saws, and use of hearing protectors. They were exposed to an equivalent continuous sound level of from 95 to 107 dB(A). The hearing level at 4000 Hz was used as a measure of NIPTS. A statistically significant difference in hearing level was found between lumberjacks with and without VWF. The findings indicate that circulatory disturbances in the fingers are associated with occupational hearing loss. The etiological mechanism for the excess NIPTS may thus be similar to that proposed for VWF, namely chronic over-excitation of the sympathetic nervous system.

RESUME: La relation entre un changement permanent du seuil auditif provoqué par le bruit et les doigts blancs dûs aux vibrations a fait l'objet d'une étude pour voir si des troubles circulatoires des doigts dûs aux vibration pourraient servir de base à une augmentation de la perte d'audition. Les sujets étudiés, 72 bûcherons en 1972 et 203 en 1978, furent regroupés selon leurs antécédents (progression des doigts blancs), leur âge, la période depuis laquelle ils utilisent des tronçonneuses et l'utilisation de protecteurs auditifs. Ils furent exposés à un niveau sonore continu équivalent entre 95 et 107 dB(A). Le niveau d'audition à 4000 Hz fut utilisé comme mesure du changement permanent du seuil auditif produit par le bruit. Une différence statistiquement significative du niveau d'audition fut constatée entre les bûcherons ayant les doigts blancs et ceux qui ne les avaient pas. Les conclusions indiquent que les troubles circulatoires des doigts sont associés à une perte d'audition professionnelle. Le mécanisme étiologique d'un changement de seuil excessif peut donc être semblable à celui qui est proposé pour les doigts blancs dûs aux vibrations, c'est-à-dire une surexcitation chronique du système nerveux sympathique.

INTRODUCTION

The development of noise-induced permanent threshold shift (NIPTS) is a long and insidious process. Years may pass before significant changes in hearing occur. The mechanisms of hair cell damage in the inner ear are not completely known, but it seems likely that over-stimulation with noise for a prolonged period of time produces vascular and metabolic changes in the hair cell structure (1). In much the same way, some workers exposed to vibration for prolonged periods develop vasospastic symptoms in the circulation of the fingers. These symptoms, often called vibration-induced white finger (VWF), are prevalent among lumberjacks after 5 to 6 years of continuous work with chain saws (2).

Vasoconstriction in the circulation of the fingers is probably mediated through the central nervous system. It is thought to arise from over-activation of the sympathetic vasoconstrictor tone, triggered by the Pacinian corpuscles which are the peripheral vibration receptors (3,4,5).

It has been proposed that the interaction of the vibration of hand-held tools with noise leads to an increase in NIPTS (6,7,2). Whole-body vibration may similarly be implicated in the development of NIPTS (8). The reason for the apparent synergistic action of vibration and noise in the etiology of NIPTS is not known. The explanation may be that vibration produces vasoconstriction in the cochlear vessels in the same way as it produces vasoconstriction in the digital arteries. To examine this hypothesis, a population of lumberjacks has been studied for a period of seven years. The subjects were grouped according to the presence of circulatory disturbances in the fingers, age, exposure to noise and their use of hearing protectors. The hearing level at 4000 Hz was used to indicate NIPTS. A more comprehensive report on the selection criteria, chain saw noise levels and the evaluation of hearing levels has been published elsewhere (9).

I SUBJECTS AND METHODS

1.1 Subjects

A typical forestry district, the parish of Suomussalmi in northeast Finland, was chosen for the location of the study. The investigation was carried out in 1972 and from 1974 to 1978, during a compulsory medical check-up of lumberjacks working for the National Board of Forestry. All men in the area who had used a chain saw a minimum of 500 h per year for at least three consecutive years were included in the study. The number of lumberjacks examined varied from year to year, due to reorganization of the work, and the retirement or resignation of workers (Table 1). Lumberjacks with known ear diseases were excluded.

1.2 Medical Examination

Prior to the examination, lumberjacks completed a questionnaire on their state of health and symptoms of the Vibration Syndrome. The medical history of each lumberjack was recorded, and a physical examination, which included inspection of the ears, was carried out. Symptoms and signs of VWF were always recorded by the same physician. All lumberjacks with a history of VWF were given a cold provocation test (5).

The diagnosis of VWF was made according to a typical history of blanching of the fingers (3,10). Other causes of finger blanching were ruled out by the medical history, by clinical examination and by routine laboratory tests. Lumberjacks who

had not experienced attacks of VWF during the two last years of the study were classified as still suffering from the condition, although we have, in other surveys, considered no attacks of VWF for two years to signify recovery (11,12).

1.3 Hearing Measurement

Hearing was tested in an acoustically treated room, where the A-weighted sound level ranged from 22 to 24 dB. The background noise of the testing room at low frequencies (500 Hz and below) exceeded the limits of permissible noise for the measurement of hearing levels of 0 dB (13), but did not exceed the limits at frequencies of 1000 Hz and above. The (occupational) noise-free period before testing ranged from 15 to 48 h. The hearing level at 4000 Hz was used to indicate NIPTS (13,14), and the mean value of the right and the left ears was obtained for each lumberjack.

1.4 Measurement of Chain Saw Noise

The noise of the eight chain saw models (from eight manufacturers) most commonly used in Finland was measured using equipment that fulfilled the requirements of IEC Standard 651, 1979, class 1 (15), and IEC 225, 1966 (16). A condenser microphone (Bruel & Kjaer 4145) was located near the ear of the operator and the noise was recorded as the saws cut wood.

The noise dose of lumberjacks was measured by a personal noise dosimeter (Wärtsilä 6074) carried during a normal workday. The readings were evaluated after every work shift. The measurements consisted of readings recorded on five workdays, and the dose was expressed in terms of the equivalent continuous sound level normalised to eight hours (L_{eq}).

1.5 Statistical Analysis

The significance of differences between the groups was separately tested using Student's t-test for independent samples. Welch's approximate t-test was applied if the sample variances differed markedly, that

Table 1. Age Distribution of Lumberjacks (percentage in parentheses). (From Ref. 9, with permission of Br J Ind Med).

Age (yrs)	Year of Examination					
	1972	1974	1975	1976	1977	1978
20-29	3 (4)	10 (10)	26 (16)	31 (18)	37 (20)	45 (22)
30-39	26 (36)	37 (37)	54 (32)	61 (34)	59 (31)	64 (32)
40-49	36 (50)	38 (38)	66 (40)	70 (38)	72 (38)	73 (36)
50-59	7 (10)	15 (15)	19 (12)	19 (10)	21 (11)	21 (10)
Total	72 (100)	100 (100)	165 (100)	181 (100)	189 (100)	203 (100)

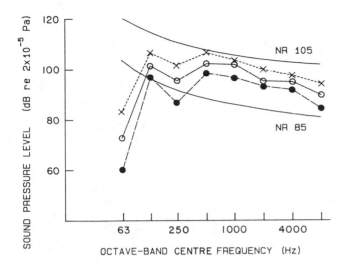

Fig. 1 Octave-band sound pressure levels at the ear when using a chain saw to cut wood. The mean spectrum (open circles) and the maximum and minimum band levels obtained from eight saws are shown. Also shown are the ISO noise rating curves NR 85 and 105. (Adapted from Ref. 9, with permission of Br J Ind Med).

is, if their ratio exceeded two or was less than one-half (17). Two-sided probability values were employed. It should be noted, however, that the requirement of independence was not completely satisfied when comparing results from different years, as some of the subjects were common to the population samples. Hence, the inferences from such statistical analyses should be regarded mainly as descriptive.

II RESULTS

2.1 Noise Measurements

The noise dose of two lumberjacks was measured during several successive days. Personal noise dose measurements over one working period gave L_{eq} values of from 95 to 107 dB(A), with a mean of 103 dB(A). The variation depended on the condition of the chain saw and the working environment.

The noise spectra of the eight most common chain saw makes are shown in Fig. 1. The mean values and the saws with highest and lowest noise spectra are shown, as are the ISO noise rating curves (NR) of 105 and 85 (18). The spectra of all saws were below NR 105, and were approximately parallel to this contour at frequencies above 250 Hz.

Both the measurements of personal noise dose and octave-band noise spectra of chain saws indicate that a risk of

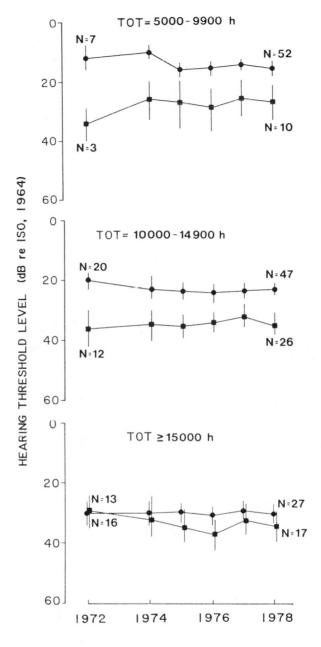

Fig. 2 Mean hearing level at 4000 Hz ± SEM for lumberjacks with VWF (squares) and without VWF (circles) in successive years, when grouped according to their total time operating chain saws (TOT). (From Ref. 9, with permission of Br J Ind Med).

developing NIPTS exists if the saws are used daily without hearing protection (19).

2.2 Hearing Evaluation

Noise-induced permanent threshold shifts were found in most lumberjacks, but

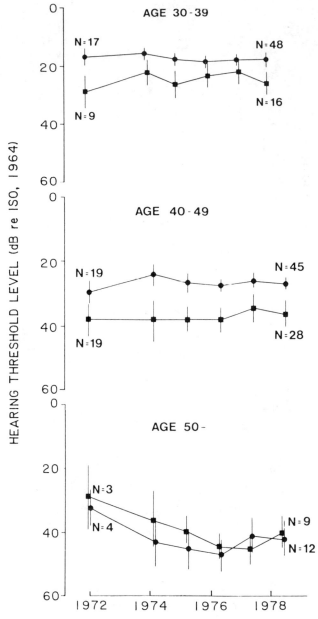

Fig 3   Mean hearing level at 4000 Hz
± SEM for lumberjacks with VWF (squares)
and without VWF (circles) in successive
years, when grouped according to age.
(From Ref. 9, with permission of Br J
Ind Med).

the variability between individuals was
great. The threshold shift at 4000 Hz was
dependent upon the amount of exposure to
noise, the age of the subject, and the use
of hearing protectors. The subjects with
VWF had a greater noise-induced threshold
shift than subjects without VWF.

Figure 2 shows the hearing level at
4000 Hz from 1972 to 1978, when the lumberjacks were grouped according to the total

chain saw operating time (TOT). The difference in hearing level between lumberjacks
with and without VWF was statistically
highly significant in the groups with from
5000 to 9900 hours and from 10 000 to
14 900 hours TOT (p<0.001 in both groups).

Figure 3 shows the hearing levels of
lumberjacks at 4000 Hz from 1972 to 1978,
grouped according to age. In the age groups
from 30 to 39 and from 40 to 49 years, the
lumberjacks with VWF consistently had
hearing levels about 10 dB greater than
those without VWF (p<0.05 and 0.01, respectively). There was no significant difference in age and use of hearing protection
between subjects with and without VWF, but
a difference in the total time of chain saw
operation was found (p<0.05) for the group
aged from 30 to 39 years (see Table 2).
Table 2 also gives the standard deviations
of the hearing levels and the total operating times for the various groups.

III   DISCUSSION

At the present rate of work, lumberjacks use chain saws continuously for about
five to six hours a day. Thus, they are, on
average, annually exposed to chain saw
noise and vibration for 1100 hours. By
1978, their accumulated chain saw operating
time ranged from 2500 to 23 500 h, with a
mean value of 11 035 h. These exposures,
on average, correspond to from 10 to 11
years of continuous exposure to chain saw
noise and vibration.

The results indicate that subjects
who have circulatory disturbances in the
fingers also have more hearing loss. To
date, however, the mechanism which causes
NIPTS is largely unknown. It is generally
agreed that changes in the vasculature and
the metabolism of the inner ear are the
immediate cause of the loss of hair cells
in the cochlea. Blood pressure and the
sympathetic nervous system are interrelated
in a complex manner in the control of blood
flow to the inner ear.

Blood pressure may well be a factor
contributing to differences between the
noise-induced hearing losses of industrial
groups (20). However, Lawrence et al. and
Perlman and Yamada were not able to show
changes in the blood flow of the stria
vascularis (21,22), nor could they show that
wide variation in carotid artery pressure
led to a decrease in oxygen concentration
within the tunnel of the organ of Corti.
No significant difference in the mean blood
pressure was found between lumberjacks with
and without VWF in this study.

The term "auto-regulation" has been
used to describe the capacity of the peripheral vascular bed to maintain constant blood
flow over a limited range of arterial
perfusion pressure and neurogenic control.
In contrast to skin circulation, which has

Table 2. Hearing Levels at 4000 Hz, in 1978, of Lumberjacks With and Without VWF, when Grouped According to Age, Chain Saw Operating Time and Use of Ear Muffs. (From Ref. 9, with permission of Br J Ind Med).

Age (yrs)			Without VWF						With VWF			
			Exposure (h)* (TOT)·10^{-2}		Hearing Level (dB)			Exposure (h)* (TOT)·10^{-2}		Hearing Level (dB)		
		N	Mean	SD	Mean	SD	N	Mean	SD	Mean	SD	
20-29	Without		15	20				49				
	With		44	19				58				
	Total	44	59	31	9	9	1	107		5		
30-39	Without		48	31				55	21			
	With		58	22				71	22			
	Total	48	105†	38	19	16	16	127†	35	26	17	
40-49	Without		69	38				70	29			
	With		58	22				65	25			
	Total	45	128	48	27	15	28	138	37	37	24	
50-	Without		68	52				63	17			
	With		63	28				71	37			
	Total	12	132	49	42	20	9	135	41	39	16	

*Values of TOT in column 4, row 1, etc. are TOT = 1500 ± 2000 h.
†p < 0.05.

a very limited ability to control circulation by auto-regulation (23), the inner ear circulation shows considerable auto-regulation (1,24). Local circulatory demands can override the systemic regulatory controls and even arterial blood flow within the inner ear can be controlled during more localized circulatory demands (24,25). Blood can be directed from areas with low energy demands to areas with high energy demands by opening and closing the capillary beds. Thus, after short-term exposure to noise, widespread compensatory changes may occur in the vascular bed of the inner ear (24).

The evidence that the autonomic nervous system may override the local control of blood flow in the membranous labyrinth is conflicting. Anatomical evidence clearly points to the presence of adrenergic axons in the arterioles of the inner ear (26,27). Perlman and Kimura and Todd et al. did not observe any changes of blood flow in the stria vascularis nor in the spiral ligament (28,29), after stimulation of the cervical sympathetic trunk and the sympathetic plexus around the vertebral arteries. Using the radiographic microsphere technique, Hultcrantz et al. showed that maximal electrical stimulation of the cervical sympathetic ganglions leads to a significant (25%) decrease of blood flow in the ipsilateral inner ear (30). Furthermore, using adrenergic agents, Suga and Snow found that the cochlear vessels are weakly controlled by the adrenergic nervous system (31). During exposure to noise, a decrease of endolymphatic oxygen concentration has been observed. Such a decrease indicates that, compared to oxygen delivery, excessive oxygen consumption occurs during intensive noise (32-34). In a cat, Maas et al. also demonstrated that sympathectomy did not noticeably influence the oxygen concentration in the three scalae (34). When the ears were exposed to loud sounds, the endolymphatic oxygen concentration decreased less quickly and recovered more quickly on the sympathectomized side than on the control side.

When animals and humans are exposed to intensive noise, the subsequent histopathologic changes show, among others, empty capillaries in the stria vascularis in areas activated by the stimulating frequency (25,35-37). These changes suggest that the mechanisms compensating for the higher oxygen demands during exposure to noise are not completely effective. Hence, during exposure to noise and vibration, it is possible that the sympathetic nervous system may override the auto-regulation of the inner ear, for example, by disturbing compensatory changes in the capillary beds during high local energy demands. Vascular changes in the inner ear circulation could result in an increase in NIPTS, and the mechanism could be analogous to that believed responsible for disturbances in finger circulation - central over-stimulation of the sympathetic nervous system induced by vibration applied to the hand (Fig. 4).

This hypothesis suggests that vasoconstrictions in the Vibration Syndrome, usually believed to be localized and limited only to finger circulation would, in fact, be generalized. It is also possible that subjects with VWF react to noise and vibration with stronger vasoconstriction in the inner ear than subjects without VWF, and so develop greater NIPTS.

Pyykkö et al.: Hearing loss

56

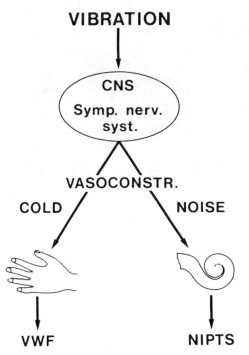

VIBRATION

CNS
Symp. nerv.
syst.

VASOCONSTR.

COLD   NOISE

VWF   NIPTS

Fig. 4 Hypothetical mechanism leading
to VWF and excess NIPTS after prolonged
exposure to vibration.

IV CONCLUSIONS

Lumberjacks who are exposed daily to
intense noise and vibration at work may
develop vasospastic symptoms in the circulation of the fingers. The same lumberjacks are also at greater risk of suffering
additional noise-induced, permanent loss of
hearing. The ability to resist the hazardous effects of noise and vibration may be
related to the sensitivity of the autonomic
nervous system to these stimuli. It may be
that vasoconstriction in the cochlear
vessels is induced in the same way as in
the peripheral circulation. Thus, the
mechanisms of the two disorders - VWF and
excess NIPTS - may be similar.

REFERENCES

1. Lawrence M. Control mechanisms of inner ear
microcirculation. Am J Otolaryngol 1980; 1:
324-333.
2. Pyykkö I. The prevalence and symptoms of
traumatic vasospastic disease among lumberjacks
in Finland: a field study. Work Environ
Health 1974; 11: 118-131.
3. Pyykkö I, Hyvärinen J. The physiological
basis of the traumatic vasospastic disease
(TVD): A sympathetic vasoconstrictor reflex

triggered by high frequency vibration. Work
Environ Health 1973; 10: 36-47.
4. Hyvärinen J, Pyykkö I, Sundberg S. Vibration
frequencies and amplitudes in the etiology of
traumatic vasospastic disease. Lancet 1973;
I: 791-794.
5. Pyykkö I. A physiological study of the vasoconstrictor reflex in traumatic vasospastic
disease. Work Environ Health 1974; 11: 170-186.
6. Taniewski M, Banaszkiewicz T. Hearing in
persons exposed to vibration. Biule Inst Med
Morskiej w Gdansku 24 1973; 3. Cited by
Sulkowski W. Noise-induced permanent threshold
shift: occupational deafness. In: Minerva
Medica, eds. Man and Noise. Turin: Minerva
Medica, 1976: 121-128.
7. Pinter I. Hearing loss of forest workers and
of tractor operators (interaction of noise
with vibration). Proc of the Int Congr on
Noise as a Public Health Problem. Washington,
DC: US Environmental Protection Agency, 1973:
315-327.
8. Sulkowski W. Noise-induced permanent thres-
hold shifts: Occupational deafness. In:
Minerva Medica, eds. Man and Noise. Turin:
Minerva Medica, 1976: 121-128.
9. Pyykkö I, Starck J, Färkkilä M, Hoikkala M,
Korhonen O, Nurminen M. Hand-arm vibration in
the etiology of hearing loss in lumberjacks.
Br J Ind Med 1981; 38: 281-289.
10. Pyykkö I. Vibration Syndrome: a review. In:
Korhonen O, ed. Vibration and Work. Helsinki:
Inst of Occup Health, 1976: 1-24.
11. Pyykkö I, Sairanen E, Korhonen O, Färkkilä M,
Hyvärinen J. A decrease in the prevalence and
severity of vibration-induced white fingers
among lumberjacks in Finland. Scand J Work
Environ Health 1978; 4: 246-254.
12. Färkkilä M, Pyykkö I. Blood flow in the contralateral hand during vibration and hand grip
contractions of lumberjacks. Scand J Work
Environ Health 1979; 5: 368-374.
13. Burns W. Noise and Man. 2nd ed. London:
John Murray, 1973.
14. Burns W, Hinchcliffe R, Littler TS. An explor-
atory study of hearing and noise exposure in
textile workers. Ann Occup Hyg 1964; 7: 323-
332.
15. International Electrotechnical Commission.
Sound Level Meters. Publication 651, 1979.
16. International Electrotechnical Commission.
Octave, Half-Octave and Third-Octave Band
Filters Intended for the Analysis of Sound and
Vibration. Publication 225, 1966.
17. Welch BL. Further note on Mrs. Aspin's tables
and on certain approximations to the tabled
function. Biometrika 1949; 36: 293-296.
18. International Organization for Standardization.
Assessment of Noise with Respect to Community
Response. Recommendation ISO/R 1996, 1971.
19. International Organization for Standardization.
Assessment of Occupational Noise Exposure for
Hearing Conservation Purposes. International
Standard ISO 1999, 1975.
20. Johnsson A, Hansson L. Prolonged exposure to
a stresful stimulus (noise) as a cause of
raised blood-pressure in man. Lancet 1977;
I: 86-87.

21. Lawrence M, Nuttall AL, Burgio P. Oxygen reserve and autoregulation in the cochlea. Acta Otolaryngol (Stockh) 1977; 83: 146-152.
22. Perlman HB, Yamada S. Autoregulation of the strial blood flow. Third Symp on the Role of the Vestibular Organs in Space Exploration. NASA SP-152. (cited by Lawrence, Ref. 1).
23. Fox RH. Effects of cold on the extremities. Proc Roy Soc Med 1968; 61· 785-707.
24. Axelsson Å, Vertes D, Miller J. Immediate noise effects on cochlear vasculature in the guinea pig. Acta Otolaryngol (Stockh) 1981; 91: 237-246.
25. Vertes D, Axelsson A, Miller J, Liden G. Cochlear vascular and electrophysiological effects in the guinea pig to 4 kHz tones of different durations and intensities. Acta Otolaryngol (Stockh) 1982. (in press).
26. Wersäll J, Densert O, Lundquist P-G. Studies on the fine structure of the inner ear vessels. In: De Lorenzo AJD, ed. Vascular Disorders and Hearing Defects. Baltimore: University Park Press, 1973.
27. Kimura RS, Ota CY. Ultrastructure of the cochlear blood vessels. Acta Otolaryngol (Stockh) 1974; 77: 231-250.
28. Perlman HB, Kimura RS. Observations of the living blood vessels of the cochlea. Ann Otol Rhinol Laryngol 1955; 64: 1176-1192.
29. Todd NE, Dennard JE, Clairmont AA, Jackson RT. Sympathetic stimulation and otic blood flow. Ann Otol Rhinol Laryngol 1974; 83: 84-91.
30. Hultcranz E. The cochlear blood flow. Uppsala Univ, 1978. PhD Thesis. (unpublished).
31. Suga F, Snow JD. Adrenergic control of cochlear blood flow. Ann Otol Rhinol Laryngol 1969; 78: 358-374.
32. Misrahy G, Shinabarger EW, Arnold JE. Changes in cochlear endolymphatic oxygen availability, action potential and microphonics during and following asphyxia, hypoxia and exposure to loud sounds. J Acoust Soc Am 1958; 30: 701-704.
33. Maass B. Tierexperimentelle Untersuchungen des sympathischen Einflussess auf die Innenohr-funktion. Dusseldorf: Habilitationsschrift, 1977.
34. Maass B, Daumgartl N, Lübbers DW. Lokale pO2- und pH2-Messungen mit Mikroazialnadelelektroden an der Basalwindung der Katzencochlea nach akuter oberer zervikaler Sympathektomie. Arch Otorhinolaryngol 1978; 211: 269-284.
35. Lawrence M, Gonzales G, Hawkins JE. Some physiological factors in noise-induced hearing loss. Am Ind Hyg Assoc J 1967; 28: 425-430.
36. Hawkins JE. The role of vasoconstriction in noise-induced hearing loss. Ann Otol Rhinol Laryngol 1971; 80: 903-913.
37. Hawkins JE. Comparative otopathology: ageing, noise, and ototoxic drugs. Adv Otorhinolaryngol 1973; 20: 125-141.

DISCUSSION

N. Olsen: Can you exclude the possibility that the saws used by the group with VWF differed from those used by the group without VWF? Also, were there differences between the noise and vibration levels experienced by the two groups?

Authors' Response: The type of chain saw used by the lumberjacks was checked each year and there was no difference between the two groups. The saws were checked in an attempt to establish why only 40% of the subjects had VWF in 1972, and why some were recovering faster than others. The life span of a chain saw in Finland is, on average, one year. The same makes of saw are used by 70% of the lumberjacks. However, the makes do change from year to year. Thus, we found no reason to claim the interaction between VWF and NIPTS depended on a particular make of chain saw. The noise and vibration levels of saws are measured by the Dept. of Agriculture and Forestry and the "worst saws" are not used in Finland.

E.S. Harris: If the primary mechanism of both NIPTS and VWF is the same and centrally mediated, one would expect VWF to be bilateral. But in chippers, it is the hand holding the chisel that is principally involved. How can this be explained?

Authors' Response: In chippers, the vibration of the chisel, which is controlled by the left hand, is about 1000 times greater than the handle held by the right hand. However, the poor coupling between the chisel and the hand reduces the vibration entering the left hand to about 3 to 4 times that entering the right hand (Färkkilä M, Starck J, Hyvärinen J, Kurppa K. Vasospastic symptoms caused by asymmetrical vibration exposure of the upper extremities to a pneumatic hammer. Scand J Work Environ Health 1978; 4: 330-335). The asymmetry of the symptoms of VWF experienced by chippers may be partly explained by the complexity of the responses of the sympathetic nervous system. As well as segmental reflexes, the response of the stellate ganglia (which control most of the sympathetic innervations of the hand) are also involved. Phenomena such as overlap of the preganglionic fibres, subliminal fringe, occlusion, and spatial and temporal summation all participate in an integrated nerve response to a specific stimulus, and may be restricted to one hand. Thus asymmetric development of VWF may result. Our plethysmographic data also support the possibility that asymmetric responses may occur. During exposure to vibration, vasoconstrictions in the ipsilateral hand were greater than in the contralateral hand (Pyykkö I, Hyvärinen J, Färkkilä MA. Studies on the etiological mechanism of the vasospastic component of the Vibration Syndrome - see elsewhere in this volume).

T. Azuma: Is there any direct evidence that noise-induced hearing loss is due to blood flow disturbances?

Authors' Response: NIPTS is considered by some investigators to be due to vascular changes within the inner ear. There are two possibilities for explaining why subjects with VWF have increased NIPTS. The vascular changes in VWF and NIPTS may occur independently from each in the same subject, or may share the same etiological mechanism. In the first case, subjects with VWF would display a greater vulnerability to noise. In the second case, both VWF and NIPTS would be triggered by "over-activation" of the sympathetic nervous system controlling the blood supply to the affected organs. There is some evidence that activation of the sympathetic nervous system may decrease cochlear blood flow. The skin circulation is known to be influenced by sympathetic nerve control. Up to now, conclusive proof for either of these mechanisms is lacking, but the balance of evidence in our opinion favours the latter possibility.

H.E. von Gierke: Two comments: First, the measurement of the noise exposure of chain saw operators usually neglects the possibility that bone-conducted "noise" is contributing to the exposure. I admit that it is hard to measure, but an effort should be made to characterize this component for various chain saws. In assessing the noise exposure from chain saws, it should be noted that the contribution from bone conduction will increase with the use of most hearing protectors.

Second, I don't believe your hypothesis concerning the similarity or even sameness of the injury mechanism for VWF and NIPTS has too much support from the available knowledge. Several investigations of this subject have been undertaken and I admit there are a few studies that could be interpreted as supporting your hypothesis. However, the overwhelming body of evidence appears to be against it. In noise-induced hearing loss,

deterioration of the vascular supply appears to occur after the primary damage to the hair cells has occurred.

Authors' Response: In all probability the vibration from chain saws does not interfere mechanically with the cochlear function and cause NIPTS in subjects with VWF. Low-frequency vibration is undoubtedly transmitted by the bones from the hands to the skull, where its intensity may be sufficient to cause vibration of the hair cells (there is about 60 dB attenuation in this path at a frequency of 100 Hz). The lumberjacks with VWF in fact used larger, hand grip (compression) forces, which allowed more vibration to be transmitted along the bones into the skull. The difference was, however, small, of the order of from 1 to 2 dB. Its practical importance is therefore questionable. The lumberjack groups were matched in age, exposure and in use of hearing protection (ear muffs). Thus, the main factor differentiating the subjects was the presence or absence of VWF.

We don't agree with your second comment. There is evidence to support the vascular etiology of hearing loss. The evidence is, however, not yet conclusive. We are not suggesting that NIPTS results solely from sympathetic over-reaction, but rather that the additional from 10 to 15 dB hearing loss in subjects with VWF may be caused by activation of the sympathetic nervous system.

Pyykkö et al.: Hearing loss

OBJECTIVE METHODS FOR
DIAGNOSIS

Vibration Perception in Persons Not Previously Exposed to Local Vibration and in Vibration-Exposed Workers

I-M. Lidström, G. Hagelthorn and N. Bjerker

ABSTRACT: Symptoms of nerve function disorders commonly occur in vibration-exposed workers. It has been difficult to find objective methods to diagnose vibration-induced injuries, particularly disorders of the peripheral nervous system. The objective of the current investigation was to establish the vibration perception thresholds of persons not previously exposed to vibration, in order to develop a method for studying nerve function in vibration-exposed workers. The perception threshold (PT) and the temporary threshold shift (TTS) were determined following exposures to various vibration frequencies, intensities, and durations. A clear relationship could be established between these variables and the TTS. When compared with the control group, the vibration-exposed group possessed permanent threshold shifts (PTS) and their TTS were significantly greater, which supports the hypothesis that a causal relationship exists between nerve function disorders and vibration exposure.

RESUME: Les symtômes de troubles nerveux fonctionnels sont communs chez les travailleurs exposés aux vibrations. Il a été difficile de trouver une méthode objective pour diagnostiquer les dommages dus aux vibrations, surtout s'il s'agit de troubles du système nerveux périphérique. L'objectif de la présente étude consistait premièrement à déterminer le seuil de perception des vibrations chez des sujets qui n'ont pas été exposés à des vibrations en vue de mettre au point une méthode applicable à l'étude de la physiologie nerveuse des travailleurs exposés aux vibrations. On a déterminé le seuil de perception (PT) et la variation temporaire du seuil (TTS) après exposition à des vibrations de fréquence, intensité et durée diverses. On a constaté qu'il existe une relation évidente entre ces variables et la TTS. On a noté, chez les travailleurs exposés aux vibrations, une variation permanente du seuil (PTS) et constaté que la TTS était supérieure de façon significative, ce qui confirme l'hypothèse voulant qu'il existe une relation de cause à effet entre les vibrations et les troubles nerveux fonctionnels.

INTRODUCTION

Symptoms of nervous disorders are common in workers exposed to vibration. Using objective methods, it has, however, been difficult to diagnose disorders of the peripheral nervous system resulting from vibration exposures. The aim of this investigation was to obtain detailed knowledge of vibration perception thresholds in persons not previously exposed to vibration, in order to provide a basis for method development for studying the function of the nervous system in workers exposed to vibration.

When a person is exposed to hand-arm vibration, as in work with vibrating, hand-held tools, there is a temporary increase in his threshold of vibration perception (TTS). Several determinations of vibration perception thresholds (PT) at different frequencies have been reported in the literature (1-10). However, no investigation has been found that elucidates how the perception threshold varies with exposure factors such as frequency, intensity, and duration. The study described here was performed to examine the effects of these variables, both separately and together.

I METHOD FOR DETERMINING PT AND TTS

The equipment used for vibration exposures and to determine thresholds of perception was an electrodynamic vibrator (one degree of freedom), with a vibrating plate specially designed to ensure no resonance within the 50-1000 Hz frequency range. A servosystem enabled a constant acceleration of the vibrator to be maintained, regardless of variations in the static loading.

A special handle designed by the Swedish Aeronautical Research Institute was fitted to the plate. The rigidity of the handle was high and the weight very low, which ensured that mechanical resonance did not occur below 1000 Hz. The handle was equipped with strain gauges in two measuring bridges, to permit compressive or tensile forces and the gripping force to be recorded. The perception threshold was determined by a procedure in which the fingertips of the right hand rested under their own weight on the vibrating plate. In this investigation, the perception threshold at each frequency was approached from below, i.e. from imperceptible to perceptible vibration, the threshold value being expressed as an acceleration. Repeated perception threshold determinations were made at each test frequency.

Following the determination of the permanent perception threshold, the subject was exposed to vibration of a given frequency and intensity for a certain period of time. To achieve this, the person was required to grip the vibrating handle with the right hand with a force of 25 N, and to pull the handle straight upwards at the same time with a force of 50 N.

Within 30 seconds of the end of the vibration exposure, the perception threshold was determined at a single frequency, in order to ascertain the value of the (temporary) perception threshold immediately after the exposure. The recovery of the perception threshold was monitored over a period of 20 minutes.

The following precautions were taken:
a) a check was made prior to the test to ensure that the skin temperature of the fingers was not below 25°C;
b) the subject was placed in a standardized position;
c) the subject was fitted with headphones emitting a masking sound during the determination of the perception threshold; and
d) the tensile and gripping forces were kept constant during the vibration exposures.

II EXPERIMENT 1: PERSONS NOT EXPOSED TO VIBRATION AT WORK

2.1 Subjects and Procedure

The object of the first part of the investigation was to study the vibration perception of 20 persons who had not been exposed to vibration at work. The persons selected were medical students, who, because of their availability, were able to participate in a long and, in some respects, fairly demanding series of experiments.

The following criteria were set for the selection of subjects:
a) age between 20 and 25 years;
b) no previous exposure to local or whole-body vibration at work;
c) anamnesis free from neurological illnesses with residual symptoms, general circulatory disorders, peripheral circulatory disorders such as Raynaud's Disease, Raynaud's Phenomenon, acrocyanosis or cutis marmorata, arthropathy with residual symptoms, and metabolic disorders;and
d) no incidence of severe trauma to the upper extremities, such as complicated fractures, or injury to the soft tissue, where there might be reason to suspect neurological or vascular injury.

The first ten men and ten women who applied to participate in the experiment conformed with these criteria. During the experimental period of between four and eight months, one of the women was forced to withdraw from the series of experiments because of lumbago-sciatica. The results obtained for this person have therefore been disregarded in the final report. All the other 19 persons completed the whole series of experiments.

The results of preliminary tests established the existence of large variations in perception thresholds between individuals. For this reason, as each of the subjects participated in all of the experiments, the individual thresholds could be used as the basis for comparison.

Each of the subjects was exposed to 53 different test cycles consisting of: a) determination of the permanent perception threshold; b) exposure to vibration; and c) determination of the temporary threshold shift.

The following variables were studied with regard to their influence on the perception threshold shift:
a) the vibration frequency to which the person was exposed. Discrete sine-wave vibrations were chosen at the following frequencies: 50, 100, 200, 400 and 800 Hz.
b) the frequency at which the person was tested. The test frequencies selected were: 50, 100, 200, 400, 600 and, sometimes, 800 Hz.
c) the intensity of exposure: the intensities involved accelerations of 20, 40 and 80 m/s^2.
d) the time of exposure: the times chosen were 2, 4 and 8 minutes.
The combinations of vibration frequency, amplitude and duration of exposure for which the TTS was determined at selected test frequencies are given in Table 1.

2.2 Results and Discussion

The mean values of the perception thresholds for the 19 persons at frequencies from 50 to 800 Hz show that the lowest threshold value was found at a frequency of

Table 1. Combinations of Vibration Frequency, Amplitude and Duration of Exposure for Which the Temporary Threshold Shift was Determined at Selected Frequencies.

Frequency of Exposure (Hz)	Amplitude of Exposure (m/s²)	50			100			200			400			600		
		2	4	8	2	4	8	2	4	8	2	4	8	2	4	8
50	20															
	40		x						x						x	
	80															
100	20					x			x			x				
	40		x		x	x			x		x	x			x	
	80				x	x			x		x	x				
200	20					x			x			x				
	40		x			x			x			x			x	
	80					x			x			x				
400	20				x	x		x	x		x	x				
	40		x		x	x	x		x		x	x	x		x	
	80				x	x	x		x		x	x	x			
800	20															
	40		x						x						x	
	80															

100 Hz (see Fig. 1). An analysis of variance of the 1292 determinations of perception threshold showed that the differences in perception between persons were greater than the differences between repeated determinations for a single person, as might be expected (Table 2).

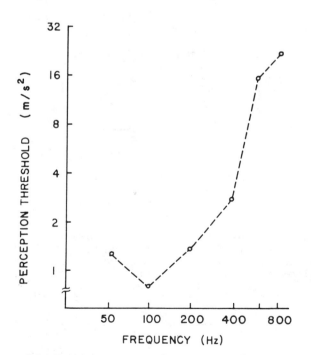

Fig. 1 Mean perception thresholds (N=19) at different frequencies.

Table 2. Permanent Threshold for Discrete Sine-Wave Vibration (Expressed in m/s²).

	Frequency (Hz)					
	50	100	200	400	600	800
Mean Value (N=19)	1.3	0.8	1.4	3.0	14.9	21.2
SD Between Individuals	0.75	0.75	1.23	3.29	15.75	20.27
SD for a given Individual	0.36	0.23	0.51	1.40	12.64	13.32

There was a significant effect of exposure frequency on the temporary shift in perception threshold, when the other variables were kept constant ($p < 0.01$). The largest TTS was observed following exposure to a frequency of 400 Hz, as can be seen from Fig. 2.

The decrease in TTS following exposure to vibration at a given frequency was found to be an almost linear function of the logarithm of time (Fig. 3).

There was also a significant difference between the TTS values at all test frequencies except 50 and 100 Hz after exposure to a single frequency, as is shown in Fig. 4 ($p < 0.01$). As in the PT determinations, the smallest scatter was observed at the 100 Hz frequency.

A clear correlation was established between TTS and the vibration amplitude to which the person was exposed. The TTS increased significantly with increasing vibration amplitude throughout the frequency range, as shown in Fig. 5 ($p < 0.01$). There

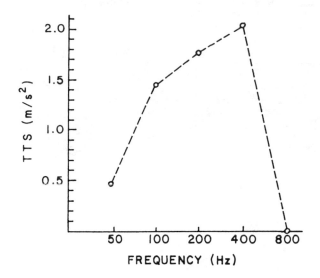

Fig. 2 Mean temporary threshold shift (N=19) after exposure to a vibration amplitude of 40 m/s^2 at frequencies of 50 to 800 Hz for 4 min.

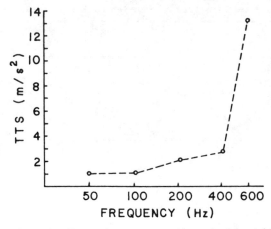

Fig. 4 Mean temporary threshold shift (N=19) at frequencies from 50 to 600 Hz after exposure to a vibration amplitude of 40 m/s^2 for 4 min at a frequency of 400 Hz.

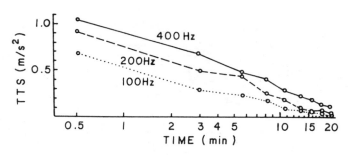

Fig. 3 Reduction in temporary threshold shift after termination of vibration exposure at different frequencies.

was also a correlation between the TTS and the exposure time, the TTS increasing with increasing exposure time. The results are summarized in Fig. 6 and are given in detail in Table 3. The recovery curve after exposure to vibration at different amplitudes and of different durations shows a greater slope the higher the TTS immediately after exposure.

A separate investigation was carried out to determine whether a shift in perception threshold can result from static loading or from fatigue during a prolonged test session. The static loading did not cause TTS, nor did prolonged testing in itself constitute a sufficient exposure to produce TTS.

In summary, this experiment established that even a very moderate exposure to vibration induces a temporary threshold shift.

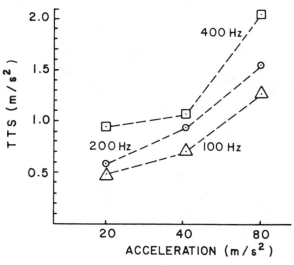

Fig. 5 Mean temporary threshold shift (N=19) after exposure to different vibration amplitudes for 4 min at frequencies of 100, 200 and 400 Hz.

The TTS observed after a short duration exposure was of a totally transient nature, and the recovery of the perception threshold followed a linear relationship with the logarithm of time. The results showed the highest reproducibility at a test frequency of 100 Hz, and the magnitude of the threshold shift was related to both the intensity and the duration of exposure. The greatest TTS was observed after exposure to a frequency of 400 Hz.

Lidström et al.: Vibration perception

Table 3. Mean Temporary Threshold Shift (N=19) Immediately After Exposure to Vibration (m/s²).

Frequency of Exposure (Hz)	Amplitude of Exposure (m/s²)	Test Frequency (Hz)								
		50	100			200	400			600
		Duration of Exposure (min)								
		4	2	4	8	4	2	4	8	4
50	40	0.8				0.47				2.52
100	20			0.49		0.89		0.75		
	40	1.01	0.38	0.69		1.46	0.86	2.32		4.86
	80		0.63	1.28		2.25	1.29	4.21		
200	20			0.58		1.03		1.87		
	40	1.04		0.92		1.81		1.68		11.68
	80			1.54		2.71		4.63		
400	20			0.95	1.33	1.76		3.18	4.42	
	40	1.09	0.51	1.07	1.86	2.07	1.54	2.63	5.73	13
	80		0.9	2.04	2.73	4.81	2.87	8.50	9.14	
800	40	0.34				-0.04				-3.44

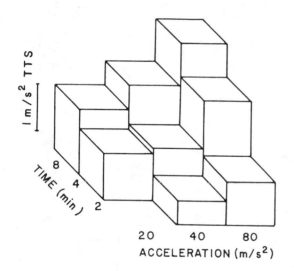

Fig. 6 Mean temporary threshold shift (N=19) after exposure to different vibration amplitudes for various exposure times at a frequency of 400 Hz.

III EXPERIMENT 2: PERSONS EXPOSED TO VIBRATION AT WORK AND CONTROLS

3.1 Subjects and Procedure

It is well known that persons exposed to vibration show not only peripheral circulatory disorders but also symptoms which suggest peripheral nerve damage. These symptoms include numbness, paresthesia, and sometimes pain in the hands and arms, especially at night. These symptoms are also exhibited by persons not exposed to vibration, and they are thus not necessarily indicative of vibration damage. In view of these difficulties in differential diagnosis, it is of interest to study the peripheral nerve function of persons exposed to vibration by an objective method, and to compare the results with those from a control group.

This investigation involved 315 persons. Of these, 160 persons had worked permanently with chain saws, rock drills, chipping hammers or grinding machines, and the remaining 155 persons constituted the controls for the respective occupational groups. The controls included persons from the same environments, which exposed the hands and arms to heavy physical work, but who had never worked with vibrating hand-tools. The persons chosen possessed an age distribution which matched that of the group exposed to vibration. The persons exposed to vibration were divided into two groups: the first consisting of 79 persons troubled by numbness, paresthesia or pain, and the second consisting of 81 persons not exhibiting these symptoms. Both groups included persons with VWF (vibration-induced white fingers). The procedure adopted in this study is described in Section I. Based on the results of the investigation of perception threshold shifts after exposure to vibration, the exposure conditions were chosen to be a vibration amplitude of 80 m/s², a duration of 8 min and a frequency of 400 Hz. The perception thresholds were measured at 100 Hz.

3.2 Results and Discussion

The results showed that the permanent perception threshold was primarily determined by factors such as skin thickness, the presence of calluses on the hands, and the person's age. The perception threshold of persons exposed to vibration, whether or not they exhibited symptoms of the peripheral nervous system, did not differ significantly from those persons who were engaged in heavy work, but who were not exposed to vibration (Fig. 7).

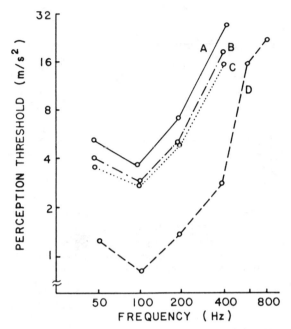

Fig. 7 Perception threshold at different frequencies. A, persons exposed to vibration with symptoms; B, persons exposed to vibration without symptoms; C, manual labourers not exposed to vibration; and D, students.

After exposure to vibration, however, the temporary threshold shift was considerably greater for the group who were exposed to vibration in their work, and who had reported symptoms, than for the other groups (see Fig. 8). The recovery time for the perception threshold was independent of the magnitude of the TTS.

IV CONCLUSIONS

The statistically significant correlation ($p < 0.01$) between the magnitude of the TTS and the occurrence of numbness/paresthesia, with or without VWF, must be interpreted both as an objective indication that nerve function disturbances are present in this group, and as support for the hypothesis that there is a causal relationship between these changes and exposure to vibration.

REFERENCES

1. Bjerker N, Kylin B, Lidström I-M. Changes in the vibratory sensation threshold after exposure to powerful vibration. Ergonomics 1972; 15: 399-406.
2. Bugard FJ. Mesure des seuils de sensation vibratoire chez l'homme. J Physiol (Paris) 1952; 44: 230-233.
3. Cadariu C, Gradina C, Constantinidis A, Marinesco V. Modifications des reaction de l'organisme chez les ouvriers exposés aux vibrations et aux bruit caracteristiques physiques differentes. XVeme Congr Int de Med du Travail 1966; 209-912.
4. Fibikar RJ. Touch and vibration sensitivity. Prod Eng 1956; 27: 177-179.
5. Ishiko N, Loewenstein WR. Effects of temperature on the generator and action potentials of a sense organ. J Gen Physiol 1961; 45: 107.
6. Miura T, Kimura K, Tominaga Y, Kimotsuki K. On the Raynaud's Phenomenon of occupational origin due to vibrating tools. Rodo Kagaku 1966; 42: 725-747.
7. Radzyukevich TM. Interrelation of temporary and permanent shifts of vibration and pain sensitivity thresholds under the effect of local vibration. News on Russian Med and Biochem 1970; 56.
8. Razumov IK, Denisov EK, Malinskaya NN, Pozdnyakova RZ. Perception thresholds of static vibration bands in man. Gig Tr Prof Zabol 1967; 5: 3-9.
9. Weitz J. Vibratory sensitivity as a function of skin temperature. J Exp Psychol 1941; 23: 21-36.

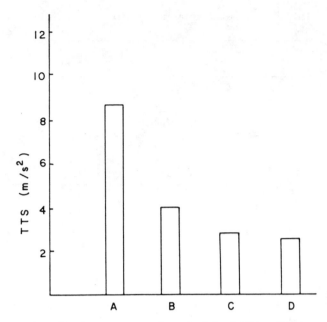

Fig. 8 Temporary threshold shift after exposure to a vibration amplitude of 80 m/s^2 for 8 min at 400 Hz. A, persons exposed to vibration with symptoms; B, persons exposed to vibration without symptoms; C, manual labourers not exposed to vibration; and D, students.

10. Yacorzynski GK, Brown M. Studies of the sensa-
    tion of vibration. 1. Variability of the
    vibratory threshold as a function of amplitude
    and frequency of mechanical vibration. J Exp
    Psychol 1941; 28: 509-516.

DISCUSSION

G. Landwehr: Your work shows that the lowest
thresholds for the perception of vibration occur in
the frequency range from 80 to 150 Hz, implying that
the fingers are most sensitive to vibration at these
frequencies. Do you think that this frequency range
is also the most harmful, a conclusion that would
be contradictory to the ISO guidelines?

Authors' Response: I think that the fingers
are most sensitive to vibrations in the frequency
range around 100 Hz, because the Pacinian corpuscles
have maximum discrimination capacity in the corresponding range, but this does not mean that it is
the most dangerous frequency.

T. Azuma: Is there any relationship between
the time constant of the exponential decay of TTS
and the frequency of vibratory stimulation?

Authors' Response: The decrease in TTS after
exposure ceased is an almost linear function of the
logarithm of time. The recovery curves for
different exposure frequencies are nearly parallel.
This means that there is a slight difference in the
recovery time between different frequencies depending upon how high the initial TTS is.

I. Pyykkö: In your conclusion, you indicated
that the reason for more pronounced TTS among
vibration-exposed workers might be a permanent disturbance in the function of the peripheral nerves.
However, your data also fit the deterioration of
the generator potential from Pacinian corpuscles,
which are the vibration receptors at these frequencies. Actually, I believe the curves showing
the perception thresholds as a function of frequency fit fatigue phenomena in Pacinian corpuscles
better. Do you have any comments?

Authors' Response: After exposure to vibration
you will find in all persons a temporary threshold
shift, the magnitude depending, among other factors
on exposure frequency, acceleration level and exposure time. The cause of the TTS may, as you
suggested, be a fatigue phenomena in the Pacinian
corpuscles. This fatigue phenomenon does not
explain the fact that persons with symptoms of
vibration injury show a changed reaction to a vibration stimulus compared with persons without symptoms.
The only reason for this nervous function disorder
is damage to the receptors within the peripheral
nerves or the CNS. There is also a possibilty of
an increase of threshold due to habituation.

Diagnosis of the Vibration Syndrome by Blood Viscosity

A. Okada, M. Ariizumi and H. Fujinaga

ABSTRACT: To investigate the hemorrhagic effects of vibration, whole blood and plasma viscosities as well as plasma cyclic nucleotides were measured in workers using vibrating tools. To examine the possibility of detecting Raynaud's Phenomenon positive subjects, the blood viscosity of chain saw workers with and without Raynaud's Phenomenon was measured at five shear rates from 230 s^{-1} to 11.5 s^{-1}. Plasma cyclic AMP and cyclic GMP levels did not differ between the workers using vibrating tools and controls. In the group with Raynaud's Phenomenon, the whole blood viscosity was significantly higher than in the group without Raynaud's Phenomenon at each shear rate. It is suggested that whole blood viscosity plays an important role in the appearance of the Vibration Syndrome, and that the investigation of blood viscosity is a useful tool for discriminating between a Raynaud's Phenomenon positive group and a negative group, between attacks.

RESUME: Afin d'étudier les effets hémorhéologiques des vibrations, on a mesuré la viscosité du sang entier et du plasma, ainsi que la teneur en nucléotides cycliques du plasma, chez des ouvriers qui se servent d'outils vibrants. Pour examiner la possibilité de dépister le phénomène de Raynaud, on a mesuré la viscosité du sang, à cinq taux de cisaillement différents compris entre 230 s^{-1} et 11,5 s^{-1}, chez des ouvriers utilisant des marteaux-piqueurs et dont certains présentaient des signes du phénomène de Raynaud. Les concentrations d'AMP cycliques et de GMP cycliques chez des ouvriers et chez des témoins utilisant des outils vibrants étaient semblables. La viscosité du sang entier était beaucoup plus élevée chez ceux qui présentaient des signes du phénomène pour chacun des taux de cisaillement. On suggère que la viscosité du sang entier dans le syndrome de vibration est un facteur important, et que l'examen de la viscosité du sang pour déceler, entre les crises, les sujets présentant des signes du phénomène de Raynaud constitue un outil utile.

INTRODUCTION

The Vibration Syndrome is an important occupational disease in Japan and presents a social problem for users of vibrating tools. The effects of vibration include various manifestations, such as peripheral vascular disturbance and damage to the peripheral nervous system, to bones, to joints and to muscles. Of these, a typical symptom is Raynaud's Phenomenon, which is the subject of the present study.

It is easy to diagnose Raynaud's Phenomenon during an attack, but it is difficult to be sure of the diagnosis when the subjects are seen between attacks. A method for the early detection of Raynaud's Phenomenon before the appearance of symptoms is clearly desirable, in order to maintain the health of workers who use vibrating tools. We have already reported the use of the cold pressor recovery index as a screening test for the discrimination of a Raynaud's Phenomenon positive group from a negative group (1). Furthermore, the application of NA-histamine iontophoresis to the detection of peripheral vascular disturbances is, in our opinion, worthy of closer examination (2). The skin temperature test is a more popular method for detecting peripheral vascular disturbances, because of its simplicity. However, it is impossible, to judge the existence of peripheral vascular disturbances by this single test.

The present paper reports investigations on the hemorrhagic aspects of workers using vibrating tools. Blood viscosity as well as plasma cyclic nucleotides have been studied to determine their usefulness for the early detection of Raynaud's Phenonenon.

I SUBJECTS AND METHOD

Thirty-four workers using vibrating tools, such as jet grinders, hand grinders, hand drills, or hand hammers, were studied. Seventeen had some subjective symptoms of numbness of the arms or pain in the arms (group with symptoms of the peripheral nerves). Fifty age-matched, healthy men were studied as controls.

In these subjects plasma cyclic AMP, cyclic GMP, and whole blood and plasma viscosity were examined.

In a second study, the whole blood and plasma viscosity of 11 chain saw workers in whom Raynaud's Phenomenon was confirmed were examined. The same tests were performed on 18 chain saw workers who were not affected by Raynaud's Phenomenon. The subjects forming both groups were almost the same in age and in duration of work. Ninety-two age-matched healthy men were used as controls in this study.

Plasma cyclic AMP and cyclic GMP levels were determined using the radio-immunological method developed by Honma et al. (3). Whole blood and plasma viscosity were measured with a Wells-Brookfield cone-plate microviscometer (model LVT) at five shear rates: 230, 115, 46, 23 and 11.5 s^{-1} (4). Statistical analyses were performed using Student's t-test.

II RESULTS AND DISCUSSION

Table 1 shows the cyclic AMP, the cyclic GMP levels and the ratio cyclic AMP/cyclic GMP, expressed in terms of the mean ± SD, for the group with subjective symptoms and for the group without subjective symptoms, both of whose members used vibrating tools. No significant difference was observed between the two groups.

The results of whole blood viscosity and plasma viscosity measured at a shear rate of 230 s^{-1} are shown in Table 2. The group with subjective symptoms possessed a significantly higher whole blood viscosity than the control group. However, in the case of plasma viscosity, the values of both groups were almost identical.

Table 3 shows the results of whole blood and plasma viscosity for the group of chain sawyers with Raynaud's Phenomenon and for the group of chain sawyers without Raynaud's Phenomenon measured at five shear rates from 230 to 11.5 s^{-1}. In the group with Raynaud's Phenomenon, the whole blood

viscosity was significantly higher at each shear rate compared with the group without Raynaud's Phenomenon. No significant differences in plasma viscosity were observed between the two groups.

From the observations of plasma cyclic AMP, cyclic GMP levels and the ratio of these two cyclic nucleotides, there were no significant differences between the group with symptoms of peripheral nerve disorders and the group without such symptoms, in workers using vibrating tools. These cyclic nucleotides are known as the "second messenger" in various hormonal reactions or in neuro-transmitting mechanisms. Changes in cyclic AMP and cyclic GMP levels may provide information on the response of the peripheral nerves to various stimuli. However, such was not found here, and further investigations are necessary to confirm the effect of vibration on these cyclic nucleotides.

High blood viscosity occurs in various diseases, such as diabetes mellitus, thrombosis or atherosclerosis, macroglobulinemia (Waldenström), malignancy, sickle cell anemia etc. It has been suggested that the change of blood viscosity is one of the important factors affecting the progression of these diseases.

George et al. showed that 20 patients with Raynaud's Disease possessed higher whole blood viscosity than 12 healthy controls (5). Furthermore, they observed higher values of plasma viscosity in these patients. On the other hand, from observations of blood viscosity in women with Raynaud's Disease, Jahnsen et al. reported that the blood viscosity in the controls was somewhat higher than in the group with Raynaud's Disease at a shear rate of 2.3 s^{-1} and a temperature of 37°C, when blood viscosity was corrected to the same haematocrit reading (6).

Turczynski et al. measured the serum viscosity and serum protein in workers exposed to mechanical vibration and noise, and found a significant rise of serum viscosity in the group with manifestations of the Vibration Syndrome (7). They suggested

Table 1. Plasma Cyclic Nucleotide Levels for 17 Workers Using Vibrating Tools With Subjective Symptoms and for 17 Workers Without Subjective Symptoms of Peripheral Nerve Disorders.

	Cyclic AMP (Mean ± SD, pmol/ml)	Cyclic GMP (Mean ± SD, pmol/ml)	Cyclic AMP/ Cyclic GMP (Mean ± SD)
Workers using vibrating tools with symptoms of peripheral nerve disturbances (N=17)	17.7 ± 2.2	5 ± 1.3	4.2 ± 2.2
Workers using vibrating tools without symptoms of peripheral nerve disturbances (N=17)	17.5 ± 2.3	4.4 ± 1.7	4.5 ± 1.3

Table 2. Mean Values (± SD) of Whole Blood and Plasma Viscosities Measured at a Shear Rate of 230 s^{-1} and a Temperature of 37°C for 17 Workers Using Vibrating Tools With Symptoms of Peripheral Nerve Disorders and 50 Controls.

	Whole Blood Viscosity (cp)	Plasma Viscosity (cp)
Workers using vibrating tools with symptoms of the peripheral nerves (N=17)	4.9 ± 0.41*	1.6 ± 0.25
Controls (N=50)	4.3 ± 0.28	1.6 ± 0.13

*$p < 0.05$ (t-test)

Table 3. Mean Values (± SD) of Whole Blood Viscosity, Plasma Viscosity and Haematocrit Measured at 37°C for 18 Chain Saw Workers Without Raynaud's Phenomenon and 11 Chain Saw Workers With Raynaud's Phenomenon.

	Viscosity (cp)										Haemato-crit (%)
	Whole Blood					Plasma					
Shear-rate (s^{-1})	230	115	46	23	11.5	230	115	46	23	11.5	
Group without Raynaud's Phenomenon (N=18)	4.59 ±0.6	5.19 ±0.81	6.76 ± 1.21	7.91 ±1.45	8.18 ±1.71	1.62 ±0.26	1.71 ±0.38	2.06 ±0.53	2.15 ±0.6	2.61 ±1.02	42.6 ± 4.3
Group with Raynaud's Phenomenon (N=11)	5.32** ±0.65	6.36** ±0.96	8.25** ±1.1	9.85** ±1.74	10.29* ± 2.57	1.71 ±0.26	1.76 ±0.4	2.20 ±0.58	2.21 ±0.6	2.74 ±0.87	44.8 ± 4.2

*$p < 0.05$ **$p < 0.01$ (t-test)

that gamma and beta globulins played the greatest role in the increase of serum viscosity in subjects with the Vibration Syndrome. In our investigations, the group with symptoms of peripheral nerve disorders showed significantly higher whole blood viscosity than the group of control subjects who had not been exposed to vibration. This suggests that an increase of whole blood viscosity may play an important role in the appearance of peripheral nerve disorders among workers using vibrating tools. Although no significant difference was observed in plasma viscosity in chain saw workers, whole blood viscosity in the group with Raynaud's Phenomenon was significantly higher than in the group without Raynaud's Phenomenon at all five shear rates examined.

Our results suggest that the measurement of blood viscosity is a useful tool for discriminating between those persons more affected and those less affected by vibration exposure. Moreover, the results indicate that whole blood viscosity may play an important role in the appearance of the vascular component of the Vibration Syndrome. In addition, the data imply that we can differentiate between a group with Raynaud's Phenomenon and a group without these symptoms between vasospasms.

Thus, an investigation of blood viscosity is of benefit in the diagnosis of the Vibration Syndrome.

REFERENCES

1. Okada A, Yamashita T, Ikeda T. Screening test for Raynaud's Phenomenon of occupational origin. Am Ind Hyg Assoc J 1972; 33: 476-82.
2. Okada A, Yamashita T, Nagano C, Ikeda T, Yachi A, Shibata S. Studies on the diagnosis and pathogenesis of Raynaud's Phenomenon of occupational origin. Br J Ind Med 1971; 28: 353-57.
3. Honma M, Satoh T, Takezawa J, Ui M. An ultra-sensitive method for the simultaneous determination of cyclic AMP and cyclic GMP in small-volume samples from blood and tissue. Biochem Med 1977; 18: 257-73.
4. Wells RE, Denton R, Merrill EW. Measurement of viscosity of biologic fluids by cone plate viscometer. J Lab Clin Med 1961; 57: 646-56.
5. George WT, Shu C, Leroy EC, Gavras I, Gavras H, Gump FE. Blood viscosity, plasma proteins, and Raynaud's Syndrome. Arch Surg 1975; 110: 1343-46.
6. Jahnsen T, Nielsen SL, Skovborg F. Blood viscosity and local response to cold in primary Raynaud's Phenomenon. Lancet 1977; II: 1001-2.

Okada et al.: Diagnosis

7. Turczynski B, Kumaszka F, Srocynski J. Serum viscosity and protein fractions, cholesterol and total lipids in workers exposed to mechanical vibration and noise. Pol Tyg Lek 1978; 33: 1029-32.

DISCUSSION

N. Olsen: You have measured the shear-rate at 37°C. However, subjects with VWF have their attacks of Raynaud's Phenomenon at temperatures lower than 37°C. Have you measured the shear-rate at lower temperatures, and, if so, what are the results for controls and for vibration-exposed subjects with and without VWF?

Authors' Response: You are correct in suggesting that the hand temperatures of vibration-exposed workers are usually lower than the body temperatures. Our blood viscosity measurements were obtained only at body temperature (37°C). It would be worthwhile studying shear rates at lower temperatures.

T. Azuma: Your results on blood viscosity are very interesting. Do you have any idea about the mechanism by which blood viscosity increased in workers with Raynaud's Phenomenon? One possible mechanism for this increase may be a reduction in the deformability of red blood cells.

Authors' Response: We are not yet able to clarify the various mechanisms involved in Raynaud's Phenomenon. As the blood viscosity of chain saw operators without Raynaud's Phenomenon was greater than that of the controls, this change in viscosity is not dependent on the mechanisms involved in the attacks associated with Raynaud's Phenomenon.

Various Function Tests on the Upper Extremities and the Vibration Syndrome

N. Harada and T. Matsumoto

ABSTRACT: For the early diagnosis of the Vibration Syndrome, peripheral circulation and sensory tests, including tests after cold water immersion, and functional capacity motor tests are widely performed on the upper extremities in Japan. Workers (N=281) exposed to three sources of vibration and controls have been examined using these function tests, and the data analyzed by principal component analysis. The function tests are shown to be of diagnostic significance as a screening test for the Vibration Syndrome. It is also suspected that peripheral circulation disturbance, sensory disturbance and motor disturbance found in the Vibration Syndrome advance independently. Inconsistencies in the findings are noted and are attributed to differences in working conditions.

RESUME: Au Japon, pour dépister le plus tôt possible le syndrome de vibration, on procède à de nombreux tests des fonctions sensorielles et de la circulation périphérique (y compris des tests après immersion dans de l'eau froide) et des tests de motricité fonctionnelle des extrémités supérieures. On a fait passer ces tests à des ouvriers (N=281) exposés à trois sources de vibrations et à des témoins, puis on a analysé les données par examen des éléments principaux. On montre l'importance diagnostique des tests comme méthode de dépistage du syndrome de vibration. On soupçonne que les troubles de la circulation périphérique, ainsi que les troubles sensoriels et les troubles moteurs qui accompagnent le syndrome de vibration progressent indépendamment. Les inconsistances ont été notées et ont été attribuées aux différentes conditions de travail.

INTRODUCTION

In 1938, health disorders due to pneumatic tool operation were first reported in Japan (1). Since then, various types of portable vibrating tools have been developed for use in industry. In 1965, the outbreak of a large number of subjects with the Vibration Syndrome among chainsaw operators in the National Forests became a nation-wide social problem. From that time, Japanese physicians have been investigating this subject actively and systematically (2).

In order to investigate the diagnosis and prevention of the Vibration Syndrome in Japan, the Japanese Association of Industrial Health organized the Committee on Vibration Hazards in 1978 (Chairman: Prof. Takamatsu). The Committee presented a report and defined the Vibration Syndrome ("vibration hazards" in the report) as follows: the health disturbances caused by vibration transmitted to the human body usually through a hand-arm system from tools, machinery or equipment. The features of the Vibration Syndrome are dependent on the site of vibratory input and the spectrum, intensity and exposure time to vibration. They are modified by working conditions such as noise, cold, weight of the tool or machine, and working posture. The principal symptoms of the Vibration Syndrome are peripheral circulation disturbance, peripheral nervous disturbance and disturbance of the musculoskeletal system. It also pointed out that central functions such as the autonomic nervous system and the endocrine system can be affected (3).

For the early diagnosis of Vibration Syndrome, it is necessary to detect the functional disorders which appear without organic changes in patients with mild disease. In Japan, peripheral circulation and sensory tests, including tests after cold water immersion, and functional capacity motor tests are widely performed on the upper extremities (4). Using these function tests, the authors examined workers exposed to vibration and control workers, and used principal component analysis for the data. The significance of these tests for screening purposes and some pathogenetic aspects of the Vibration Syndrome are discussed in this paper.

I SUBJECTS AND METHODS

The total number of subjects examined was two hundred and eighty-one. Of these, sixty-nine were operators of leg-type rock-drills in a zinc mine; forty-one were chipping-hammer operators in an iron foundry; one hundred were motorcycle mailmen; and seventy-one were controls without occupational exposure to vibration but who worked in the same places as the workers exposed to vibration. Age, period of exposure to vibration, and the number of workers with a history of Raynaud's Phenomenon are given in Table 1.

The working conditions of the three groups exposed to vibration were as follows. The vibration acceleration values, about 30 G (rms) for both the rock-drill and the chipping-hammer, and about 2 G (rms) for the motorcycle, exceeded the exposure limits proposed by the ISO (5). The work place temperatures were 17 to 20°C in all seasons for the rock-drill group, -2 to 2°C in winter for the chipping-hammer group, and -2 to 8°C in winter for the motorcycle group.

The following function tests were performed on the upper extremities. The peripheral circulatory function was assessed by the skin temperature of the third finger and the value of the nail press test on the middle finger. The nail press test evaluates the recovery time of normal colour after pressing the nail strongly for ten seconds (6). Sensory function was assessed by pain threshold and the vibratory sense threshold of the middle finger at 125 Hz. Pain threshold was measured by means of weighted needles and determined by the weight applied. Motor function was evaluated by grasping power, pinching power of the thumb and middle finger, and tapping ability of the middle finger for thirty seconds. As for the provocative cooling test, one hand of a subject was immersed to the wrist in a stirred water bath at 10°C for ten minutes. The peripheral circulatory function and sensory function were recorded immediately after immersion and again

recorded after five and ten minutes. All the tests were conducted from December to April and the room temperature was maintained at 20°C.

Twenty-five variables were selected from the results of the examination and subjected to principal component analysis. All values of skin temperature (except those before and immediately after immersion), of the nail press test, and of pain threshold, were adjusted logarithmically to normalize the distribution. From the correlation matrix computed among these twenty-five variables, the principal components were extracted and rotated according to the Varimax procedure. After that, the factor scores for each subject were computed.

II RESULTS

The means and standard deviations of the function tests for each group are shown in Table 2. Both the rock-drill group and the chipping-hammer group had significantly lower functional capacity than the control group on the basis of skin temperature, the nail press test (except the variables before immersion of these two tests), pain threshold, vibratory sense threshold and grasping power. The motorcycle group had significantly lower functional capacity than the control group on the basis of skin temperature, the nail press test, vibratory sense threshold after immersion, pinching power and tapping ability.

Four principal components whose factor loadings are shown in Table 3 were extracted by analyzing the data of the control group. Because factor loading is the correlation coefficient between the principal component and the variables, the four principal components can be referred to as peripheral circulation (skin temperature and nail press test), pain sensation, vibratory sensation and motor function (grasping power, pinching power and tapping ability). About 62.2% of the variance in the twenty-five variables are explained by these four principal components.

The three principal components shown in Table 4 were obtained from the analyses of the groups exposed to vibration. Though the rock-drill group's first and second

Table 1. Number of Subjects, Their Age and Period of Exposure to Vibration.

	N	Age (yrs) Mean	Age (yrs) SD	Exposure (yrs) Mean	Exposure (yrs) SD
Rock-drill operators	69 (40)	42.4	5.5	12.8	6.5
Chipping-hammer operators	41 (18)	45.3	6.3	10.7	7.5
Motorcycle riders	100 (27)	37.8	10.1	11.5	5.6
Control workers	71	38.7	9.5		

( ): Number of subjects with history of Raynaud's Phenomenon.

Table 2. Results of the Function Tests on the Upper Extremities.

		Rock-drill Mean	SD	Chipping-hammer Mean	SD	Motorcycle Mean	SD	Control Mean	SD
Skin temperature (°C)	[A]	30	3.5	28.7	3.4	28.1	3.1 **	29.8	3.2
	[B]	10.7	0.6 **	11.3	1.8	10.8	0.7 **	11.3	1
$(\log_{10}(°C-10))$	[C]	0.74	0.23*	0.74	0.25*	0.73	0.15**	0.83	0.19
	[D]	0.94	0.23	0.9	0.26	0.89	0.17**	1.01	0.19
Nail press test	[A] R.	0.2	0.11**	0.33	0.13	0.48	0.16**	0.3	0.15
	[A] L.	0.22	0.12**	0.34	0.16	0.48	0.16**	0.29	0.15
	[B]	0.57	0.26*	0.65	0.24**	0.7	0.19**	0.48	0.17
$(\log_{10}(s))$	[C]	0.53	0.28*	0.62	0.26**	0.66	0.2 **	0.43	0.2
	[D]	0.42	0.25	0.58	0.26**	0.64	0.24**	0.39	0.2
Pain threshold	[A] R.	0.66	0.43**	0.77	0.34**	0.32	0.35	0.35	0.41
	[A] L.	0.69	0.48**	0.71	0.34**	0.25	0.39	0.31	0.42
	[B]	1.03	0.35**	0.93	0.42**	0.51	0.44	0.53	0.45
$(\log_{10}(g))$	[C]	0.89	0.39**	0.88	0.33**	0.34	0.38	0.39	0.44
	[D]	0.81	0.44**	0.85	0.32**	0.29	0.38	0.28	0.4
Vibratory sense threshold	[A] R.	15	9.5 **	9	6.6 **	5.3	7.3	5	7.7
	[A] L.	14.4	10.2 **	8.7	7.5 **	4.6	6.5	3.9	8.5
	[B]	30.3	8.9 **	28.1	7.9 **	27.1	9.2 **	19.5	7.4
(dB)	[C]	23.1	9.8 **	22.1	10.5 **	21.8	8.7 **	12.9	7.4
	[D]	19.5	9.8 **	18.2	11.6 **	19.1	9.1 **	9.8	8.4
Grasping power	R.	39.1	7 **	37.4	6.3 *	50.7	7.6 **	46	8.8
(kg)	L.	36.6	6.1 **	36.8	6.4 **	48.9	7.2 **	43.7	8.3
Pinching power	R.	6.8	2.4	7	2.8	5.7	1.9 *	6.5	2.1
(kg)	L.	6.7	2.4	7.2	2.5	5.4	1.9 **	6.4	2.1
Tapping ability	R.	135.3	18.3	133.2	15	129.2	19.4 **	139.3	21.4
	L.	124.9	17.4	123.9	16.4	120	18.3 *	127.7	20.1

[A]: Before immersion, [B]: Immediately after immersion, [C]: Five minutes after immersion, [D]: Ten minutes after immersion.
*p < 0.05, **p<0.01: Statistical significance compared with Controls.

principal components were the reverse of the other groups, the three groups were alike in the structure of the principal components. The three principal components were peripheral circulation (skin temperature and nail press test), sensory function (pain threshold and vibratory sense threshold), and motor function (grasping power, pinching power and tapping ability). Pain sensation and vibratory sensation, unlike the results of the control group, were not separated. These three principal components explained 58.2% of the total variance for the rock-drill group, 59.2% for the chipping-hammer group and 52.1% for the motorcycle group.

Table 5 shows the relationship between Raynaud's Phenomenon and factor score. For age and years of exposure, there were no significant differences between the subjects with or without a history of Raynaud's Phenomenon. Larger factor scores for subjects with a history of Raynaud's Phenomenon were observed in the principal components, referred to as peripheral circulation and sensory function in the rock-drill group, and peripheral circulation in the chipping-hammer group. The differences between subjects with Raynaud's Phenomenon and those without are statistically significant in some cases.

Table 6 shows the relationship between numbness of fingers and factor score. Larger factor scores for subjects with the symptom of finger numbness were observed in the principal component referred to as sensory function in the rock-drill group and the motorcycle group. The differences are again statistically significant. These observations indicate the hypofunctions relating to Raynaud's Phenomenon or to the numbness of fingers.

III DISCUSSION

For the diagnosis of the Vibration Syndrome, some attempts were previously made to induce Raynaud's Phenomenon by immersing the upper extremities in cold water (7,8). However, such a test is considered to be inadequate because Raynaud's Phenomenon could not be induced in 100% of the subjects. Also, an abnormal vasoconstriction reflex might be intensified by this procedure. In this study, the three groups exposed to vibration showed lower functional capacity than the control group for most of the

Harada et al.: Function tests

Table 3. Factor Loadings Computed by Principal Component Analysis of the Control Group.

			PC 1	PC 2	PC 3	PC 4
Skin	[A]		-0.67	0	-0.08	-0.28
temperature	[B]		-0.5	0.07	-0.11	-0.04
	[C]		-0.72	-0.26	-0.24	-0.28
	[D]		-0.74	-0.23	-0.31	-0.32
Nail Press	[A]	R.	0.71	-0.22	-0.23	-0.09
test		L.	0.68	-0.31	-0.21	-0.12
	[B]		0.72	-0.14	0.06	-0.17
	[C]		0.78	-0.04	0.14	-0.07
	[D]		0.75	-0.02	0.08	-0.09
Pain	[A]	R.	-0.03	0.73	-0.03	-0.11
threshold		L.	-0.06	0.77	0.03	-0.16
	[B]		-0.31	0.78	0.06	0.04
	[C]		-0.06	0.85	0.11	0.15
	[D]		0.01	0.87	0.17	0.08
Vibratory	[A]	R.	-0.18	-0.06	0.85	-0.12
sense		L.	-0.23	0.09	0.87	-0.09
threshold	[B]		0.27	0.05	0.55	-0.09
	[C]		0.33	0.2	0.78	-0.04
	[D]		0.35	0.12	0.77	0.11
Grasping power		R.	0.37	0.02	-0.07	0.61
		L.	0.41	-0.01	0.02	0.59
Pinching power		R.	-0.24	-0.38	-0.13	0.46
		L.	-0.26	-0.26	-0.16	0.49
Tapping ability		R.	0.04	0.03	-0.04	0.85
		L.	-0.19	0.12	0.01	0.78
Factor contribution			5.38	3.82	3.38	2.97

R - right hand; L - left hand.
For explanation of [A], [B], [C], [D] see footnote to Table 2.

variables of the function tests on the upper extremities. In addition, the analyses of factor scores of the groups exposed to vibration demonstrate that these function tests reflect the symptoms of Raynaud's Phenomenon. It is therefore believed that these function tests are of diagnostic significance as a screening test for the Vibration Syndrome.

From the analyses of the groups exposed to vibration, three principal components were obtained. Because the principal components are independent of each other, it is suspected that peripheral circulation disturbance, sensory disturbance and motor disturbance found in the Vibration Syndrome are not secondary to the other disturbances but develop independently of each other. The vibratory sensation after cold water immersion proved to have a relatively large factor loading on the principal component referred to as peripheral circulation; but this is probably attributed to the effect of skin temperature on vibratory sensation (9).

A different order of principal components was observed in the groups exposed to

vibration: the first principal component was peripheral circulation in the chipping-hammer group and the motorcycle group, but sensory function in the rock-drill group. This is considered to be due to the different environmental temperatures during work in winter, which were lower for the chipping-hammer group and the motorcycle group than for the rock-drill group. This coincides with the observation that the values of skin temperature and the nail press test were lowest in the motorcycle group, followed by the chipping-hammer group. The motorcycle group showed no statistical differences in the examinations of pain sensation and vibratory sensation except for the variables after immersion, presumably because of lower vibration exposure than the other two groups. In motor tests, a lower functional capacity for grasping was found in the rock-drill group and the chipping-hammer group, but for pinching and for tapping in the motorcycle group. This is conceivably due to differences in the handling of tools and machines. Further work is needed to resolve this matter.

Harada et al.: Function tests

Table 4. Factor Loadings Computed by Principal Component Analysis of the Groups Exposed to Vibration.

			Rock-drill			Chipping-hammer			Motorcycle		
			PC 1	PC 2	PC 3	PC 1	PC 2	PC 3	PC 1	PC 2	PC 3
Skin temperature	[A]		-0.1	-0.59	0.19	-0.82	-0.3	-0.13	-0.75	0.04	0.15
	[B]		0.21	-0.49	0.04	-0.19	-0.13	-0.21	-0.59	0.1	0.05
	[C]		-0.22	-0.88	-0.13	-0.89	-0.16	-0.09	-0.72	-0.19	0.06
	[D]		-0.22	-0.89	-0.11	-0.9	-0.18	-0.1	-0.77	-0.15	0.02
Nail press test	[A]	R.	-0.03	0.52	-0.39	0.29	-0.1	0.04	0.39	-0.14	-0.01
		L.	0.11	0.36	-0.46	0.66	0.23	0.15	0.52	-0.12	0.03
	[B]		0.19	0.68	0.19	0.57	0.02	0.16	0.69	-0.18	-0.09
	[C]		0.22	0.79	0.27	0.71	0.06	0.18	0.8	-0.08	-0.05
	[D]		0.21	0.75	0.17	0.85	0.05	0.16	0.8	-0.14	-0.02
Pain threshold	[A]	R.	0.79	0.17	-0.16	0.26	0.79	-0.01	-0.28	0.44	-0.11
		L.	0.84	0.08	-0.1	0.08	0.74	0.19	-0.27	0.55	0.03
	[B]		0.85	0.15	-0.01	-0.02	0.85	-0.03	-0.08	0.68	-0.18
	[C]		0.88	0.12	0.01	-0.06	0.79	-0.02	-0.16	0.78	-0.16
	[D]		0.88	0.24	0.05	0.23	0.85	0.2	-0.15	0.84	-0.2
Vibratory sense threshold	[A]	R.	0.68	-0.23	-0.34	0.19	0.5	-0.06	0.07	0.61	-0.04
		L.	0.6	-0.06	-0.38	0.4	0.6	-0.01	0.19	0.66	-0.06
	[B]		0.51	0.42	-0.28	0.59	0.45	-0.07	0.53	0.62	-0.02
	[C]		0.68	0.51	-0.17	0.79	0.47	0.01	0.64	0.5	-0.05
	[D]		0.69	0.47	-0.17	0.82	0.47	0.01	0.69	0.52	-0.09
Grasping power		R.	-0.31	0.22	0.47	0.11	0.02	0.85	0.11	-0.09	0.77
		L.	-0.28	0.27	0.5	-0.02	-0.02	0.83	0.03	-0.07	0.79
Pinching power		R.	-0.07	0.24	0.65	0.44	0.07	0.62	0.07	-0.35	0.6
		L.	-0.11	0.16	0.64	0.38	0.07	0.74	-0.09	-0.29	0.61
Tapping ability		R.	0.01	-0.10	0.64	0.1	0.08	0.68	-0.25	-0.07	0.6
		L.	-0.09	-0.17	0.65	-0.03	-0.09	0.6	-0.27	0.13	0.59
Factor contribution			6.11	5.29	3.16	6.65	4.74	3.41	5.79	4.38	2.84

R - right hand; L - left hand.
For explanation of [A], [B], [C], [D] see footnote to Table 2.

Table 5. Relation Between Raynaud's Phenomenon and Factor Score of the Groups Exposed to Vibration.

Group	Raynaud's Phenomenon	N	Age (yrs) Mean	SD	Exposure (Yrs) Mean	SD	FS 1 Mean	SD	FS 2 Mean	SD	FS 3 Mean	SD
Rock-	(+)	40	41.9	5	13.4	6.5	0.31	0.83**	0.28	1.07**	0.01	1.12
drill	(-)	25	43.2	6.6	12.2	6.9	-0.44	1.1	-0.46	0.75	-0.03	0.88
Chipping-	(+)	18	44.3	5.5	13.3	6.6	0.6	0.85**	0.17	1.12	0.22	0.92
hammer	(-)	22	46.5	6.7	8.8	7.7	-0.5	0.87	-0.12	0.92	-0.12	1.03
Motor-	(+)	27	39.5	10.7	11.3	5.9	0.22	1.14	0.29	1.08	0.15	0.22
cycle	(-)	73	37.2	9.9	11.6	5.5	-0.08	0.94	-0.11	0.96	-0.05	0.94

*p < 0.05, **p < 0.01: Statistical significance compared with the subjects without history of Raynaud's Phenomenon.

In the chipping-hammer group and the motorcycle group, FS 1, FS 2 and FS 3 are referred to as peripheral circulation, sensory function and motor function, respectively. In the rock-drill group, they are referred to as sensory function, peripheral circulation and motor function, respectively.

The smaller N's for the rock-drill group and the chipping-hammer group are due to partial lack of data for some subjects.

Table 6. Relation Between Numbness of Fingers and Factor Score for the Groups Exposed to Vibration.

Group	Numbness of Fingers	N	Age (Yrs) Mean	SD	Exposure (Yrs) Mean	SD	FS 1 Mean	SD	FS 2 Mean	SD	FS 3 Mean	SD
Rock-drill	(+)	31	42.7	5.4	12.9	6.9	0.46	0.7 **	0.11	1.16	0.11	1.12
	(−)	37	42.1	5.7	12.7	6.2	−0.4	1.04	−0.08	0.85	−0.07	0.92
Chipping-hammer	(+)	24	44.4	6.4	10.5	7.4	−0.03	0.85	0.02	1.04	0.05	0.92
	(−)	17	46.6	6.1	11	7.8	0.04	1.22	−0.03	0.97	−0.07	1.12
Motor-cycle	(+)	40	39.3	11.2	11.6	5.9	0.14	0.9	0.29	1.09*	0	0.94
	(−)	60	36.8	9.3	11.5	5.4	−0.1	1.06	−0.2	0.89	− 0	1.05

See footnote to Table 5.

IV CONCLUSIONS

The function tests on the upper extremities, including immersion in cold water, have been shown to reflect the effect of vibration exposure and the symptoms of Raynaud's Phenomenon. In consequence, they are considered to be of diagnostic significance as a screening test for the Vibration Syndrome. From principal component analyses of the groups exposed to vibration, it is suspected that peripheral circulation disturbance, sensory disturbance and motor disturbance found in the Vibration Syndrome advance independently of each other. Differences in the findings between the three groups have been recognized and are attributed to variations in the working conditions, particularly in exposure to cold and/or to vibration.

REFERENCES

1. Murakosi H. On the health disturbances due to pneumatic tool operation. Rinsho Igaku 1938; 26: 506-8. (in Japanese).
2. Yamada S. Prevention of the vibration hazards caused by chain-saw operation in Japan. Proc VIII-th World Cong on the Prevention of Occup Accidents and Disease. 1977; 2: 664-6.
3. Shindou Shougai Iinkai. Report of the committee on vibration hazards of the Japan Association of Industrial Health. 1980. (in Japanese).
4. Labour Standards Bureau, Japanese Ministry of Labour. Criteria for recognition as vibration hazards. Jpn Med J 1977; 2774: 95-7. (in Japanese).
5. International Organization for Standardization. Principles for the measurement and the evaluation of human exposure to vibration transmitted to the hand. Draft International Standard ISO/DIS 5349, 1979.
6. Yamada S. Primary factors for the occurrence of white waxy changes of the finger in vibration hazards with presentation of the nail press test. Jpn J Ind Health 1972; 14: 529-41. (in Japanese with English abstract).
7. Agate JN. An outbreak of cases of Raynaud's phenomenon of occupational origin. Br J Ind Med 1949; 6: 144-63.
8. Jepson RP. Raynaud's phenomenon in workers with vibratory tools. Br J Ind Med 1954; 11: 180-5.
9. Weitz J. Vibratory sensitivity as a function of skin temperature. J Exp Psychol 1941; 28: 21-36.

DISCUSSION

D.E. O'Connor: Your paper indicates that certain function tests were able to discriminate between the control group and the vibration exposed groups. I would like to ask if the variances of the distributions encountered would allow you to discriminate between individuals? In other words, could any of the function tests be used as an objective test for vibration disease in an individual?

Authors' Response: We have attempted discriminant analyses using 25 variables of these function tests. The analyses correctly classified subjects with a history of Raynaud's Phenomenon in the groups exposed to vibration as compared to the control group in 90 to 98% of cases. We therefore think that these function tests are useful to discriminate patients from healthy workers individually.

Approche Electromyographique pour l'Evaluation de l'Astreinte Due aux Vibrations sur le Système Main-Bras: Validation de la Méthodologie

J. P. Bakirzade, N. Di Renzo et L. Roure

RESUME: Dans le but d'évaluer l'astreinte musculaire, nous avons mis au point des traitements statistiques du signal électromyographique (EMG). Afin de valider ces méthodes, on a effectué une étude systématique sur six sujets développant une charge constante grâce à la contraction isométrique du muscle biceps brachii. Les calculs de la valeur rms, de la fréquence moyenne et médiane, des coefficients d'aplatissement et de dissymétrie effectués sur la densité spectrale de puissance du signal EMG prouvent que l'astreinte musculaire est quantifiable du fait des changements significatifs de l'évolution temporelle et fréquentielle de l'activité myoélectrique. Par ailleurs, on présente deux tests permettant d'estimer les résultats expérimentaux. En outre, on a vérifié l'indépendance de la répartition fréquentielle du spectre de l'EMG avec le niveau de contraction musculaire et son lien en fin d'expérimentation. La méthode est en cours d'application pour différentes contraintes vibratoires appliquées au système main-bras.

ABSTRACT: In order to evaluate muscular stress, statistical methods for processing the electromyographic (EMG) signal have been developed. These methods have been validated by a systematic study on six subjects, who established a constant load through isometric contraction of the biceps brachii muscle. Calculation of the rms value, mean and median frequencies, flattening and skewness coefficients of the power spectral density (DSP) of the EMG signal shows that muscular stress can be quantified, because significant changes in the frequency and time history of the myoelectric activity occur. Two tests for estimating the experimental results are described. In addition, the independence of the frequency content of the EMG with the muscular contraction level and their link at the end of the experimentation have been verified. The method is being tested for various vibratory forces applied to the hand-arm system.

INTRODUCTION

Dans le cadre de l'étude des effets neuro-musculaires des vibrations mécaniques sur l'homme, on s'intéresse à l'activité électrique de la musculature striée impliquée dans le système main-bras. L'analyse du signal électromyographique (EMG), par un traitement approprié, peut être utilisée comme étant un indice de l'état physiologique des muscles testés. L'astreinte liée aux vibrations peut être décelée par une éventuelle fatigue électro-physiologique local. Ainsi, l'objet de cette étude est de définir des méthodes de traitement statistique quantifiant la fatigue électrophysiologique dans le cas de contraction isométrique. Ces méthodes pourront être appliquées à toute contrainte physique entraînant une astreinte musculaire importante.

Toute activité organique comporte une limitation dans le temps due à l'activité elle-même. Dans le cas de l'activité musculaire, on parle de fatigue électro-physiologique ou de fatigue locale. Ce phénomène physiologique empêche le maintien à son niveau initial de la force développée par le sujet et existe quel que soit le type d'activité musculaire (statique ou dynamique). D'après certains auteurs, il est probable que la fatigue est due à un manque d'apport vasculaire local entraînant des changements dans la conduction des courants transmembranaires (1).

Au cours de la fatigue locale, on constate des phénomènes mécaniques et électromyographiques.

a) Phénomènes mécaniques: la force maximale développée par le sujet diminue. De plus, il lui est impossible de maintenir cette force maximale. On peut dire que la fatigue altère la performance mécanique du sujet (2).

b) Phénomènes électromyographiques: la fatigue locale modifie l'amplitude (analyse temporelle) et la fréquence (analyse fréquentielle) du signal EMG. Pour une force développée constante, l'amplitude du signal EMG augmente en fontion du temps (3). On observe également un accroissement de la valeur moyenne et de la valeur efficace (valeur rms) du signal EMG.

Depuis un certain nombre d'années, l'analyse fréquentielle est considérée comme une méthode d'évaluation de la fatigue électrophysiologique (4). Actuellement, les traitements du signal les plus récents qui utilisent la transformée de Fourier confirment les résultats des différents chercheurs étudiant l'astreinte musculaire (3,5-8). Ainsi, du point de vue fréquentiel, on constate des modifications du spectre de puissance du signal EMG au cours de la fatigue locale. De nombreux chercheurs ont montré un déplacement de l'énergie du spectre vers les basses fréquences (3,5-8), ainsi qu'une augmentation de cette énergie. L'étude de la fatigue par l'électromyographie de surface peut s'effectuer en calculant la fréquence "médiane" du spectre de puissance du signal EMG. Des travaux montrent que cette fréquence, partageant le spectre de puissance en deux parties d'énergie égale, décroît linéairement avec le temps (7). La complexité du système neuro-musculaire rend difficile l'interprétation de ces résultats expérimentaux. Néanmoins, les modifications des phénomènes électriques ont été interprétées par certains auteurs. Ainsi, Viitasalo et Komi affirment que le recrutement des unités motrices évolue en fonction du temps (9). De nouvelles unités motrices sont activées pour maintenir la performance mécanique. Dans certains cas, on observe une diffusion de l'activité musculaire. Cette diffusion signifie que le niveau de contraction de certains muscles fixateurs augmente avec la fatigue. Par ailleurs, les unités motrices ont des fréquences de décharge de plus en plus synchronisées les unes par rapport aux autres (10). Actuellement, les résultats d'autres recherches montreraient que les mécanismes, tels que la rotation des unités motrices actives, le recrutement et la synchronisation ne sont pas nécessaires pour expliquer le déplacement du spectre vers les basses fréquences, ainsi que l'augmentation de l'énergie de ce même spectre de puissance. Ainsi, la diminution de la vitesse de propagation du potentiel d'action musculaire paraît suffisante pour interpréter les changements de la densité spectrale de puissance (DSP) du signal EMG (1,3).

I PROTOCOLE EXPERIMENTAL

Afin de vérifier les affirmations contenues dans la littérature concernant les modifications spectrales du signal EMG lors de la fatigue électrophysiologique,

nous avons défini un protocole expérimental le plus simple possible permettant de confirmer les assertions suivantes.
1) Le déplacement vers les basses fréquences de la densité spectrale de puissance du signal EMG d'un muscle fatigué.
2) L'indépendance de la repartition fréquentielle de l'EMG non fatigué avec son niveau de contraction (valeur rms de l'EMG).

On étudie sur 6 sujets jeunes en bonne santé et plutôt sportifs l'activité du muscle biceps brachii en contraction isométrique. Le sujet est assis sur une chaise, l'épaule en appui sur le dossier. La partie supérieure du bras est dans le prolongement du corps et l'avant-bras est positionné selon l'axe horizontal. Au niveau du poignet, le sujet exerce une force mesurée par un capteur de force à jauge de contrainte (sédème A 100) relié à un pont d'extensométrie (sédème TS 105). Ce capteur est fixé à une plate-forme lestée par l'intermédiaire de ridoirs permettant un ajustement de la position du système. La tension électrique de sortie de l'auxiliaire de mesure préalablement étalonnée est mesurée et visualisée par un voltmètre numérique calculateur. La tâche du sujet consiste à maintenir une force constante de 12,5 daN jusqu'à l'épuisement. Pour celà, il contrôle sa force par l'intermédiaire de l'affichage numérique du voltmètre calculateur.

On pose deux électrodes de surface sur la partie la plus ventrue du muscle biceps brachii en contraction et une électrode de masse sur le front du sujet. Le poignet est en position de supination. Au cours de ces expérimentations, les muscles fléchisseurs du coude tels que le Brachioradialis et le Brachialis peuvent être éventuellement actifs. En tout état de cause et particulièrement pendant une période de fatigue musculaire, les muscles fixateurs de l'épaule peuvent aussi perturber l'expérimentation en relayant l'activité du muscle biceps Brachii. On enregistre sur bande magnétique (Schlumberger EPI II), d'une part, la force développée par le sujet et, d'autre part, l'activité myoélectrique par l'intermédiaire d'un amplificateur différentiel.

Dans cette étude concernant l'isométrie, nous avons choisi une valeur inférieure à la force maximale développée mais suffisamment importante afin que les modifications spectrales du signal EMG, si elles existent, apparaissent le plus rapidement possible.

II TRAITEMENT DU SIGNAL

2.1 Analyse spectrale du signal EMG

La difficulté de quantifier la performance mécanique associée au signal myoélectrique d'un groupe musculaire en activité rend difficile l'utilisation de l'analyse temporelle. De plus,

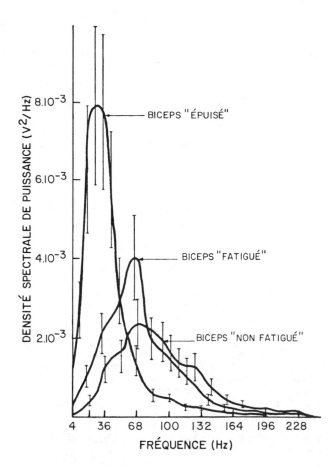

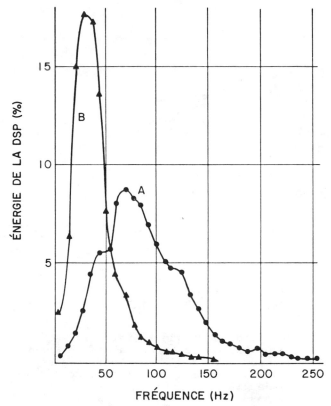

Fig. 1 Exemple d'évolution temporelle de la DSP du signal EMG d'un muscle biceps brachii en contraction iso-métrique. Le sujet maintient une charge de 12,5 daN. En outre, on indique, pour un niveau de confiance de 95%, les limites de l'erreur (traits verticaux) d'une classe sur quatre du spectre de puissance. Les conditions d'analyse sont les suivantes: fréquence d'échantillonnage 512 Hz, finesse d'analyse 8 Hz et nombre de moyennes 60.

l'indépendance de la répartition des fréquences avec le niveau de contraction de l'EMG semble nous indiquer que l'analyse spectrale est un traitement du signal per-tinent pour mettre en évidence la fatigue locale (3,5,7).

Le signal EMG est traité grâce à un analyseur de Fourier (PDP11-1923 Time Series System). La DSP du signal EMG est définie comme étant le produit de la transformée de Fourier du signal EMG par sa quantité con-juguée. Ce calcul a été effectué en langage TSL à partir d'un algorithme utilisant la transformation de Fourier discrète définie par:

$$F(S) = \frac{1}{N} \sum_{t=o}^{t=N-1} f(t)e^{-2j\pi St/N} \quad (1)$$

Fig. 2 Energies de la DSP du signal EMG exprimées en pourcentage: courbe A début de l'essai - sujet non fatigué; courbe B fin de l'essai - sujet épuisé physiquement. Ce graphe correspond à celui de la fig. précédente.

avec S la fréquence, N le nombre d'échan-tillons, f(t) le signal temporel, t le temps et F(S) la transformée de Fourier discrète. La densité spectrale de puissance du signal EMG est alors estimée selon la formule:

$$DSP(s) \sim F(s).F(s)* \quad (2)$$

avec F(s)* la quantité complexe conjuguée de la transformée de Fourier F(s). Pour analyser au mieux le signal EMG, on doit justifier le choix des conditions d'analyse dont les principales sont la gamme de fré-quence et la fréquence d'échantillonnage du signal, le type de fenêtre, l'intervalle de fréquence ou résolution, et le nombre de moyennes.

2.1.1 Gamme de fréquence et fréquence d'échantillonnage

Des analyses préliminaires de la DSP du signal EMG montrent que la répartition fréquentielle n'est jamais la même d'un sujet à l'autre. Néanmoins, les mêmes

Bakirzade et al.: L'astreinte musculaire

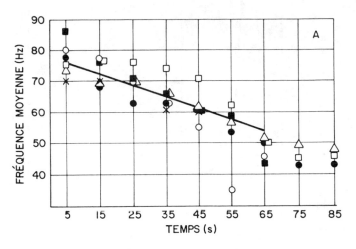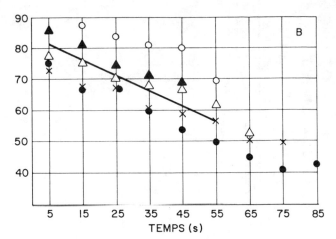

Fig. 3 Evolution temporelle de la fréquence moyenne du spectre de puissance de l'EMG.
Ajustement linéaire des données expérimentales: A Biceps droits - fréquence moyenne
= -0,465 t + 80,4:   r = -0,866; B Biceps gauches - fréquence moyenne = -0,458 t + 83,8:
r = -0,759.

analyses indiquent que les fréquences ne
dépassent pas quelques centaines de Hertz.
Des considérations d'ordre énergétique nous
ont donc fait choisir une fréquence maximum
unique de 256 Hz. Pour satisfaire aux
conditions minimums définies par le
théorème de Shannon, la fréquence d'échantillonnage du signal EMG est au moins égale
à deux fois la fréquence maximale du même
signal, soit 512 Hz (11).

2.1.2 Intervalle de fréquence ou résolution

La résolution est fonction de la
finesse du résultat recherché; en ce qui
nous concerne, on a surtout cherché à
quantifier un déplacement global de la DSP
du signal EMG avec la fatigue. Une trop
grande finesse de résolution n'est pas
nécessaire; une résolution de 8 Hz, en-
trainant une estimation de la DSP par un
ensemble de 32 valeurs discrétes, nous a
paru suffisante.

2.1.3 Type de fenêtre

Le signal échantillonné et numérisé
est multiplié par une fonction mathématique
appelée fenêtre temporelle. De par
l'étendue des fréquences du signal, nous
avons utilisé une fenêtre dite de Hanning.
Cette fenêtre permet de s'affranchir d'une
erreur liée à la troncature de l'échantillonnage du signal (11).

2.1.4 Nombre de moyennes

L'analyseur de Fourier affiche la
courbe d'une DSP résultante issue du calcul
de N = 60 moyennes. Chacune des valeurs

des 32 classes de cette DSP résultante
correspond à la moyenne arithmétique des
valeurs correspondantes par chaque spectre
de puissance. Ce nombre de moyennes est
très important si l'on veut faire une
estimation statistique des résultats obtenus.
Bien que nous ayons utilisé une fenêtre de
Hanning, on considérera que le nombre de
degrés de liberté de la DSP est égal à deux
fois le nombre de moyennes.

En réalité, le choix des conditions
d'analyse est un compromis entre le souhait
d'obtenir la connaissance la plus fine
possible du spectre fréquentiel et la
contrainte de ne pas avoir un temps de
calcul global T trop important, ce qui
limite ainsi le nombre de moyennes et, en
conséquence, la signification statistique
des résultats (fonction du nombre de degrés
de liberté 2N). En d'autres termes, le
temps, T, doit être court pour les deux
raisons suivantes: la non stationnarité
du signal EMG (qui évolue avec la fatigue)
et la rapidité avec laquelle les sujets
s'épuisent physiquement.

Des études préliminaires sur la DSP du
signal EMG nous permettent d'affirmer que,
quel que soit le muscle étudié, le spectre
de puissance est plutôt dissymétrique avec
une distribution de l'énergie à droite et
aplati avec une forte concentration de son
énergie dans les basses fréquences. Ainsi,
le calcul de plusieurs paramètres carac-
térisant la DSP est intéressant pour rendre
compte d'une éventuelle évolution de la
répartition fréquentielle du signal EMG de
surface.

Les données brutes du spectre de
puissance ont été visualisées puis imprimées
sur ruban. Ensuite, ces rubans ont été
relus par le lecteur d'un calculateur

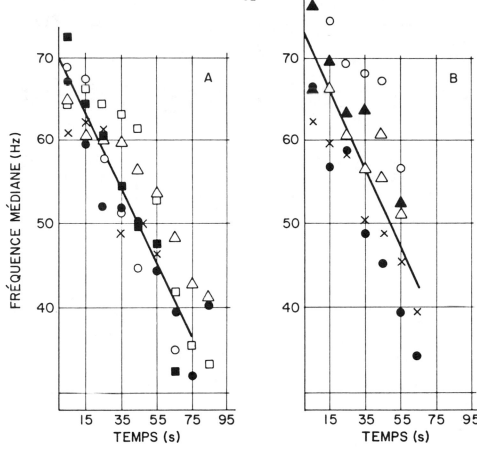

Fig. 4 Evolution temporelle de la fréquence médiane du spectre de puissance de l'EMG. Ajustement linéaire des données expérimentales: A Biceps droits - fréquence médiane = 0,443 t + 69,7: r = -0,847; B Biceps gauches - fréquence médiane = -0,472 t + 73,8: r = -0,797.

(Hewlett Packard 3000). Enfin, les résultats numériques mis en mémoire dans le calculateur ont été traités par un programme qui effectue les traitements suivants.

1) La fréquence "moyenne" du spectre de puissance; on la définit par:

$$F_M = \sum_{i=j}^{i=k} S_i \cdot DSP_{(i)} / \sum_{i=j}^{i=k} DSP_{(i)} \quad (3)$$

avec S_i la fréquence centrale de chaque classe i de la DSP (j, k dépendent du filtrage choisi par l'expérimentateur) et $DSP_{(i)}$ l'énergie contenue dans chaque classe i de la DSP.

2) La fréquence "médiane" du spectre de puissance; on la définit par:

$$F_{Med} = S_p + \left\{ \left(\sum_{i=j}^{i=k} DSP_i \right) / 2 - \sum_{i=j}^{i=p-1} DSP_i \right\} \cdot C / DSP_p \quad (4)$$

où
S_p = fréquence médiane non interpolée

telle que $\sum_{i=j}^{i=p} DSP_i < \left(\sum_{i=j}^{i=k} DSP_i \right) / 2$,

$\sum_{i=j}^{i=k} DSP_i$ = énergie totale du spectre de puissance,

$\sum_{i=j}^{i=p-1} DSP_i$ = énergie du spectre de puissance contenue dans toutes les classes inférieures à la classe de la fréquence médiane non interpolée,

DSP_p = énergie contenu dans la classe de la fréquence médiane non interpolée,

C = intervalle en hertz d'une classe du spectre de puissance.

3) Le coefficient de "dissymétrie" du spectre de puissance; on le définit par:

$$C_D = m_3 / (m_2)^{3/2} \quad (5)$$

avec le moment spectral d'ordre r

$$m_r = \sum_{i=j}^{i=k} DSP_i (S_i - A)^r / \sum_{i=j}^{i=k} DSP_i \quad (6)$$

Bakirzade et al.: L'astreinte musculaire

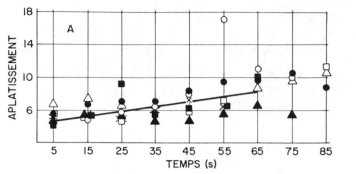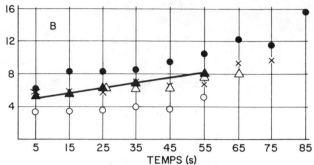

Fig. 5 Evolution temporelle du coefficient spectral d'aplatissement de l'EMG. Ajustement linéaire des données expérimentales: A Biceps droits - coefficient d'aplatissement
= 0,071 t + 4,48: r = 0,633; B Biceps gauches - coefficient d'aplatissement = 0,06 t
+ 4,7: r = 0,556.

où A peut prendre les valeurs suivantes:
zéro pour obtenir le moment non centré;
fréquence moyenne du spectre ainsi, on
calcule le moment centré; fréquence médiane
de la DSP; et mode de la DSP.

Les calculs de ce coefficient (12),
nous renseignent sur la dissymétrie du
spectre de puissance autour de la fréquence
"moyenne" (A = fréquence "moyenne"), la
fréquence "médiane" (A = fréquence
"médiane") et du "mode" (A = "mode").
4)   Le coefficient "d'aplatissement"; on
le définit par:

$$C_A = m_4 / (m_2)^{4/2} \qquad (7)$$

Les calculs de ce coefficient nous
renseignent sur l'aplatissement du spectre
de puissance autour de chacune des valeurs
de A précédemment citées (12).

Les paramètres précédents ont été
définis de manière analogue à celle dont
sont habituellement définis les paramètres
statistiques classiquement utilisés tels
que valeur moyenne, médiane, etc., à cette
différence prés: au lieu d'utiliser la
densité de probabilité pour calculer les
différents moments, on a utilisé la densité
spectrale de puissance de ce signal. Les
paramètres ainsi obtenus, appelés fréquence
"moyenne", fréquence "médiane", etc., ne
sont pas des caractéristiques d'amplitude
du signal mais des caractéristiques
spectrales.

2.2 Erreur statistique des résultats
     expérimentaux

La question générale qui se pose devant
une série de résultats expérimentaux est de
savoir si les différences observées sont
dues au hasard (fluctuations d'échantillonnage) ou sont liées à des phénomènes réels.
En ce qui concerne la DSP du signal EMG,

on peut calculer l'erreur des résultats
expérimentaux par différents outils
statistiques.

Bendat et Piersol ont montré que
l'erreur statistique normalisée, lors d'une
mesure de densité spectrale de puissance,
est liée à la largeur de bande B (Hertz) ou
intervalle de fréquence et au temps
d'intégration du signal T(seconde) par la
formule (11):

$$\varepsilon_r = 1/\sqrt{B.T} \qquad (8)$$

Cela signifie que pour une DSP mesurée,
l'erreur du à la différence entre la DSP
vraie et la DSP mesurée est comprise entre
±2ε pour un niveau de confiance de 95%
(cette formule est valable pour ε < 0,2).

Nous avons élaboré un test statistique
permettant de juger si la différence entre
deux fréquences "moyennes" est effective ou
bien si elle peut s'expliquer simplement
par des fluctuations d'échantillonnage.
Des considérations théoriques (voir annexe)
nous ont permis, pour un spectre de puissance donné, d'approcher l'écart-type de la
fréquence "moyenne" estimée $\hat{F}_m$ selon

l'eqn A19. Ainsi, pour un même sujet, on
calcule aux temps t_1 et t_2 les fréquences
"moyennes" F_{m_1} et F_{m_2} d'écarts-types

respectivement σ_1 et σ_2.

Les méthodes statistiques classiques
de comparaison des valeurs moyennes peuvent
alors nous dire si on peut admettre, et
avec un niveau de confiance donné, l'hypothèse suivant laquelle les fréquences
"moyennes" estimées $\hat{F}_{m_1}$ et $\hat{F}_{m_2}$ provien-

draient de DSP différentes. Le test statis-
tique peut être unilatéral ($\hat{F}_{m_2} < \hat{F}_{m_1}$) ou

bilatéral ($F_{m_2} \neq F_{m_1}$). On utilise pour cela

la variable centrée réduite définie par (12):

Bakirzade et al.: L'astreinte musculaire

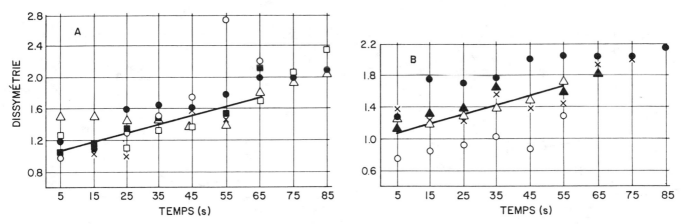

Fig. 6 Evolution temporelle du coefficient spectral de dissymétrie de l'EMG. Ajustement linéaire des données expérimentales: A Biceps droits - coefficient de dissymétrie
= 0,0134 t + 1,03: r = 0,745; B Biceps gauches - coefficient de dissymétrie = 0,012 t
+ 1,04: r = 0,614.

$$Z = (\hat{F}_{m_1} - \hat{F}_{m_2})/\sigma(\hat{F}_{m_1} - \hat{F}_{m_2})$$

$$= (\hat{F}_{m_1} - \hat{F}_{m_2})/(\hat{\sigma}_1^2 + \hat{\sigma}_2^2)^{\frac{1}{2}} \qquad (9)$$

Selon l'hypothèse d'une répartition gaussienne et pour un niveau de confiance de
95%, ce test aboutit aux conclusions
suivantes:

$$F_{m_2} < F_{m_1} \text{ si } Z > 1,645 \text{ (test unilatéral)}$$

$$F_{m_2} \neq F_{m_1} \text{ si } Z > 1,95 \text{ (test bilatéral)}$$

$$(10)$$

III RESULTATS

3.1 Evolution temporelle de la DSP du
signal EMG lors d'une contraction
isométrique

L'évolution temporelle du spectre
fréquentiel de l'EMG, exprimée en valeur
brute (fig. 1) ou ramenée à une énergie
constante (fig. 2), confirme le déplacement
de la DSP vers les basses fréquences. On
constate que les traitements statistiques
varient de façon monotone jusqu'au moment
où le sujet ne peut plus assurer le maintien de la charge. Néanmoins, les valeurs
des "moments spectraux", calculées par
rapport au mode, sont très fluctuantes.
Etant donné que la valeur modale n'est pas
issue d'un calcul incluant toutes les
classes de la DSP, on comprend le peu
d'intérêt qu'il nous apporte. La similitude

de l'évolution des "moments spectraux",
calculés par rapport aux fréquences moyenne
et médiane, nous ont conduit à étudier
uniquement les coefficients d'aplatissement
et de dissymétrie par rapport à la fréquence
moyenne. On remarque que ces coefficients
semblent évoluer linéairement dans le temps.
L'ajustement des données expérimentales,
par une droite de régression, semble prouver
que les différents paramètres calculés
évoluent linéairement dans le temps. Les
fréquences "moyenne" (fig. 3) et "médiane"
(fig. 4) diminuent de plus de 40% alors que
les coefficients d'aplatissement (fig. 5)
et de dissymétrie (fig. 6) augmentent en
fonction du temps. Du point de vue de
l'information qu'ils nous donnent, ces
traitements de signal semblent équivalents.
A l'opposé des quatre traitements
précédents, l'évolution temporelle de la
valeur rms du spectre de l'EMG (fig. 7) ne
suit pas un ajustement linéaire. En effet,
l'augmentation de la valeur rms, en fonction
du temps, est précédée par une période de
stabilité.
Le calcul de l'erreur de Bendat et
Piersol nous montre que, en début d'expérimentation, les différences significatives
se situent surtout dans les basses fréquences
(fig. 1). En fin d'expérimentation, le
calcul de l'erreur normalisée pour chaque
classe de la DSP donne des différences
significatives pour tout le spectre
(fig. 1). L'utilisation du second test, qui
détermine la significativité de la différence
de deux fréquences "moyennes", nous indique
qu'un écart de quelques hertz permet
d'affirmer la non responsabilité des fluctuations d'échantillonnage dans les variations constatées.

Bakirzade et al.: L'astreinte musculaire

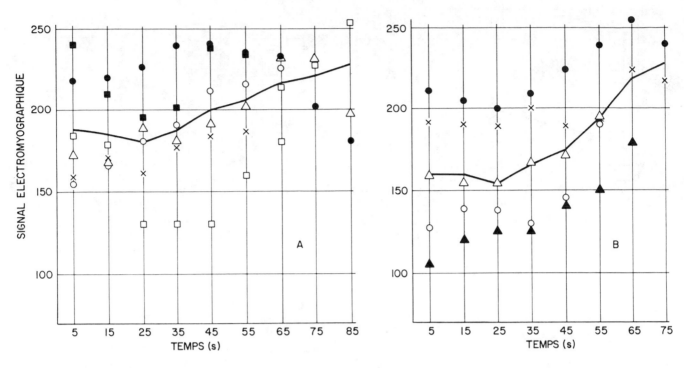

Fig. 7 Evolution temporelle de la valeur rms du signal EMG: A biceps droits; B biceps gauches.

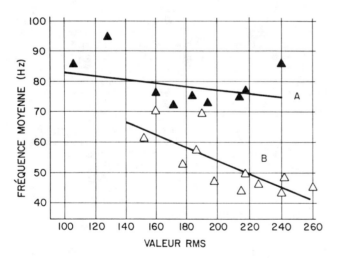

Fig. 8 Evolution de la fréquence "moyenne" de la DSP du signal EMG en fonction de la valeur rms du même signal (11 essais biceps droits ou gauches). Courbe A: début d'expérimentation (corrélation non significative) - fréquence moyenne = -0,0616 EMG$_{rms}$ + 89,7: 0 < r (niveau de confiance de 95%) <0,782. Courbe B: fin d'expérimentation (corrélation significative) - fréquence moyenne = -0,187 EMG$_{rms}$ + 90,2: -0,143 < r (niveau de confiance de 95%) <0,914.

3.2 Indépendance de la répartition spectrale de l'énergie du signal EMG avec le niveau de contraction du muscle biceps brachii

Après avoir vérifié le déplacement du spectre de l'EMG vers les basses fréquences, on a cherché l'existence d'une éventuelle corrélation entre la fatigue locale et le niveau de contraction musculaire. On a ajusté deux droites de régression, la première représente l'évolution au temps t = 5 s de la fréquence moyenne du spectre en fonction de la valeur rms de l'EMG (courbe A de la fig. 8), la seconde (courbe B de la fig. 8) reprend les mêmes paramètres mais calculés pour le dernier spectre de chaque expérimentation (le muscle est à l'état d'épuisement).

Au temps 5 secondes, les résultats ne semblent pas mettre en évidence une corrélation entre la fréquence moyenne et la valeur rms de l'EMG. Par contre, en fin d'expérimentation, on constate que l'évolution de la fréquence moyenne suit sensiblement celle de la valeur rms.

IV DISCUSSION

Les résultats que nous avons obtenus vérifient le déplacement spectral de l'EMG vers les basses fréquences avec la fatigue. La quantification spectrale de l'EMG, par le calcul de la fréquence "moyenne" et de

Bakirzade et al.: L'astreinte musculaire

85

la fréquence "médiane", ainsi que le calcul des coefficients de "dissymétrie" et "d'aplatissement" semble évoluer linéairement en fonction du temps. Il apparaît que l'on puisse considérer ces traitements de la DSP du signal EMG comme des indices d'évaluation de la fatigue électrophysiologique. En outre, on présente deux méthodes de calcul permettant d'estimer statistiquement les résultats expérimentaux. Dans le premier test, on utilise le calcul de l'erreur normalisée sur chaque classe de la DSP du signal EMG de surface. Le second test reprend le calcul précédent de l'erreur normalisée pour obtenir l'écart-type de la fréquence "moyenne" du spectre de puissance du signal EMG. Il semblerait que le second test statistique soit le plus intéressant car la méthode de calcul tient compte de l'énergie de chaque classe du spectre de puissance.

Quant à l'interprétation des résultats, deux thèses sont en présence, la première théorie privilégie le contrôle de la fatigue électrophysiologique par le système nerveux central et périphérique. Dans ce cas, les déplacements du spectre de puissance sont dus à des modifications de l'activité des unités motrices.

Ainsi, par de simples considérations statistiques, Blinowska et Col ont montré que les décharges des potentiels d'actions musculaires ne sont pas décorrélées entre elles, mais synchronisées (10). Les mêmes auteurs affirment que la décomposition en fréquence du signal électrique d'une unité motrice semble être affectée par les variations de son niveau d'activité et par la présence de décharges doubles. De plus, une plus ou moins grande synchronisation des unités motrices influe sur les valeurs de l'énergie de la DSP dans les basses fréquences. La DSP du signal EMG semblerait donc être fonction du recrutement spatio-temporel et de la synchronisation des unités motrices (6,10). Blinowska et Col suggèrent que l'augmentation de l'énergie du spectre de puissance du signal EMG, constatée lors de la fatigue, s'explique par le fait que les décharges des différentes unités motrices actives tendent à se synchroniser.

La seconde théorie ne tient pas compte des mécanismes de graduation de la contraction musculaire. Lindstrom et Col considèrent que les variations du recrutement spatio-temporel et la synchronisation des unités motrices n'expliquent pas les modifications spectrales accompagnant la fatigue électrophysiologique. En effet, on sait que le niveau d'activité d'un muscle non fatigué en contraction isométrique, essentiellement contrôlé par le système nerveux central et périphérique (13), est indépendant de la quantification de la DSP du signal EMG (7). Ainsi, l'évaluation de la fatigue électrophysiologique n'est pas toujours corrélée avec la valeur rms du

signal EMG. Il a été également démontré qu'à partir d'une fréquence de décharge qui est rapidement atteinte, le recrutement temporel n'a pas d'influence sur la DSP du signal EMG. Des expériences prouvent qu'un déficit en oxygène transforme les processus chimiques musculaires aérobiques en processus anaérobiques (7). Il s'ensuit une accumulation d'acide lactique et de différents métabolites. Ces variations de concentration chimiques diminuent la vitesse de conduction des potentiels d'actions musculaires. Par conséquent, la diminution de cette vitesse de propagation serait la principale cause du déplacement spectral du signal EMG.

Le développement de la fatigue électrophysiologique serait uniquement sous le contrôle de phénomènes locaux. La diminution des fréquences "moyennes" et "médianes" est attribuée à l'accroissement de la durée du potentiel d'action musculaire. De la même manière, l'accroissement des coefficients "d'aplatissement" et de "dissymétrie" peut être lié à la diminution de la vitesse de conduction des phénomènes électriques se propageant le long de la fibre musculaire active.

Les résultats auxquels nous avons abouti ne nous permettent pas d'opter pour l'une ou l'autre théorie. Néanmoins, il semble que le recrutement spatio-temporel (valeur rms) du signal EMG, qui n'est pas corrélé en début d'expérimentation avec la fatigue électrophysiologique, le soit en fin d'expérimentation.

V CONCLUSION

Cette méthode de quantification de la fatigue électrophysiologique pourrait avoir de nombreuses applications dans des domaines autres que la contraction volontaire isométrique. Cette méthode a plusieurs avantages. Premièrement, elle pourrait indiquer l'état de fatigue dans lequel se trouve le groupe musculaire étudié. De plus, ce type de traitement serait utilisable pour toute analyse ergonomique d'un système homme-machine où les activités musculaires sont prédominantes (maintien postural prolongé, contrainte vibratoire intense, etc.). Enfin, les changements quantifiés du signal myoélectrique fournissent un éventuel critère de tolérance à toute contrainte impliquant une astreinte musculaire. Compte tenu des résultats obtenus, les méthodes de traitement que nous avons développées sont actuellement utilisées dans le laboratoire afin de quantifier les effets musculaires de différentes contraintes vibratoires appliquées au système main-bras.

BIBLIOGRAPHIE

1. Lindstrom L, Magnusson R, Petersen I. Muscular fatigue and action potential conduction velocity

changes studied with frequency analysis of EMG signals. Electromyography 1970; 4: 341-356.

2. Scherrer J, Monod H. Physiologie de la musculature squelettique chez l'homme. Dans: Kayser, ed. Système nerveux et muscle. Tome 2, 1976.

3. Lindstrom L, Kadefors L, Peterson I. An electromyographic index for localized muscle fatigue. J Appl Physiol 1977; 43: 750-754.

4. Kadefords R, Kaiser E, Peterson I. Dynamic spectrum analysis of myo-potentials and with special reference to muscle fatigue. Electromyography 1968; 8: 39-73 .

5. Gross D, Grassino A, Ross WRD, Macklen PI. Electromyogram pattern of diaphragmatic fatigue. J Appl Physiol 1979; 46: 1-7.

6. Komi PV, Tesch P. EMG frequency spectrum, muscle structure and fatigue during dynamic contractions in man. Eur J Appl Physiol 1979; 42: 41-50.

7. Petrofsky IS, Lind AR. Frequency analysis of surface electromyography during sustained

8. Schweitzer TW, Fitzgerald IW, Bowden IA, Lynnes Davies P. Spectral analysis of human inspiratory diaphramatic electromyograms. J Appl Physiol 1979; 46: 152-165.

9. Viitasalo JHT, Komi PV. Signal characteristics of EMG during fatigue. Europ J Appl Physiol 1977; 37: 111-121.

10. Blinowska A, Verroust J, Cannet G. An analysis of synchronization and double discharge effects of low frequency electromyographic power spectra. Electromyogr Clin Neurophysiol 1980; 20: 465-480.

11. Bendat JS, Piersol AS. Random Data: Analysis and Measurement Procedures. New York: Wiley Interscience, 1971.

12. Spiegel MR, Théorie et applications de la statistique. (Série Schaum) McGraw Hill, 1978.

13. Maton B. Etude périphérique de l'organisation du mouvement volontaire. Centre national de la recherche scientifique (Paris), 1975. Thèse de D ès S. (inédit).

isometric contraction. Eur J Appl Physiol 1980; 43: 173-182.

ANNEXE

L'analyse spectrale d'un signal aléatoire et stationnaire n'est, en pratique, jamais exacte. On obtient une densité spectrale de puissance estimée, $\hat{DSP}_{(S_i)}$, pour des conditions d'analyse où la résolution et le temps d'intégration ont des valeurs finies. On aurait la densité spectrale de puissance exacte, $DSP_{(S_i)}$, pour un temps d'intégration infini et une résolution infiniment petite. L'erreur $\varepsilon_{(S_i)}$ introduite par l'estimation de la DSP est donnée par:

$$\varepsilon_{(S_i)} = \hat{DSP}_{(S_i)} - DSP_{(S_i)} \qquad (A1)$$

Quand l'erreur $\varepsilon_{(S_i)}$ est inférieuré à 0,2 (11), la distribution statistique de la variable aléatoire $\varepsilon_{(S_i)}$ est sensiblement gaussienne et centrée. L'écart-type de cette variable est égal à:

$$\sigma_{\varepsilon(S_i)} = DSP_{(S_i)}/(B.T)^{\frac{1}{2}} \qquad (A2)$$

que l'on peut estimer par:

$$\hat{\sigma}_{\varepsilon(S_i)} = \hat{DSP}_{(S_i)}/(B.T)^{\frac{1}{2}} \quad . \qquad (A3)$$

De plus, on admet que les différentes erreurs $\varepsilon_{(S_j)}, \ldots, \varepsilon_{(S_p)}, \ldots, \varepsilon_{(S_k)}$ sont décorrélées entre elles. Une estimation F_m de la fréquence "moyenne" $\hat{F}_m$ est donnée par:

$$\hat{F}_m = \sum_{i=j}^{i=k}(S_i.\hat{DSP}_{(S_i)})/\sum_{i=j}^{i=k}\hat{DSP}_{(S_i)} \qquad (A4)$$

avec S_i la fréquence de la classe i et $DSP_{(S_i)}$ l'énergie contenue dans la classe i de fréquence S_i (j, k dépendent des conditions de filtrage choisies par l'expérimentateur).

$$\hat{F}_m = \left(\sum_{i=j}^{i=k}S_i.DSP_{(S_i)} + \varepsilon_1\right)/\left(\sum_{i=j}^{i=k}DSP_{(S_i)} + \varepsilon_2\right) \qquad (A5)$$

avec:

$$\varepsilon_1 = \sum_{i=j}^{i=k}S_i.\varepsilon_{(S_i)} \qquad (A6)$$

$$\varepsilon_2 = \sum_{i=j}^{i=k}\varepsilon_{(S_i)} \quad . \qquad (A7)$$

Or:

$$F_m = \sum_{i=j}^{i=k}(S_i.DSP_{(S_i)})/\sum_{i=j}^{i=k}DSP_{(S_i)} \quad . \qquad (A8)$$

La différence des fréquences "moyennes" $\hat{F}_m$ et F_m est égale à:

$$\hat{F}_m - F_m = \frac{\sum S_i.DSP_{(S_i)}+\varepsilon_1}{\sum DSP_{(S_i)}+\varepsilon_2} \quad \frac{\sum S_i.DSP_{(S_i)}}{\sum DSP_{(S_i)}} \qquad (A9)$$

$$\hat{F}_m - F_m = \frac{\sum DSP_{(S_i)}.\varepsilon_1 - \sum S_i.DSP_{(S_i)}.\varepsilon_2}{\sum DSP_{(S_i)}\left(\sum DSP_{(S_i)}+\varepsilon_2\right)} \qquad (A10)$$

d'où

$$\hat{F}_m - F_m \sim (\varepsilon_1 - F_m \cdot \varepsilon_2) / \sum_{i=j}^{i=k} DSP_{(S_i)} \quad . \tag{A11}$$

Comme les distributions des erreurs ε_1 et ε_2 sont centrées, la différence $\hat{F}_m - F_m$ est centrée et de variance égale à:

$$\text{Variance} = \frac{E\{(\varepsilon_1 - F_m \varepsilon_2)^2\}}{|\sum DSP_{(S_i)}|^2} \tag{A12}$$

avec $E(X) =$ espérance mathématique de la variable aléatoire X. Or

$$E\{(\varepsilon_1 - F_m \varepsilon_2)^2\} = E\{\varepsilon_1^2 + \varepsilon_2^2 \cdot F_m - 2F_m \cdot \varepsilon_1 \cdot \varepsilon_2\}$$

$$= E\{\varepsilon_1^2\} + F_m^2 \cdot E\{\varepsilon_2^2\} - 2F_m \cdot E\{\varepsilon_1 \cdot \varepsilon_2\} \tag{A13}$$

avec

$$E\{\varepsilon_1^2\} = \sum S_i^2 \cdot \sigma_{\varepsilon(S_i)}^2$$

$$E\{\varepsilon_2^2\} = \sum \sigma_{\varepsilon(S_i)}^2 \tag{A14}$$

$$E\{\varepsilon_1 \cdot \varepsilon_2\} = \sum S_i \cdot \sigma_{\varepsilon(S_i)}^2$$

alors

$$E\{(\varepsilon_1 - F_m \cdot \varepsilon_2)^2\} = \sum S_i^2 \cdot \sigma_{\varepsilon(S_i)}^2 + F_m \cdot (\sum \sigma_{\varepsilon(S_i)}^2)$$

$$- 2F_m (\sum S_i \cdot \sigma_{\varepsilon(S_i)}^2) \quad . \tag{A15}$$

Or, on a:

$$F_m = (\sum S_i \cdot DSP_{(S_i)}) / \sum DSP_{(S_i)} \tag{A16}$$

$$\sigma_{\varepsilon(S_i)} = DSP_{(S_i)} / (B.T)^{\frac{1}{2}} \quad . \tag{A17}$$

Ainsi, la variance de la différence $(\hat{F}_m - F_m)$ est égale à:

$$V_{ar}(\hat{F}_m - F_m) = \frac{1}{B.T(\sum DSP_{(S_i)})^4} \cdot [(\sum S_i^2 \cdot DSP_{(S_i)}^2)$$

$$\cdot (\sum DSP_{(S_i)})^2 + (\sum DSP_{(S_i)}^2)$$

$$\cdot (\sum S_i \cdot DSP_{(S_i)})^2 - 2(\sum S_i \cdot DSP_{(S_i)}^2)$$

$$\cdot (\sum S_i \cdot DSP_{(S_i)}) \cdot (\sum DSP_{(S_i)})] \quad . \tag{A18}$$

En conséquence, l'écart-type de la différence $(\hat{F}_m - F_m)$ peut être estimé par:

$$\hat{\sigma}(\hat{F}_m - F_m) = \frac{1}{(B.T)^{\frac{1}{2}} \cdot [\sum D\hat{S}P_{(S_i)}]^2} \cdot [(\sum S_i^2 \cdot D\hat{S}P_{(S_i)}^2)$$

$$\cdot (\sum D\hat{S}P_{(S_i)})^2 + (\sum D\hat{S}P_{(S_i)}^2) \cdot (\sum S_i \cdot D\hat{S}P_{(S_i)})$$

$$- 2(\sum S_i \cdot D\hat{S}P_{(S_i)}) \cdot (\sum S_i \cdot D\hat{S}P_{(S_i)})$$

$$\cdot (\sum D\hat{S}P_{(S_i)})]1/2 \quad . \tag{A19}$$

Cette estimation $\hat{\sigma}(\hat{F}_m - F_m)$ permet de tester sur un sujet, aux temps t_1 et t_2, l'hypothèse que les deux spectres de puissance correspondant ont la même fréquence "moyenne" selon cette hypothèse et en admettant que les fluctuations spectrales sont décorrélées entre les instants t_1 et t_2, on obtient:

$$E\{\hat{F}_{m_1} - \hat{F}_{m_2}\} = 0$$

$$V_{ar}(\hat{F}_{m_1} - \hat{F}_{m_2}) \sim \hat{\sigma}_1^2 + \hat{\sigma}_2^2 \tag{A20}$$

$$\sigma(\hat{F}_{m_1} - \hat{F}_{m_2}) \sim (\hat{\sigma}_1^2 + \hat{\sigma}_2^2)^{\frac{1}{2}}$$

On peut alors effectuer le test classique de différence de deux valeurs moyennes en utilisant la variable réduite Z définie par eqn 9.

Bakirzade et al.: L'astreinte musculaire

MEASUREMENT OF VIBRATION ENTERING THE HAND

Measurement of Vibration Coupled to the Hand-Arm System

G. Rasmussen

ABSTRACT: Some of the difficulties encountered measuring vibration are reviewed, with emphasis on filtering techniques and detector integrating times. A light-weight, finger-held transducer mount has been developed to facilitate the measurement of hand-transmitted vibration at the origin of the coordinate system specified by ISO/DIS 5349. The physical characteristics and performance of the mount are described. Of particular interest is its transmissibility, which is close to unity at all frequencies of concern for hand-arm vibration.

RESUME: On examine certaines des difficultés que pose la mesure des vibrations et plus particulièrement les techniques de filtrage et les temps d'intégration des détecteurs. On a mis au point un support de transducteur léger, ajustable sur un doigt pour faciliter la mesure des vibrations des mains à l'origine du système coordonné spécifié par la norme ISO/DIS 5349. On décrit les caractéristiques physiques et l'efficacité du dispositif. Ce dernier point est particulièrement intéressant, car, aux fréquences qui importent dans l'étude des vibrations des mains, son efficacité est presque totale.

INTRODUCTION

Techniques for measuring the vibration exposure of the hand-arm system have for many years left much to be desired. Exposure data have frequently lacked adequate description of the instrumentation. There have also been difficulties in mounting a transducer to monitor hand-transmitted vibration at the origin of the coordinate system for the hand specified by the ISO (1). With the introduction of digital techniques increasing the capability for data processing, it has become necessary to describe more fully the parameters being measured, and the instrumentation and experimental methods being used.

These subjects are reviewed in this paper, and the design and performance of a novel transducer mount is reported.

I INSTRUMENTATION CHARACTERISTICS

1.1 General Considerations

Vibration acceleration is measured in units of metres per second, per second (m/s^2), usually in 1/3 octave frequency bands (or possibly 1/1 octave bands), over the frequency range of interest. The root mean square value (rms) is usually determined. The level of vibration may also be quoted in dB re 1 $\mu m/s^2$, as defined in the ISO Vocabulary on Shock and Vibration and

the ISO Standard 1683 (2,3). This is particularly useful when quoting overall frequency-weighted acceleration levels, where the relation of the measure to units of m/s^2 is less evident due to the frequency weighting.

The use of filter networks with characteristics standardized by both national and international conventions ensures that the power spectra measured by different instruments will be comparable (4,5). However, the use of power spectral density obtained from a Fourier spectrum requires further definition, in order to ensure that comparisons with existing data from standardized 1/3 octave filters will be meaningful (see Fig. 1).

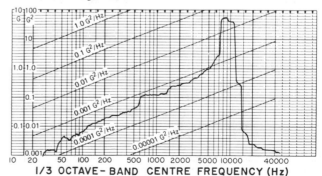

1/3 OCTAVE- BAND CENTRE FREQUENCY (Hz)

Fig. 1 Comparison of a 1/3 octave power spectrum with contours of equal power spectral density.

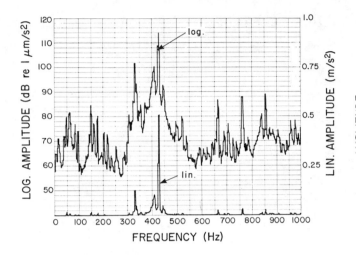

Fig. 2 Comparison of linear and logarithmic amplitude scales.

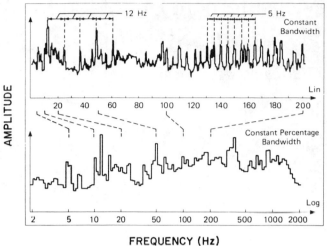

Fig. 3 Comparison of linear and logarithmic frequency scales, and of the use of constant bandwidth and constant percentage bandwidth filters.

It should be noted that no fundamental incompatibility exists between the use of digital and any other data gathering techniques. However, the alternatives for presenting data based on the measurement of power spectral density suggest the need for standardization of bandwidth, of sampling rate, etc. For example, will the spectral density of a pure sinusoid (with zero bandwidth) be considered to be of infinite magnitude, when its magnitude as determined by a real filter will be defined by the filter bandwidth? Vibration data, in relation to their influence on man, are most conveniently reported on logarithmic scales, while other data may sometimes be more usefully expressed in other forms (see Figs. 2 and 3).

The time constant involved in detecting the level of a signal is also of great importance. Human reaction time constants of from 0.8 to 2 s have been proposed for whole-body vibration by the ISO (6). Others argue that 125 ms is the correct time constant for the evaluation of human reaction to shock. Certainly, the upper limiting frequency of 80 Hz for fatigue-decreased proficiency indicates that a time constant faster than 12 ms should be used to measure peak amplitudes. Similarly, a time constant of less than 1 ms should be chosen to measure the peak amplitudes of hand-arm vibration, as the upper limiting frequency in this case is 1000 Hz.

1.2 Filters

There are various techniques for filtering signals available. Traditional analogue discrete filters consist of fixed frequency filters either switched sequentially or coupled in parallel. The use of sequential switching requires the signal to be steady for a time significantly greater than that

employed for analysis, to ensure that the averaged band levels are independent of the choice of time origin (7). This tends to be rather time consuming and is not well suited to the variability of vibrations experienced by man. Parallel analogue filters also have shortcomings, principally in the detector response which may introduce errors when analysing rapidly varying signals.

In contrast, Fast Fourier Processors analyse signals occurring within a given time period. It is important to realize that these "blocks of data" represent an approximation if a continuously varying signal is analysed. The use of the Hanning or other time-varying weighting functions may reduce the collection of data in real time unless sophisticated techniques like scan-averaging are used (8). Also, the eventual synthesis of 1/3 or 1/1 octave bands often contains further approximations. An accurate and non-compromised digital filter and detector can be realized, however, that allows data collection at very fast rates with no loss of integration time, either linear or exponential, and maintains a chosen confidence level (see Fig. 4).

The use of narrow filters normally results in a large amount of data for each measurement. In contrast, a single number measure is desirable for legal and statistical purposes. One method of simplification suggested in standards is the use of overall frequency-weighting networks. Such networks have been proposed for the measurements of hand-arm vibration (see Fig. 5). Some standards also consider exposure time and level (see, for example, Ref. 6),

Rasmussen: Measurement of vibration

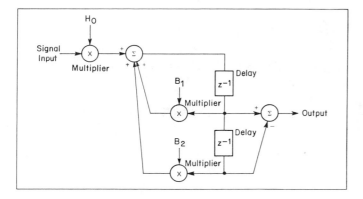

Fig. 4 Block diagram of a 2-pole digital filter.

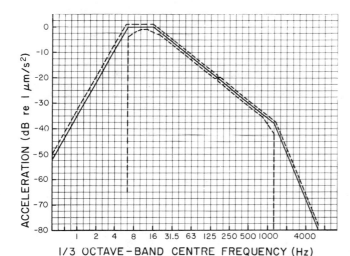

Fig. 5 Frequency weighting for hand-arm vibration filter.

thus giving exposures or vibration doses in percentages, for up to 24 hours. The use of overall weighting networks is suited to such applications.

1.3 Detector Integrating Times

The introduction of digital techniques has also encouraged linear integration over a fixed time interval. A 60 s interval has been proposed for use when circumstances permit, as it covers many needs. From this, the crest factor may be defined as the ratio of the peak amplitude to the 60 second rms value. Using a definition such as this enables values of the crest factors of different instruments to be compared.

The instrument designer must still, however, decide on the use of linear or exponential averaging during the measurement time interval. The differences between the averages recorded by these two methods can be significant, as is illustrated in Fig. 6.

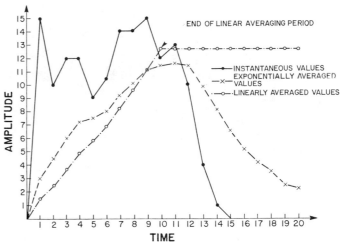

Fig. 6 Comparison of linear and exponential averaging.

The root mean square acceleration is defined as:

$$a_{rms} = \{\frac{1}{T} \int_0^T a^2(t)dt\}^{\frac{1}{2}} , \qquad (1)$$

where $a(t)$ is the instantaneous acceleration at time t. This equation implies linear time averaging over a period, T, of 60 s. The acceleration level is given by:

$$L_{eq} = 20 \log\{\frac{a_{rms}}{a_o}\} \qquad (2)$$

where a_o is the reference acceleration, which is usually 1 $\mu m/s^2$.

On the other hand, exponential time averaging requires:

$$a_{rms} = \{\frac{1}{\tau} \int_{-\infty}^T a^2(t) e^{-(T-t)/\tau}dt\} \qquad (3)$$

where τ = 1 s for hand-arm vibration. (To obtain the maximum rms acceleration of a single shock, a time constant of 135 ms has been proposed.)

For the summation of component accelerations a_X, a_Y, and a_Z, on orthogonal axes X, Y and Z, it has been proposed that the identity:

$$a_{combined} = \{a_X^2 + a_Y^2 + a_Z^2\}^{\frac{1}{2}} \qquad (4)$$

be formed, and that any level more than 10 dB below the highest component be disregarded.

Rasmussen: Measurement of vibration

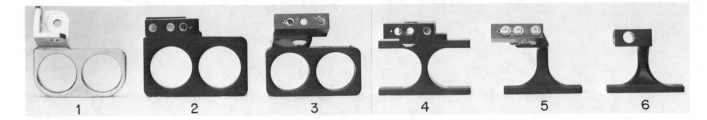

Fig. 7 Photographs of six transducer mounts

II TRANSDUCER MOUNTS

The selection and mounting of a transducer to monitor the vibration coupled to the hand present several problems of mensuration, as is evident from the following quotation from the Draft International Standard ISO/DIS 5349 (1).

"The vibration pick-up must be small and light enough for the specific application. Its cross-axis sensitivity must be at least 20 dB below the sensitivity in the axis to be measured."

"The measurements in the three axes shall be made at, or clearly related to, the surface of the hand where the energy enters the body. If the hand of the person is in direct contact with the vibrating surface of the hand grip, the transducer should be fastened to the vibrating structure. If a resilient element is being used between the hand and the vibrating structure (for example, a cushioned handle), it is permissible to use a suitable mount for the transducer (for example, a thin, suitably formed metal sheet) placed between the hand and the surface of the resilient material. In either case, care must be taken that the size, shape and mounting of the transducer or of the special transducer support do not significantly influence the transfer of vibration to the hand. Care must also be taken when mounting the transducer that the transfer function is flat up to 1500 Hz for all three directions."

"For signals with a very high crest factor, for example those obtained from percussive tools, special precautions must be taken to avoid overloading any part of the system. Correct choice of the transducer is essential in this case. It may be possible to use a mechanical filter with a suitable calibrated linear transfer function to reduce the crest factor of these signals.

The proposed method for the case of a resilient element between the hand and the

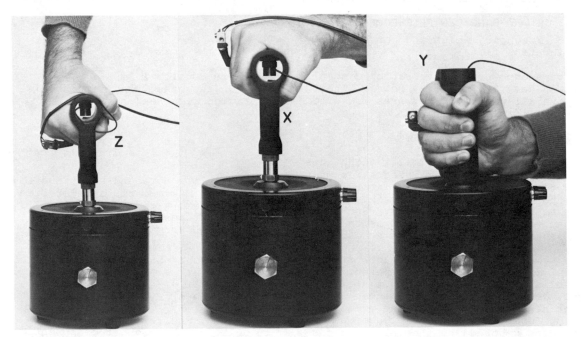

Fig. 8 Photograph showing transducer mount #6 held between the fingers, which in turn are gripping the vibrating handle.

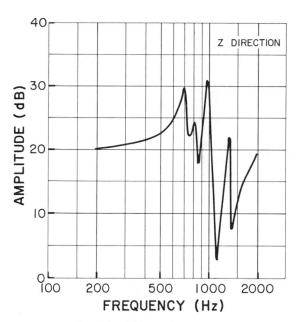

Fig. 9 Frequency response of mount #1
with Bruel & Kjaer accelerometer #4375.

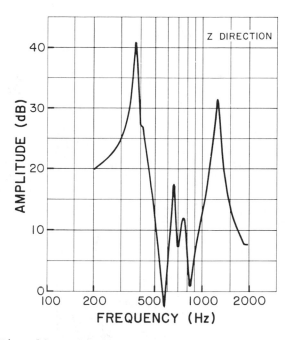

Fig. 10 Frequency response of mount #2
with special triaxial accelerometer.

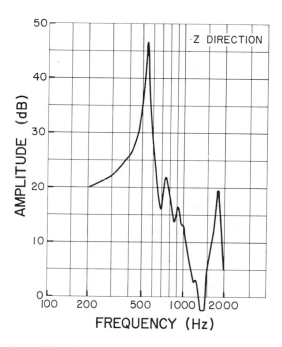

Fig. 11 Frequency response of mount #3
with special triaxial accelerometer.

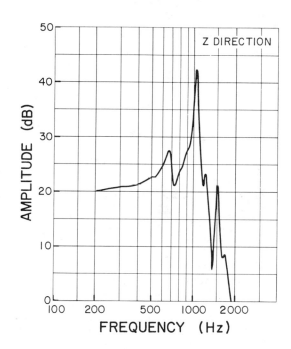

Fig. 12 Frequency response of mount #4
with special triaxial accelerometer.

vibrating structure is not satisfactory
for all conditions, particularly in the
case of thin cushions mainly affecting the
transfer of higher frequencies. In such
cases it might be prefereable to make the
measurements with the transducer rigidly

attached to the handle or structure and to
report separately the type, thickness,
physical properties and estimated attenuation achieved by the cushioning material."
    "Although characterization of the
vibration exposure currently uses the

Rasmussen: Measurement of vibration

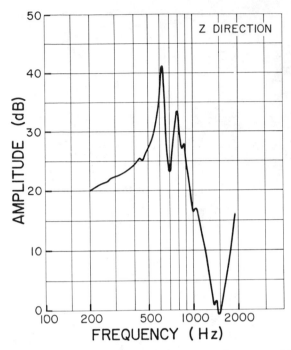

Fig. 13 Frequency response of mount #5 with special triaxial accelerometer.

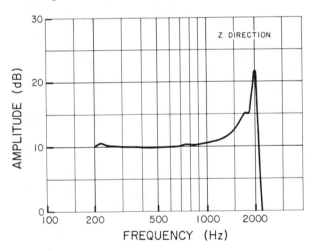

Fig. 14 Frequency response of mount #6 with Bruel & Kjaer accelerometer #4375.

acceleration (velocity) transmitted to the hand as the primary quantity, it is reasonable to assume that the biological effects might depend to a large extent on the energy transmitted. This energy depends on the coupling of the hand-arm system to the vibration source and consequently on the grip pressure applied and the magnitude and direction of the static force...... It must be realized that changes in coupling can affect considerably the vibration exposure measured."

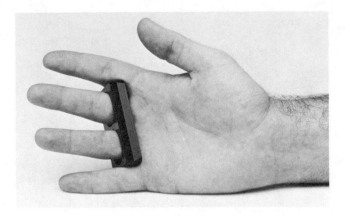

Fig. 15 Photograph of two-ringed mount (#1 to 3) showing finger separation.

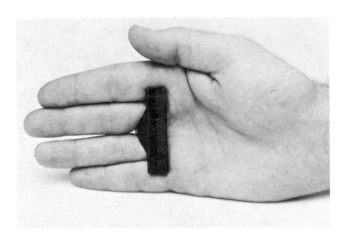

Fig. 16 Photograph of mount held between two fingers (#4 to 6).

In order to meet these requirements, a special transducer mount has been developed with the following design goals:
a) The frequency response of the mount should be flat from 5 Hz to above 1200 Hz;
b) The mount should represent a minimum dynamic load to the hand;
c) It should be easily installed and measure as close as possible to the standardized reference point (the origin of the coordinate system for the hand), on both right and left hands (1);
d) It should reflect the grip strength used; and
e) It should never underestimate the energy transmitted to the hand from the handle.
A series of mounts have been constructed. They are shown in Fig. 7. Each is slipped over two fingers like a double ring (#1-3), or held between two fingers (#4-6). In each case, the part in contact with the

Rasmussen: Measurement of vibration

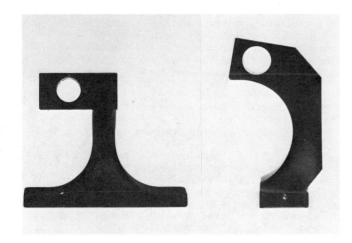

Fig. 17   Photographs of transducer mount #6: front and side views. Note scales are different.

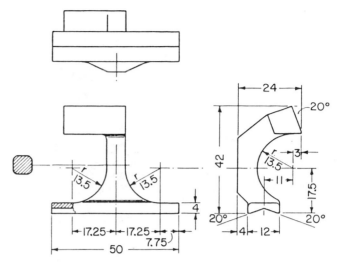

Fig. 18   Working drawing of transducer mount (dimensions in mm): manufactured from magnesium or aluminium alloy.

palm of the hand is held against the vibrating surface.

The frequency responses of these transducer mounts were determined by holding a handle attached to a vibration exciter. Measurements in the directions of the coordinate axes specified in Ref. 1 were obtained by careful orientation of the hand, as shown in Fig. 8. Note that the accelerometer is positioned close to the specified origin of the coordinate system, the head of the third metacarpal bone. Results for the Z direction are given in Figs. 9 to 14.

Except for version #6, the mounts failed to fulfill the requirements for one or more of the following reasons: poor frequency response (see Figs. 9 to 13); separation of the fingers by the mount, leading to variations in performance with the size of the hand (compare Figs. 15 and 16); resonance peaks within the frequency band of interest; and a potential safety hazard to the user, through the possibility of hooking onto objects. Mount #6 represents a good compromise on all these points and is shown in detail in Figs. 17 and 18. The view of the mount when looking along the length of the fingers is shown to the left of Fig. 17.

Properly described in terms of its maximum weight, overall dimensions and performance, it is hoped that a transducer mount similar to that described may serve as the basis for standardization of the measurement of vibration coupled to the hand.

ACKNOWLEDGEMENTS

The permission of the Standards Council of Canada, under authority of the International Organization for Standardization, to reproduce extracts from Draft International Standard ISO/DIS 5349 (1979) is gratefully acknowledged.

REFERENCES

1.   International Organization for Standardization. Principles for the Measurement and the Evaluation of Human Exposure to Vibration Transmitted to the Hand. Draft International Standard ISO/DIS 5349, 1979.

2.   International Organization for Standardization. Vibration and Shock Vocabulary. ISO 2041, 1975.

3.   International Organization for Standardization. Preferred Reference Quantities for Acoustic Levels. Draft International Standard ISO/DIS 1683.2, 1976.

4.   International Electrotechnical Commission. Octave, Half-Octave and Third-Octave Band Filters Intended for the Analysis of Sounds and Vibrations. IEC 225, 1966.

5.   See, for example, American National Standards Institute. American Standard Specification for Octave, Half-Octave and Third-Octave Band Filter Sets. ANSI S1.11, 1971.

6.   International Organization for Standardization. Guide for the Evaluation of Human Exposure to Whole-Body Vibration. ISO 2631, 1978.

7.   Randall RB. Application of B&K Equipment to Frequency Analysis. Naerum: Bruel & Kjaer, 1977.

8.   Thrane N. The discrete Fourier transform and FFT analysers. In: Technical Review. Naerum: Bruel & Kjaer 1979; 1: 3-25.

DISCUSSION

A.J. Brammer: What is the cross-axis sensitivity of transducer mount #6?

Author's Response: When held firmly onto a
cylindrical rod, the transverse sensitivity from
the Z or X directions to the Y direction is less
than 10%.

M.J. Griffin: What is the weight of the transducer mount with accelerometer attached?

Author's Response: The weight of mount #6
alone is 18 g when made of aluminium, and 12 g
when made of magnesium. The triaxial accelerometer
weighted 10 g and the uniaxial accelerometer weighted
0.65 g.

Do you agree that a mount of this type can
easily distort the measurement of the effectiveness
of a vibration-isolation system between the hand
and a handle, since the mechanical impedance of the
mount may be large compared to the impedance of
the relevant part of the hand.

Author's Response: For normal hand grips, the
distortion is believed to be minimal.

H.R. Martin: While I support the view that
levels in dBs be used as a measure of hand-arm
vibration, it is important to establish clearly the
reference level. The use of 1 G, 1 m/s^2 and other
values is found in the literature, and often the
reference value is not published. Would the author
comment on the preferred reference for hand-arm
vibration, and on how people can be encouraged to
use this value?

Author's Response: The internationally proposed
reference value for acceleration is 1 μm/s^2 (ISO/DIS
1683.2).

Method for Measuring the Vibration of Impact Pneumatic Tools

D. E. O'Connor and B. Lindquist

ABSTRACT: Accurate measurement of the vibration of pneumatic, percussive hand
tools has long been a problem. The large-amplitude, repeated impacts often cause
non-linear transduction within piezoelectric accelerometers, leading to erroneous
measures of tool vibration. A "back-to-back" test has been developed to compare
two measuring systems subjected to the same impacts. Two undamped piezoelectric
accelerometers were mounted rigidly on opposing faces of a solid metal block
welded to the handle of a chipping hammer. The transducers studied were general
purpose accelerometers (delta shear construction) mounted on a mechanical filter
and a shock accelerometer (compression construction). By comparing the frequency
spectra produced by the two measuring systems, it was found that the shock accelerometer performed unsatisfactorily. A correct measure of the vibration of chipping hammers was obtained only by using an accelerometer mounted on a low-pass
mechanical filter.

RESUME: La mesure exacte des vibrations produites par les outils manuels
pneumatiques et à percussion pose des problèmes depuis longtemps. Les impacts
répétés de grande amplitude provoquent souvent une transduction non linéaire
dans les accéléromètres piezoélectriques, ce qui fausse la mesure des vibrations
de l'outil. Un essai "dos-à-dos" a été mis au point pour comparer deux dispositifs de mesure soumis aux mêmes impacts. Deux accéléromètres piezoélectriques
non amortis ont été fixés aux faces opposées d'un bloc de métal massif soudé à la
poignée d'un marteau-piqueur. Les transducteurs étudiés étaient des accéléromètres
polyvalents (à montage transversal en triangle) placés sur un filtre mécanique
et un accéléromètre de choc (à montage en compression). En comparant les spectres
de fréquence produits par les deux dispositifs de mesure, on a découvert que
l'accéléromètre de choc fonctionnait mal. On ne pouvait obtenir une mesure exacte
des vibrations des marteaux-piqueur qu'en utilisant un accéléromètre monté sur un
filtre mécanique passe-bas.

INTRODUCTION

It has been known for many years that
the operation of vibrating pneumatic tools
may lead to vibration-induced disorders of
the hand (1). More recently, difficulties
associated with the measurement of the
vibration of these and other percussive
tools have become apparent. Frood,
Hempstock and O'Connor, and Kitchener have
all reported non-linear effects in accelerometers during impulse measurements (2-4).
The phenomenon, often described as the
problem of DC (or zero) shifts, has been
the subject of a study by a subcommittee of
PNEUROP, the European Committee of Manufacturers of Compressors, Vacuum Pumps and
Pneumatic Tools, in association with research workers from the Inst. National de
Recherche et de Sécurité (France) and the
Univ. of Salford.

The primary purpose of the PNEUROP
work was to assess the use of shock accelerometers and mechanical filters for the
measurement of the vibration of pneumatic
chipping hammers. Several experiments were
conducted using 'back-to-back' tests and
the results are reported in this paper.
Further information on this work can be
found in Ref. 5.

I REVIEW OF THE PROBLEM

The vibration of a working percussive
tool, e.g. a chipping hammer, presents a
very complex measuring problem. The impacts
are normally in the range 100 to 1000 km/s^2,
depending on the design and working conditions of the tool. The frequency spectrum
of these impacts extends from approximately
zero to above the natural frequency of the

accelerometer, with the highest intensities occurring at frequencies over 10 kHz. In contrast, the frequencies of interest for human exposure to vibration are below 1 kHz, and at these low frequencies the intensities are in the range 1 to 10 m/s^2. This means that a measuring system consisting of a shock accelerometer plus a suitable pre-amplifier has to respond to signal levels that range in amplitude by up to 120 dB (i.e. 10^6) before the first electronic filtering can be performed.

Measuring equipment available today with that large dynamic range is rare; hence, strange results have been reported. In the majority of cases, errors caused by sudden changes in the DC signal level have been noticed - a phenomenon commonly known as a DC shift. These unwanted signals can be caused by a number of different mechanisms, such as preamplifier hysteresis, input overload, input noise, generation of signals in the transducer connecting cable (triboelectric effects) and fatigue fracture of its centre conductor. In addition, the internal mechanical assembly and the piezoelectric material of the measurement transducer can cause DC shifts. The existence of this phenomenon has been known for a number of years but no satisfactory theory has yet been offered for its origin. Most of the sources external to the accelerometer can be avoided by careful selection of instruments and measurement procedure. However, non-linear effects leading to DC shifts have been observed in all piezoelectric measurement devices, especially those of high sensitivity, and are probably due to the severe stresses on the piezoelectric material and to situations where resonance in the accelerometer contributes to the stress. Other explanations include reorientation of the crystal domains in the piezoelectric material, hysteresis due to internal or external losses, irreversible deformations or slippage between the metal and piezoelectric interfaces, and output due to heat generated through internal movements in the transducer. Probably one or more of these mechanisms dominate, depending on the particular design of the transducer. As all occur within the accelerometer during the process of transduction, any measurement error so introduced cannot be subsequently removed by electronic signal processing.

Subjective tests indicate that zero shifts of the order of 1% of the peak amplitude can hardly be avoided when impacts with accelerations exceeding 100 000 m/s^2 are encountered. To illustrate the significance of this, the following numerical example is given.

We assume that measurements are performed with a preamplifier lower limiting frequency (LLF) of 3 Hz and that a 1% zero shift is produced when a shock acceleration of 300 km/s^2 is applied. This will produce a single zero-shift pulse with a 3 km/s^2 step and a decay rate determined by the 3 Hz LLF, which has a frequency spectrum whose amplitude decreases with increasing frequency, f (i.e. proportional to 1/f). In the 31.5 Hz third-octave filter band, the zero-shift pulse will produce an amplitude component of approximately 100 m/s^2, (i.e. approximately 3.5% of the step).

Single pulses of this nature, but of random amplitude, occur and are associated with each impact; these contain a frequency content similar to a single pulse, starting from DC but with reduced amplitude. If 10% of the single zero-shift pulse amplitude is now assumed, the measured response in the 31.5 Hz third-octave filter will be 10 m/s^2, corresponding to most of the values observed. In the third-octave bands with centre frequencies at 8 and 16 Hz, the effect of repeated zero shifts is usually more pronounced (Licht T, personal communication).

1.1 Potential Solution - A Mechanical Filter

One method for avoiding most of these problems, when only low-frequency signals are of interest, is to mount the accelerometer on a mechanical filter. A mechanical filter is basically a well-damped spring which, together with the mass of an accelerometer, forms a one-degree-of-freedom system. The acceleration transmitted through the filter can therefore be assumed to be constant from zero up to frequencies near its mechanical resonance (around 5 kHz), where a few decibels increase in amplitude may occur. At higher frequencies, the transmissibility decreases by 13 dB/octave (i.e. 100 times/decade). A typical transmission characteristic is shown in Fig. 1, where it can be seen that the response of the accelerometer is significantly reduced at its resonance, which occurs at about 40 kHz (to -1 dB).

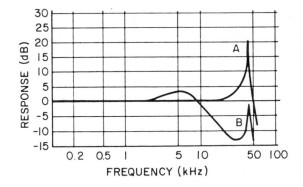

Fig. 1 Typical frequency response of: A, undamped piezoelectric accelerometer; and B, same accelerometer mounted on a low-pass mechanical filter.

O'Connor et al.: Impact measurement

By mounting the mechanical filter between the accelerometer and the vibrating surface, the acceleration levels will be reduced by more than 10 dB at high frequencies and the zero shifts by a factor of more than 100. This suggests that normal accelerometers can be employed and that the dynamic range required is greatly reduced. The purpose of the experiment described in this report has been to demonstrate that, in practice, this is the case.

A few limitations are incurred due to the size and temperature dependence of the mechanical filter. For example, its performance may be influenced by vibration in directions other than that designed for transmitting vibration. It is also important that the accelerometer be mounted according to the manufacturer's instructions. In particular, the accelerometer and mechanical filter should be firmly attached to a plane surface on the handle or to a suitable clip connected rigidly to the handle.

II THE EXPERIMENT

It had been thought that shock accelerometers, which are designed to measure very high acceleration levels, would not suffer from non-linear effects when recording the vibration of pneumatic tools. The question arose as to how to test these accelerometers and also accelerometers mounted on mechanical filters for non-linear behaviour. To this end, 'back-to-back' tests were performed. Two accelerometers were mounted rigidly on opposing (parallel) faces of a solid metal block which was welded to the handle of a chipping hammer. The mounting is illustrated in Fig. 2, where it can be seen that the direction of measurement was parallel to the direction of the blows. The signals from each transducer were conditioned by

a charge amplifier and subsequently recorded on a multi-channel instrumentation tape recorder.

The philosophy of the 'back-to-back' test is as follows. If the two accelerations recorded are different, then one or both is incorrect. If they are the same, then they are either both correct or both incorrect. For both systems to give the same incorrect measurement, then both systems must have gone non-linear in an identical way. This is very unlikely for two mechanically different accelerometers mounted in different ways, so that one can assume that if the two accelerations are the same, then they are correct.

The signals from the two transducers (vibration waveforms in the time domain), which were recorded simultaneously, were analysed to obtain rms accelerations in the one-third octave bands with centre frequencies from 16 to 1000 Hz. Care was taken to average data from the same section of the tape recording, that is, corresponding segments of the time domain signals. In order to compare the resulting frequency spectra, the difference in level for each one-third octave band was calculated (in dB) from:

$$\text{Level Difference (dB)} = 20 \log (A_1/A_2) \quad (1)$$

where A_1 and A_2 are the one-third octave-band rms accelerations recorded by the two accelerometers.

III RESULTS

The tests were performed with a pneumatic chipping hammer as illustrated in Fig. 2. The transducers were general purpose accelerometers (delta shear construction) mounted on a low-pass mechanical filter and a shock accelerometer (compression construction) designed for the measurement of shocks with peak amplitudes of up to 1 000 000 m/s^2.

Figure 3 shows the difference spectrum obtained when two general purpose

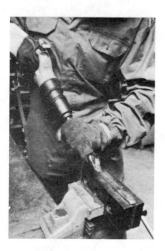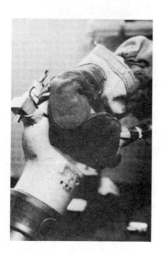

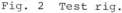
Fig. 2 Test rig.

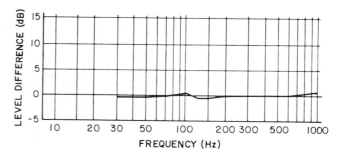

Fig. 3 Difference spectrum obtained from a back-to-back test with two general purpose accelerometers and low-pass mechanical filters.

O'Connor et al.: Impact measurement

accelerometers mounted on mechanical filters were compared. The two signals are
clearly substantially the same.

Figure 4 shows the results of a
comparison between a general purpose accelerometer mounted on a mechanical filter
and a shock accelerometer attached directly
to the metal block. Figure 5 shows a
comparison between the same two systems
when the pneumatic tool was fitted with a
round-ended piece and was hammering a
surface. In both cases the shock accelerometer gives higher levels and, clearly,
the difference is substantial at frequencies
below 100 Hz.

Figure 6 shows the difference spectrum
between two shock accelerometers mounted
directly on the block in the back-to-back
configuration. The comparison reveals a
considerable discrepancy between the two
transducers and strongly suggests that
neither of them is behaving in a linear
manner. Several laboratories produced results similar to those shown in Figs. 3-6.

One laboratory compared the vibration
spectra recorded by a shock accelerometer,
and a general purpose accelerometer mounted
on a mechanical filter as a function of the
air pressure fed to the pneumatic tool.

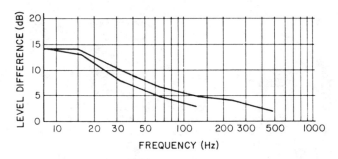

Fig. 4 Difference spectra obtained
from a back-to-back test with a general
purpose accelerometer mounted on a
mechanical filter and a shock accelerometer. Data from two laboratories.

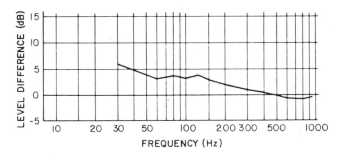

Fig. 5 Difference spectrum for the two
measuring systems of Fig. 4 when the
tool was fitted with a round end for
hammering.

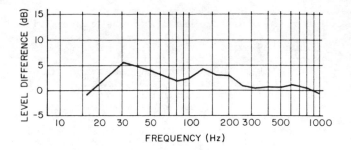

Fig. 6 Difference spectrum obtained
from a back-to-back test with two shock
accelerometers.

The results of this investigation are shown
in Table 1. When the air pressure was less
than 200 kPa, the difference in vibration
for the band containing the blow frequency
(determined by the repetition rate of the
tool) was negligible. As the air pressure
is increased above 200 kPa, the difference
between the accelerations recorded increases
substantially. It would appear, therefore,
that non-linear behaviour only appears when
the peak accelerations exceed a critical
value, which occurred in this experiment
when the feed pressure exceeded 200 kPa.

Table 1. Comparison Between Two Measuring Systems
in Back-to-Back Tests as a Function of Air
Pressure Fed to the Chipping Hammer. Values are
for the One-Third Octave-Band Containing the
Impact Frequency.

Pressure (kPa)	Shock Accelerometer	Accelerometer with mechanical filter	Difference dB
50	30	30	0
100	67	67	0
200	85	79	0.7
300	145	124	1.4
400	251	156	4
500	396	198	6
600	531	318	4.5

RMS Acceleration (m/s^2)

IV CONCLUSIONS

It would appear that the shock accelerometers when attached directly to a
chipping hammer behave in a non-linear
manner, and so produce acceleration values
that are in excess of those actually occurring on the tool. The two general purpose
accelerometers mounted back-to-back on
mechanical filters gave substantially the
same spectra, and this suggests that the
signals obtained were correct. Investigations using different accelerometers,

O'Connor et al.: Impact measurement

different mechanical filters and different preamplifiers indicate that as long as the transducer is mounted on a mechanical filter which adequately reduces the peak acceleration levels at high frequencies, then the resulting vibration spectra will be correct.

It is possible that there are commercially available accelerometers that do not exhibit this non-linear behaviour. It is strongly recommended that no accelerometer be relied upon to function properly when subjected to extreme accelerations, similar to those generated by many percussive tools, unless its linearity has been demonstrated, perhaps by a back-to-back test.

During these investigations, it was found that correct one-third octave-band spectra for the vibration of a common pneumatic tool could be obtained only when an accelerometer was mounted on a low-pass mechanical filter. This filter has the added advantage of providing attenuation of vibration at frequencies above about 2000 Hz, thus reducing the dynamic range of the signal being recorded. It is recommended that such a mechanical filter be used for all measurements of vibration where mass loading is not a problem.

REFERENCES

1. Agate JN, Druett HA. A study of portable vibrating tools in relation to the clinical effects which they produce. Br J Ind Med 1947; 4: 167-174.
2. Frood ADM. Test methods and some of the problems involved in measuring the vibration of hand-held pneumatic tools. In: Wasserman DE, Taylor W, Curry MG, eds. Proc of the Int Occup Hand-Arm Vibration Conf. Cincinnati, OH: Dept of Health and Human Services, 1977. (NIOSH publication no. 77-170): 146-152.
3. Hempstock TI, O'Connor DE. Evaluation of human exposure to hand-transmitted vibration. In: Wasserman DE, Taylor W, Curry MG, eds. Proc of the Int Occup Hand-Arm Vibration Conf. Cincinnati, OH: Dept of Health and Human Services, (NIOSH publication no. 77-710): 129-135.
4. Kitchener R. The measurement of hand-arm vibration in industry. In: Wasserman, DE, Taylor W, Curry MG, eds. Proc of the Int Occup Hand-Arm Vibration Conf. Cincinnati, OH: Dept of Health and Human Services, 1977. (NIOSH publication no. 77-170): 153-159.
5. European Committee of Manufacturers of Compressors, Vacuum Pumps and Pneumatic Tools.

Vibrations in Pneumatic Hand Tools: Investigations on Hand-Held Percussive Tools. (Copies available from British Compressed Air Society, 8 Leicester Street, London WC2H 7BL, England).

DISCUSSION

A.G. Taylor: What variation in third-octave band levels could result from instrument tolerances? Authors' Response: Less than ±0.5 dB.

G. Rasmussen: We have found the hand-held accelerometer mount described elsewhere in this volume most suitable for measuring the vibration of impact pneumatic tools. High frequencies are not transmitted into the mount, or the accelerometer, as it is only held in contact with, and not rigidly attached to, the vibrating surface. A comparison of chipping-hammer vibration measured with this device and with an accelerometer mounted on a low-pass mechanical filter (attached to a welded stud) is shown in the diagram. It can be seen that the acceleration recorded at low frequencies by the transducer on the hand-held mount is less than that recorded by the other measuring system. This is possibly due to a further reduction in non-linear effects.

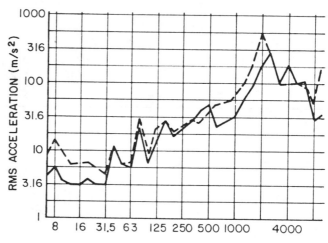

Fig. D1 Comparison between one-third octave-band spectra at the handle of a chipping hammer obtained with the hand-held mount (solid curve), and with an accelerometer mounted on a mechanical filter (dashed curve).

O'Connor et al.: Impact measurement

The Transmission of Vibration to the Hand and the Influence of Gloves

M. J. Griffin, C. R. Macfarlane and C. D. Norman

ABSTRACT: Experimental measurements of the effect of inter-subject variability, vibration amplitude, grip force, push and pull forces and posture (arm angle) on the apparent mass of the hand at frequencies between 10 and 1000 Hz are reported. Alternative experimental methods for measuring the transmission of vibration through gloves are compared under controlled conditions. The application of one method to a prototype glove shows that the attenuation of high frequency vibration from tool handles is possible. The prediction of glove transmissibility from a knowledge of the dynamic characteristics of the hand and glove material is discussed.

RESUME: On rapporte des mesures expérimentales de l'effet de la variabilité d'un sujet à l'autre, de l'amplitude des vibrations, de la force de l'étreinte, des forces de poussée et de traction et de la posture (angle du bras) sur la masse apparente de la main à des fréquences comprises entre 10 et 1000 Hz. On compare plusieurs méthodes expérimentales pour déterminer à quel point les vibrations traversent des gants lors d'expériences effectuées sous stricte surveillance. L'application d'une méthode à un gant prototype démontre qu'il est possible d'atténuer les vibrations haute fréquence des poignées d'outils. On discute comment prédire la transmissibilité du gant lorsqu'on connaît les caractéristiques dynamiques de la main et du matériau du gant.

INTRODUCTION

Many factors determine the severity of hand-arm vibration exposures. Reductions in the vibration hazard might, therefore, be achieved by many different methods. Isolation of the hand from vibration is one method which, although widely mentioned, is not widely adopted as a preventive measure. The use of gloves to reduce the transmission of vibration to the hand has been considered in several countries (1-16). It can be shown that the isolation provided by gloves will depend on both the dynamic properties of the hand-arm system and those of the material used in the construction of the gloves.

This paper initially presents some measures of the dynamic response of the hand-arm system to vibration. Alternative methods of measuring the transmission of vibration through materials to the fingers and hand are next compared. The application of these methods to the measurement and prediction of glove transmissibility is then considered.

I FACTORS AFFECTING THE DYNAMIC RESPONSE OF THE HAND AND ARM

1.1 Variables

The dynamic response of a system is commonly measured by either the ratio of the amount of movement to the force at the same or different points in the system, or the ratio of the movements at different points in the system. These alternative measures yield impedance-like or transmissibility-like quantities; the former are listed in Table 1.

Table 1. Common Measures of Dynamic Response.

Apparent Mass	$= \dfrac{\text{Force}}{\text{Acceleration}}$	$= \dfrac{1}{\text{Inertance}}$
Mechanical Impedance	$= \dfrac{\text{Force}}{\text{Velocity}}$	$= \dfrac{1}{\text{Mobility}}$
Dynamic Stiffness	$= \dfrac{\text{Force}}{\text{Displacement}}$	$= \dfrac{1}{\text{Receptance}}$

Griffin et al.: Dynamic response

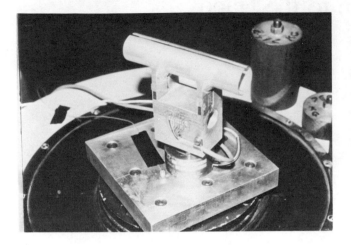

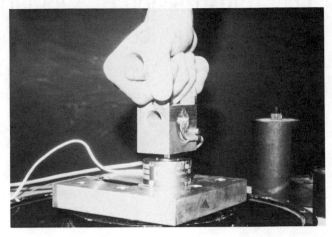

Fig. 1 Handle used to measure hand-
arm apparent mass, hand grip forces
and hand push forces.

Fig. 2 Hand gripping handle used for
hand-arm apparent mass studies.

The studies of gloves reported below
primarily employed mechanical impedance.
For practical convenience, the studies of
the factors affecting the dynamic response
of the hand and arm were conducted using
apparent mass. With single frequency excitation and response, the conversion to
impedance requires that the modulus of the
apparent mass be multiplied by $2\pi f$, where
f is the frequency. Although phase was
measured in both series of studies, the
results will be discussed elsewhere.

The principal variables that might be
expected to affect the measured dynamic
response of the hand are: a) inter-subject
variability, b) vibration amplitude,
c) grip force, d) push and pull forces, and
e) arm angle. A handgrip was developed to
allow both control and quantification of
these variables, so that they could be
studied systematically.

1.2 Methods

The aluminium handle shown in Figs. 1
and 2 was developed for this study (17).
It had a mass of 0.68 kg and was designed
so that the grip force on the split tubular
handle would be indicated by strain gauges
mounted on cantilevers supporting the tube.
This grip was calibrated by mounting the
handle on one side and hanging known weights
around the upper half of the tube. In the
experiments, the base of the handle was
screwed to a Kulite TC 2000-500 load cell
secured to a vertically orientated Derritron
VP85 electrodynamic vibrator. The first
handle resonance occurred at approximately
2120 Hz and the measured apparent mass of
the handle alone deviated by less than 10%
over the frequency range, up to 1000 Hz.

The experiments were conducted with
discrete sinusoidal excitation at the
twenty-one, preferred, third-octave band
centre frequencies from 10 to 1000 Hz. At
each frequency, the apparent mass of the
hand and handle combination was calculated
from the modulus of force (indicated by the
load cell) divided by the modulus of the
acceleration (indicated by an accelerometer
located beside the load cell). The apparent
mass of the hand was determined by sub-
tracting the apparent mass of the handle
measured at the same frequency.

1.3 Results

1.3.1 Inter-Subject Variability

The apparent mass was determined for
the right hands of the six male subjects
whose relevant physical characteristics are
listed in Table 2. The subjects were seated
adjacent to the apparatus so that they could
grip the tubular handle comfortably in their
right hands, with their lower arm both
horizontal and parallel to the x axis of
the body. The vertical vibration was in
the X axis of the hand (18). The rear
surface of the hand was uppermost with
fingers and thumb beneath the tube. They
were required to maintain a constant grip
force (46 N) and zero push force, during
vibration of 2.5 m/s^2 (rms) at each frequency from 10 to 1000 Hz.

Figure 3 shows the mean value of the
apparent mass measured from the six subjects
(plus and minus one standard deviation).
In the present study, the individual results
generally fell well within a 2:1 range, with
the greatest difference occurring at around
80 and 100 Hz. The apparent mass reached
a maximum of about 1 kg in the range 10 to
32 Hz, falling rapidly to a mean of about
0.15 kg at 50 Hz and then increasing to
approximately 0.3 kg at frequencies between 80 and 100 Hz. Above 500 Hz, the

Table 2. Anthropometric Data for Subjects.

Subject Number	Height m	Weight kg	Hand Circumference m	Hand Length m	Distance from tip of middle finger to the acromion process in the shoulder m
1	1.78	82.3	0.222	0.19	0.844
2	1.83	66.2	0.216	0.18	0.775
3	1.8	64.5	0.255	0.21	0.777
4	1.7	53.9	0.215	0.18	0.736
5	1.82	62.3	0.21	0.2	0.81
6	1.79	80.1	0.228	0.19	0.755

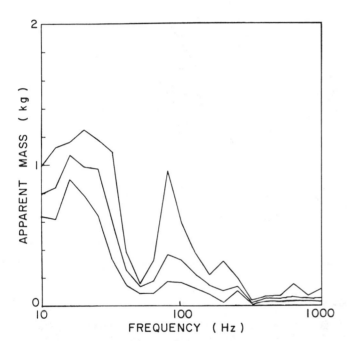

Fig. 3 Mean value (±SD) of hand-arm apparent mass for 6 subjects: X axis, 46 N grip force.

apparent mass was generally below 0.05 kg and was not easily measured with reliability.

Figure 4 shows the data for each subject presented in order of increasing hand size (hand length × hand circumference). It can be seen that there is some evidence that larger hands are associated with increased apparent mass at low frequencies.

1.3.2 Vibration Level

An experiment identical to that reported in Section 1.3.1 was conducted at three vibration levels: 2.5, 4 and 6 m/s^2 (rms). The results from one subject, shown

in Fig. 5, illustrate that only slight changes in apparent mass occurred with this change of level.

1.3.3 Grip Force

Using the same posture, with zero push force and a vibration level of 5 m/s^2 (rms), the effect of varying grip force from zero (loose hold on handle) to 186 Newtons is shown in Fig. 6.

At most frequencies, the apparent mass increases with increasing grip force, up to 92 Newtons. Further increases in grip force increased the apparent mass in the frequency range from 31.5 to 63 Hz and from 125 to 250 Hz, but the apparent mass decreased at frequencies below 31.5 Hz and around 100 Hz. Even after excluding the zero grip condition, the range of values for the subject shown in Fig. 6 was generally much greater than those obtained at constant grip with six subjects. For example, at 40 and 200 Hz the change in apparent mass from a grip of 46 to 186 Newtons was almost 10:1.

1.3.4 Arm Angle

The effect of varying the arm angle from the posture adopted in previous experiments, with zero push force and a 46 N grip force, is shown in Fig. 7. As the arm angle increased from horizontal (0°) to vertical (90°), the greatest change in apparent mass occurred at frequencies below 20 Hz. Increasing the angle to 45° reduced the apparent mass by more than a half at these frequencies. However, further increases to 90° caused the arm to couple more effectively with the vibrating system and this greatly increased the apparent mass, up to 2 kg (more than double that at 0°).

1.3.5 Push-Pull Forces

Figure 8 shows the change in apparent mass due to exerting push and pull forces of 85 N while gripping the handle with a force of 46 N. These data were obtained by

Griffin et al.: Dynamic response

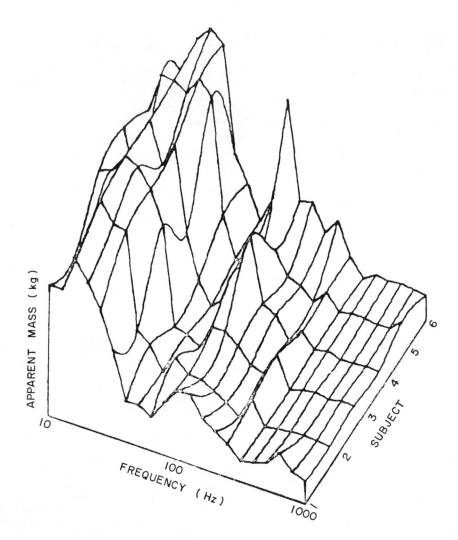

Fig. 4 Inter-subject variability in hand-arm apparent mass: X axis, 46 N grip
force. Data are in order of hand size from smallest, 1, to largest, 6.

the subject standing with his shoulder over
the handle and with his arm straight and
vertical. In this position the apparent
mass at low frequencies is much increased -
values in the range 2.5 to 5.5 kg were
obtained for all three push-pull forces at
frequencies of 16 Hz and below.

At frequencies less than about 100 Hz,
a zero push force resulted in the lowest
apparent mass and a push force of 85 N
generally produced the greatest apparent
mass. However, in the range 160 to 500 Hz,
a pull force of 85 N resulted in an apparent mass greater than the push force.

1.4 Discussion

Although the apparent mass was affected by all variables investigated, it
appears that grip force, push force and
arm angle may be the most important. The
full range of the many postures used with

tools was not studied but it is likely that
the above factors will prove important
under most conditions.

The range of inter-subject variability
in hand-arm apparent mass was probably
reduced in the experiment by controlling
posture, and grip and push forces. When
using power tools, these factors may be
expected to vary considerably between and
within individuals and give rise to a far
wider range of inter-subdect variability.

Apparent mass (impedance, etc.) are
quantities for which large values may not
necessarily be detrimental. Their variation
will affect the transmission of vibration
into the hand (e.g. as measured by absorbed
energy) and also determine the degree to
which some form of isolation (e.g. a glove)
may reduce the transmission of vibration
to the hand. The absolute values of
apparent mass reported here are of primary
value in illustrating the general frequency

Griffin et al.: Dynamic response

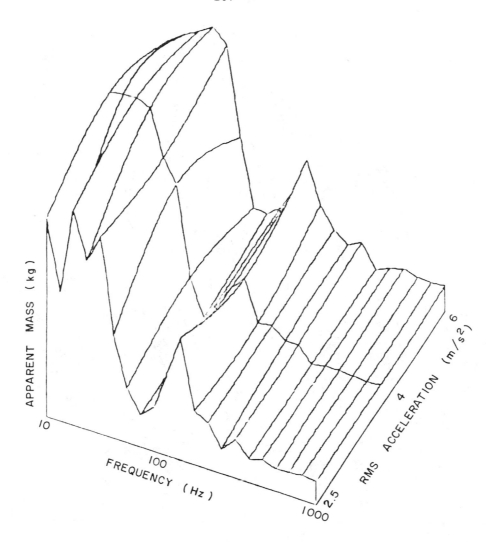

Fig. 5 Effect of vibration amplitude on hand-arm apparent mass: X axis, 46 N grip force.

dependence and the importance of posture, grip and push force on the dynamic response of the hand and arm.

II THE TRANSMISSIBILITY OF GLOVES

The results presented above show clearly that the hand does not respond as a rigid mass. If this is assumed in either the measurement of the transmissibility of glove material or the prediction of glove transmissibility, large errors are likely. The large reduction in apparent mass of the hand from 20 to 50 Hz increases the difficulty of isolating the higher frequencies from the hand.

Although some empirical knowledge of the dynamic response of the hand is essential for the determination of glove transmissibility, two alternative approaches

are possible. Glove transmissibility may be either measured or predicted. Measurements require the determination and verification of a satisfactory method, and predictions require some knowledge and assumptions concerning both the glove material and the hand-arm system dynamic properties.

The objective of the studies reported here was to determine a method for measuring the transmissibility of glove-like materials. Preliminary investigations indicated that the transmissibility of existing gloves should be measured as a function of frequency, up to 1000 Hz. However, in view of the dominant vibration frequencies most commonly found on the handles of tools associated with vibration white finger (19), it was considered that the response to 500 Hz was sufficient for

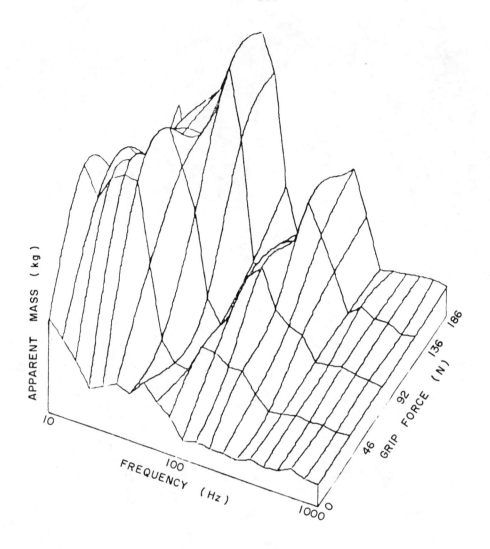

Fig. 6 Effect of grip force on hand-arm apparent mass: X axis.

studying potentially useful anti-vibration gloves.

2.1 Measurement Methods

2.1.1 Subjective Methods

Vibration thresholds at various frequencies (or equivalent-comfort contours) could be determined with and without a glove - the difference in the two curves may then indicate the attenuation provided by the glove. This method is used for assessing the acoustic attenuation provided by hearing protectors, for example, but has several disadvantages for use with gloves. For example, when wearing a glove, the vibration may be distributed over a very different area of the hand and fingers, and high vibration levels, which produce intense sound levels, are required at high frequencies. The various sources of intra-subject variability, in particular the difficult task of judging high frequencies, the need to use discrete frequencies (or narrow frequency bands) and the time-consuming nature of the experiment, determined that this method be not pursued. With care, however, subjective methods may be valuable for measurements at low frequencies.

2.1.2 Measurement with a Rigid Mass

Consider a mass or hand compressing some glove material secured to a vibrating surface. Using mechanical impedance theory based on four-pole parameters (20), it can be shown that the free velocity transmissibility, V_{12}^f, through the glove material is (21):

$$V_{12}^f = z_{12}^b z_1^{2f} / (z_2^{3f} z_1^{2f} + z_{12}^b z_{12}^f) \quad (1)$$

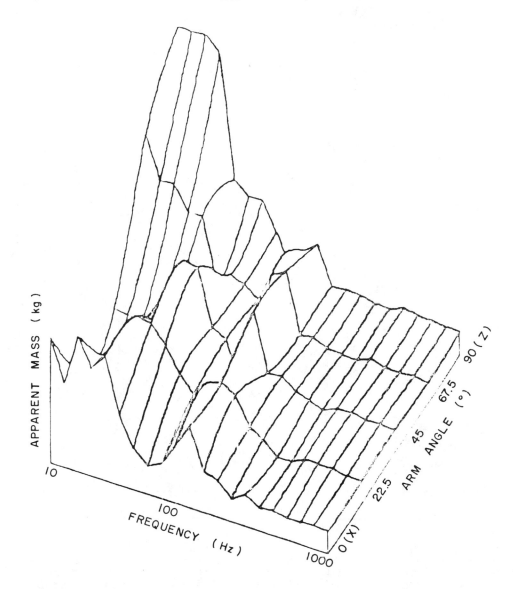

Fig. 7 Effect of arm angle on hand-arm apparent mass (46 N grip force).

where

V_{12}^f = velocity transmissibility through the material,

z_{12}^b = blocked transfer mechanical impedance of the glove material,

z_1^{2f} = free point mechanical impedance of the glove material,

z_2^{3f} = free point mechanical impedance of the 'mass' or 'hand', and

z_{12}^f = free transfer mechanical impedance of the glove material.

Only the parameter z_2^{3f} will vary, depending on whether a mass or hand compresses the glove material. Since the results in Section 1 show that the apparent mass and, therefore, the mechanical impedance of the hand cannot be represented by a rigid mass, it follows that no constant, rigid mass load can produce glove transmissibilities similar to those occurring with a human hand.

2.1.3 Measurement of Transmissibility

The ratio of the acceleration on the handle side of a glove to the acceleration on the hand side of a glove may be used to measure its transmissibility. The principal difficulty is that the size and mass of currently available accelerometers are not insignificant in comparison to the fingers within a glove. Two alternative methods for mounting accelerometers were explored.

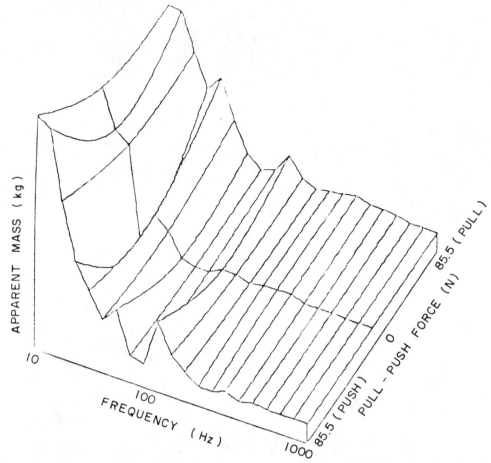

Fig. 8 Effect of push-pull force on hand-arm apparent mass: Z axis-46 N grip force.

The first method used a small cylindrical aluminium ring (internal diameter 17 mm, external diameter 22 mm, length 1 cm), weighing 3.5 g, with two flattened outside surfaces. An accelerometer (mass 1 g) was secured to one of these surfaces; then, with the ring over the distal phalanx of the index finger, the 1 square cm area of the outer flattened surface was pressed against a material sample. This is called the "ring method" (see Fig. 9).

The second method involved mounting an accelerometer on some part of the finger or hand. In studies of the transmission of vibration to the fingers, a small light-weight accelerometer (Knowles BU-1771-DE or Bruel & Kjaer 8307), weighing approximately 0.5 g, was secured by wax to the nail of the index finger (see Fig. 10). In studies of the transmission of vibration to the hand, a Bruel & Kjaer type 8307 accelero-meter was attached to the skin over the knuckle of the middle finger (i.e. over the metacarpophalangeal joint of the second digit), see Fig. 11. In both cases the orientation of the accelerometer and hand were arranged so that the sensitive axis of the accelerometer was parallel to the

direction of the applied vibration. With this method, the transmissibility from the vibrating surface to the finger (or hand) mounted accelerometer was determined both with and without the glove material. The ratio of the two transmissibilities then defined the quotient transfer function of the glove material.

2.2 Results

2.2.1 Comparison of Methods

Using the finger grip apparatus shown in Figs. 9 and 10, an experiment was con-ducted in which the transmission of vibra-tion through two thicknesses (3 mm and 9 mm) of material was measured by both of the methods described in Section 2.1.3, for six subjects applying two grip forces (5 and 15 N) (15). A swept frequency (sine wave) source of vibration was used.

Figure 12 shows examples of the quotient transfer functions determined by the ring-mounted and fingernail-mounted accelerometer methods. In all cases, data from the ring-mounted method exhibited a lower resonance frequency and appreciably

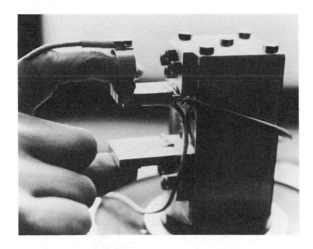

Fig. 9 Ring method of measuring the transmission of vibration to the finger using the finger-grip apparatus.

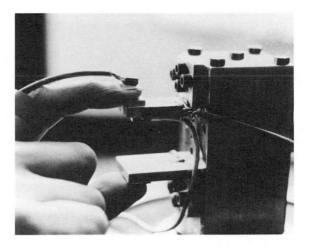

Fig. 10 Fingernail method of measuring the transmission of vibration to the finger using the finger-grip apparatus.

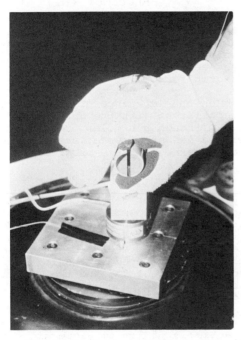

Fig. 11 Method of measuring the vibration transmitted through the hand when using the hand-grip apparatus.

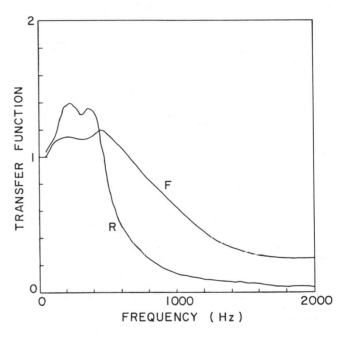

Fig. 12 Mean quotient transfer functions (moduli) for 3 mm thick material measured with a ring-mounted (R) and a fingernail-mounted (F) accelerometer. Data from 6 subjects and for a 5 N finger-grip force.

greater attenuation at higher frequencies. Additional studies with rings weighing more than 3.5 g showed that the maximum transmissibility occurred at decreasing frequencies with increasing mass. It was concluded that the 3.5 g ring had a mass large compared to the active mass of the finger at frequencies above about 300 Hz, and that it could not be used to measure glove transmissibility above about 100 Hz.

An accelerometer mounted on the finger-nail may also affect the dynamic response of the finger. However, its effect may be lessened by the calculation of the quotient transfer function, the use of an accelerometer less than one-tenth the weight of the ring mount and the fact that the transmissibility of the fingernail is near unity

Griffin et al.: Dynamic response

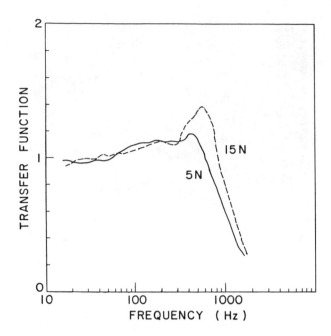

Fig. 13 Mean quotient transfer functions
(moduli) for 3 mm thick material when
finger grip forces of 5 N and 15 N are
employed. Data from 6 subjects with a
fingernail-mounted accelerometer.

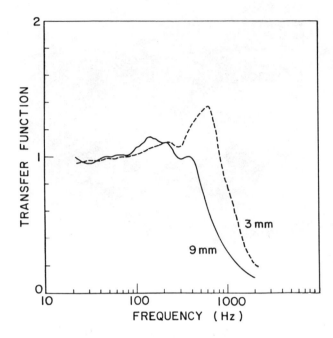

Fig. 14 Mean quotient transfer functions
(moduli) for 3 mm and 9 mm thick material.
Data from 6 subjects with a fingernail-
mounted accelerometer using a 15 N
finger-grip force.

over much of the frequency range. A miniature accelerometer mounted on the index
fingernail was therefore used in subsequent experiments with the finger-grip
apparatus.

2.2.2 Effect of Finger-Grip Force

Figure 13 shows the mean quotient
transfer functions obtained for a 3 mm
thick sample of material from six subjects
with two grip forces (5 and 15 N), using
a fingernail mounted accelerometer. The
data suggest that the stronger grip force
compressed the material so as to increase
its stiffness and hence its resonance
frequency. For this thickness and type of
material, increased grip force therefore
reduces further the slight isolation that
might be obtained at high frequencies.

It was also found that the transmissibility of the finger alone only changed
significantly with grip force at frequencies
above 1000 Hz.

2.2.3 Effect of Material Thickness

Figure 14 shows the mean effect on the
transmissibility of two material thicknesses
(3 mm and 9 mm), obtained from measurements
on six subjects using a 15 N grip force. A
three-fold increase in the material thickness may be expected to reduce its stiffness to one-third and so tend to reduce the
resonance frequency by approximately $1/\sqrt{3}$,

depending on the impedance of the finger.
This is consistent with the data shown in
Fig. 14. Although a similar trend was
found with a 5 N grip force, the magnitude
of the difference was less predictable.

2.2.4 Prototype Anti-Vibration Glove

A prototype anti-vibration glove was
constructed from a common lightweight glove
with ∿2 mm thick chrome leather palm and
finger faces, and a cotton material back.
Pieces of 12 mm thick medium-hardness, open-
cell rubber were adhered to the leather palm
and fingers of the glove, and two 1.5 cm
square pieces to the base of the first and
second digits (see Fig. 15). A single
5×1.5 cm rectangular piece was attached
across the base of both the third and fourth
digits, a similar 5×1.5 cm piece along the
thumb, and two pieces, one 12×3.5 cm and
the other 7×3.5 cm, across the palm. The
outer edges of each piece of rubber was cut
so as to allow a virtually unimpeded grip
by the empty hand. There was no rubber
over the extremities of the fingers.

The static stiffness of the rubber
material was determined from load/compres-
sion curves obtained by applying a force of
up to 68 N to a 10 mm by 20 mm sample. Over
the range of pressures employed (less than
5×10^4 Pa), the material sample was approximately linear with a stiffness of approximately 1.5×10^4 N/m. (The effective stiffness of this type of material varies with

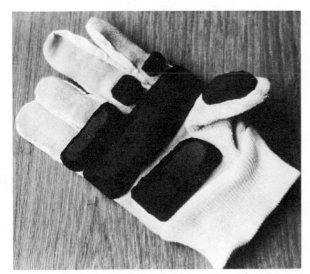

Fig. 15   Prototype anti-vibration glove.

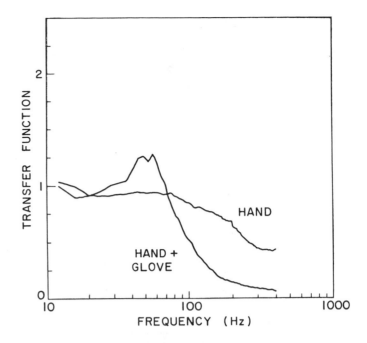

Fig. 16   Comparison of mean transmissibility through the hand and through the gloved hand. Data from 8 subjects using a 46 N push force.

sample size and compressive force, and for this sample became non-linear above about 12 N.) The damping ratio of the material was determined from the logarithmic decrement measured by dropping an accelerometer, secured to a weight, onto a 12×7.5 cm sample of material. A mean damping ratio of 0.11 was determined, from which a mean equivalent viscous damping coefficient of 30 Nm/s was calculated using the measured natural frequency and stiffness.

Figures 16 and 17 show the transmissibility through the hand to the knuckle with and without the glove when a 46 and 90 N push force were applied. The quotient transfer functions in Fig. 18 show that there was 20 to 30% amplification of vibration around 50 Hz for both push forces, but attenuation at all frequencies above about 75 Hz. At frequencies above 120 Hz, there was more than 50% attenuation. The mean and standard deviation from measurements on eight subjects are shown in Fig. 19 for a push force of 45 N.

These results show that the prototype glove provided attenuation which might be beneficial for operators of some tools. However, other transfer functions, different material thickness, sizes and locations would be required in many cases. It is therefore desirable to develop a method of predicting the transfer functions of glove-like materials from a knowledge of their physical properties.

2.3   Prediction Methods

Many alternative methods of predicting glove transfer functions could be developed. Two of the more attractive methods are to use a) lumped parameter models of the glove, hand and arm; and b) the measured dynamic properties of the hand and glove.

2.3.1   Predictions from Lumped Parameter Models of Glove, Hand and Arm

It has already been noted that a single-degree-of-freedom model in which the hand is represented by a rigid mass cannot usefully predict glove transmissibility. The next most simple model is a two-degrees-of-freedom system in which the hand is represented by a single mass-spring-damper system supported by a similar mass-spring-damper system representing the glove.

By selecting values of 1 g, 2×10^4 N/m and 30 Ns/m for the material and 10 g, 2×10^4 N/m and 30 Ns/m for the hand, it was possible to obtain a reasonable empirical fit to the measured transmissibility to the fingernail of a subject participating in the experiment described in Section 2.1.3 (see Fig. 20). These model parameters were then used to predict the transmissibility through the material alone. This prediction is compared with the measured quotient transfer function in Fig. 21.

The measured and predicted data in Fig. 21 suggest that this simple method may have some value. However, hand impedance is not well represented by a single-degree-of-freedom model and, more important, is highly variable, depending on the factors discussed in Section 1. A more powerful, though more complex, prediction method might be based on the stiffness and damping of the material combined with the measured impedance of the hand.

Griffin et al.: Dynamic response

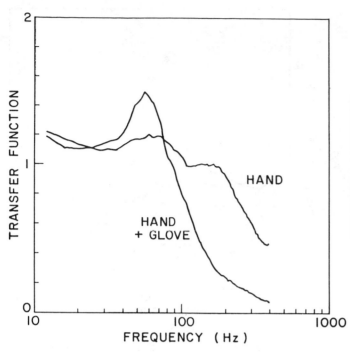

Fig. 17 Comparison of mean transmissibility through the hand and through the gloved hand. Data from eight subjects using a 90 N push force.

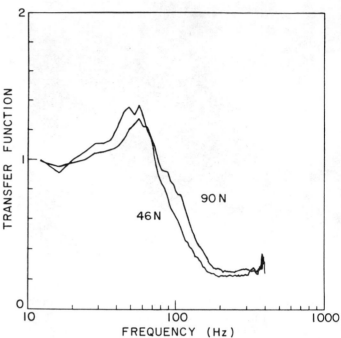

Fig. 18 Mean glove quotient transfer function (moduli). Data from eight subjects using a 46 N and a 90 N push force.

2.3.2 Predictions Using the Measured Dynamic Properties of the Hand and Glove

Depending on the assumptions made, several alternative mathematical procedures for predicting glove transmissibility from impedance quantities are available. Many predictions of the data shown in Figs. 16 to 18 have been attempted. For some subjects, it has been possible to obtain good estimates of glove transmissibility from the measured hand impedance. However, this has not always been the case and further analysis is required to determine the reasons for the discrepancies and to decide which assumptions are valid.

There is a need for a prediction procedure which is both accurate and simple. It will be important that the measures or models of hand-arm impedance used in the predictions are appropriate for the conditions in which a glove is to be used.

III CONCLUSIONS

The dynamic response of the hand-arm system is dependent on the subject, his posture, hand grip, and push-pull force. These factors may therefore also influence the transmission of vibration through gloves. A technique for determining glove transfer functions has been evolved and

appears to provide reliable data. In addition, a prototype glove has been developed to demonstrate that attenuation of high frequency vibration is possible.

The design of anti-vibration gloves requires simple procedures for predicting their transfer functions. The procedures must define both the method of measuring the relevant physical properties of the glove material, and how they may be used to predict the vibration isolation (and amplification) of a glove when worn on the hand. Such predictions must encompass the wide range of hand-arm dynamic responses that occur when a glove is used with a vibratory tool.

Since gloves tend to increase the vibration level at low frequencies and decrease the level at high frequencies, it is necessary to make assumptions concerning the relative importance of different vibration frequencies to assess their performance. If, for example, a frequency weighting corresponding to the limits defined in currently proposed standards is used, it is possible to assess gloves by means of the following relation:

$$\text{Glove Isolation Effectiveness } \% = \frac{\left\{\int_{f=8}^{f=1000} G_{hh}(f)s^2(f)df\right\}^{\frac{1}{2}}}{\left\{\int_{f=8}^{f=1000} G_{gg}(f)s^2(f)df\right\}^{\frac{1}{2}}} \times 100 \quad (2)$$

Griffin et al.: Dynamic response

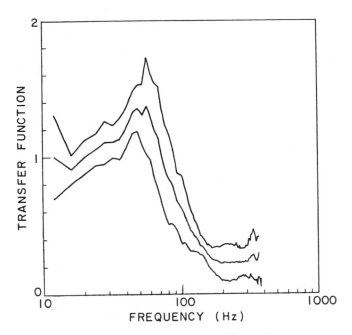

Fig. 19 Mean value (±SD) of the glove quotient transfer function (modulus). Data from eight subjects using a 45 N push force.

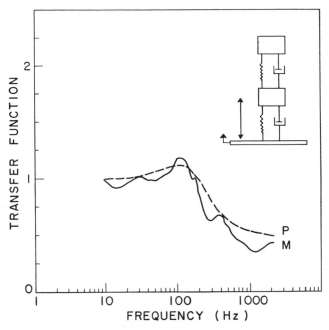

Fig. 21 Comparison of measured (M) and predicted (P) material transfer functions (moduli) using the two-degrees-of-freedom model shown and the index finger.

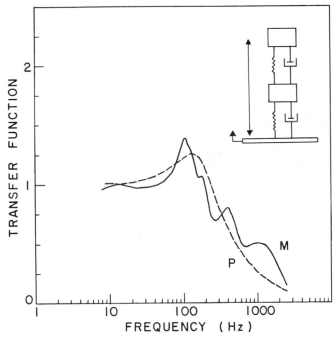

Fig. 20 Comparison of measured (M) and fitted (P) transmissibility to the fingernail of the index finger using the two-degrees-of-freedom model shown.

where $G_{hh}(f)$ is the power spectral density of vibration entering the hand, $G_{gg}(f)$ is the power spectral density of vibration entering the glove, and $S(f)$ is the hand-arm frequency weighting function. The above equation also demonstrates the importance of the frequency of the vibration on the tool to the evaluation of the isolation provided by a glove. Using the measurement procedures defined here, this mathematical expression may be used to assess the suitability of existing gloves for use with any tool. Alternatively, the concept may be included in a simple prediction procedure, so that measures of the properties of a glove, combined with data on the spectral content of the vibration, can be used to predict glove isolation effectiveness.

REFERENCES

1. Miwa T. Studies in hand protectors for portable vibrating tools, 1: measurements of the attenuation effect of porous materials. Ind Health (Japan) 1964; 2: 95-105.
2. Miwa T. Studies of hand protectors for portable vibrating tools, 2: simulations of porous elastic materials and their applications to hand protectors. Ind Health (Japan) 1964; 2: 106-123.

Griffin et al.: Dynamic response

3. Konecny F, Vejdelkova V. Individual protection against the noise and vibration associated with working with pneumatic tools. Rudy 1969; 17: 50-54.
4. Cvizba J. Vibration-damping handles. Ohrana truda i social'noe strahovanie 1971; 6: 40.
5. USSR Standard. System of Safety Engineering. Means of Personal Protections of Hands from Vibration. Method of Efficiency Definition. GOST 18728, 1973.
6. USSR Standard. System of Standards on Safety Engineering. Means for Personal Protection of Hands from Vibration. General Technical Specification. GOST 12.4.002-74, 1974.
7. Suggs CW. Modelling of the dynamic characteristics of the hand-arm system. In: Taylor W, ed. The Vibration Syndrome. London; Academic Press, 1974: 169-186.
8. Mikulinskji AM, Radzjukevic TM, Scjmam LS. A method of laboratory evaluation of vibration-protection devices for tools vibrating at high frequencies. Gig Sanit 1974; 4: 75-78.
9. Vlkova L, Pachner P, Danickova H, Kocianova M. Occupational traumatic vasoneurosis when stitching engine blocks. Pracov Lek 1974; 26: 374-377.
10. Cempel C. Criteria on the minimum dynamical effects for the operator's hand-tool system. Zagadnienia Drgan Nieliniowych 1975; 16: 165-171.
11. Cundiff JS. Energy dissipation in human hand-arm exposed to random vibration. J Acoust Soc Am 1976; 59: 212-214.
12. Krause P, Popov K. Investigation on the lessening of vibration action with an elastic coating on the hand grip of a motor chain saw. Ergonomische Berichte 1977; 15: 14-18.
13. Tattermusch W. The Effectiveness of Vibration Safety Gloves and Elastic Handgrip, Including Analytical and Measurement Technique Methods for their Determination. Zentralinstitut für Arbeitsschutz beim Staatssekretariat für Arbeit und Löhne (ZIAS) Report 784, 1978.
14. Miwa T, Yonekawa Y, Kanada K. Vibration isolators for portable vibrating tools, part 4: vibration isolation gloves. Ind Health (Japan) 1979; 17: 141-152.
15. Macfarlane CR. The vibration response of gloves and the human hand and arm. United Kingdom Informal Group Meeting on Human Response to Vibration. Royal Aircraft Establishment, Farnborough, 1979. (unpublished).
16. Macfarlane CR. Anti-vibration gloves and the dynamic response of the human hand-arm. United Kingdom Informal Group Meeting on Human Response to Vibration. Univ. College, Swansea, 1980. (unpublished).
17. Norman CD. Dynamic response of the hand-arm. Univ. of Southampton, 1979. MSc Thesis. (unpublished).
18. International Organization for Standardization. Principles for the Measurement and the Evaluation of Human Exposure to Vibration Transmitted to the Hand. Draft International Standard ISO/DIS 5349, 1979.
19. Griffin MJ. Hand-arm vibration standards and dose-effect relationships. In: Brammer AJ, Taylor W, eds. Vibration Effects on the Hand and Arm in Industry. New York: Wiley, 1982.
20. Molloy CT. Use of four-pole parameters in vibration calculation. J Acoust Soc Am 1957; 29: 843-853.
21. Crede CE, Ruzicka JE. Theory of vibration isolation. In: Harris CM, Crede CE, eds. Shock and Vibration Handbook. New York: McGraw Hill, 1976.

DISCUSSION

R.A. Willoughby: In my opinion, some key parameters have been disclosed concerning the design requirements for systems to attenuate hand-arm vibration. It appears from several studies that the frequency range of interest is 50 to 200 Hz (where most vasoconstriction occurs); the apparent mass of the hand is about 0.1 kg; typical hand grip forces are approximately 25 N; and the vibration direction is commonly axial to the forearm. Do these values define reasonable design parameters, or are there others that need to be identified?

Authors' Response: Over the frequency range 50 to 200 Hz the apparent mass of the hand will depend on hand posture, grip and push forces and intersubject variability but is likely to be approximately 0.2 kg. It seems highly desirable to design so as to minimize grip force in all situations. The arm angle in relation to the principal axis of vibration appears to be most important at low frequencies. Vibration below about 25 Hz may be associated with bone and joint injury rather than VWF, and the avoidance of situations in which this vibration acts along the arm seems desirable.

P. Lord: Could you comment on how the apparent stiffness of the hand is influenced by the factors you examined?

Authors' Response: The measures used in this work were apparent mass and mechanical impedance. The dynamic stiffness may be estimated from the relations shown in Table 1. The effects on dynamic stiffness of inter-subject variability, posture, grip and push forces will be similar to the effects on apparent mass. However the influence of vibration frequency will be different.

Three- and Four-Degrees-of-Freedom Models of the Vibration Response of the Human Hand

D. D. Reynolds and R. J. Falkenberg

ABSTRACT: Three- and four-degrees-of-freedom, lumped parameter models have been developed for the vibrational response of the human hand. Numerical curve-fitting techniques were employed to establish model parameters that correlated best with the measured dynamic compliance of the human hand in the frequency range from 5 to 1000 Hz. Experimental values for the dynamic compliance were obtained in a field study of 75 foundry workers. The fit to the experimental data was generally better with the four-degrees-of-freedom model, though the predicted dynamic compliance is still inaccurate at frequencies of less than 20 Hz in the Z direction. The parameters of both models can be related to the main physiological structures of the hand, and suggest that the hand and arm are effectively decoupled at frequencies above approximately 70 Hz.

RESUME: Des modèles à paramètres composés à trois et quatre degrés de liberté ont été mis au point pour décrire la réaction de la main humaine aux vibrations. Les techniques numériques d'ajustage de courbes ont été utilisées pour établir les paramètres du modèle qui corrélaient le mieux avec la souplesse dynamique de la main humaine dans la gamme des fréquences de 5 à 1000 Hz. Des valeurs expérimentales de la souplesse dynamique ont été obtenues dans une étude sur le terrain de 75 travailleurs de fonderie. La correspondance aux données expérimentales était généralement supérieure dans le cas du modèle à quatre degrés de liberté, bien que la souplesse dynamique prédite soit toujours imprécise à des fréquences inférieures à 20 Hz dans la direction Z. Les paramètres des deux modèles peuvent être reliés aux principales structures physiologiques de la main et indiquent que la main et le bras sont effectivement découplés à des fréquences supérieures à environ 70 Hz.

INTRODUCTION

Vibration-induced health problems are common among workers who use hand-held tools, such as chain saws, chipping hammers, and grinders. One of the most important is Raynaud's Phenomenon of occupational origin, or vibration-induced white finger (VWF), a disorder that becomes progressively more severe with continuing exposure (1). In order to develop meaningful standards for exposure of the hand to vibration, both the vibration of hand tools and the response of the hand-arm system when coupled to a tool must be better understood. The purpose of this paper is to discuss the development of more accurate models for the vibration response of the human hand-arm system.

Past investigators have used measurements of transmissibility and mechanical impedance to study the characteristics of the hand-arm system. To obtain the transmissibility, the transfer function between the acceleration at the driving point and at other locations is measured (2,3). Previous studies have shown that vibration entering the hand is confined primarily to the hands and fingers at frequencies above 100 Hz. In studies of the mechanical impedance of the hand, the driving point acceleration and force are measured and the dynamic compliance (displacement/force) computed. Several investigators have used the latter method (4-12), and some of the most comprehensive studies have been conducted by Reynolds, Keith, and Basel.

One of the major limitations of previous investigations has been the small number of subjects, so that the results may not be representative of the population at large. Most studies have been carried out in universities and the measurements have generally been on student populations. In

Table 1. Mean Values for the Dynamic Compliance of the Hand Obtained when Gripping the Large Handle with a Force of 25.4 N.

1/3 Octave-Band Centre Frequency (Hz)	X Direction $10^5 \cdot$X/F (m/N)	Phase (°)	Y Direction $10^5 \cdot$X/F (m/N)	Phase (°)	Z Direction $10^5 \cdot$X/F (m/N)	Phase (°)
6.3	53.3	50	31.2	46.9	27.8	58.5
8	37.6	48.7	21.6	54.2	17.6	60
10	27.6	48.2	16.7	65.5	12.2	59.9
12.5	20.3	46.3	15.1	62	8.66	69.3
16	13.8	40.4	10.8	51.5	7.9	61.7
20	9.48	35	6.42	54	5.7	48.6
25	6.22	31.7	4.01	68.5	3.18	47.7
31.5	3.83	32.5	3	87.9	1.7	64.3
40	2.57	34.9	2.92	98.4	1.36	84
50	1.75	35.5	2.71	97.3	1.3	87.4
63	1.11	39.1	2.4	93.9	1.11	89.2
80	0.653	56.2	0.205	87.3	0.999	91.2
100	0.511	70.4	1.51	86.9	0.926	83.3
125	0.442	75	1.15	89.6	0.751	69.4
160	0.376	75.9	0.911	89.2	0.509	57.4
200	0.32	70.8	0.751	84.5	0.315	55.3
250	0.259	63.7	0.591	81	0.2	62.7
315	0.178	58.5	0.435	80.5	0.138	69.9
400	0.116	59.3	0.352	73.4	0.109	73.3
500	0.078	61.3	0.254	62.8	0.087	71.5
630	0.0515	62.9	0.158	53.4	0.0642	67.5
800	0.0334	67.2	0.0974	45.7	0.0441	66
1000	0.0297	68.9	0.0582	31.4	0.0337	53.7

Values of X/F in column 2, row 1, etc. are X/F = 53.3×10^{-5}, etc.

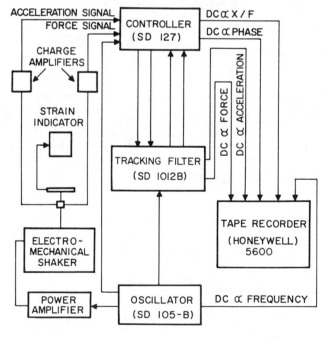

Fig. 1 Block diagram of the displacement mobility data acquisition system.

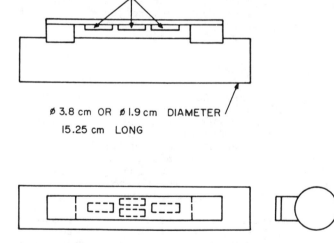

Fig. 2 Handle instrumented with strain gauges.

this investigation, dynamic compliance measurements were made on 75 foundry workers who use pneumatic chipping hammers and grinders, as part of a multidisciplinary

Reynolds et al.: Models of the hand

Table 2. Mean Values for the Dynamic Compliance of the Hand Obtained when Gripping the Small Handle with a Force of 25.4 N.

1/3 Octave-Band Centre Frequency (Hz)	X Direction $10^5 \cdot X/F$ (m/N)	Phase (°)	Y Direction $10^5 \cdot X/F$ (m/N)	Phase (°)	Z Direction $10^5 \cdot X/F$ (m/N)	Phase (°)
6.3	74.1	57.3	68.2	46	37	57.9
8	52.9	55	51.2	43.1	23.3	56
10	37.6	53.5	37.9	33.7	16	55.1
12.5	28.6	50.7	23.2	31.3	11.3	61.8
16	19.5	49	12.8	41.1	9.01	53.6
20	14.3	48.9	8.82	53	5.98	47
25	10.9	46.9	6.66	63.4	3.55	48.8
31.5	7.96	39.8	5.29	69.5	2.05	62.6
40	5.47	31.9	4.03	73.1	1.56	81.4
50	3.35	27	3.14	80.4	1.35	95
63	1.98	29.8	2.56	89.9	1.32	109
80	1.17	40.2	2.2	89.9	1.47	109
100	0.788	48.5	1.76	91.5	1.4	93
125	0.555	57.4	1.4	94.2	1.1	75.5
160	0.396	68.3	1.12	96.2	0.717	65.2
200	0.307	75.8	0.916	96.2	0.442	64.6
250	0.25	81.3	0.765	96.5	0.283	71.6
315	0.205	83.4	0.651	93.3	0.197	81.1
400	0.167	82.1	0.55	84.7	0.162	85.5
500	0.129	79.6	0.419	74.6	0.133	83.9
630	0.0974	73.6	0.282	67.3	0.108	76
800	0.0674	62.3	0.184	60.1	0.0781	60.4
1000	0.0429	49.3	0.13	48.9	0.0496	42.6

Values of X/F in column 2, row 1, etc. are $X/F = 74.1 \times 10^{-5}$, etc.

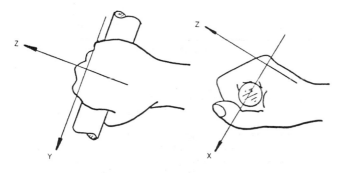

Fig. 3 Coordinate system for the hand-arm system.

field study of several hundred workers using pneumatic hand tools (13).

Three- and four-degrees-of-freedom models of the driving-point dynamic compliance of the hand were then investigated. The three-degrees-of-freedom model provided improved values for the parameters of the model developed by Keith and Reynolds (10, 11). An examination of their work revealed an error in the computer programme. Even though this error has led to a revision of the model, the present investigation has verified that their conclusions are essentially correct. The four-degrees-of-freedom model was developed to obtain a more accurate fit to the compliance data from human hands.

I DYNAMIC COMPLIANCE MEASUREMENTS

A block diagram of the apparatus used for these measurements is shown in Fig. 1. The foundry workers were asked to grasp an instrumented handle, which was then vibrated by an electro-mechanical shaker. The linkage between the handle and the shaker contained a force transducer and an accelerometer (impedance head). To measure grip force, the handle was instrumented with a narrow beam to which strain gauges were attached, as shown in Fig. 2. The beam was calibrated by applying a force at the centre of the span using a point-loading device. The workers wore their usual work clothing during the experiment, so that any influence of clothing on the response of the hand-arm system was typical of that occurring during normal working conditions. Two handles were used: a 3.8 cm diameter "large" and a 1.9 cm diameter "small" handle, to simulate the handle and chisel respectively, of a pneumatic chipping hammer. The large handle was tubular with a 0.64 cm

Reynolds et al.: Models of the hand

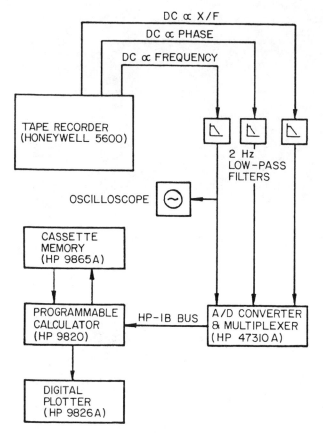

Fig. 4 Data analysis system.

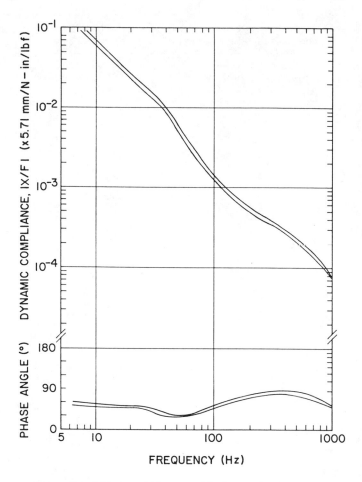

Fig. 5 90% confidence limits of the dynamic compliance (magnitude and phase) from 75 foundry workers: X direction, 25.4 N force gripping the 1.9 cm diameter handle.

wall thickness and the small handle was solid. Both were constructed of aluminium, to achieve low mass.

The workers were instructed to grasp the large or small handle in the manner they would normally hold the handle or chisel of a chipping hammer. The subjects maintained their grip force at a predetermined constant level throughout the test. To help them achieve this, the workers were permitted to watch a voltmeter that displayed the output of the handle-mounted strain gauges. A grip force of 25.4 N was used, which is typical of that used by the chippers and grinders in their work.

The handle was vibrated in a single direction while the frequency was varied continuously from 5 to 1000 Hz. The sweep rate of the sweep-frequency oscillator, a Spectral Dynamics (SD) type 105A, was maintained at the same value for all tests. The mass of the vibrating handle was electronically cancelled by a special circuit on the mechanical impedance transfer function measurement controller (SD 127 MZ/TFA).

Six measurements were conducted on each subject, in three orthogonal directions, with each handle. The coordinate system used is shown in Fig. 3 and is almost identical to that proposed by the ISO (14), differing only in that the Y and Z

directions are rotated slightly to align them with the axes of the handle.

The signals from the force transducer and accelerometer were fed into the mechanical-impedance transfer-function measurement system. The ratio between the displacement and force amplitudes, X/F, the phase angle between the displacement and the acceleration, and the frequency of the signal were produced by this apparatus. These signals were recorded on magnetic tape using a multi-channel FM tape recorder: real-time plots of X/F and phase as a function of frequency were also obtained. Calibration information was recorded on tape at the start of each day and consisted of a frequency sweep from 5 to 1000 Hz when a known reference mass was attached to the shaker. The values of X/F for the reference mass at 5 Hz and a phase angle of zero, and at 151 and 1000 Hz and a phase angle 180 degrees were also recorded. This information was used for scaling the data during the digitization process, which employed a

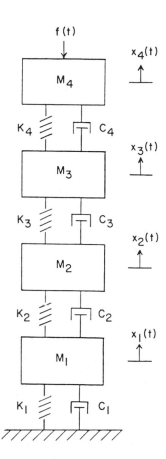

Fig. 6 Conceptual schematic of a four-degrees-of-freedom mass-spring-damper system.

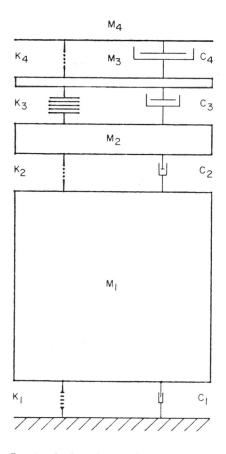

Fig. 7 Scaled schematic representation of the four-degrees-of-freedom model: X direction, 25.4 N palm grip of the 1.9 cm diameter handle.

Hewlett Packard (HP) 9820A calculator and the peripheral equipment shown in Fig. 4. The programme for digitizing the data was started manually at the beginning of each recorded frequency sweep, at which time the low-pass filtered analogue signals (X/F, phase and frequency) were sampled in rapid succession and stored in the calculator memory. The programme was terminated automatically when 1000 Hz was reached. The digital data were then recorded onto magnetic tape (cassette) data files for storage.

The X/F data were sampled at sequential frequencies, but the digitized frequencies were not always the same for each data file. To obtain values for X/F and phase at the preferred 1/3 octave-band centre frequencies, a spline function was used to interpolate between these frequencies (15). The calculated function was compared with the analogue curves recorded at the time of the X/F and phase measurements, to ensure that the reconstructed curves were the same as those originally measured.

The mean and 90% confidence limits of the dynamic compliance, |X/F| and phase

angle, were then calculated at each 1/3 octave-band centre frequency for the 75 foundry workers. Figure 5 shows a typical set of curves for the X direction obtained with the 1.9 cm diameter handle. Tables 1 and 2 list the mean values as a function of the 1/3 octave-band centre frequencies between 6.3 and 1000 Hz, for the three orthogonal directions and two handle diameters.

II THE MODEL

The hand and arm form a very complex, continuous, nonhomogeneous system consisting of skin, muscle, bone, etc., and an accurate model must contain all these components. However, past investigations have shown that the hand-arm system can be modeled as a lumped-parameter, mass-excited system. In other words, it can be represented by a number of discrete masses, linear springs and viscous dampers. The accuracy of such a model will be related to its complexity, that is, to the number of discrete elements employed. In previous

Reynolds et al.: Models of the hand

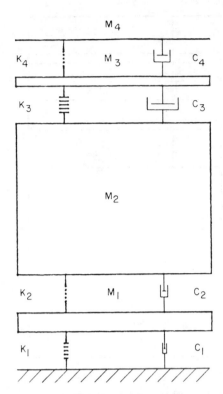

Fig. 8 Scaled schematic representation of the four-degrees-of-freedom model: Y direction, 25.4 N palm grip of the 1.9 cm diameter handle.

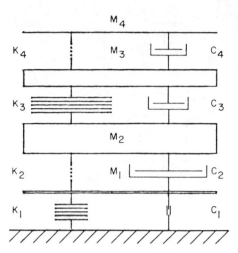

Fig. 9 Scaled schematic representation of the four-degrees-of-freedom model: Z direction, 25.4 N palm grip of the 1.9 cm diameter handle.

M_1 - M_4, the four springs are K_1 - K_4, the four viscous resistances are C_1 - C_4, and the displacements of masses M_1 - M_4 as a function of time are $x_1(t)$, $x_2(t)$, $x_3(t)$ and $x_4(t)$, respectively.

The solution of these equations, which yields the displacement amplitude of mass #4, X_4, when driven by a harmonic force $f(t)$ of amplitude F, is given in the Appendix. Here it is shown that the driving point dynamic compliance may be written in terms of an amplitude:

$$\left|\frac{X_4}{F}\right| = (G_9^2 + H_9^2)^{\frac{1}{2}} \qquad (5)$$

and a phase angle:

$$\theta = \tan^{-1}(H_9/G_9) , \qquad (6)$$

where G_9 and H_9 are defined by eqns. A56 and A57.

A computer programme was then written to calculate the driving-point dynamic compliance frequency response from 5 Hz to 1000 Hz and to construct a Bode plot. In order to describe fully the response and transmissibility of the hand-arm system, it was necessary to examine the dynamic compliance of all four masses. The remaining three transfer dynamic compliances were developed in a similar manner to X_4/F using Cramer's Rule, and computer programmes were written to construct Bode plots of the frequency response functions.

III RESULTS AND DISCUSSION

The results of this study differ somewhat from the results of earlier attempts

analyses, one-, two- and three-degrees-of-freedom models have been developed by fitting the parameters of the models to measurements of dynamic compliance and phase, by trial and error. Because of the errors found in the three-degrees-of-freedom model reported in the literature (11), results are presented here for both three- and four-degrees-of-freedom models. However, in view of the similarity of the models, only the analytical development of the latter is discussed.

A four-degrees-of-freedom mass-excited system is shown schematically in Fig. 6. From force equilibrium, the equations of motion are:

$$M_4\ddot{x}_4(t) + C_4\dot{x}_4(t) - C_4\dot{x}_3(t) + K_4x_4(t) - K_4x_3(t) = f(t) \qquad (1)$$

$$M_3\ddot{x}_3(t) + (C_4+C_3)\dot{x}_3(t) - C_3\dot{x}_2(t) - C_4\dot{x}_4(t) + (K_4+K_3)x_3(t)$$
$$-K_3x_2(t) - K_4x_4(t) = 0 \qquad (2)$$

$$M_2\ddot{x}_2(t) + (C_3+C_2)\dot{x}_2(t) - C_3\dot{x}_3(t) - C_2\dot{x}_1(t) + (K_3+K_2)x_2(t)$$
$$-K_3x_3(t) - K_2x_1(t) = 0 \qquad (3)$$

$$M_1\ddot{x}_1(t) + (C_2+C_1)\dot{x}_1(t) - C_2\dot{x}_2(t) + (K_2+K_1)x_1(t)$$
$$-K_2x_2(t) = 0 . \qquad (4)$$

In these equations, the four masses are

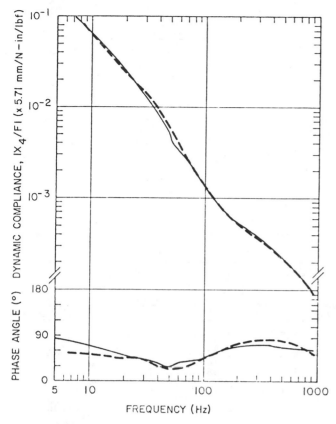

Fig. 10 Comparison of the measured
driving-point dynamic compliance, magnitude and phase, (dashed curve) with
predictions of the four-degrees-of-
freedom mechanical model (solid curve):
X direction, 25.4 N palm grip of the
1.9 cm diameter handle.

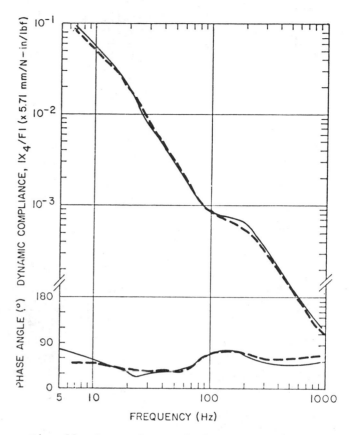

Fig. 11 Comparison of the measured
driving-point dynamic compliance, magnitude and phase, (dashed curve) with
predictions of the four-degrees-of-
freedom mechanical model (solid curve):
X direction, 25.4 N palm grip of the
3.8 cm diameter handle.

at modeling the hand-arm system, but they
are in general agreement with subjective
assessments and measurements of its transmissibility reported elsewhere (3,6,8,16).
These studies revealed that vibration
entering the hand is transmitted as far as
the shoulder, and can be felt in the forearm region at frequencies between 19 and
85 Hz. Thus, at frequencies below 100 Hz,
a large portion of the hand-arm system is
in motion. The same effects are seen in
the four-degrees-of-freedom model.

The three-degrees-of-freedom lumped-
parameter model of Keith showed that the
hand-arm system could be approximated by a
model weighing, at most 0.36 kg (10). The
values of the parameters reported by Keith
are, however, slightly inaccurate due to a
programming error. Previous work by other
investigators also indicated that the hand-
arm system contained a mass of less than
0.5 kg (5,7). These studies demonstrated
that the observed hand-arm compliance did

not involve the entire hand-arm system but,
rather, only local effects in the hand.
The three-degrees-of-freedom model reported
here is very insensitive to the value of
M_1, which can vary from small to relatively
large values without changing the dynamic
compliance curves. Our results give possible maximum weights to the hand-arm
system of 2.24 kg in the vertical (X) direction, 0.85 kg in the axial (Y) direction,
and 0.28 kg in the horizontal (Z) direction.
These weights suggest that the measured
driving-point dynamic compliance involves
the response of the arm as well as the
hand. However, the total weight of the
model can be significantly reduced (in the
range of values reported by previous investigators) without changing the system
response, by decreasing the value of M_1.

A listing of the parameters for the
three-degrees-of-freedom model is given in
Tables 3 to 5. The fit of the model to the
dynamic compliance data was better for the

Reynolds et al.: Models of the hand

Table 3. Three-Degrees-of-Freedom Model Parameters for the X Direction.

Handle Diameter (cm)	1.91	1.91	1.91	3.81	1.91	1.91
Grip Type	Finger	Palm	Palm	Palm	Finger	Palm
Grip Force (N)	8.9	8.9	25.4	25.4	35.6	35.6
M_1 (kg)	1.75	1.75	1.75	1.75	1.75	1.75
M_2 (kg)	0.105	0.298	0.21	0.368	0.175	0.263
M_3 (kg)	0.053	0.053	0.053	0.114	0.035	0.061
$10^{-5} \cdot K_1$ (N/m)	1.75	1.75	1.75	1.75	1.75	1.75
K_2 (N/m)	175	175	175	175	175	175
$10^{-5} \cdot K_3$ (N/m)	2.45	1.23	1.75	1.23	3.5	2.98
C_1 (N·s/m)	350	350	350	350	158	175
C_2 (N·s/m)	54.3	52.5	43.8	52.5	70.1	78.8
C_3 (N·s/m)	105	158	175	175	193	175

1) Values of K_1 and K_3 in column 1, etc. are $K_1 = 1.75 \times 10^5$ and $K_3 = 2.45 \times 10^5$
2) For definition of grip type see Ref. 11.

Table 4. Three-Degrees-of-Freedom Model Parameters for the Y Direction.

Handle Diameter (cm)	1.91	1.91	1.91	3.81	1.91	1.91
Grip Type	Finger	Palm	Palm	Palm	Finger	Palm
Grip Force (N)	8.9	8.9	25.4	25.4	35.6	35.6
M_1 (kg)	0.018	0.018	0.018	0.018	0.018	0.018
M_2 (kg)	0.14	0.351	0.526	0.789	0.105	0.351
M_3 (kg)	0.012	0.009	0.011	0.044	0.009	0.009
$10^{-4} \cdot K_1$ (N/m)	1.75	4.38	7.88	7.88	4.38	2.63
K_2 (N/m)	175	175	175	175	175	175
$10^{-4} \cdot K_3$ (N/m)	2.63	1.75	1.75	2.19	7.88	3.06
C_1 (N·s/m)	123	613	35	17.5	613	876
C_2 (N·s/m)	52.5	52.5	35	52.5	70.1	70.1
C_3 (N·s/m)	43.8	52.5	87.6	87.6	70.1	70.1

1) Values of K_1 and K_3 in column 1, etc. are $K_1 = 1.75 \times 10^4$ and $K_3 = 2.63 \times 10^4$, etc.
2) For definition of grip type see Ref. 11.

Table 5. Three-Degrees-of-Freedom Model Parameters for the Z Direction.

Handle Diameter (cm)	1.91	1.91	1.91	3.81	1.91	1.91
Grip Type	Finger	Palm	Palm	Palm	Finger	Palm
Grip Force (N)	8.9	8.9	25.4	25.4	35.6	35.6
M_1 (kg)	0.018	0.018	0.018	0.018	0.018	0.018
M_2 (kg)	0.105	0.14	0.158	0.175	0.131	0.158
M_3 (kg)	0.044	0.061	0.053	0.088	0.061	0.061
$10^{-4} \cdot K_1$ (N/m)	7.88	10.5	24.5	28	14	24.5
K_2 (N/m)	175	175	175	175	175	175
$10^{-5} \cdot K_3$ (N/m)	1.4	1.75	2.98	5.25	2.8	2.8
C_1 (N·s/m)	105	87.6	70.1	175	105	70.1
C_2 (N·s/m)	175	210	263	210	228	263
C_3 (N·s/m)	70.1	96.3	140	245	114	140

1) Values of K_1 and K_3 in column 1, etc. are $k_1 = 7.88 \times 10^4$ and $k_3 = 1.4 \times 10^5$, etc.
2) For definition of grip type see Ref. 11.

Reynolds et al.: Models of the hand

Table 6. Four-Degrees-of-Freedom Model Parameters for the X Direction.

Handle Diameter (cm)	1.91	1.91	1.91	3.81	1.91	1.91
Grip Type	Finger	Palm	Palm	Palm	Finger	Palm
Grip Force (N)	8.9	8.9	25.4	25.4	35.6	35.6
M_1 (kg)	1.75	1.75	1.75	1.75	1.75	1.75
M_2 (kg)	0.123	0.351	0.28	0.438	0.175	0.351
M_3 (kg)	0.088	0.088	0.088	0.175	0.14	0.14
M_4 (kg)	0.0018	0.0018	0.0018	0.0018	0.0018	0.0018
$10^{-4} \cdot K_1$ (N/m)	35	3.5	17.5	3.5	35	3.5
K_2 (N/m)	175	175	175	175	175	175
$10^{-5} \cdot K_3$ (N/m)	3.5	2.63	3.15	1.75	7.88	5.25
K_4 (N/m)	1750	1750	1750	1750	1750	1750
C_1 (N·s/m)	35	52.5	35	52.5	35	52.5
C_2 (N·s/m)	52.5	52.5	42	43.8	52.5	78.8
C_3 (N·s/m)	105	193	298	175	175	245
C_4 (N·s/m)	473	525	525	876	473	525

1) Values of K_1 and K_3 in column 1, etc. are $K_1 = 3.5 \times 10^5$ and $K_3 = 3.5 \times 10^5$
2) For definition of grip type see Ref. 11.

Table 7. Four-Degrees-of-Freedom Model Parameters for the Y Direction.

Handle Diameter (cm)	1.91	1.91	1.91	3.81	1.91	1.91
Grip Type	Finger	Palm	Palm	Palm	Finger	Palm
Grip Force (N)	8.9	8.9	25.4	25.4	35.6	35.6
M_1 (kg)	0.175	0.175	0.175	0.175	0.175	0.175
M_2 (kg)	0.158	0.473	1.4	1.4	0.351	1.23
M_3 (kg)	0.0175	0.0175	0.088	0.088	0.026	0.026
M_4 (kg)	0.0018	0.0018	0.0018	0.0018	0.0018	0.0018
$10^{-4} \cdot K_1$ (N/m)	1.3	0.876	3.5	2.6	8.8	2.6
K_2 (N/m)	175	175	175	175	175	175
$10^{-4} \cdot K_3$ (N/m)	5.3	4.4	8.8	5.3	16	8.8
K_4 (N/m)	1750	1750	1750	1750	1750	1750
C_1 (N·s/m)	140	263	17.5	140	263	140
C_2 (N·s/m)	87.6	70.1	52.5	87.6	70.1	87.6
C_3 (N·s/m)	70.1	70.1	280	140	158	123
C_4 (N·s/m)	140	140	140	263	140	140

1) Values of K_1 and K_3 in column 1, etc. are $K_1 = 1.3 \times 10^4$ and $K_3 = 5.3 \times 10^4$
2) For definition of grip type see Ref. 11.

X and Y directions than for the Z direction. In the Z direction, the phase agreement was poor below about 40 Hz and above about 400 Hz, and the amplitude agreement was poor below 20 Hz. In the Y direction, the predicted phase angle and amplitude were in agreement with the observed values, except at frequencies above 200 Hz where the calculated phase angle is high. In the X direction, the amplitude agreement is good throughout the spectrum and the phase angle agreement is good between 20 and 200 Hz.

These findings suggest that a four-degrees-of-freedom system may be needed to improve the agreement between a biodynamic model of the hand and arm and measurements on people.
Tables 6 to 8 give the parameters of the four-degrees-of-freedom model. Figures 7 to 9 are scaled schematic drawings of the results. The fit of the model to the dynamic compliance data was generally better in all three directions than for the three-degrees-of-freedom model. The agreement between the prediction of amplitude and phase angle

Reynolds et al.: Models of the hand

Table 8. Four-Degrees-of-Freedom Model Parameters for the Z Direction.

Handle Diameter (cm)	1.91	1.91	1.91	3.81	1.91	1.91
Grip Type	Finger	Palm	Palm	Palm	Finger	Palm
Grip Force (N)	8.9	8.9	25.4	25.4	35.6	35.6
M_1 (kg)	0.0175	0.0175	0.0175	0.0175	0.0175	0.0175
M_2 (kg)	0.07	0.28	0.28	0.351	0.175	0.351
M_3 (kg)	0.105	0.158	0.158	0.351	0.158	0.351
M_4 (kg)	0.0018	0.0018	0.0018	0.0018	0.0018	0.0018
$10^{-5} \cdot K_1$ (N/m)	1.1	1.9	3.5	5.3	2.6	4.9
K_2 (N/m)	175	175	175	175	175	175
$10^{-5} \cdot K_3$ (N/m)	3	5.3	8.8	11	7.9	11
K_4 (N/m)	175	175	175	175	175	175
C_1 (N·s/m)	140	105	1.8	1.8	140	1.8
C_2 (N·s/m)	438	876	701	701	701	1051
C_3 (N·s/m)	17.5	140	350	350	87.6	263
C_4 (N·s/m)	245	315	315	525	315	315

1) Values of K_1 and K_3 in column 1, etc. are $K_1 = 1.1 \times 10^5$ and $K_3 = 3 \times 10^5$
2) For definition of grip type see Ref. 11.

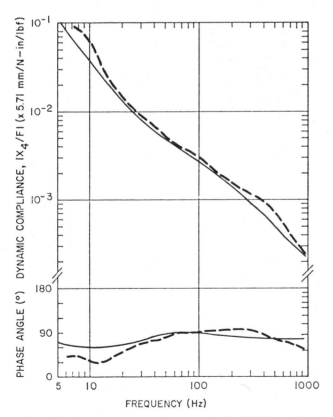

Fig. 12 Comparison of the measured driving-point
dynamic compliance, magnitude and phase, (dashed
curve) with predictions of the four-degrees-of-
freedom mechanical model (solid curve): Y
direction, 25.4 N palm grip of the 1.9 cm diameter handle.

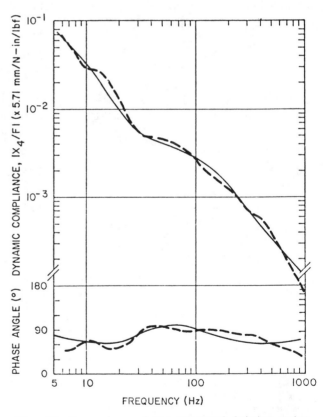

Fig. 13 Comparison of the measured driving-point
dynamic compliance, magnitude and phase, (dashed
curve) with predictions of the four-degrees-of-
freedom mechanical model (solid curve): Y
direction, 25.4 N palm grip of the 3.8 cm diameter handle.

Reynolds et al.: Models of the hand

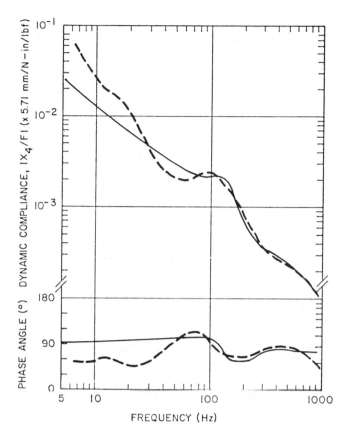

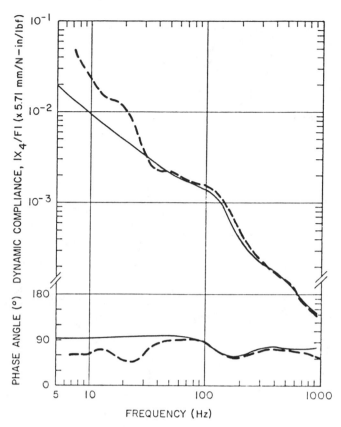

Fig. 14 Comparison of the measured
driving-point dynamic compliance, magnitude and phase, (dashed curve) with
predictions of the four-degrees-of-
freedom mechanical model (solid curve):
Z direction, 25.4 N palm grip of the
1.9 cm diameter handle.

Fig. 15 Comparison of the measured
driving-point dynamic compliance, magnitude and phase, (dashed curve) with
predictions of the four-degrees-of-
freedom mechanical model (solid curve):
Z direction, 25.4 N palm grip of the
3.8 cm diameter handle.

at low frequencies and the human data is
still poor in the Z direction. This
suggests that a five-, or more, degrees-of-
freedom model may be needed to describe
accurately the response of the hand-arm
system in this direction. Figures 10 to 15
show a comparison of the measured driving-
point dynamic-compliance components of the
hand-arm system and the four-degrees-of-
freedom mechanical model for a 25.4 N palm
grip and both handle diameters.

A little understanding of the physiology of the hand is required to appreciate
the significance of the model parameters.
The outer tissue of the fingers and hand
are composed of very dense, closely packed
cells in layers forming the epidermis and
dermis. Beneath the dermis is the subcutaneous tissue, where most of the veins,
arteries, and arterioles carrying blood and
fluids to and from the hand and fingers,
and the nerve endings in the hand and
fingers are located. The elastic bond
between the subcutaneous tissue and dermis

is fairly strong even though the former is
less dense. The muscles lie below the
subcutaneous tissue and the elastic bond
between them and the subcutaneous tissue is
very weak.

The four-degrees-of-freedom model for
the X direction consists of a large mass
M_1, with a relatively strong elastic
coupling to the ground, and three smaller
masses, M_2, M_3, and M_4. The elastic coupling between M_2 and M_3 is very strong, and
M_3 is coupled to M_4 by a spring of average
stiffness and a strong damping element.
It thus appears that M_4 and M_3 represent
the masses of the dermis and epidermis, and
K_4 and C_4 represent the stiffness and
damping associated with these tissues. The
strong coupling between the dermis and subcutaneous tissue is represented by K_3 and
C_3, so that M_2 represents the mass of the
subcutaneous tissue, and K_2 and C_2 the weak
elastic coupling between the subcutaneous
tissue and muscle. Hence M_1 probably represents the muscle mass of the hand, and

Reynolds et al.: Models of the hand

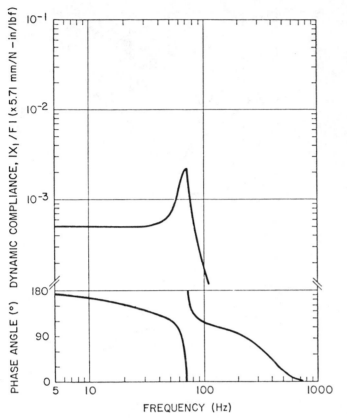

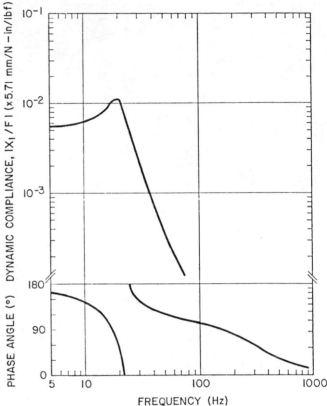

Fig. 16 Dynamic compliance (magnitude and phase) at mass #1 of the four-degrees-of-freedom mechanical model: X direction, 8.9 N finger grip of the 1.9 cm diameter handle.

Fig. 17 Dynamic compliance (magnitude and phase) at mass #1 of the four-degrees-of-freedom mechanical model: X direction, 8.9 N palm grip of the 1.9 cm diameter handle.

K_1 and C_1 the coupling between the muscle and bones. The magnitude of M_1 suggests that structures within the arm may also be included.

This interpretation of the model and the transmissibility studies imply that M_1 should vibrate only at low frequencies. The transfer dynamic compliance of M_1 rapidly decreases at frequencies above 80 Hz with the finger grip (Fig. 16), and above 30 Hz with the palm grip (Fig. 17). The transfer compliances also indicate that relative motion occurs between M_1 and M_2 throughout the frequency range, and between M_2 and M_3, and M_3 and M_4 at high frequencies. Thus at frequencies of less than 70 to 80 Hz for the finger grip, and 20 to 50 Hz for the palm grip, energy is transmitted into the arm from the hand, but at high frequencies the hand becomes decoupled from the arm, so that the vibration remains within the hand. This confirms the results of transmissibility studies and previous modeling work.

In the four-degrees-of-freedom model for the Y direction, M_1 is coupled to ground

by a spring of average stiffness. M_2 is a very large mass and is coupled to M_1 by a very weak spring, K_2. M_3 and M_4 are smaller masses; M_3 is coupled to M_2 by a comparatively stiff spring, and the coupling between M_3 and M_4 is weak. As in the previous case, M_4 and M_3 are believed to represent the masses of the dermis and epidermis, with K_4 and C_4 being the associated stiffness and damping of these tissues. M_2 represents the mass of the subcutaneous tissue and M_1 the muscle mass of the hand. K_3 and C_3 then represent the strong coupling between the skin and subcutaneous tissue, and K_2 and C_2 represent the weak coupling between the subcutaneous tissue and muscle.

The four-degrees-of-freedom model for the Z direction consists of a small mass M_1 coupled to ground by a stiff spring, a larger mass M_2 coupled to M_1 by a very weak spring, and two masses, M_3 and M_4, coupled to M_2 by a strong spring, and coupled to each other by a weak spring and large damper. As before, it is believed that M_4 and M_3 represent the masses of the epidermis and dermis, M_2 represents the mass of the subcutaneous tissue, and M_1 the muscle mass.

The results of this study also reveal an increase in the mass of the model system for the palm grip compared to the finger grip. In the X, Y and Z directions, the increase occurs in M_2, which is taken to represent the subcutaneous tissue. Trends in other parameters were not evident, though there seemed to be an increase in system mass with increasing grip force. Increasing the handle diameter was found to increase the mass of M_2, M_3, and M_4 in the X and Z directions, but had little effect on the model parameters in the Y direction.

IV CONCLUSIONS

1. The agreement between the measured and predicted driving-point dynamic compliance is better in the X and Y directions than in the Z direction, for both the three- and four-degrees-of-freedom models.
2. For the three-degrees-of-freedom model, the measured and predicted phase angles are in good agreement between 20 and 200 Hz in the X direction, between 40 and 400 Hz in the Z direction and above 20 Hz in the Y direction; and the amplitudes are in good agreement from 5 to 1000 Hz in the X and Y directions and above 20 Hz in the Z direction.
3. The fit to the experimental data is generally better in all three directions with the four-degrees-of-freedom model; however, the predicted phase angle and amplitude are still inaccurate at frequencies below 20 Hz in the Z direction.
4. The parameters of both models can be related to the physiology of the hand-arm system. In the three-degrees-of-freedom model, M_3 represents the mass of the dermis and epidermis, M_2 the mass of the subcutaneous tissue, and M_1 the muscle mass of the hand. In the four-degrees-of-freedom model, M_4 and M_3 represent the masses of the dermis and epidermis, M_2 again represents the mass of the subcutaneous tissue, and M_1 the muscle mass of the hand.
5. At frequencies of less than 70 to 80 Hz with the finger grip and 20 to 50 Hz with the palm grip, vibration entering the hand is transmitted to the arm, but at higher frequencies the hand becomes decoupled from the arm.

ACKNOWLEDGEMENTS

The research reported in this paper was carried out under NIOSH Contract No. 210-77-0165, while Dr. D.D. Reynolds was an Associate Professor in the Dept. of Mechanical Engineering at the Univ. of Pittsburg.

REFERENCES

1. In: Wasserman DE, Taylor W, Curry MG, eds. Proc of the Int Occup Hand-Arm Vibration Conf. Cincinnati, OH: Dept of Health and Human Services, 1977. (NIOSH publication no. 77-170).
2. Suggs CW. Modelling of the dynamic characteristic of the hand-arm system. In: Taylor W, ed. The Vibration Syndrome. London: Academic Press, 1974: 169-186.
3. Reynolds DD, Angevine EN. Hand-arm vibration, part II: vibration transmission characteristics of the hand-arm system. J Sound Vib 1977; 51: 255-265.
4. Dieckmann D. Ein mechanisches modell fur das schwengungserregte hand-arm system des menschen. Int Z Angew Physiol Einschl Arbeitsphysiol 1957; 17: 125-132.
5. Abrams CF. A study of the transmission of high frequency vibration in the human arm. North Carolina State Univ, 1968. MS Thesis. (unpublished).
6. Abrams CF, Suggs CW. Chain saw vibration: isolation and transmission through the human arm. Oral paper, Am Soc Agricultural Engineers. West Lafayette In: 1969. (unpublished).
7. Reynolds DD, Soedel W. Dynamic response of the hand-arm system to a sinusoidal input. J Sound Vib 1967; 21: 339-353.
8. Reynolds DD, Jokel CR. Hand-arm vibration - an engineering approach. Am Ind Hyg Assoc J 1974; 35: 613-622.
9. Jokel CR. Modelling the hand-arm system's response to vibration. Univ of Texas, 1973. MS Thesis. (unpublished).
10. Keith RH. An analytical model of the vibration characteristics of the hand-arm system. Univ of Texas, 1975. MS Thesis. (unpublished).
11. Reynolds DD, Keith RH. Hand-arm vibration, part I: analytical model of the vibration response characteristic of the hand. J Sound Vib 1977; 51: 237-253.
12. Basel RA. Hand tool vibration and vibration energy transmitted to the hands of pneumatic chipping hammer and pneumatic grinder operators during foundry casting cleaning operations. Univ of Pittsburgh, 1980. MS Thesis. (unpublished).
13. Wasserman D, Reynolds DD, Behrens V, Taylor W, Samueloff S, Basel R. Vibration White Finger Disease in US Workers Using Pneumatic Chipping and Grinding Hand Tools II: engineering testing. Cincinnati OH: Dept of Health and Human Services, 1981. (NIOSH publication no. 82-101).
14. International Organization for Standardization. Principles for the Measurement and the Evaluation of Human Exposure to Vibration Transmitted to the Hand. Draft International Standard ISO/DIS 5349, 1979.
15. Grenville TNE. Spline functions, interpolations and numerical quadrature. In: Ralston A, Wilf HS, eds. Mathematical Methods for Digital Computers. New York: Wiley, 1967.
16. Reynolds DD, Standlee KG, Angevine EN. Hand-arm vibration, part III: subjective response characteristics of individuals to hand-induced vibration. J Sound Vib 1977; 51: 267-282.

Reynolds et al.: Models of the hand

APPENDIX: SOLUTION OF THE EQUATIONS OF MOTION

The driving point dynamic compliance of the four-degree-of-freedom model can be obtained from the equations of motion in the following way. Assume harmonic force and displacement solutions of the form,

$$f(t) = Fe^{j\omega t} \tag{A1}$$

$$x_i(t) = X_i e^{j\omega t} \tag{A2}$$

$$\dot{x}_i(t) = j\omega X_i e^{j\omega t} \tag{A3}$$

$$\ddot{x}_i(t) = -\omega^2 X_i e^{j\omega t} \tag{A4}$$

where i = 1, 2, 3, 4. The equations of motion then become, in matrix form,

$$-\omega^2 e^{j\omega t}
\begin{vmatrix}
M_1 & 0 & 0 & 0 \\
0 & M_2 & 0 & 0 \\
0 & 0 & M_3 & 0 \\
0 & 0 & 0 & M_4
\end{vmatrix}
\begin{vmatrix}
X_1 \\ X_2 \\ X_3 \\ X_4
\end{vmatrix}
+ j\omega e^{j\omega t}
\begin{vmatrix}
(C_2+C_1) & -C & 0 & 0 \\
-C_2 & (C_3+C_2) & -C_3 & 0 \\
0 & -C_3 & (C_4+C_3) & -C_4 \\
0 & 0 & -C_4 & C_4
\end{vmatrix}
\begin{vmatrix}
X_1 \\ X_2 \\ X_3 \\ X_4
\end{vmatrix}$$

$$+ e^{j\omega t}
\begin{vmatrix}
(K_2+K_1) & -K_2 & 0 & 0 \\
-K_2 & (K_3+K_2) & -K_3 & 0 \\
0 & -K_3 & (K_4+K_3) & -K_4 \\
0 & 0 & -K_4 & K_4
\end{vmatrix}
\begin{vmatrix}
X_1 \\ X_2 \\ X_3 \\ X_4
\end{vmatrix}
= e^{j\omega t}
\begin{vmatrix}
0 \\ 0 \\ 0 \\ F
\end{vmatrix} \tag{A5}$$

or,

$$\begin{vmatrix}
[-\omega^2 M_1 + j\omega(C_2+C_1) + (K_2+K_1)] & -j\omega C_2 - K_2 & 0 & 0 \\
-j\omega C_2 - K_2 & [-\omega^2 M_2 + j\omega(C_3+C_2) + (K_3+K_2)] & -j\omega C_3 - K_3 & 0 \\
0 & -j\omega C_3 - K_3 & [-\omega^2 M_3 + j\omega(C_4+C_3) + (K_4+K_3)] & -j\omega C_4 - K_4 \\
0 & 0 & -j\omega C_4 - K_4 & [-\omega^2 M_4 + j\omega C_4 + K_4]
\end{vmatrix}
\begin{vmatrix}
X_1 \\ X_2 \\ X_3 \\ X_4
\end{vmatrix}
=
\begin{vmatrix}
0 \\ 0 \\ 0 \\ F
\end{vmatrix} \tag{A6}$$

Cramer's rule may now be used to solve for the driving point displacement, X,

$$X = \frac{DET\ A}{DET\ B} \tag{A7}$$

where:

$$DET\ A =
\begin{vmatrix}
[K_1 + K_2 + j\omega(C_1+C_2) - \omega^2 M_1] & -(K_2 + j\omega C_2) & 0 & 0 \\
-(K_2 + j\omega C_2) & [K_2 + K_3 + j\omega(C_2+C_3) - \omega^2 M_2] & -(K_3 + j\omega C_3) & 0 \\
0 & -(K_3 + j\omega C_3) & [K_3 + K_4 + j\omega(C_3+C_4) - \omega^2 M_3] & 0 \\
0 & 0 & -(K_4 + j\omega C_4) & F
\end{vmatrix} \tag{A8}$$

and

$$DET\ B =
\begin{vmatrix}
[K_1 + K_2 + j\omega(C_1+C_2) - \omega^2 M_1] & -(K_2 + j\omega C_2) & 0 & 0 \\
-(K_2 + j\omega C_2) & [K_2 + K_3 + j\omega(C_2+C_3) - \omega^2 M_2] & -(K_3 + j\omega C_3) & 0 \\
0 & -(K_3 + j\omega C_3) & [K_3 + K_4 + j\omega(C_3+C_4) - \omega^2 M_3] & -(K_4 + j\omega C_4) \\
0 & 0 & -(K_4 + j\omega C_4) & [K_4 + j\omega C_4 - \omega^2 M_4]
\end{vmatrix} \tag{A9}$$

For simplicity, these expressions are simplified to:

$$DET\ A =
\begin{vmatrix}
D_1 + j\,E_1 & D_2 + j\,E_2 & 0 & 0 \\
D_2 + j\,E_2 & D_3 + j\,E_3 & D_4 + j\,E_4 & 0 \\
 & D_4 + j\,E_4 & D_5 + j\,E_5 & 0 \\
0 & 0 & D_6 + j\,E_6 & F
\end{vmatrix} \tag{A10}$$

and

$$DET\ B = \begin{vmatrix} D_1 + j E_1 & D_2 + j E_2 & 0 & 0 \\ D_2 + j E_2 & D_3 + j E_3 & D_4 + j E_4 & 0 \\ 0 & D_4 + j E_4 & D_5 + j E_5 & D_6 + j E_6 \\ 0 & 0 & D_6 + j E_6 & D_7 + j E_7 \end{vmatrix} \quad (A11)$$

where,

$$D_1 = K_1 + K_2 - \omega^2 M_1 \quad (A12)$$

$$D_2 = -K_2 \quad (A13)$$

$$D_3 = K_2 + K_3 - \omega^2 M_2 \quad (A14)$$

$$D_4 = -K_3 \quad (A15)$$

$$D_5 = K_3 + K_4 - \omega^2 M_3 \quad (A16)$$

$$D_6 = -K_4 \quad (A17)$$

$$D_7 = K_4 - \omega^2 M_4 \quad (A18)$$

$$E_1 = \omega(C_1 + C_2) \quad (A19)$$

$$E_2 = -\omega C_2 \quad (A20)$$

$$E_3 = \omega(C_2 + C_3) \quad (A21)$$

$$E_4 = -\omega C_3 \quad (A22)$$

$$E_5 = \omega(C_3 + C_4) \quad (A23)$$

$$E_6 = -\omega C_4 \quad (A24)$$

$$E_7 = \omega C_4 \quad (A25)$$

Expanding the first determinant, eqn. A10, and simplifying gives:

$$DET\ A = (D_1+jE_1)\{F[D_3D_5-D_4^2-E_3E_5+E_4^2+j(D_3E_5+D_5E_3-2E_4D_4)]\}-(D_2+jE_2)\{F[D_2D_5-E_2E_5+j(D_2E_5+D_5E_2)]\} \quad (A26)$$

or,

$$DET\ A = F(D_1 + jE_1)(G_1 + jH_1) - F(D_2 + jE_2)(G_2 + jH_2) \quad (A27)$$

where,

$$G_1 = D_3D_5 - D_4^2 - E_3E_5 + E_4^2 \quad (A28)$$

$$H_1 = D_3E_5 + D_5E_3 - 2E_4D_4 \quad (A29)$$

$$G_2 = D_2D_5 - E_2E_5 \quad (A30)$$

$$H_2 = D_2E_5 + D_5E_2 . \quad (A31)$$

Now, further simplifying this expression gives:

$$DET\ A = F[D_1G_1 - E_1H_1 - D_2G_2 + E_2H_2 + j(D_1H_1 + E_1G_1 - D_2H_2 - E_2G_2)] \quad (A32)$$

or,

$$DET\ A = F(G_3 + jH_3) \quad (A33)$$

where,

$$G_3 = D_1G_1 - E_1H_1 - D_2G_2 + E_2H_2 \quad (A34)$$

$$H_3 = D_1H_1 + E_1G_1 - D_2H_2 - E_2G_2 . \quad (A35)$$

In a similar manner, DET B, eqn. A11, may be reduced to:

$$DET\ B = (D_1+jE_1)\{(D_3+jE_3)[D_5D_7-E_5E_7+j(D_5E_7+D_7E_5)-D_6^2+E_6^2-j2D_6E_6]-(D_4+jE_4)[D_4D_7-E_4E_7+j(D_4E_7+D_7E_4)]\}$$

$$-(D_2+jE_2)\{(D_2+jE_2)[D_5D_7-E_5E_7+j(D_5E_7+D_7E_5)-D_6^2+E_6^2-j2D_6E_6]\} \quad (A36)$$

or,

$$DET\ B = (D_1+jE_1)[(D_3+jE_3)(G_4+jH_4)-(D_4+jE_4)(G_5+jH_5)]-(D_2+jE_2)[(D_2+jE_2)(G_4+jH_4)] \quad (A37)$$

where,

$$G_4 = D_5D_7 - E_5E_7 - D_6^2 + E_6^2 \quad (A38)$$

$$H_4 = D_5E_7 + D_7E_5 - 2D_6E_6 \quad (A39)$$

$$G_5 = D_4D_7 - E_4E_7 \quad (A40)$$

$$H_5 = D_4E_7 + D_7E_4 . \quad (A41)$$

Further expansion and simplification gives:

$$DET\ B = (D_1+jE_1)[D_3G_4-E_3H_4+j(D_3H_4+E_3G_4)-D_4G_5+E_4H_5-j(D_4H_5+E_4G_5)]-(D_2+jE_2)[D_2G_4-E_2H_4+j(D_2H_4+E_2G_4)] \quad (A42)$$

or,

$$DET\ B = (D_1 + jE_1)(G_6 + jH_6) - (D_2 + jE_2)(G_7 + jH_7) \quad (A43)$$

where,

$$G_6 = D_3G_4 - E_3H_4 - D_4G_5 + E_4H_5 \quad (A44)$$

$$H_6 = D_3H_4 + E_3G_4 - D_4H_5 - E_4G_5 \quad (A45)$$

$$G_7 = D_2G_4 - E_2H_4 \quad (A46)$$

$$H_7 = D_2H_4 + E_2G_4 . \quad (A47)$$

Finally,

$$\text{DET } B = D_1 G_6 - E_1 H_6 + j(D_1 H_6 + E_1 G_6) - D_2 G_7 + E_2 H_7 - j(D_2 H_7 + E_2 G_7) \tag{A48}$$

or,   where,

$$\text{DET } B = G_8 + jH_8 \tag{A49}$$

$$G_8 = D_1 G_6 - E_1 H_6 - D_2 G_7 + E_2 H_7 \tag{A50}$$

$$H_8 = D_1 H_6 + E_1 G_6 - D_2 H_7 - E_2 G_7 \ . \tag{A51}$$

Now, the driving point displacement may be written:

$$X_4 = \frac{\text{DET } A}{\text{DET } B} = \frac{F(G_3 + jH_3)}{G_8 + jH_8} \ . \tag{A52}$$

Similarly, the driving point dynamic compliance may be written:

$$\frac{X_4}{F} = \frac{G_3 + jH_3}{G_8 + jH_8} \frac{(G_8 - jH_8)}{(G_8 - jH_8)} = \frac{G_3 G_8 + H_3 H_8 + j(H_3 G_8 - H_8 G_3)}{G_8^2 + H_8^2} \tag{A53}$$

or,   or,

$$\frac{X_4}{F} = \frac{G_3 G_8 + H_3 H_8}{G_8^2 + H_8^2} + j \ \frac{H_3 G_8 - H_8 G_3}{G_8^2 + H_8^2} \tag{A54}$$

$$\frac{X_4}{F} = G_9 + jH_9 \tag{A55}$$

where,   and

$$G_9 = \frac{G_3 G_8 + H_3 H_8}{G_8^2 + H_8^2} \tag{A56}$$

$$H_9 = \frac{H_3 G_8 - H_8 G_3}{G_8^2 + H_8^2} \ . \tag{A57}$$

The driving point dynamic compliance may now be expressed in terms of an amplitude:

$$\left| \frac{X_4}{F} \right| = (G_9^2 + H_9^2)^{\frac{1}{2}} \tag{A58}$$

and phase angle: $\theta = \tan^{-1}(H_9/G_9) \ . \tag{A59}$

DISCUSSION

E. Rivin: How do vibration amplitude and a person's fatigue influence the parameters of the model?

Authors' Response: The model only takes into account the physical parameters associated with the hand-arm system. It does not include nor can it predict subjective or physiological response of the hand to vibration.

The model assumes that the hand and arm behave as a linear elastic system. In general this is not true; the system is probably non-linear. However, the dynamic compliance predicted by the model usually falls within the spread of experimental data from human subjects. The model thus gives a fairly accurate indication of the response of the hand to vibration provided the vibration levels are not excessive. For exceptionally high levels of vibration, the non-linear characteristics of the hand-arm system may become important. The model may not then be valid, and may require modification.

It is not believed that fatigue will have any direct effect on the model parameters. However, fatigue may influence how an individual clasps a tool handle, and grip force and type have been shown to affect the model parameters.

I. Pyykkö: We have found that significant increases in grip force produce only small increases in vibration level at the elbow, irrespective of frequency (Pyykkö I, Färkkilä M, Toivanen J, Korhonen O, Hyvärinen J. Transmission of vibration in the hand-arm system with special reference to changes in compressive force and acceleration Scand J Work Environ Health 1976; 2: 87-95). Thus, grip force may not be an important determinant of the transfer of vibration in the hand-arm system. Could you comment on what your model studies reveal on this subject?

Authors' Response: The model predicts and measurements confirm that low frequency vibration (<10 Hz) entering the hand travels to the shoulder. As frequency is increased, subjects perceive vibration to travel less distance up the arm until, above 100 Hz, it appears to be localized in the hand. At even higher frequencies, vibration is confined to the fingers in contact with the vibrating source.

At frequencies much less than 100 Hz, the grip force will probably not affect the vibration energy transmitted beyond the wrist. However, at higher frequencies, when vibration is localized in the hand and fingers, the coupling between the hand and the vibrating source increases with increasing grip force. The net result is that as grip force is increased, even though the vibration levels may not increase, the energy directed into the hand increases. This could result in an increase in physiological damage to the fingers.

Energy Entering the Hands of Operators of Pneumatic Tools Used in Chipping and Grinding Operations

D. D. Reynolds, D. E. Wasserman, R. Basel and W. Taylor

ABSTRACT: This paper presents a method for calculating the energy levels entering the hands of operators who use vibrating hand tools. The data are from a
comprehensive, multidisciplined, field study of several hundred chipper and
grinder workers who use pneumatic tools. The results indicate that, for a frequency range of 6.3 to 1000 Hz, the work per unit time transmitted to the hand
from the handle of chipping hammers was as much as 1.57×10^2 J/s, and even more
from the chisel. For pneumatic grinders, the work per unit time was of the order
of 4.2×10^{-2} J/s over the same frequency range. The methods used to determine
the energy transmitted to the hand are discussed in detail.

RESUME: On présente une méthode pour calculer l'énergie transmise aux mains
pendant l'utilisation d'un outil vibrant. Les données proviennent d'une étude
multidisciplinaire détaillée réalisée sur le terrain et portant sur plusieurs
centaines d'ouvriers travaillant avec des marteaux-piqueurs et des meules. On a
constaté que pour une fréquence variant de 6,3 à 1000 Hz, le travail par unité
de temps transmis à la main pouvait atteindre $1,57 \times 10^2$ J/s dans le cas du manche
des marteaux-piqueurs et encore plus dans le cas du ciseau; cette valeur étant de
l'ordre de $4,2 \times 10^{-2}$ J/s dans le cas des meules. On commente de façon détaillée
les méthodes qui ont servi à mesurer l'énergie transmise aux mains.

INTRODUCTION

Much discussion has centred around
the desirability of deriving a single number
measure for assessing the vibration of hand-
held power tools. Lidström has conducted a
study of groups of workers employed exclusively as rock drillers, chisellers and
grinders, and shown that vibration-induced
white finger (VWF) depends on the amount of
vibrational energy incident on the hand from
tool operation (1). It was found that the
groups had the same relative ranking when
ranked both according to the percentage of
individuals in each group who contracted
symptoms of VWF, and the energy per unit
time (power) entering the hand.

The Lidström energies are single value
measures of exposure. While this single
number measure is convenient to use, it has
been well established in the literature
that the response of the hand-arm system
to vibration is frequency dependent. The
equal sensation contours reported by Miwa

show this (2), as do mechanical impedance
models and test data presented by Reynolds
and Keith, Suggs and Mishoe, and others
(3-5). Energy frequency spectra are thus
needed to help determine the role of vibration frequency in the development of VWF.

As a result of the Hand-Arm Vibration
Conference sponsored by the National
Institute for Occupational Safety and Health
(NIOSH) in 1975, a large, multidisciplinary
field study of pneumatic chipping hammer and
grinder operators was undertaken. References 6 to 9 discuss the background to
the study, the worker population investigated, and the acceleration measurements on
the pneumatic chipping hammers and grinders.
References 6, 7, 10 and 11 discuss the
measurement of the dynamic compliance of
the hands of 75 foundry workers investigated
during the NIOSH study, and the development
of four-degrees-of-freedom models of the
human hand and arm. This paper combines
the results of the tool acceleration measurements reported elsewhere in this volume

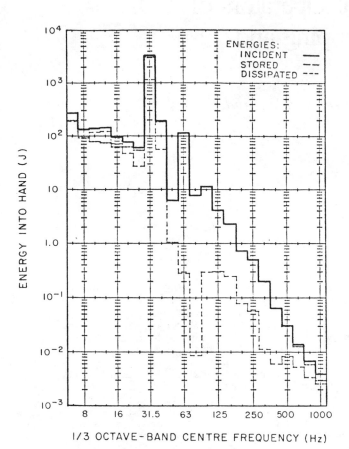

Fig. 1 RMS amplitude of instantaneous energy directed into the hand from the chisel of chipping hammer A used to clean castings. Slot chipping on nodular cast iron at full throttle.

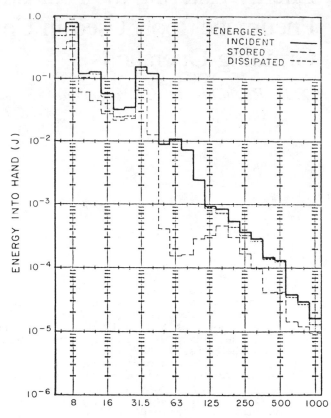

Fig. 2 RMS amplitude of instantaneous energy directed into the hand from the handle of chipping hammer A used to clean castings. Slot chipping on nodular cast iron at full throttle.

and dynamic compliance measurements, to determine the energy frequency spectra and the energy per unit time (power) spectra of some of the tools. Single number energy per unit time (power) data are presented for all tools in the NIOSH study, with comments on how this information may be used for possible single number ratings of hand-held power tools.

I DERIVATION OF ENERGY EQUATIONS

To measure the total energy incident on the hand-arm system, Lidström used a specially designed handle equipped with force transducers and accelerometers (1). In many measurements, there is concern that the measuring device will alter the characteristics of the system being studied. In this instance, the handle was designed with low mass and high stiffness, to reduce the possibility of distortion due to resonance effects. Other factors that may

affect the measurement are size, shape and surface finish of the handle, not only because they may influence the measurement, but also because they may affect an operator's reaction to the tool.

An alternate approach to direct force measurement is to calculate the force using the input displacement and the driving point dynamic compliance, X/F, determined for the hand-arm system. The driving point dynamic compliance may be measured experimentally using a vibration exciter attached to an instrumented handle. The displacement may be found by integrating acceleration twice with respect to time. If the driving point dynamic compliance is experimentally determined for three mutually orthogonal directions, then the force transmitted from a vibrating tool to the hand-arm system may be established by measuring the acceleration of the tool handle in the same three mutually orthogonal directions. Since the corresponding displacement may be derived from this acceleration, the

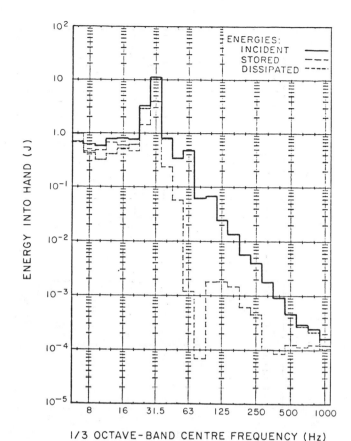

Fig. 3   RMS amplitude of instantaneous energy directed into the hand from the chisel of chipping hammer D used to shape propeller blades.   Chipping on Ni-Al bronze at 1/2 to 3/4 throttle.

appropriate force may be determined using displacement and compliance data.

The instantaneous energy incident on the hand-arm system is:

$$E(t) = \overline{F} \cdot \overline{X} \quad . \qquad (1)$$

Let

$$\overline{F} = F \cos(\omega t) \qquad (2)$$

$$\overline{X} = X \cos(\omega t + \phi) \quad , \qquad (3)$$

where F and X are the amplitudes of force and displacement, respectively, ω is the circular frequency in radians per second, and ϕ is the phase angle between force and displacement (in radians).

Since the force and displacement are measured in the same direction, the spatial angle between the vectors is zero.   Thus, the dot product is a simple product of the time varying magnitudes, or:

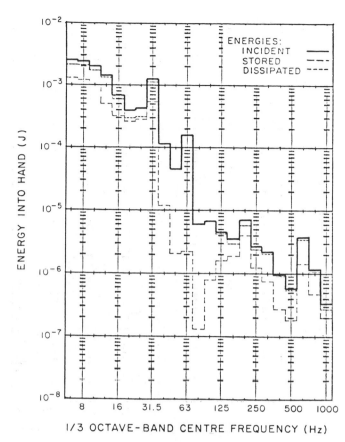

Fig. 4   RMS amplitude of instantaneous energy directed into the hand from the handle of chipping hammer D used to shape propeller blades.   Chipping on Ni-Al bronze at 1/2 to 3/4 throttle.

$$E(t) = FX \cos(\omega t) \cos(\omega t + \phi)$$

$$= \frac{FX}{2} \{\cos(\phi) + \cos(2\omega t + \phi)\} \quad . \qquad (4)$$

Now by the definition of dynamic compliance (F/X):

$$\overline{F} = \overline{X}(F/X) = \frac{\overline{X}}{(X/F)} \quad . \qquad (5)$$

Acceleration is given in terms of the displacement by:

$$\ddot{\overline{X}} = \frac{d^2\overline{X}}{dt^2} = \frac{d}{dt} \{-\omega X \sin(\omega t + \phi)\}$$

$$= -\omega^2 X \cos(\omega t + \phi): \qquad (6)$$

Let

$$\ddot{\overline{X}} = \ddot{X} \cos(\omega t + \phi) \qquad (7)$$

so that

$$X = \frac{-\ddot{X}}{\omega^2} \quad . \qquad (8)$$

Reynolds et al.:   Energy levels

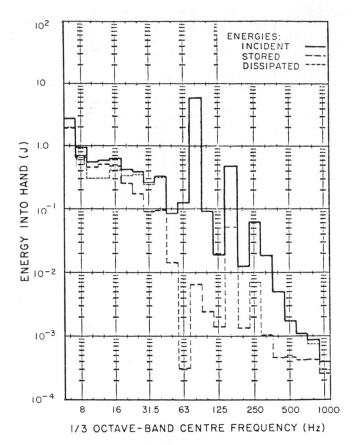

Fig. 5 RMS amplitude of instantaneous
energy directed into the hand from the
chisel of small chipping hammer used to
carve limestone. Chipping hammer
operated at full throttle.

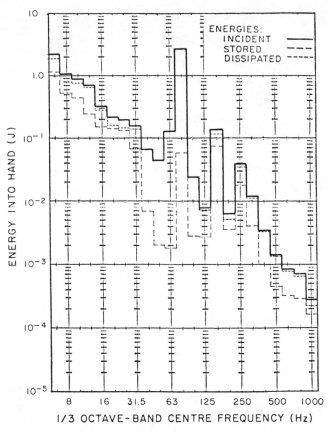

Fig. 6 RMS amplitude of instantenteous
energy directed into the hand from the
handle of small chipping hammer used to
carve limestone. Chipping hammer
operated at full throttle.

Now, combining eqns. 4, 5, and 8, the
instantaneous energy incident on the hand-
arm system in a given direction is:

$$E(t) = \frac{\ddot{X}^2}{2\omega^4(X/F)} \{\cos(\phi)+\cos(2\omega t+\phi)\} \ . \quad (9)$$

It can be seen that the instantaneous
energy has an average value due to the cos
(ϕ) term and a time varying component due
to the cos ($2\omega t+\phi$) term. The amplitude of
the time varying component is:

$$|E| = \frac{\ddot{X}^2}{2\omega^4(X/F)} \quad . \quad (10)$$

This quantity has physical significance
in that it may be obtained using existing
instrumentation. (With Lidström's instrumentation, this quantity is the product of
the force and integrated acceleration.)
The energy might also be obtained using an
analogue computer simulation of the hand-
arm system, based on an analytical model
of the hand and arm, and the measured

tool handle acceleration. In this paper,
the energy is calculated using (digital)
data for dynamic compliance of the hand,
and frequency spectra for the tool handle
accelerations.

The dynamic compliance of the hand
(X/F) is a complex quantity, having both
real and imaginary parts. In complex
notation, dynamic compliance is expressed
in terms of an amplitude and a phase angle:

$$(X/F) = |X/F|e^{j\phi} \ . \quad (11)$$

The phase angle is defined as:

$$\phi = \tan^{-1} \frac{Im(X/F)}{Re(X/F)} \ , \quad (12)$$

where ϕ is the phase shift between the displacement and the force, as before.

Substituting eqn. 11 into 10, the
amplitude of the instantaneous energy
becomes:

Reynolds et al.:   Energy levels

$$|E| = \frac{\ddot{X}^2}{2\omega^4 |X/F| e^{j\phi}} = \frac{\ddot{X}^2 e^{-j\phi}}{2\omega^4 |X/F|} \qquad (13)$$

or

$$|E| = \frac{\ddot{X}^2}{2\omega^4 |X/F|} \{\cos(\phi) - j\sin(\phi)\} . \qquad (14)$$

The amplitude of the incident energy given in eqn. 14 is a complex quantity having both real and imaginary parts. It can be shown that the amplitude of the energy dissipated $|E_D|$ in the hand and arm due to damping or other dissipative mechanisms in the hand and arm is the imaginary part of eqn. 14, or (6-8):

$$|E|_D = \frac{\ddot{X}^2 \sin\phi}{2\omega^4 |X/F|} . \qquad (15)$$

The amplitude of the energy $|E|_S$ that is stored in the hand as kinetic and/or potential energy, and constantly transferred back and forth between the hand and a vibrating handle, is the real part of eqn. 14, or (6-8):

$$|E|_S = \frac{\ddot{X}^2 \cos\phi}{2\omega^4 |X/F|} . \qquad (16)$$

Lidström determined the quantity of energy transferred to the hand-arm system from a vibrating power tool over a given period of time. This may be expressed as the work done on the hand-arm system over a specified period of time by the tool. Now work is defined as:

$$W = \int \overline{F} \cdot d\overline{X} . \qquad (17)$$

If force and displacement are given by eqns. 2 and 3, $d\overline{X}$ is:

$$d\overline{X} = \frac{d\overline{X}}{dt} dt = -\omega X \sin(\omega t + \phi) dt . \qquad (18)$$

Substituting eqns. 2, 5, 8 and 18 into eqn. 17 yields:

$$W = -\int_o^t \frac{\ddot{X}^2}{\omega^3 (X/F)} \cos(\omega t) \sin(\omega t + \phi) dt \qquad (19)$$

or

$$W = \frac{-\ddot{X}^2}{2\omega^3 |X/F|} \times$$

$$[\sin(\phi)t - \frac{1}{2\omega} \{\cos(2\omega t + \phi) - \cos(\phi)\}] \qquad (20)$$

It can be seen that the cosine terms in eqn. 20 drop out if t is chosen to correspond to a whole number of complete cycles. Then the amplitude of the work per unit time is given by:

$$\left|\frac{W}{t}\right| = \frac{\ddot{X}^2 \sin(\phi)}{2\omega^3 |X/F|} \qquad (21)$$

From eqns. 15 and 21, the relationship between the amplitude of the instantaneous dissipated energy and the amplitude of the work per unit time is

$$\left|\frac{W}{t}\right| = \omega |E_D| . \qquad (22)$$

II RESULTS AND DISCUSSION

A complete discussion of the pneumatic tools and the work conditions under which measurements were made is contained in Refs. 8 and 9. These papers provide details of the accelerometer mounts, and their location and orientation. The coordinate system employed to define the X, Y and Z vibration components is consistent with that proposed in the Draft International Standard ISO/DIS 5349, 1979 (12), and is shown in Fig. 4 of Ref. 9.

2.1 Instantaneous Energy

2.1.1 Chipping Hammers

Four different Type 2 pneumatic chipping hammers (designated chipping hammers A, B, C and D) and a small chipping hammer, for carving limestone, were investigated. For the Type 2 chipping hammers, two different types of chipping operations were studied. One was slot chipping. This is a typical chipping operation used in the cleaning of castings in automotive type foundries. The hammer is operated at full throttle and the point of the chisel is usually directed straight into (or perpendicular to) the casting being cleaned. This is probably the most severe type of chipping. The second was a chipping operation used in the forming of propeller blades for ships. For this operation, the chipping hammer is operated at 1/2 to 3/4 throttle, and the chisel is positioned so that it can cut out a path of metal usually 0.1 inch deep by 0.75 inch wide.

Figures 1 through 6 show the 1/3 octave-band instantaneous energy levels for the chisels and handles of selected chipping hammers, calculated from eqns. 10, 15 and 16. Each figure contains plots of the total incident energy (eqn. 10), the stored kinetic and potential energy (eqn. 16), and the dissipated energy (eqn. 15). The energy levels are expressed in Joules (J).

Figures 1 and 2 are typical instantaneous energy levels for slot chipping. Figures 3 and 4 are typical instantaneous energy levels for the chipping operations used in the forming of ship propeller blades. Figures 5 and 6 are typical instantaneous energy levels encountered in limestone carving. A complete set of energy data for all the chipping hammers investigated in the NIOSH study is contained in Refs. 6 to 8.

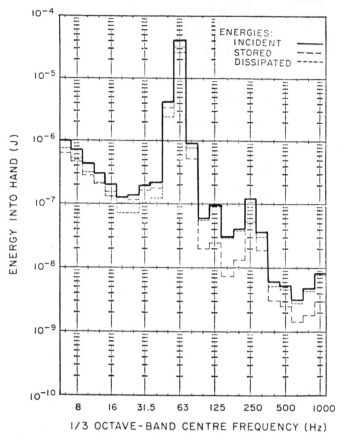

Fig. 7 RMS amplitude of instantaneous energy directed into the hand from a horizontal grinder with coarse radial wheel: Right hand, X direction.

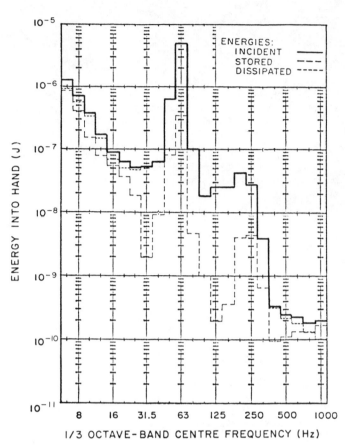

Fig. 8 RMS amplitude of instantaneous energy directed into the hand from a horizontal grinder with coarse radial wheel: Right hand, Y direction.

The highest energies for the chisels were found at the chipper operating frequencies. Approximately 3000 J was obtained at 31.5 Hz for the chisel of chipping hammer A. The second peak at 63 Hz is approximately 100 J, while the third peak at 100 Hz is 10 J. The incident energies for the chisel of chipping hammer A are in excess of 60 J at all frequencies below 31.5 Hz. In contrast, the maximum chisel energies for hammer D are 1.8 J and 10 J, when chipping at 1/2 to 3/4 throttle on mild B steel and Ni-Al bronze, respectively. Both peaks for hammer D occur at 31.5 Hz. The maximum energy contribution for the chisel of the small limestone chipper is approximately 6 J at 80 Hz. It can be seen that over a very substantial portion of the frequency range, the energy levels for the chisel of hammer A are much higher than the highest peaks for the chisels of the other hammers.

The handle instantaneous energy levels are all much lower than the levels for the chisels. For chipping hammer A, the handle

energy level at 31.5 Hz is reduced by a factor of 10 000 from the chisel level. In general, the energy levels are reduced by 1000. A reduction of 1000 is also experienced between the chisel and handle energies of hammer D when chipping on both mild B steel and on Ni-Al bronze. For the small limestone chipper, the reduction between the chisel and handle energies is only a factor of 10.

An interesting observation is that the instantaneous energy levels for slot chipping are of nearly the same magnitude for all the chipping hammer handles. In general, the energy levels for hammers A and B are nearly equal. The levels for the small limestone chipper and for hammer D are comparable. Both are somewhat higher than the levels for hammers A and B. The energy levels for hammer C are somewhat less than those of the other hammers.

On the other hand, the energy levels for hammer D chipping at 1/2 to 3/4 throttle on mild B steel and on Ni-Al bronze are comparable, but are at least a factor of

Reynolds et al.: Energy levels

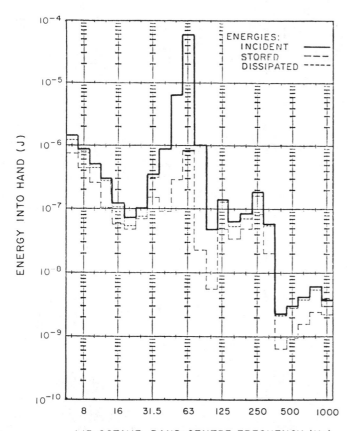

Fig. 9 RMS amplitude of instantaneous
energy directed into the hand from a
horizontal grinder with coarse radial
wheel: Right hand, Z direction.

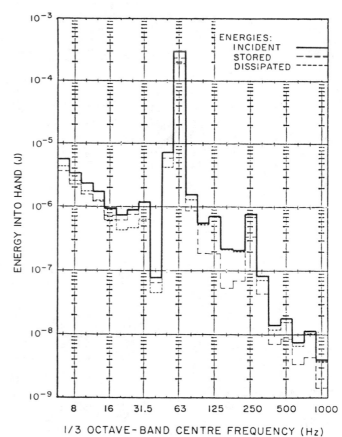

Fig. 10 RMS amplitude of instantaneous
energy directed into the hand from a
horizontal grinder with coarse radial
wheel: Left hand, X direction.

100 less than for slot chipping. This
points out once again the importance of
testing the actual operation and not just
the material. Chipping hammer D, when slot
chipping at full throttle, produced some of
the highest handle energy levels; yet, for
example, when operated at 1/2 to 3/4
throttle chipping on mild B steel and Ni-Al
bronze, the levels were much lower. Thus,
when measuring the energy or acceleration
of hand held tools, it is desirable to
obtain data while the tool is operating as
nearly as possible under actual working
conditions.

Another interesting aspect of the
handle instantaneous energy data is that
the maximum energy levels occurred at
either 6.3 or 8 Hz, and not at the principal
striking frequency of the tool, for all of
the chipping hammers except the small limestone chipper. For the last mentioned, the
energy peak at 80 Hz is slightly higher
than at 6.3 Hz. As a general rule, for all
of the handle and chisel data, the magnitudes of the instantaneous energy levels

decrease sharply as the frequency increases.
The slope of this trend is approximately
-15 dB/octave, although peaks do occur at
the principal striking frequencies and their
harmonics. These observations tend to
indicate that the majority of the instantaneous energy transmitted to the hand-arm
system from the chisels and handles of the
chipping hammers is contained in the lower
frequencies, say 125 Hz and below. It is
also significant to note that, for both
handles and chisels, the total incident
energy is essentially dissipated or absorbed
in the hand at frequencies of 31.5 Hz and
above.

2.1.2 Grinders

Figures 7 through 12 show typical 1/3
octave-band instantaneous energy levels for
the horizontal grinder shown in Fig. 2 of
Ref. 9. A complete set of instantaneous
energy data for all the grinders in the
NIOSH study is given in Refs. 6 to 8. The
grinder energy levels are much less than

Reynolds et al.: Energy levels

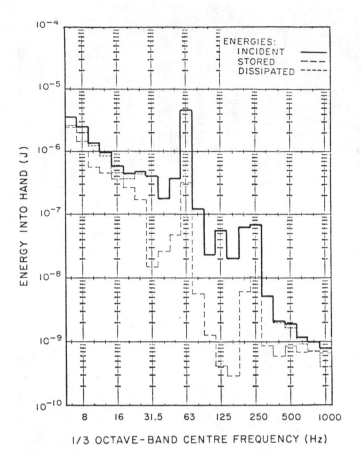

Fig. 11 RMS amplitude of instantaneous energy directed into the hand from a horizontal grinder with coarse radial wheel: Left hand, Y direction.

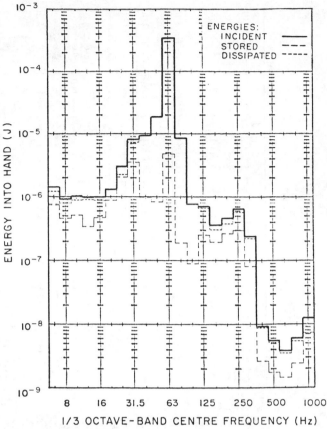

Fig. 12 RMS amplitude of instantaneous energy directed into the hand from a horizontal grinder with coarse radial wheel: Left hand, Z direction.

those of the chipping hammers. The energies for hammer D chipping on mild B steel and Ni-Al bronze are 10 to 100 times larger than the grinder energies at most frequencies. For the horizontal grinder with the coarse radial wheel and flared cup wheel, some energy peaks are comparable to the energy levels of hammer D at the same frequency. However, the grinder peaks are always much less than the chipping hammer handle peaks.

The maximum grinder energy level is 3.3×10^{-4} J, which occurs at 63 Hz for the left handle of the horizontal grinder, with the coarse radial wheel (Z direction). All of the coarse radial wheel spectra have the largest peak at 63 Hz. The largest energy levels for the horizontal grinders generally occur at some principal frequency, which seems to vary with the type of grinding wheel used. For the coarse radial wheel, the principal frequency occurs at 63 Hz; the fine radial wheel has large peaks at 31.5 Hz, and the principal frequency for

the flared cup wheel is 40 Hz. The vertical grinder, with the sanding pad, has a peak at 40 Hz in each spectrum. However, for the right handle and for the Z direction of the left handle, the maximum energy levels occur at 6.3 Hz.

All of the grinder energy data tend to have higher energy levels at low frequencies. With the exception of the peak at the principal frequency, the energy levels decrease with increasing frequency. As with the chipping hammers, this indicates that the majority of the energy from the grinders incident on the hand and arm is contained in the lower frequencies.

The energy levels for the horizontal grinders with the coarse radial wheel and flared cup wheel are of comparable magnitude. The energies for the horizontal grinder with the fine radial wheel and the vertical grinder with the sanding pad are comparable, and are slightly less than those of the coarse radial wheel and the flared cup wheel. The energy levels of

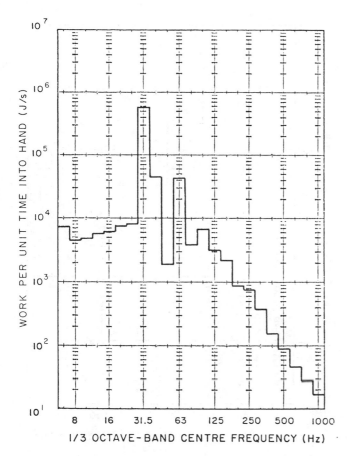

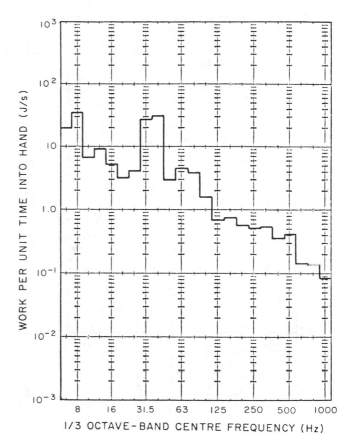

Fig. 13 RMS amplitude of work per unit time directed into the hand from the chisel of chipping hammer A used to clean castings. Slot chipping on nodular cast iron at full throttle.

Fig. 14 RMS amplitude of work per unit time directed into the hand from the handle of chipping hammer A used to clean castings. Slot chipping on nodular cast iron at full throttle.

the left handle of the horizontal grinder are somewhat higher than those of the right handle. This is probably because on the horizontal grinder the left hand is closer to the grinding wheel.

The horizontal grinder Y direction energy levels are considerably less than the X and Z direction levels. The opposite is true for the vertical grinder. The vertical grinder Y direction energy levels are, in contrast, slightly higher than those for the X and Z directions. Note also that the general energy levels for the vertical grinder in the Y direction are comparable to the general levels for the horizontal grinder, when fitted with the coarse radial and flared cup wheels.

2.2 Energy Dissipated Per Unit Time

An examination of all the curves for instantaneous energy indicates that most of the energy incident upon the hand is contained in the lower frequencies

(frequencies below the fundamental operating frequency of the tool), and is dissipative in nature (i.e., it is either dissipated in, or absorbed by, the hand and arm). Equations 21 and 22 show that there is a relation between the amplitude of the instantaneous energy dissipated and the amplitude of the work done per unit time (power). An investigation by Lidström indicates that a correlation exists between the incidence of VWF in rock chiselers and grinders, and the power directed into their hands (1).

The instantaneous energy data seem to imply that low frequency vibration may be the primary cause of VWF. This is contrary to the results of many investigations, which tend to indicate that vibration in the mid frequency region (40 Hz to 600 Hz) is the primary cause of VWF (13).

Figures 13 to 19 show the work (energy) per unit time that corresponds to the instantaneous dissipated energy in Figures 1 through 12. An examination of the work per unit time frequency spectra indicates

Reynolds et al.: Energy levels

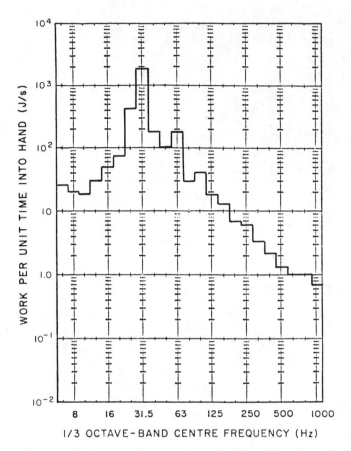

Fig. 15 RMS amplitude of work per unit time directed into the hand from the chisel of chipping hammer D used to shape propeller blades. Chipping on Ni-Al bronze at 1/2 to 3/4 throttle.

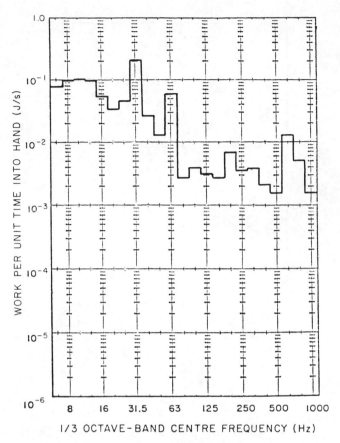

Fig. 16 RMS amplitude of work per unit time directed into the hand from the handle of chipping hammer D used to shape propeller blades. Chipping on Ni-Al bronze at 1/2 to 3/4 throttle.

that the general slope of these plots (neglecting peaks at the tool operating frequencies) is substantially less than that of the corresponding instantaneous energy spectra. Thus, the work per unit time plots indicate that more energy is absorbed into the hands in the mid frequency range and at the operating frequency than is indicated by the instantaneous energy plots. This tends to support the results of the investigations already mentioned. This observation, together with the results of Lidström, suggests that the parameter to be considered when measuring the vibration levels on hand tools is the work (or energy) per unit time (power).

The cumulative work per unit time, or power, in the 1/3 octave frequency bands from 6.3 to 1000 Hz for the pneumatic chipping hammers and grinders investigated during the NIOSH study, and for the proposed ISO exposure guidelines, are listed in Tables 1 to 4. As would be expected, the highest energies are for the chipping

hammer chisels, though the accuracy of these results must be questioned owing to the acceleration data used in their derivation (for a discussion of the potential errors in the chisel acceleration measurements, see Ref. 9).

The ranking of the various chipping hammers by handle power is quite different from the ranking by chisel power, and the power values are generally much lower. The cumulative work per unit time for the handle of the small limestone chipper is more than 10 times the value for the handle of hammers A and B. Surprisingly, the work per unit time for hammer D slot chipping is almost 30% greater than the value for hammer A. As in the case of the instantaneous energies, it is apparent that the energy transferred to the hand-arm system from the handles of the small chipping hammers is substantially more than from larger hammers operating under similar conditions.

The cumulative work done per unit time by the handle of chipping hammer C is much

Table 1. Work Per Unit Time for Chipping Hammers.

Chipping Hammer, Transducer Location, & Operation	Work Per Unit time (J/s)
A, Slot Chipping	
Handle	1.57×10^2
Chisel	7.23×10^5
B, Slot Chipping	
Handle	1.56×10^2
C, Slot Chipping	
Handle	3×10^1
D, Slot Chipping	
Handle	2.04×10^2
D, Chipping Ni-Al bronze	
Handle	8.52×10^{-1}
Chisel	3.18×10^3
D, Chipping Mild B Steel	
Handle	2.28
Chisel	1.08×10^3
Small Limestone Hammer	
Handle	1.99×10^3
Chisel	4.14×10^3

Table 2. Work Per Unit Time for the Horizontal Grinders.

Tool and Vibration Component		Work Per Unit Time (J/s)
Coarse Radial Wheel		
Right Hand	X	1.21×10^{-2}
	Y	2.57×10^{-3}
	Z	2.71×10^{-2}
	Total	4.17×10^{-2}
Left Hand	X	8.13×10^{-2}
	Y	2.94×10^{-3}
	Z	1.51×10^{-1}
	Total	2.35×10^{-1}
Fine Radial Wheel		
Right Hand	X	1.84×10^{-3}
	Y	1.12×10^{-3}
	Z	3.62×10^{-3}
	Total	6.58×10^{-3}
Left Hand	X	4.95×10^{-3}
	Y	6.99×10^{-4}
	Z	1.84×10^{-2}
	Total	2.41×10^{-2}
Flared Cup Wheel		
Right Hand	X	4.44×10^{-3}
	Y	1.93×10^{-2}
	Z	1.79×10^{-2}
	Total	4.16×10^{-2}
Left Hand	X	1.31×10^{-2}
	Z	4.62×10^{-2}
	Z	6.67×10^{-2}
	Total	1.26×10^{-1}

Table 3. Work Per Unit Time for the Vertical Grinder.

Tool and Vibration Component		Work Per Unit Time (J/s)
Sanding Pad		
Right Hand	X	2.51×10^{-3}
	Y	4.52×10^{-3}
	Z	1.29×10^{-3}
	Total	8.32×10^{-3}
Left Hand	X	1.89×10^{-3}
	Y	8.58×10^{-3}
	Z	1.01×10^{-2}
	Total	2.06×10^{-2}

Table 4. Work Per Unit Time for the Exposure Guidelines Proposed by ISO/DIS 5349, 1979 (Ref. 12).

Exposure Duration and Vibration Component		Work Per Unit Time (J/s)
8 Hours		
Large Handle	X	3.48×10^{-1}
	Y	2.53×10^{-1}
	Z	4.4×10^{-1}
	Total	1.04
Small Handle	X	2.35×10^{-1}
	Y	1.54×10^{-1}
	Z	3.29×10^{-1}
	Total	7.17×10^{-1}
30 Minutes		
Large Handle	X	8.71
	Y	6.33
	Z	1.1×10^1
	Total	2.6×10^1
Small Handle	X	5.88
	Y	3.84
	Z	8.22
	Total	1.79×10^1

less than by hammers A and B. The lowest values were found for the handle of hammer D chipping at 1/2 to 3/4 throttle on Ni-Al bronze and mild B steel. The value for chipping on mild B steel is approximately three times that for Ni-Al bronze. Apparently, material may be a significant factor in determining the cumulative work done per unit time by the handle.

The power levels at the grinders' handles are much lower than that of the handle of chipping hammer D. Even the largest value for all three directions on one hand is approximately 25% of the value for hammer D chipping on Ni-Al bronze. The largest total power level for one hand is for the left hand of the horizontal grinder with the coarse radial wheel. For this case, the left hand value is approximately six times that for the right hand. For other grinding combinations, the total power entering the left hand is approximately three times the right hand value. The

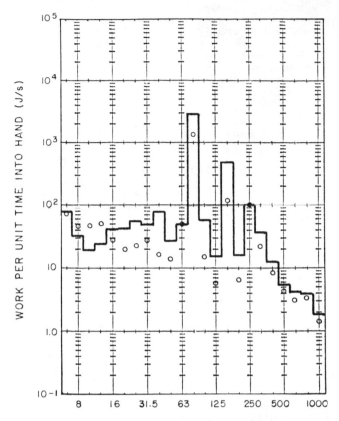

Fig. 17 RMS amplitude of work per unit time directed into the hand by the small chipping hammer used to carve limestone. Chipping hammer operated at full throttle: Chisel, continuous line; handle, open circles.

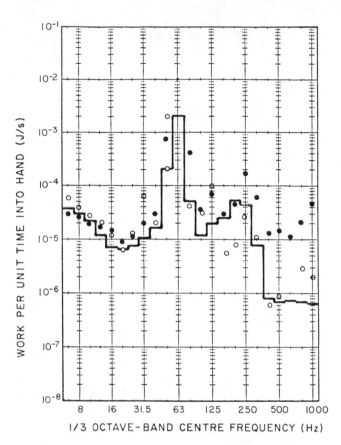

Fig. 18 RMS amplitude of work per unit time directed into the hand from a horizontal grinder with coarse radial wheel: Right hand; Y direction, continuous line; X direction, closed circles; Z direction, open circles.

horizontal grinder with the flared cup wheel has power levels approximately equal to those for the coarse radial wheel. Similarly, the horizontal grinder with the fine radial wheel has values roughly equal to those for the vertical grinder with the sanding pad. For the horizontal grinder, the Z direction component is usually the largest and the X direction the smallest. The total power entering the right hand is always larger than that entering the left.

Lidström's results for rock chiseling and grinding are 2.7 J/s and 0.07 J/s, respectively. The rock chiseling data were measured for chipping hammer handles only, and are consistent with the handle data in Table 1 for chipping on Ni-Al bronze or mild B steel. The grinding data are also consistent with the data in Tables 2 and 3.

III CONCLUSIONS

1. The highest energy levels for the chisels of chipping hammers occurred at the fundamental operating frequency.
2. The vibration energy levels on the handles of chipping hammers were substantially less than on the chisels. For chipping hammers used to clean castings, reductions of a factor of 1000 or greater were experienced between the chisel and handle. For small limestone chippers, this reduction was a factor of 10.
3. The highest handle energy levels occurred at the lowest frequencies analysed, 6.3 and 8.0 Hz.
4. The grinder instantaneous energy levels were less than the chipping hammer handle energies by a factor of 10 to 100.
5. The work per unit time (power) plots indicate that most of the energy that is absorbed into the hands is in the mid frequency range of 40 to 600 Hz, and at the fundamental operating frequencies of the pneumatic tools.
6. The results of this investigation tend to imply that the important parameter to be

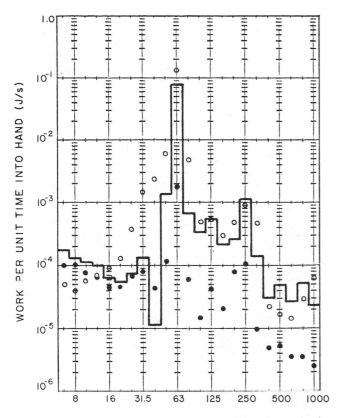

Fig. 19 RMS amplitude of work per unit time directed into the hand from a horizontal grinder with coarse radial wheel: Left hand; X direction, continuous line; Y direction, closed circles; Z direction, open circles.

considered when measuring the vibration of hand tools is the work per unit time (power).

7. The overall power levels measured on chipping hammer handles and on pneumatic grinders during this investigation agree fairly well with the results reported by Lidström.

ACKNOWLEDGEMENTS

The research reported in this paper was carried out under NIOSH Contact No. 210-77-0165, while Dr. D.D. Reynolds was an Associate Professor in the Dept. of Mechanical Engineering at the Univ. of Pittsburgh.

DISCLAIMER

Mention of commercially available services, apparatus, instrumentation, devices, products, or proposed standards does not constitute endorsement by the National Institute for Occupational Safety and Health.

REFERENCES

1. Lidström I-M. Vibration injuries in rock drillers, chiselers and grinders. In Wasserman DE, Taylor W, Curry MG, eds. Proc of the Int Occup Hand-Arm Vibration Conf. Cincinnati, OH: Dept of Health and Human Services, 1977. (NIOSH publication no. 77-170): 77-83.
2. Miwa T. Evaluation methods for vibration effect, part 3. Measurement of threshold and equal sensation contours on hand for vertical and horizontal sinusoidal vibrations. Ind Health (Japan) 1967; 5: 213-220.
3. Reynolds DD. Vibration interaction of the human hand-arm system with vibration power tools (especially chain saws). Purdue Univ, 1972. PhD thesis. (unpublished).
4. Reynolds DD, Keith RH. Hand-arm vibration, part I: analytical model of the vibration response characteristics of the hand. J Sound Vib 1977; 51: 237-253.
5. Suggs CW, Mishoe JW. Hand-arm vibration: implications drawn from lumped parameter models. In Wasserman DE, Taylor W, Curry MG, eds. Proc of the Int Occup Hand-Arm Vibration Conf. Cincinnati, OH: Dept of Health and Human Services, 1977. (NIOSH publication no. 77-170): 136-141.
6. Basel RA. Hand tool vibration and vibration energy transmitted to the hands of pneumatic chipping hammer and pneumatic grinder operators during foundry casting cleaning operations. Univ of Pittsburgh, 1980. MS thesis. (unpublished).
7. Reynolds DD, Basel RA. Hand Tool Vibration and Vibration Energy Transmitted to the Hands of Pneumatic Chipping Hammer and Pneumatic Grinder Operators during Foundry Casting Cleaning Operations. Final Report, NIOSH contract 210-77-0165 (unpublished).
8. Wasserman DE, Reynolds DD, Behrens V, Taylor W, Samueloff S, Basel RA. Vibration white finger disease in US workers using pneumatic chipping and grinding hand tools II: engineering testing. Cincinnati, OH: Dept of Health and Human Services, 1981. (NIOSH publication no. 82-101).
9. Reynolds DD, Wasserman DE, Basel RA, Taylor W, Doyle TE, Asbury W. Vibration acceleration measured on pneumatic tools used in chipping and grinding operations. In Brammer AJ, Taylor W, eds. Vibration Effects on the Hand and Arm in Industry. New York: Wiley, 1982.
10. Falkenberg RJ. Analytical models of the vibration characteristics of the hand-arm system. Univ of Pittsburgh, 1980. MS thesis. (unpublished).
11. Reynolds DD, Falkenberg RJ. Three- and four-degrees-of-freedom models of the vibration response of the human hand. In: Brammer AJ, Taylor W, eds. Vibration Effects on the Hand and Arm in Industry. New York: Wiley, 1982.

Reynolds et al.: Energy levels

12. International Organization for Standardization.
    Principles for the Measurement and the Evalua-
    tion of Human Exposure to Vibration Transmitted
    to the Hand. Draft International Standard
    ISO/DIS 5349, 1979.
13. Griffin MJ. Vibration Injuries of the Hand and
    Arm: Their Occurrence and the Evolution of
    Standards and Limits. London: Her Majesty's
    Stationery Office, 1980. (Health and Safety
    Executive Research Paper 9).

DISCUSSION

E. Rivin: Is it a correct conclusion that
grinders do not cause VWF due to the fact reported
in your paper that their vibrational energy is about
three orders of magnitude less than that of chipping
hammers?

Authors' Response: Yes and no. The data
relates to a foundry with very good maintenance
procedures. NIOSH found vibration levels of
grinders 25 to 50 times higher and a VWF prevalence
of approximately 47% in another foundry. (For
further details see NIOSH report no HHE 80-189-870).

M. Morin: This paper tends to demonstrate
that grinders are far better tools than chippers in
terms of vibration. However, it has been noted
that the vibration of grinders can become worse with
use. It seems to me important that this aspect of
the problem should be recognized, so that it can be
appreciated that grinders may not necessarily be a
good alternative to chippers.

I. Pyykkö: I would like to ask you whether the
measurement of the energy spectrum of vibration is
sufficient. Vibration is transmitted in the hand-
arm system in a well documented manner. Up to now,
we have measured the transfer of energy, both from
the handles of tools and in the hand-arm system as a
power spectrum. Now the impulses from a pneumatic
tool are of very short duration and reach large
peak amplitudes, and it is possible that the power
spectrum is not representative of the biological
effects of vibration. The tissues may well react
not only to energy dissipation, but also to the
vibration impulses or shocks (as many receptors
react to shocks). Should we not therefore also
think of other methods of analysing vibrations,
such as measuring how quickly the levels change,
or determining the characteristics of the vibration
impulses?

Authors' Response: These could be important
areas for investigation.

OCCUPATIONAL EXPOSURE TO VIBRATION

Vibration Syndrome in Workers Using Pneumatic Chipping and Grinding Tools

V. Behrens, W. Taylor and D. E. Wasserman

ABSTRACT: A total of 385 subjects in two grey iron foundries and one shipyard foundry, representing all workers using pneumatic chipping and grinding tools, together with a control population, were surveyed for the signs and symptoms of the Vibration Syndrome. The results of a questionnaire and a general medical examination (to exclude all other causes of white fingers) showed that in the two grey iron foundries, the median latency of tingling was seven months, numbness nine months, and blanching 17 months. The prevalence of VWF was 47%. By comparison, the results in the shipyard foundry showed mean latencies of 9.1 years for tingling, 12 years for numbness, 16.8 years for blanching, with a VWF prevalence of 19%. Vibration measurements on the chipping and grinding tools, whilst engaged on the work processes, proceeded simultaneously and have been reported elsewhere.

RESUME: Un nombre total de 385 sujets travaillant dans des fonderies de fonte grise et une fonderie de chantier naval, représentant tous les travailleurs utilisant des outils pneumatiques pour le burinage et le meulage, ainsi qu'une population témoin, furent examinés pour déceler les signes et les symptômes du syndrome des vibrations. Les résultats d'un questionnaire et un examen médical général (pour exclure toutes les autres causes des doigts blancs dûs aux vibrations) indiquaient que dans les deux fonderies de fonte grise, la latence médiane était de sept mois pour le picotement, de neuf mois pour l'engourdissement et de 17 mois pour le blanchissement. La prévalence des doigts blancs dûs aux vibrations était de 47%. Par contre, les résultats dans la fonderie du chantier naval indiquaient des latences moyennes de 9,1 ans pour le picotement, 12 ans pour l'engourdissement et 16,8 ans pour le blanchissement, et une prévalence des doigts blancs dûs aux vibrations de 19%. Des mesures des vibrations produites par les outils de burinage et de meulage, pendant leur utilisation pour les diverses opérations, furent entreprises simultanément et ont été décrites ailleurs.

INTRODUCTION

Workers using certain vibrating hand tools are known to risk the development of vascular and neurological disorders of the fingers, hands, and arms variously called the Vibration Syndrome, vibration-induced white finger (VWF), Raynaud's Phenomenon of Occupational Origin, and traumatic vasospastic disease. In recent years, the majority of epidemiological investigations have reported on forestry workers who have used gasoline-powered chain saws in, for example, Australia (1), Canada (2), Czechoslovakia (3), Finland (4), Japan (5), New Zealand (6), Norway (7), Poland (8), Sweden (9), and in the United Kingdom (10). Other investigators have reported on the Vibration Syndrome among workers using pneumatic hand tools, such as rock drills (11), grinders (11-15), chipping hammers (11, 14-19) and jack-leg type drills (20-22).

There have been few investigations of the Vibration Syndrome in the U.S.A. In 1918, Hamilton (16), Rothstein (23), and Leake (24) reported on the Syndrome among stonecutters using air hammers (pneumatic chipping hammers) to cut limestone in Indiana. In 1946, Dart described adverse effects on the hands of workers using high speed pneumatic and electric tools in the aircraft industry (25). In 1964, Ashe and Williams studied the Syndrome in hard rock miners (26). Despite world-wide recognition of the hazards of vibrating hand tools, Pecora concluded in 1960 from a questionnaire sent to physicians that Raynaud's Phenomenon of Occupational Origin "may have become an uncommon occupational disease approaching extinction in this country" (27).

The National Institute for Occupational Safety and Health (NIOSH) initiated a vibration research programme in 1973, with onsite surveys of work sites with sources of vibration exposure (28). From this survey, it was estimated that 1.2 million workers are exposed to occupational hand-arm vibration in the U.S.A. In 1975, NIOSH held an international, occupational, hand-arm vibration

Table 1. Differential Diagnosis for Raynaud's Phenomenon (From Ref. 10, with Permission of W. Taylor and P.L. Pelmear).

Primary Raynaud's Disease Secondary Raynaud's Phenomenon	Constitutional White Finger
1. Connective Tissue Disease	a. Scleroderma b. Systemic Lupus Erythematosus c. Rheumatoid Arthritis d. Dermatomyositis e. Polyarteritis Nodosa f. Mixed Connective Tissue Disease
2. Trauma i. Direct to Extremities	a. Following injury, fracture or operation b. Of occupational origin (vibration) c. Frostbite and Immersion Syndrome
ii. To Proximal Vessels by Compression	a. Thoracic outlet syndrome (cervical rib, scalenus anterior muscle) b. Costoclavicular and hyperabduction syndromes
3. Occlusive Vascular Disease	a. Thromboangiitis obliterans b. Arteriosclerosis c. Embolism d. Thrombosis

4. Dysglobulinemia	a. Cold hemagglutination syndrome
	   - Cryoglobulinaemia
	   - Macroglobulinaemia

5. Intoxication	a. Acro-osteolysis b. Ergot c. Nicotine
6. Neurogenic	a. Poliomyelitis b. Syringomyelia c. Hemiplegia

conference (29). Recommendations from experts at this conference were used to design the protocol for the NIOSH Pneumatic Chippers and Grinders Vibration Study. The multidisciplinary study consisted of medical, physiological and engineering investigations. This paper presents a part of the epidemiological results, from a questionnaire and medical examination. Complete results of the epidemiological study will be published elsewhere (30). The vibration levels measured on the tools during normal operation, and the energy entering the workers' hands are reported elsewhere in this volume (31, 32). They are also the subject of a separate NIOSH report (33).

I METHODS

1.1 Data Collection

Companies in the U.S.A., with more than 50 pneumatic chipping and grinding workers, were asked to participate voluntarily in the study. Two foundries and one shipyard agreed to participate. All workers at these foundries and shipyard who were using Type 2 pneumatic chipping hammers (from various manufacturers) and pneumatic grinders, together with unexposed or potential control workers, were invited to volunteer as subjects. A total of 385 workers were surveyed and examined, representing all the pneumatic

Table 2. Percentage (Number) of Workers With, and Without, Confounding Exposure Histories and/or Medical Conditions in Total Study Population (385 persons).

	Primary Raynaud's Disease	Other Confounding Medical Conditions	No Confounding Medical Conditions
Exposed Group	1% (3)	7% (27)	53% (205)
Control Group	1% (3)	2% (6)	16% (63)
Confounded Exposure History	1% (4)	2% (9)	17% (65)

Table 3. Stage Assessment for Vibration-Induced White Finger (After Ref. 10, with Permission of W. Taylor and P.L. Pelmear).

Stage	Condition of Digits	Work and Social Interference
00	No tingling, numbness or blanching of digits.	No complaints.
0T	Intermittent tingling.	No interference with activities.
0N	Intermittent numbness.	No interference with activities.
0TN	Intermittent tingling and numbness.	No interference with activities.
01	Blanching of one or more fingertips with or without tingling and numbness.	No interference with activities.
02	Blanching of fingers beyond tips, usually confined to winter.	Slight interference with home and social activities. No interference at work.
03	Extensive blanching of digits. Frequent episodes summer as well as winter.	Definite interference at work, at home and with social activities. Restriction of hobbies.
04	Extensive blanching, most fingers. Frequent episodes summer and winter.	Occupational changed to avoid further vibration exposure because of severity of signs and symptoms.

Note: Complications are not used in this grading.

chipping and grinding workers at these work sites during the time of the surveys. Some workers who were not using vibrating hand tools on the job were also examined and included as potential control subjects. The workers were examined in a mobile medical trailer and an engineering van brought to the work sites.

The volunteers participated in the following procedures:
1) informed consent;
2) a questionnaire administered by trained interviewers;
3) a general medical examination;
4) sensory tests of the hands and fingers;
5) a special medical history and finger examination to diagnose the Vibration Syndrome;
6) three objective tests: a) X-rays of the hands and fingers, for the detection of bone cysts, bone density and bone/tissue ratios; b) esthesiometry (depth sense and two-point discrimination); and c) photocell plethysmography.
7) engineering tests to measure vibration acceleration and energy impinging on the hands.
Only the results of the questionnaire and medical examinations (items 2, 3 and 5) are presented in this paper. The former included complete histories of; a) occupational and hobby tool use; b) health in relation to the Vibration Syndrome; and c) tobacco and alcohol consumption. A general medical examination was performed by a physician and used to detect medical conditions which may confound diagnosis of the

Syndrome. The study physician (WT) performed the examination for VWF.

1.2 Diagnosis of VWF

There are many causes of Raynaud's Phenomenon which is characterized by neurological symptoms, especially abnormal tingling and numbness of the fingers, hands and even arms, and vascular symptoms, primarily temporary loss of blood circulation in the fingers (i.e. finger blanching or "white finger"). Some of the medical conditions and environmental exposures associated with Raynaud's Phenomenon are listed in Table 1. Persons with signs and symptoms of Raynaud's but without a causative medical condition or environmental exposure are diagnosed as Primary Raynaud's Disease. Workers with Raynaud's Phenomenon attributable to any cause other than vibration and those with Primary Raynaud's Disease have been excluded. Hence, only those workers with Raynaud's Phenomenon attributable to the vibration exposure from chipping and grinding tools have been included in the analysis.

1.3 Data Analysis

Some of the questionnaire data and all of the medical data were coded by hand from the original forms. All questionnaire and medical data were keypunched, verified, formed into SAS data sets (34), computer edited and, for important analysis variables, all verified by hand. SAS programmes were

Table 4. Prevalence of Vibration White Finger Stages in Foundry and Shipyard Populations.

VWF Stages	Controls Foundries and Shipyard N=63	Vibration Foundries N=147		Exposed Shipyard N=58	
00	100%	17%		36%	
0T		9%		11%	
0N		7%	36%	17%	45%
0TN		20%		17%	
01		20%		9%	
02		22%	47%	5%	19%
03		5%		5%	

Table 5. Latencies of Tingling, Numbness and Blanching.

	Foundries Median (yrs)	Mean (yrs)	Shipyard Median (yrs)	Mean (yrs)
Latency of Tingling Stages 0T,0TN,01,02,03	0.6 (N=94)	1.8	4.2 (N=21)	9.1
Latency of Numbness Stages 0N,0TN,01,02,03	0.8 (N=80)	2.2	9.5 (N=26)	12.0
Latency of Blanching Stages 01,02,03	1.4 (N=69)	2.0	16.5 (N=11)	16.8

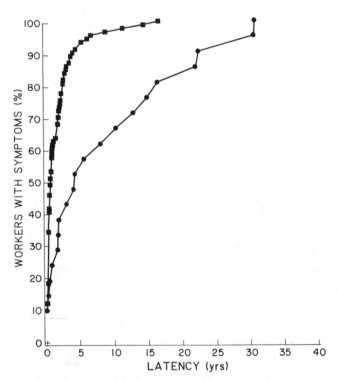

Fig. 1 Cumulative distribution showing the latency of tingling in foundry and shipyard workers using chipping hammers (data shown by squares and circles, respectively).

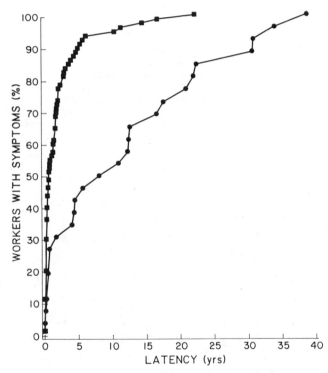

Fig. 2 Cumulative distribution showing the latency of numbness in foundry and shipyard workers using chipping hammers (data shown by squares and circles, respectively).

used to perform statistical analyses.

A selection model was developed and the computer programmed to place workers into vibration exposed and control groups. The exposed group included a worker who met the following criteria:
a)   Has a current job title (i.e. at the time of the survey) which was one of the eleven designated for workers who use pneumatic chipping hammers on the job.
b)   Cannot have used on his current job a vibrating hand tool, such as a jack hammer or gasoline-powered chain saw, that could confound the vibration exposure. (For a complete discussion of the criteria for confounding vibration exposures, see Ref. 30.)
c)   Cannot have used a different vibrating hand tool on a job previous to the current job, except when the current job has been held for 12 months or more, and the total duration of the confounding vibration exposures on previous jobs was four months or less.

Behrens et al.: Chipping and grinding

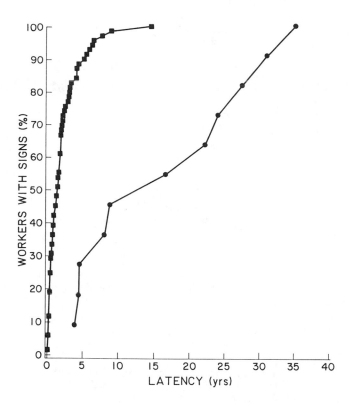

Fig. 3 Cumulative distribution showing
the latency of blanching in foundry
and shipyard workers using chipping
hammers (data shown by squares and
circles, respectively).

d)   Cannot have used vibrating hand tools
during off-the-job hours (i.e. as a hobby
tool).

The criteria for inclusion in the
control group were as follows:
a)   Must never have used any type of
vibrating hand tool (pneumatic, electric,
gasoline-powered or otherwise) on his
current job or any previous job, including
all part-time, military and full-time
employment.
b)   Cannot have used gasoline-powered chain
saws or any pneumatic hand tools during
off-the-job hours (i.e. as hobby tools).
By applying these criteria, controls had no
occupational exposure to hand-arm vibration
and insignificant hobby tool exposure.

The project medical doctors reviewed
questionnaire data and medical examination
data for each worker without knowledge of
the worker's exposure classification, and
identified cases of Primary Raynaud's
Disease and Secondary Raynaud's Phenomenon
attributable to causes other than vibration.
In this way, workers with medical conditions
that confound a diagnosis of the Vibration
Syndrome were identified. Table 2 shows
the percentage of workers in the total study
population who did, and did not, have confounding hand-arm exposure histories and/or
confounding medical conditions. The results

presented apply only to those 268 exposed
and control workers who did not have confounding exposure or medical histories.

II   RESULTS

Diagnosed cases of VWF were staged
according to an assessment system developed
by Taylor and Pelmear (10,35), shown in
Table 3. The prevalence of these Stages
in the foundry and shipyard population are
shown in Table 4. As expected, no control
workers had Raynaud's Phenomenon after
exclusion of workers with confounding
medical conditions.

The latent period for the Vibration
Syndrome is defined as the time from the
first occupational exposure to hand-arm
vibration until the onset of symptoms of
the Syndrome. For this study, the starting
date of the earliest job using a pneumatic
chipping hammer was designated the beginning
of hand-arm vibration exposure. The times
from this date until the onset of tingling,
numbness or blanching were the latency
periods for these symptoms and signs. Onset
dates of these symptoms and signs and the
beginning and ending dates for jobs were
recorded on the questionnaire. Table 5
gives the mean and median latencies for
tingling, numbness and blanching in the
foundry and shipyard populations. Figures
1, 2 and 3 give the cumulative distributions
for the onset of these signs and symptoms
in the population groups.

Workers in the study population were
asked fourteen questions during their interviews concerning the degree of: 1) pain or
aching in the fingers, hand and arms (four
questions); 2) manual impairment (four
questions); and 3) occurrence of symptoms
during off-the-job activities (six questions). These questions and the mean percentage of affirmative answers by VWF Stage
are given in Table 6. The proportion of
positive answers to these questions increased with increasing severity of the
Stage. In all cases, Stage 03 had the
greatest proportion of positive responses.
Stage 02 was next, except for questions
about pain and aching in the fingers, hands
and arms. For these questions the percentage with Stage 0TN was slightly greater.
Stages 0TN and 01 had similar proportions
of positive responses to these questions,
except that the responses in Stage 0TN were
always somewhat greater than those in
Stage 01. The controls and exposed workers
without the Vibration Syndrome had insignificant proportions of affirmative answers.
For all fourteen questions, the chi square
test for homogenity and trend was statistically significant (p<0.01).

Figure 4 shows the relationship between the vibration white finger staging
and the number of years exposed to the
vibration from chipping. The association
between increasing years on jobs using a

Table 6. Mean Percentage of Workers Answering "Yes" to Questions About Symptoms in the Hands and Arms; Manual Impairment; and Symptoms During Activities.

Questions (See Legend Below)	Controls 00 N=63	Vibration Exposed 00 N=46	Vibration White Finger Stage OT N=20	ON N=20	OTN N=39	01 N=34	02 N=36	03 N=10
A. 4 Questions: Symptoms in Hands and Arms	4	14	36	21	56	39	53	60
B. 4 Questions: Manual Impairment	2	6	14	11	21	18	36	48
C. 5 Questions: Symptoms During Activities	0	3	14	8	29	18	38	54
D. 1 Question: Trouble Sleeping Due to Symptoms	0	4	10	5	28	26	36	40

Legend: A. Do you ever have pain or aching in your wrists? Do you ever have pain or aching in your elbows? What about aching in your fingers? How about pain in your hands?

B. Do you have difficulty doing any of the following activities? Doing fine work? Fastening buttons? Handling or picking up coins? Distinguishing between hot and cold objects?

C. Do you have pain, tingling or numbness in your hands or fingers when you do any of the following things? Travelling to work? Washing your car? Watching sports outdoors? Playing games? Doing other hobbies?

D. Have you had trouble sleeping because of numbness or tingling in your hands or fingers?

chipping hammer, the numeric variable, and increasing severity of VWF Stage becomes statistically significant when the numeric variable is transformed into a categorical variable and the Stages are grouped together in order to increase the cell sizes (p<0.001). These tests were performed separately for the foundry and shipyard populations using Kendal's TAU-B measure of association (36).

III DISCUSSION

The prevalence of VWF is often quoted in the literature as evidence of the extent or severity of the Vibration Syndrome in a population. This unit, however, without first establishing a cohort of known vibration exposure time is misleading. The latency of VWF signs (e.g. blanching) and symptoms (e.g. numbness, tingling or both) represents the severity or amount of vibration energy entering the hand from any working process. This factor together with the vibration exposure time of the workers will determine the magnitude of the Vibration Syndrome hazard in any given population. The mean latency of blanching is the traditional measure of the severity of the Syndrome. For this study the mean latencies of the neurological symptoms - tingling and numbness - have been added. A further addition has been the median latencies.

Figures 1, 2 and 3 show sharp increases in the cumulative percentage of workers with comparatively shorter latencies up to the median, 50 percentile, in the foundry population, and the 30 percentile in the shipyard population. After these points, the functions level off due to outliers with relatively longer latencies. These graphs indicate, at least for the foundry populations, that the median may be a more meaningful measure of the latency of vibration signs and symptoms than the mean.

The study results show that the median latencies of signs and symptoms in the foundry population are very short, ranging from seven months for tingling, to one year and five months for blanching, with numbness after nine months. Consequently, the prevalences of both neurological Stages (36%) and blanching Stages (47%) were high in the foundry population (see Table 4). By comparison, the mean latencies of neurological symptoms in the shipyard population are long (9.1 yrs for tingling and 12 yrs for numbness), and the latency of blanching encompasses half a working life time (16.8 years). The prevalence of blanching Stages at the shipyard (19%), was lower than at the foundries, as expected. The full interpretation of the differences between foundry and shipyard populations requires

Behrens et al.: Chipping and grinding

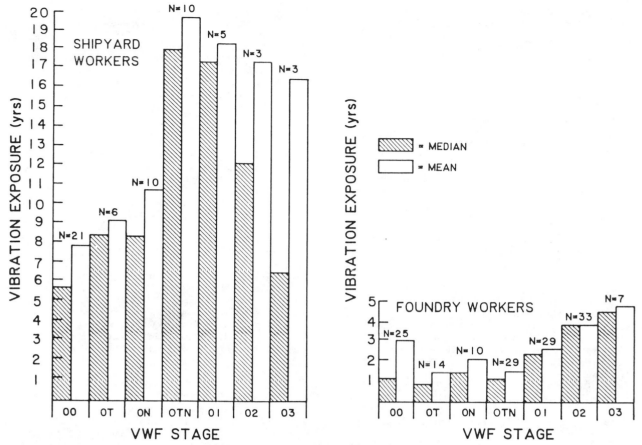

Fig. 4 Relation between the duration of employment involving operation of a chipping hammer and the Stage of VWF.

extensive engineering and industrial hygiene measurements reported elsewhere, and is beyond the scope of this paper.

All foundry workers with sufficient vibration exposure time had advanced into the blanching Stages of the Vibration Syndrome (see Fig. 4). In contrast, workers at Stage OTN in the shipyard population have not shown blanching symptoms, although they have been exposed for a sufficiently long time interval. This observation may explain, in part, the relatively high prevalence (45%) of workers with neurological Stages at the shipyard. The different pathology - the foundries with the emphasis on the arterial system and the shipyards with the neurological signs and symptoms (tingling and numbness) - suggests that the vibration is acting independently on the hand-arm tissue systems (arteries and nerves). It also suggests that the rate at which energy is introduced into the hand is one factor in the destructive processes. In both populations there was a statistically significant association between vibration exposure time using pneumatic chipping hammers and the severity of VWF, assessed by Stage classification.

DISCLAIMER

Mention of commercially available services, apparatus, instrumentation, devices, products, or proposed standards does not constitute endorsement by the National Institute for Occupational Safety and Health.

REFERENCES

1. Grounds MD. Raynaud's phenomenon in users of chain saws. Med J Aust 1964; 1: 270-272.
2. Laroche G. Traumatic vasospastic disease in chain saw operators. Can Med Assoc J 1976; 115: 1217-1221.
3. Huzl F, Stolarik R, Mainerova J, Jankova J, Sykora J. Damage due to vibrations when felling timbers by power saws. Pracov Lek 1971; 23: 7-15.
4. Pyykkö I. The prevalence and symptoms of traumatic vasospastic disease among lumberjacks in Finland. Work Environ Health 1974; 11: 118-131.
5. Matsumoto T, Yamada S, Harada N. A comparative study of vibration hazards among operators of vibrating tools in certain industries. Arh Hig Rada Toksikol 1979; 30: 701-707.

6. Allingham PM, Firth RD. The vibration syndrome. NZ Med J 1972; 76: 317-321.

7. Hellstrom B, Stensvold I, Halvorsrud JR, Vik T. Finger blood circulation in forest workers with Raynaud's phenomenon of occupational origin. Int Z Angew Physiol 1970; 29: 18-28.

8. Rafalski H, Bernacki K, Switonick T. The diagnostics and epidemiology of vibration disease and hearing impairment in motor sawyers. In: Wasserman DE, Taylor W, Curry MG, eds. Proc of the Int Occup Hand-Arm Vibration Conf. Cincinnati, OH: Dept of Health and Human Services, 1977. (NIOSH publication no. 77-170): 84-88.

9. Axelsson SA. Progress in solving the problem of hand-arm vibration for chain saw operators in Sweden, 1967 to date. In: Wasserman DE, Taylor W, Curry MG, eds. Proc of the Int Occup Hand-Arm Vibration Conf. Cincinnati, OH: Dept of Health and Human Services, 1977. (NIOSH publication no. 77-170): 218-224.

10. Taylor W, Pelmear PL, eds. Vibration White Finger in Industry. London: Academic Press, 1975.

11. Lidström I-M. Vibration injury in rock drillers, chiselers and grinders. In: Wasserman DE, Taylor W, Curry MG, eds. Proc of the Int Occup Hand-Arm Vibration Conf. Cincinnati, OH: Dept of Health and Human Services, 1977. (NIOSH publication no. 77-170): 77-83.

12. Mikulinskii AM. The effect of vibration of various ranges of high frequency on some physiological functions of the organisms of working men. Gig Tr Prof Zabol 1967; 11: 48-50.

13. Agate JN, Druett HA, Tombleson JBL. Raynaud's phenomenon in grinders of small metal castings. Br J Ind Med 1946; 3: 167-174.

14. Bovenzi M, Petronio L, Marino FD. Epidemiologic survey of shipyard workers exposed to hand-arm vibration. Int Arch Occup Environ Health 1980; 46: 251-266.

15. Asanova TP. Vibration disease among workers using portable power tools in Finnish shipyards. In: Korhonen O, ed. Vibration and Work: Proc of the Finnish-Soviet-Scandinavian Vibration Symposium. Helsinki: Inst of Occup Health, 1976: 52-62.

16. Hamilton A. A study of spastic anemia in the hands of stonecutters. Washington: Government Printing Office, 1918. (Bull US Bureau of Labor Statistics, no. 236: Ind Accidents and Hygiene Series, no. 19): 53-66.

17. Hunter D, McLaughlin AIC, Perry KMA. Clinical effects of the use of pneumatic tools. Br J Ind Med 1945; 2: 10-16.

18. Suzuki H. Vibration syndrome of vibrating tool users in a factory of steel foundry. Jpn J Ind Health 1978; 20: 261-268. (in Japanese).

19. Matsumoto T, Harada N, Yamada S, Kobayaski F. On vibration hazards of chipping hammer operators in an iron foundry. Jpn J Ind Health 1981; 23: 51-60 (in Japanese).

20. Matsumoto T, Yamada S, Hisanaga N, Harada N, Kaneda K. On vibration hazards in rock drill operators of a metal mine. Jpn J Ind Health 1977; 19: 256-265 (in Japanese).

21. Iwata H. Effects of rock drills on operators. Part 2. Survey and examination of Raynaud's phenomenon cases. Ind Health (Japan) 1968; 6: 37-58.

22. Chatterjee DS, Petrie A, Taylor W. Prevalence of vibration-induced white finger in fluorspar mines in Weardale. Br J Ind Med 1978; 35: 208-218.

23. Rothstein T. Report of the physical findings in eight stonecutters from the limestone region of Indiana. Washington: Government Printing Office, 1918. (Bull US Bureau of Labor Statistics, no. 236: Ind Accidents and Hygiene Series, no. 19): 67-96.

24. Leake JP. Health hazards from the use of the air hammer in cutting Indiana limestone. Washington: Government Printing Office, 1918. Bull US Bureau of Labor Statistics, no. 236: Ind Accidents and Hygiene Series, no. 19: 100-113.

25. Dart EE. Effects of high speed vibrating tools on operators engaged in the aeroplane industry. Occup Med 1946; 1: 515-550.

26. Ashe WF, Williams N. Occupational Raynaud's II. Arch Environ Health 1964; 9: 425-433.

27. Pecora LJ, Udel M, Christman RP. Survey of current status of Raynaud's phenomenon of occupational origin. Am Ind Hyg Assoc J 1960; 21: 80-83.

28. Wasserman DE, Badger DW, Doyle TE, Margolies L. Industrial vibration - an overview. J Am Soc Safety Eng 1974; 19: 38-43.

29. In: Wasserman DE, Taylor W, Curry MG, eds. Proceedings of the Occup Hand-Arm Vibration Conf. Cincinnati, OH: Dept of Health and Human Services, 1977. (NIOSH publication no. 77-170).

30. Wasserman DE, Taylor W, Behrens V, Samueloff S, Reynolds D. Vibration White Finger Disease in US Workers Using Pneumatic Chipping and Grinding Hand Tools. I-Epidemiology. Cincinnati, OH: Dept of Health and Human Services, 1982 (NIOSH publication no. 82-118).

31. Reynolds DD, Wasserman DE, Basel R, Taylor W, Doyle TE, Asburry W. Vibration acceleration measured on pneumatic tools used in chipping and grinding operations. In: Brammer AJ, Taylor W, eds. Vibration Effects on Hand and Arm in Industry. New York: Wiley, 1982.

32. Reynolds DD, Wasserman DE, Basel R, Taylor W. Energy entering the hands of operators of pneumatic tools used in chipping and grinding operations. In: Brammer AJ, Taylor W, eds. Vibration Effects on Hand and Arm in Industry. New York: Wiley, 1982.

33. Wasserman DE, Reynolds D, Behrens V, Taylor W, Samueloff S, Basel R. Vibration White Finger Disease in US Workers Using Pneumatic Chipping and Grinding Tools. II-Engineering Testing. Cincinnati, OH: Dept of Health and Human Services, 1981. (NIOSH publication no. 82-101).

34. SAS Institute Inc. SAS User's Guide. Cary, North Carolina: Statistical Analysis System Inc, 1979.

35. Taylor W, ed. The Vibration Syndrome. London: Academic Press, 1974.

36. Agresti A, Agresti BF. Statistical methods for the social sciences. San Francisco: Dellen Publishing Co, 1979.

DISCUSSION

M. Färkkilä: My question concerns the staging of VWF. How can you be sure that tingling in the fingertips is a sign of forthcoming VWF and not of neuropathy?

Authors' Response: The Taylor-Pelmear VWF Stage classification is essentially clinical. It is based on the subject's description of his signs and symptoms and his impairment at work, at home, and in his leisure-hobby activities found at the time of the clinical examination. With regard to the question, no examiner can be certain that a vibration exposed worker complaining of tingling in his hands and/or fingers will proceed to blanching of the fingers (Stages 1, 2 or 3). All our data (from 1968) show that in the majority of chain saw operators, tingling is an early symptom, and that given sufficient additional vibration exposure the arterial system will ultimately become affected. This is dependent on: a) the vibration level of the stimulus being introduced into the hands from the saw; and b) the total exposure time. In epidemiological terms, this is seen in over 90% prevalences of finger blanching in some of our chain saw operator populations. The data in this paper indicate a shorter latent interval for both tingling and numbness than for blanching. From the shipyard data it would appear that the vibration stimulus is acting independently on the neurological and arterial systems. The Taylor-Pelmear classification does not rule out that tingling and numbness (especially numbness) may co-exist with blanching. In our surveys, when subjects get to Stages 2 and/or 3 the predominant complaint is the number and severity of blanching attacks, with the interference of these attacks in their enjoyment of life (referred to by MacCallum as "the quality of living"). In these subjects, the neurological damage, although undoubtedly present, is secondary to the arterial system degeneration, first producing sensitivity to cold and finally obliterating the lumen of the vessels. With increasing vibration exposure, there is increasing arterial damage. The Stage classification merely indicates increasing damage to neurological and arterial systems (together with functional impairment).

A Longitudinal Study of the Vibration Syndrome in Finnish Forestry Workers

I. Pyykkö, O. S. Korhonen, M. A. Färkkilä,
J. P. Starck and S. A. Aatola

ABSTRACT: A longitudinal study of the Vibration Syndrome (VS) in forest workers has been conducted from 1972 (118 subjects) to 1980 (197 subjects). The prevalence of vibration-induced white finger (VWF) was 40% in 1972, when the mean latent period was 5600 h (SD=2500 h). A gradual decline in the prevalence of VWF has since occurred, to 7% in 1980, and the severity of VWF has decreased significantly. Paresthesia of the hands and arms also decreased from 78% to 40% during this period. No correlation was found between the severity of VWF and peripheral nerve symptoms. A separate study of 81 forest workers, who had used only saws with vibration-isolated handles, revealed that 28% had symptoms of paresthesia and 16% had VWF. No single, satisfactory, objective test for the VS or method for establishing the impairment of sufferers has been found.

RESUME: Une étude longitudinale du syndrome de vibration chez des travailleurs forestiers a été effectuée entre 1972 (118 sujets) et 1980 (197 sujets). La prévalence des doigts blancs dûs aux vibrations (VWF) était de 40% en 1972, alors que la période latente moyenne était de 5600 h (SD=2500 h). Une baisse progressive (à 7% en 1980) de la prévalence des doigts blancs a eu lieu depuis et la gravité des doigts blancs a diminué de façon significative. La paresthésie des mains et des bras a également diminué de 78% à 40% au cours de cette période. Aucune corrélation n'a pu être établie entre la gravité des doigts blancs et des symptômes nerveux périphériques. Une autre étude de 81 travailleurs forestiers, qui n'avaient utilisé que des scies avec poignées antivibrations, a révélé que 28% avaient des symptômes de paresthésie et 16% avaient des doigts blancs. Aucun test objectif, satisfaisant et unique pour le syndrome de vibration ni aucune méthode pour déterminer l'affaiblissement des victimes n'ont été trouvés.

INTRODUCTION

Many surveys have confirmed the connection between the vibration of hand-held tools and disturbances in the circulation of the fingers (see, for example, Refs. 1-4). Other evidence suggests that vibration may also cause symptoms in the peripheral nerves, muscles, bones and joints (5). All these symptoms are part of a disease entity, known as the Vibration Syndrome (6,7). The different symptoms of the Vibration Syndrome may occur together or independently from each other (8), perhaps indicating different etiological mechanisms.

The most prominent component of the Vibration Syndrome is periodic ischemic attacks affecting the fingers, provoked by cold weather, known as Traumatic Vasospastic Disease (TVD) (9), or Vibration-Induced White Finger (VWF) (6). Peripheral nerve symptoms have also been reported, e.g.

numbness, paresthesia and pain in the arms and hands (10,11). These symptoms can disturb sleep, waking the worker and forcing him to massage his hands (12). Weakness of grip has been reported (13-16), but has not been verified as a component of the Syndrome, despite careful examination (17,18).

The chain saws of the early 1950's were cumbersome and their use was limited to two to three hours per day (19). They were infrequently associated with the Vibration Syndrome. By the early 1960's, modification of the chain saw allowed its use for the limbing of trees, and, as a result, the work time was increased to five or six hours per day (12,20). Some time after the introduction of these saws, an alarming increase in the number of men with vasospastic symptoms occurred.

The prevalence of VWF among the forest workers of Finland in the late 1960's and early 1970's was from 40 to 60% (21,22).

Similar figures were reported during the same period from Scandinavia, Australia and Britain (18,20,23,24).

Since 1969, technical changes in the engine and the introduction of devices to dampen vibration have reduced the acceleration of chain saw handles from 60 to 350 m/s^2, to about 30 to 70 m/s^2 (25-27). Our earlier reports (14,28), and preliminary reports from Britain (29), indicate a significant decrease in the incidence of the Vibration Syndrome is taking place, which could be attributed to the decreased vibration.

A longitudinal study was undertaken to determine the current prevalence and any changes in the Vibration Syndrome during the years 1972 to 1980 among a stable population of Finnish Forest Workers. Preliminary reports from the survey were published in 1972 and 1975 (12,28).

I SUBJECTS AND METHODS

The study was carried out in connection with compulsory medical examinations in North Eastern Finland during the winters of 1972 and 1975 to 1980. All forest workers working for the National Board of Forestry in the parish of Suomussalmi were examined. The study focussed on full-time forest workers. Only those workers who had used a chain saw for not less than 500 h per year during three consecutive years were included. The number of Forest Workers studied and their age distribution in the different years are shown in Table 1.

1.1 Evaluation of the Vibration Syndrome

Prior to examination, the forest workers completed a questionnaire about their state of health, their use of medication and their symptoms of the Vibration Syndrome. A routine medical examination was carried out by the same physician on all occasions, with special emphasis on symptoms and signs suggesting the Vibration Syndrome. The severity of VWF was evaluated by an index (TVD index) each year (12). If more than two years had passed since the

last attack of VWF, the subject was considered to have recovered.

Each year, a subjective evaluation of the presence and severity of symptoms of the Vibration Syndrome, and any occupational disability they caused, was requested. In addition, an evaluation of other symptoms known to cause disability in lumberjacks, such as back and neck problems, was also requested. In 1975, the medical history was repeated and the percentage disability caused by different symptoms was compared with annual earnings, and with annual sick leave (compensated by the Social Insurance Institution).

1.2 Objective Measurements

A cold provocation test was performed on all subjects with a history of white fingers and on a control group of forest workers who were randomly selected each year. The temperature of the testing room was maintained at 18 to 22°C. The lumberjacks submerged their arms up to the shoulders in water at 13 to 15°C while gripping metal cylinders. Cold, wet towels from a water bath at 13 to 15°C were laid across their bare shoulders and changed every 15 seconds. After 15 minutes, the provocation was interrupted, and alterations in the colour of the skin were checked. Whiteness of a finger persisting for more than one minute was regarded as positive evidence of Raynaud's Phenomenon.

During the annual medical examination, other measurements were carried out. Finger plethysmography and skin temperature measurements recorded in 1972 and 1975 have been published elsewhere (30,31). The vibration perception threshold of the finger pad at different frequencies and the temporary increase in threshold with vibration exposure (TTS) were measured between 1977 and 1979 (with and without ischemia of the upper arm) (32,33). In addition, the grip strengths of the lumberjacks with and without simultaneous vibration exposure were measured from 1977 to 1979: the results of this study have been published elsewhere (34,35).

Table 1. Age Distribution of Lumberjacks Studied in Different Years (Percentages in Parentheses).

Age (yrs)	Year of Examination						
	1972	1975	1976	1977	1978	1979	1980
20-29	32 (27)	45 (24)	31 (18)	37 (20)	45 (22)	49 (23)	47 (22)
30-39	48 (41)	57 (30)	61 (34)	59 (31)	64 (32)	60 (29)	65 (30)
40-49	34 (29)	76 (41)	70 (38)	72 (38)	73 (36)	77 (37)	77 (35)
50-59	4 (3)	9 (5)	19 (10)	21 (11)	21 (10)	24 (11)	28 (13)
Total	118 (100)	187 (100)	181 (100)	189 (100)	203 (100)	210 (100)	217 (100)

II RESULTS

2.1 Prevalence, Latency and Subjective Complaints of VWF

In 1972, 52 (40%) of 118 forest workers gave a history of Raynaud's Phenomenon. During the follow-up period, the prevalence of VWF has fallen steadily (Fig. 1). The prevalence of VWF among the 197 forest workers in 1980 was 7%. Since 1972, only three new subjects have been disabled by VWF. In one case, the disorder resulted from the thoracic outlet syndrome.

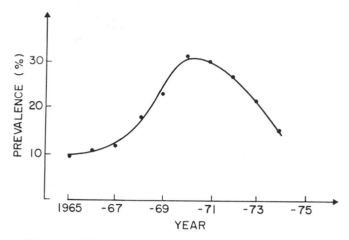

Fig. 2 The percentage prevalence of VWF among forest workers in the years 1965-1974. The number of lumberjacks was 137 in 1965 and increased (almost linearly) to 187 in 1975. (From Ref. 28, with permission of Scand J Work Environ Health).

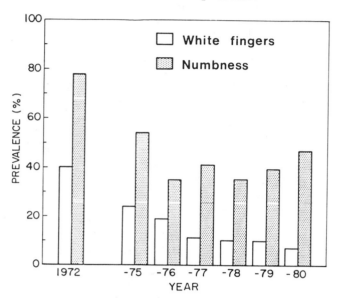

Fig. 1 The percentage prevalence of VWF and numbness of the hands and arms among lumberjacks in the years 1972 to 1980.

The history of attacks among the 187 forest workers complaining of VWF in 1975 was analysed retrospectively. After 1965, attacks of VWF started to become more common among forest workers; a peak value was reached in 1970 (Fig. 2). Since then, the incidence of VWF has been decreasing.

The mean latency for the development of VWF determined in 1975, when the annual work rate was about 1300 h per year, is shown in Fig. 3. VWF occurred, on average, after four to five years of full-time use of a chain saw. It must be stressed that the latent period of onset of VWF in our study reflects the effect of the second generation of chain saws which did not possess vibration-isolated handles, not the presently used third generation saws (first generation saws were large and cumbersome). According to the most recent subjective evaluation, one of the 13 subjects with VWF in 1980 regarded it as a major handicap at work, although 16% considered it slightly disabling (Table 2).

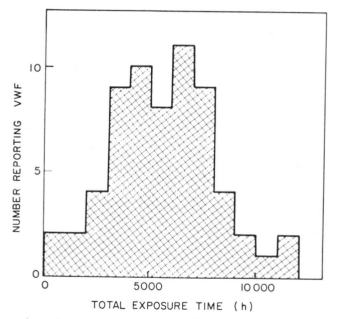

Fig. 3 The latent periods of VWF reported by 64 (of 187) lumberjacks, in 1975. (From Ref. 28, with permission of Scand J Work Environ Health).

Table 3 shows the occurrence of VWF during different work phases, as reported in the survey of 1972. It occurred most often on the way to and from work, and most commonly while riding motorcycles. Since 1972, the motorcycle has been replaced by the (heated) car as the means of transport to and from work (Fig. 4). This may be an important factor influencing the rapid

Table 2. The Subjective Disability Caused by the Vibration Syndrome and Other Symptoms Reported by 217 Lumberjacks in 1980.

Symptom	Number	Slight Disability	Considerable or Severe Disability
VWF	13	2	1
Paresthesia of hands and arms	93	7	2
Decreased muscle force	33	10	2
Pain or stiffness in the back	102	37	26

Table 3. Occurrence of Attacks of VWF (N=47).

Activity	N	%
Travelling to or from work	16	34
During sawing	13	28
During pauses between sawing	4	8
Irregularly during different work activities	14	30
Total	47	100

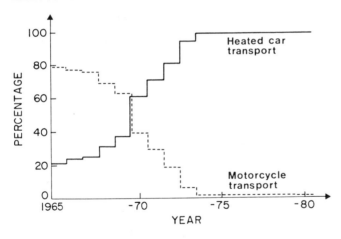

Fig. 4 Transportation used by forest workers to and from work in different years.

decline in the prevalence of VWF in the middle of the 1970's. Another may have been the weather, which was mild in the early 1970's. In our experience, very cold weather most frequently provokes attacks of VWF, although we have observed no increase in the prevalence of VWF during recent cold winters.

2.2 Prevalence and Subjective Evaluation of Numbness

Numbness of the hands occurred among 78% of the forest workers in 1972, more commonly in subjects with VWF. The numbness began, on average, a year later than the first attack of VWF and was not related to the severity of VWF. Numbness of the hands and arms occurred especially at night (Table 4), and was disturbing to subjects who were awakened, in some cases several times, and were forced to rub and shake their hands. From 1972 to 1976, a significant reduction in the prevalence of this symptom was observed (see Fig. 1). It has now reached a plateau of about 40%, and is more than expected among workers not exposed to vibration (30%) (36).

Table 4. Occurrence of Numbness of the Hands and Arms in 1972 (N=118).

Symptoms	N	%
No numbness	26	22
Numbness only during work	21	18
Numbness during work and/or at night	71	60
Total	118	100

According to the lumberjacks' own estimate, numbness of the hands was the most disabling component of the Vibration Syndrome in 1975, when considerable occupational disability was reported by 21% of the men with the symptom. In 1980 the corresponding figure was 2% (Table 2.).

2.3 Muscle Fatigue

Muscle fatigue has been analysed systematically since 1975, when it was realised that the symptom was a component of the Vibration Syndrome. In 1975, a history of excessive muscle fatigue was present among 19% of lumberjacks. In subjective evaluations, 20% of these forest workers considered it a cause for major disability at work. In 1980, the symptom was present in 17% of all lumberjacks, and regarded as a major cause of occupational disability by 6% of men with this symptom.

2.4 Vibration Syndrome in Subjects Exposed Only to the Vibration of A/V Chain Saws

Eighty-one forest workers who live in different parts of Finland, and are employed by a large forest company, were examined in 1975. They had used only modern chain saws equipped with vibration-isolated handles (third generation saws). The age distribution of these subjects is shown in

Pyykkö et al.: Finnish lumberjacks

Table 5. Age Distribution of 81 Lumberjacks Exposed Only to the Vibration of A/V Chain Saws.

Age (yrs)	N	%
<29	68	84
30-39	9	11
40-49	4	5
>50	0	0
Total	81	100

Table 5. VWF was present in 16% of these lumberjacks, and numbness of the hands and arms in 29%.

2.5 Objective Tests

In most years all lumberjacks with a history of VWF were subjected to a cold provocation test. Figure 5 shows the percentage of positive test results each year in a group of 44 subjects with VWF at the commencement of our studies. The results reveal a decrease in the number of positive tests, which is in agreement with the decreasing prevalence of VWF.

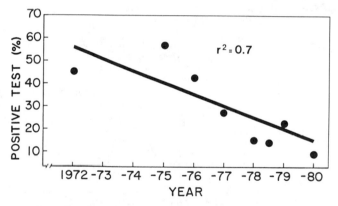

Fig. 5 Results of the cold provocation test, in different years, on 44 forest workers initially suffering from VWF.

Table 6 shows the results of the cold provocation test in the survey of 1975 when done twice during the day. The cold provocation test was positive on first application for only 45% of the forest workers with a history of VWF. When the test was repeated, the number of positive results increased to 67%. If the test was repeated after an interval of 6 h instead of 2 or 4 h, the result of the second test was significantly more often positive than the first. Thus, the effectiveness of the cold provocation test can be improved by repeating the test the same day, preferably following an interval of six hours.

Table 6. Number of Positive Results for Two Consecutive Cold Provocation Tests on 64 Lumberjacks with a History of VWF, in 1975.

Cold Provocation	Positive	
	N	%
First test	29	45
Second test	37	58
Total	43	67

No correlation was found between vasoconstrictions measured during exposure to vibration and the results of the cold provocation test. Furthermore, forest workers without VWF could also react to vibration or cold with strong vasoconstriction. As used by us, finger-pulse plethysmography did not assist in the diagnosis.

Figure 6 shows the psycho-physical vibration detection thresholds of the distal pad of the third finger on the left hand. No statistically significant differences exist between subjects with different components of the Vibration Syndrome and symptomless forest workers exposed to an equal amount of vibration. There was a statistically significant difference in the TTS of the perception thresholds reported by subjects with VWF or with muscle fatigue, and control subjects (see Fig. 7). There was no statistically significant difference, however, between control subjects and subjects with paresthesia of the hands and arms.

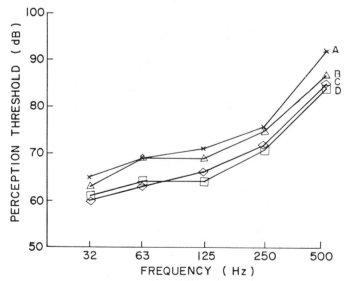

Fig. 6 Psycho-physical vibration detection thresholds: A, for 18 subjects with decreased muscle force; B, for 30 subjects with VWF; C, for 24 subjects with paresthesia of the hand and arm; and D, for 46 symptomless forest workers (dB re 0.0005 m/s^2).

Pyykkö et al.: Finnish lumberjacks

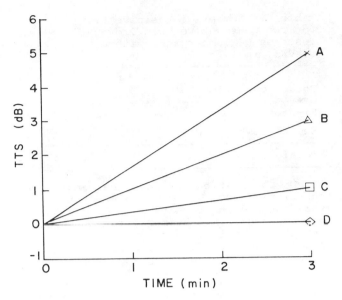

Fig. 7 Temporary threshold shift at 250 Hz after exposure to vibration at this frequency for 3 min: A, for 9 subjects with a history of decreased muscle force; B, for 30 subjects with VWF; C, for 22 subjects with paresthesia of the hand and arm; and D, for 49 symptomless forest workers (dB re 0.0005 m/s^2).

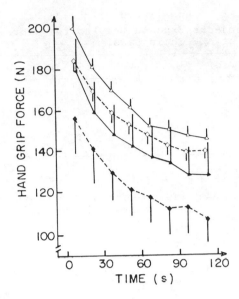

Fig. 8 Muscle fatigue curves without (open symbols) and with (closed symbols) vibration exposure for subjects with no history of the Vibration Syndrome (the triangles), and for subjects with a history of diminished grip force (the diamonds), during repeated maximal grip force-relaxation task. Mean values and SEM (in one direction).

Muscle fatigue and muscle force were normal in forest workers with VWF, whereas the latter was reduced in subjects with a history of numbness of the hands and/or a history of excessive muscle fatigue (Fig. 8). In addition, exposure to vibration further decreased muscle force in forest workers with a history of numbness of the hands and/or decreased muscle force, but not in normal subjects or in forest workers with VWF only.

III DISCUSSION

The wood forest products industry plays an important role in the economic life of Finland, and provided employment for 135 000 professional forest workers in 1966 (37). Because of advances in technology and organization, this number has been decreasing in recent years. At present there are only about 25 000 active forest workers, but it has been estimated that in 1985 there will still be some 20 000 forest workers in Finland (37).

Since the early 1970's, the reported number of vibration-induced health problems has been decreasing because of the falling prevalence of the Vibration Syndrome, and because fewer men are now working in

forestry. The decrease is not evident from the official records of cases of the Vibration Syndrome accepted as occupational disease for the years 1963 to 1979 (Table 7). There are several reasons for the low number of approved cases of the Vibration Syndrome, some of which are associated with the state of the national economy; more important reasons are the minor degree of disability caused by the Vibration Syndrome, and a lack of awareness of the Syndrome among practicing physicians.

Even in the scientific community there is a diversity of opinion about whether VWF and numbness of the hands are of the same

Table 7. Recorded Cases of the Vibration Syndrome as an Occupational Disease in Finland.

1963	1
1968	4
1969	5
1971	47
1972	60
1973	102
1974	83
1975	172
1976	188
1977	103
1978	91
1979	79

origin (6,11,8,38), and whether muscle fatigue is an individual component of the Vibration Syndrome (35). There is also a widespread belief that significant bone degeneration occurs in the Vibration Syndrome. Like some other investigations (18,39), the present studies do not support this opinion. It is therefore necessary to discuss each of the components of the Vibration Syndrome.

3.1 Vascular Disorders

Vascular disorders involving periodic blanching of the fingers, which closely resemble those of Raynaud's Disease, are the most prominent symptoms of the Vibration Syndrome. In the forest workers we examined, the vasoconstriction usually lasted from 5 to 15 minutes. Recovery was achieved by massage or warmth.

The vasoconstriction in our subjects did not show any tendency to progress to gangrenous changes of the digits, which have been occasionally described (40,41).

A separate study verified that the changes in prevalence observed among the limited number of forest workers at Suomussalmi reflected changes occurring throughout Finland (28). Five hundred and one forest workers who live in different parts of Finland were contacted. According to the results of self-administered questionnaires, VWF was present in 201 (40%) of the 501 forest workers in 1975; during the following years, 111 (of 201) with VWF indicated an improvement.

There is still debate concerning whether the Vibration Syndrome is reversible or not. Agate, using a self-administered questionnaire, found that a few workers reported their first attack of VWF some months after they had stopped working with vibrating tools (42). In 36% of workers who already had VWF, the vascular disturbances were claimed to have progressed rather than to have improved after the cessation of work. Other evidence, however, suggests that the vascular component of the Vibration Syndrome is reversible. Stewart and Goda observed that five years after the cessation of work involving vibration exposure, 30% of the workers no longer experienced attacks of VWF (36). Among lumberjacks operating chain saws in Sweden, a six year follow-up showed that a prevalence of VWF had decreased from 48 to 38% (43). In England, a similar study indicated improvement among lumberjacks in recent years (29, 44).

Thus, the reversibility of VWF seems to be established. However, a prolonged period is required before the abnormal reactivity of the peripheral vessels subsides (45,46), and the structural changes of the vessel walls regress (9,41,47). In the present study, the recovery period is similar to the latent interval.

One factor influencing the apparent course of VWF in our study is the increase in the use of heated cars for transportation to and from work, and elsewhere. If the men who experienced attacks of VWF while riding motorcycles to and from work were to resume riding to work, they might still experience attacks. As an indication of this possibility, we sometimes found a positive cold provocation test in men who have not had a single attack of VWF for five years. Thus, some of these men have not really "recovered"; rather, they do not "experience attacks", which indicates that under appropriate conditions they may still suffer from vasospasms. The milder winters in the beginning of the 1970's might also be a contributing factor in the reduced prevalence of white fingers, but this improvement may be only temporary.

3.2 Numbness of the Hands and Arms

Numbness of the hands and arms occurs in vibration-exposed subjects to a significantly greater extent than in workers not exposed to vibration (15,16,36). In 1972, the symptom was prevalent in 80% of forest workers in this study who were exposed to chain saw vibration, which is greater than the 30% prevalence reported in non-exposed subjects (36). According to Marshall et al. (38), peripheral neuropathy in the vegetative system as well as the somato-sensory nerves leads to the Vibration Syndrome. By measuring the conduction velocities of the peripheral nerves, Seppäläinen showed that occupational exposure to vibration may lead to peripheral neuropathy (11). In the present study, forest workers with VWF showed symptoms of peripheral neuropathy more often than subjects without VWF. However, the observation that neuropathy in forest workers bears no relation to the severity of the vascular component, and may occur independently, suggests separate mechanisms for these two components. They should therefore be evaluated separately.

The prevalence of numbness of the hands and arms has also been decreasing during recent years. Because the symptom is expected in about 30% of subjects not exposed to vibration, there is only a 10% increase of this symptom in vibration-exposed workers in 1980. Calculated in this way, the decreased prevalence of numbness of the hands and arms is close to the decreased prevalence of VWF.

3.3 Muscle Force

The data on the prevalence of extensive muscle fatigue in the hands and arms of forest workers, which occurs among 14 to 35% of the subjects, suggests that occupational exposure to vibration is the reason for inadequate muscle contraction (14-16). Since Bannister and Smith showed that the use of vibrating tools is associated with a significant decrease in manipulative dexterity (48), it seems that the muscular weakness is at least partly due to a disturbance of the fine control of the hand muscles. Furthermore, Färkkilä (34), and Färkkilä et al. (35), demonstrated objectively that exposure to vibration leads to a significant decrease in muscle force of the hands, and that the decrease is more advanced in subjects with a history of muscle weakness.

The effect of vibration on muscle tissue and muscle contraction is not well understood. The finding of Lung and Sivertsson that the reaction of denervated muscle tissue to vibration is to relax (49), indicates that vibration might interfere with muscle contraction by splitting the cross linkage between actin and myocin. In an intact muscle, a momentary decrease in muscle force is also observed when the muscle or tendon is exposed to vibration (35). This kind of decrease probably results in a simultaneous inhibition of agonistic and antagonistic muscles through the tonic vibration reflex, which is activated by distension of the muscle spindles during vibration (30,35,50,51).

The findings of atrophy in the thenar and interosseous muscles, reported by Teleky (5), are difficult to relate to the dynamic changes of muscle force. The atrophy is a late result of extensive neural degeneration in the hand and arm.

Very often, however, the same subjects who showed extensive symptoms of neuropathy also had decreased muscle strength. In our experiments, subjects with signs of peripheral neuropathy were also found to have significantly decreased muscle force. In a preliminary study, a correlation seemed to exist between the decrease in muscle force and nerve conduction velocity (26). Hence, it seems possible that degeneration in the nerves which innervate the muscles could be the immediate cause of excessive muscle fatigue.

There has been only a slight decrease in the prevalence of muscle fatigue among forest workers during our longitudinal study. One explanation might be that heavy and strenuous work might partly influence the development of muscle fatigue. During the study a temporary decrease in working hours was observed. The annual saw operating time decreased from 1300 h in the early 1970's to 1100 h in the late 1970's, but is now increasing. Furthermore, recovery from this symptom may not be evident because of ageing of the subjects (35).

3.4 Disability Caused by the Vibration Syndrome

The Vibration Syndrome consists of different symptoms which can occur together or separately. Thus, in order to classify the occupational handicap, all the different components need to be analysed and included. In addition to occupational disability, interference with recreation and leisure time activities should be taken into consideration. It is difficult to assess the handicap caused by VWF in a subject who is unable to swim, fish, or sail even in the heat of summer. Also paresthesia of the hands and arms that regularly awakes the sufferer, in some cases several times during the same night, can be very annoying. Similarly, impaired manipulative dexterity must be considered (some of our subjects were even unable to change a lamp at home).

The handicap caused by finger blanching has been studied by means of a questionnaire. Grounds was the first to report that, in spite of the high prevalence of Raynaud's Phenomenon, none of the forest workers questioned considered the disability sufficient to give up his job (53). Kylin and Lidström found that VWF appeared to cause little or moderate disability in 45% of 453 forest workers, whereas in 55% the disease was not a handicap (20). During the last five years, the severity of the disease among lumberjacks seems to have decreased (28,44). Most of the forest workers who still had attacks of VWF at Suomussalmi in 1980 found the symptoms mild, and none described them as causing difficulties or disability.

In contrast, peripheral nerve symptoms can be severe, and may cause a loss of wages and considerable handicap among forest workers and industrial workers, as stressed by Klimková-Deutschová (10).

Information on the disability caused by decreased muscle strength is contradictory. Helström and Lange Anderson did not find any observable changes in the muscle strength of lumberjacks who used chain saws, in comparison to non-users (18). In Suomussalmi, weakening of grip force caused considerable disability in some lumberjacks, even to the extent that earnings were reduced.

The official rating of the occupational disability caused by the Vibration Syndrome varies between different countries. In Norway and Sweden, a proved secondary Raynaud's Phenomenon with adequate exposure to vibration is enough for a diagnosis of occupational disease. In contrast, in Finland, a subject has to show signs of the involvement of at least two organ systems. In England, VWF has only recently been recommended for compensation as a Prescribed Disease (Stage 3 in Taylor's Classification (52)). Thus a great need exists for the development of universally acceptable standards for the handicap associated with the Vibration Syndrome, which include interference with both social and occupational activities. A uniform method of staging different symptoms and severity has not yet been discovered, though two indices for VWF have been proposed (12,52). Unfortunately, the limits between different symptoms and Stages are often based on subjective interpretation by both the vibration-exposed worker and the examining physician, and in consequence the indices are more suitable for research purposes than for assessing disability.

3.5 Objective Tests for the Vibration Syndrome

A cold provocation test is easy to interpret even under primitive conditions. It also seems to correlate positively with the number of affected digits (12,42). A negative result in the test, however, does not exclude the possibility of Raynaud's Phenomenon. The percentage of positive tests in men with a history of VWF appears to range from 40 to 95% (12,42,54), and the results of the test can be different if it is repeated. Among the forest workers at Suomussalmi, for example, repetition of the test increased the percentage of positive results from 45 to 67%. Measurement of the recovery time of digital blood flow for individuals greatly enhances the positive results of the test, as recently indicated by Juul and Nielsen (54). In contrast, plethysmography of the digits as well as angiography of the hands and arms have not yet proved to be suitable methods for the diagnosis of VWF (30,35,55,56).

Hopf's method of measuring the conduction velocity of nerve fibres is reliable in estimating the injuries to the peripheral nerves (11). The disadvantage of this method is its high sensitivity and lack of specificity, since polyneuropathies are frequently found among workers not exposed to vibration (21). The equipment is also cumbersome and requires a trained operator even under laboratory conditions.

The psycho-physical vibration detection threshold test and tactile discrimination test are widely used (52,57,58). However, a significant difference in the perception of vibration between normal and vibration-exposed subjects, and in subjects with different components of the Vibration Syndrome, has not been found. These observations are in agreement with the results of some other investigators (59). Because of the wide variation in sensory discrimination of vibration, this test should probably be used only to supplement other diagnostic techniques. The same criticism applies to tactile discrimination tests.

Measurements of the maximal hand grip force and the fatigue of the grip force during a two minute interval reveal differences between non-symptomatic and symptomatic groups of forest workers (31,34). However, there is a wide range in the results from individuals, and other factors including injuries to, and rheumatic or arthritic pains of, the hands and arms can also influence the hand grip. In addition, the motivation of subjects influences the reliability of the test results in some cases. The test can be used, as can most, to provide additional information for the diagnosis of the Vibration Syndrome.

IV CONCLUSIONS

The common use of chain saws in the 1960's caused a gradual increase in the Vibration Syndrome and in occupational disability among forest workers; the latent period of VWF was about five years. The highest morbidity in Finland was reached in 1970. In 1972, 40% of the lumberjacks in one forestry district had VWF, but in 1980 the prevalence had decreased to 7%. A similar peak and decrease in the prevalence of numbness of the hands and arms was also observed.

There is, so far, no simple objective test for the evaluation of the Vibration Syndrome. This is a major difficulty in the evaluation of individual cases. At present, it seems likely that the different components of the Syndrome, e.g. VWF, numbness of the hands and arms, and muscle fatigue, may arise independently. Individual tests for each of the components of the Vibration Syndrome should therefore be performed.

REFERENCES

1. Loriga G. Il lavoro con i martelli pneumatici. Boll inspett lavoro 2: 35, 1911, cited by Hasan. Biomedical aspects of low frequency vibration: A selective review. Work Environ Health 1970; 7: 19-45.

2. Hamilton A. A study of spastic anemia in the hands of stonecutters. Washington: Government Printing Office, 1918. (Bull US Bureau of Labor Statistics, no. 236: Ind Accidents and Hygiene Series, no. 19). (cited by Agate, Ref. 41).

3. Hamilton A. A vasomotor disturbance in the finger of stonecutters. Int Arch Gewerbepat Gewerbehyg Health 1930; 1: 348-358.

4. Dart EE. Effect of high speed vibrating tools on operators engaged in the airplane industry. JOM 1946; 1: 515-550.

5. Teleky L. Pneumatic tools. Occup Health Saf 1938; 1: 1-12.

6. Taylor W. Introduction. In: Taylor W. ed. The Vibration Syndrome. London: Academic Press, 1974: 1-12.

7. Korhonen O, Pyykkö I, Starck J, Toivanen J. Hand Transmitted Vibration: Vibration Disease. Norms and Measuring Methods. Katsauksia 24. Helsinki: Inst Occup Health, 1978: 1-69. (in Finnish).

8. Pyykkö I. Vibration syndrome: a review. In: Korhonen O ed. Vibration and Work. Helsinki: Inst Occup Health, 1976: 1-24.

9. Gurdjian ES, Walker LW. Traumatic vasospastic disease of the hand (white fingers). JAMA 1945; 129: 668-672.

10. Klimkovà-Deutschovà E. Neurologische Aspekte der Vibrationskrankheit. Int Arch Gewerbepat Gewerbehyg 1966; 22: 297-305. (in German).

11. Seppäläinen A-M. Peripheral neuropathy in forest workers: a field study. Work Environ Health 1972; 9: 106-111.

12. Pyykkö I. The prevalence and symptoms of traumatic vasospastic disease among lumberjacks in Finland. Work Environ Health 1974; 11: 118-131.

13. Pyykkö I. A Review on the Health Hazard Caused by Vibration. Helsinki: Inst Occup Health, 1975; 35-48. (in Finnish).

14. Pyykkö I, Sairanen E, Korhonen O, Färkkilä M, Ojala J-P, Ruokonen E. Vibration disease among the forest workers. Suom Laakaril 1976; 31: 2791-2797. (in Finnish).

15. Matsumoto K, Itoh N, Kasamatsu T, Iwata H. A study on subjective symptoms based on total operating time of chain saw. Jpn J Ind Health 1977; 19: 1, 22-28. (in Japanese).

16. Korhonen O, Nummi J, Nurminen M, Nygård K, Soininen H, Wiikeri M, Metsätyöntekijä. Osa 2: Terveys Verrattuna Ammatissa Toimivan Väestön Terveyteen. Työterveyslaitoksen tutkimuksia 126. Helsinki: Inst Occup Health, 1977. (in Finnish).

17. Iwata H. Effects of rock drills on operators: II. Survey and examination of Raynaud's phenomenon. Ind Health (Japan) 1968; 6: 37-46.

18. Hellström B, Lange Andersen K. Vibration injuries in Norwegian forest workers. Br J Ind Med 1972; 29: 255-263.

19. Aho K. Method of Measuring the Vibration of Chain Saws and Evaluating the Results. Helsinki: Finnish Research Inst of Engineering in Agriculture & Forestry, 1971. (Vakola Report no 8): 1-19.

20. Kylin B, Lidström I-M. Hälso-och miljöunder-Sökning Bland Skogsarbetare. AI-rapport. Stockholm: Arbetsmedicinska Institutet, 1968; 44-62.

21. Seppäläinen A-M. Neurophysiological detection of vibration syndrome in the shipbuilding industry. In: Korhonen O. ed. Vibration and Work. Helsinki: Inst Occup Health, 1976; 63-71.

22. Kumlin T, Wiikeri M, Sumari P. Radiological changes in carpal and metacarpal bones and phalanges caused by chain saw vibration. Br J Ind Med 1973; 30: 71-73.

23. Barnes R, Longley EO, Smith ARB, Allen JG. Vibration disease. Med J Aust 1969; 1: 901-905.

24. Taylor W, Pearson J, Kell RL, Keighley GD. Vibration syndrome in forestry commission chain saw operators. Br J Ind Med 1971; 28: 83-89.

25. Taylor W, Pelmear PL, Hempstock TI, O'Connor DE, Kitchner R. Correlation of epidemiological data and the measured vibration. In: Taylor W, Pelmear PL, eds. Vibration White Finger in Industry. London: Academic Press, 1975; 123-133.

26. Pyykkö I, Seppäläinen A-M, Futatsuka M, Starck J, Korhonen O, Färkkilä M. The decrease in

muscle force is correlated with decrease in peripheral nerve function in vibration syndrome. (in preparation).

27. Starck J, Aatola S, Hoikkala M, Färkkilä M, Korhonen O, Pyykkö I. Chain saw vibration: effects of age of the saw and the repeatability of measurements. In: Brammer AJ, Taylor W, eds. Vibration Effects on the Hand and Arm in Industry. New York: Wiley, 1982.

28. Pyykkö I, Sairanen E, Korhonen O, Färkkilä M, Hyvärinen J. A decrease in the prevalence and severity of vibration-induced white fingers among lumberjacks in Finland. Scand J Work Environ Health 1978; 4: 246-254.

29. Taylor W, Pelmear PL, Pearson JCG. A longitudinal study of Raynaud's phenomenon in chain saw operators. In: Taylor W, Pelmear PL eds. Vibration White Finger in Industry. London: Academic Press, 1975: 15-20.

30. Pyykkö I. A physiological study of the vasoconstrictor reflex in traumatic vasospastic disease. Work Environ Health 1974; 11: 170-186.

31. Färkkilä M, Pyykkö I. Blood flow in the contralateral hand during vibration and hand grip contractions of lumberjacks. Scand J Work Environ Health 1979; 5: 368-374.

32. Starck J, Färkkilä M, Aatola S, Pyykö I, Korhonen O. Vibration syndrome and vibration in pedestal grinding. Br J Ind Med (to appear).

33. Aatola S, Starck J, Pyykkö I, Färkkilä M, Korhonen O. Vibration detection threshold of lumberjacks. Proc Int Symp on Protection of Workers Against Vibration. Geneva: Int Labor Office (to appear).

34. Färkkilä M. Grip force in vibration disease. Scand J Work Environ Health 1978; 4: 159-166.

35. Färkkilä M, Pyykkö I, Korhonen O, Starck J. Vibration-induced decrease in the muscle force in lumberjacks. Eur J Appl Physiol 1980; 43: 1-9.

36. Stewart AM, Goda DF. Vibration syndrome. Br J Ind Med 1970; 27: 19-27.

37. Heikinheimo L, Heikinheimo M, Lehtinen L, Reunala A. Finnish lumberjacks. Porvoo: Werner Söderström Oy, 1972: 1-142. (in Finnish).

38. Marschall J, Poole EB, Reynard WA. Raynaud's phenomenon due to vibrating tools. Lancet 1954; I: 1151-1156.

39. James PB, Yates JR, Pearson JG. An investigation of the prevalence of bone cysts in hands exposed to vibration. In: Taylor W, Pelmear PL, eds. Vibration White Finger in Industry. London: Academic Press, 1975; 43-51.

40. Blair HM, Hadington JT, Lynch PJ. Occupational trauma, Raynaud phenomenon, and sclerodactylia. Int Arch Environ Health 1974; 28: 80-81.

41. Walton KW. The pathology of Raynaud's phenomenon of occupational origin. In: Taylor W, ed. The Vibration Syndrome. London: Academic Press, 1974: 109-119.

42. Agate JN. An outbreak of cases of Raynaud's phenomenon of occupational origin. Br J Ind Med 1949; 6: 144-163.

43. Thulesius O. Methods for the evaluation of peripheral vascular function in the upper extremities. Acta Chir Scand 1976; Suppl 465: 53-54.

44. Taylor W, Pearson JCG, Keighley GH. A longi-
    tudinal study of Raynaud's phenomenon in chain
    saw operators. In: Wasserman DE, Taylor W,
    Curry MG, eds. Proc of the Int Occup Hand-Arm
    Vibration Conf. Cincinnati, OH: Dept of Health
    and Human Services, 1977. (NIOSH publication
    no. 77-170): 69-76.
45. Lewis T. Vascular Disorder of the Limbs. 2nd
    ed. London: MacMillian, 1949.
46. Hyvärinen J, Pyykkö I, Sundberg S. Vibration
    frequencies and amplitudes in the aetiology of
    traumatic vasospastic disease. Lancet 1973;
    I: 791-794.
47. Ashe WF, Cook WT, Old JW. Raynaud's phenomenon
    of occupational origin. Arch Environ Health
    1962; 5: 333-343.
48. Banister PA, Smith FM. Vibration induced white
    fingers and manipulative dexterity. Br J Ind
    Med 1972; 29: 264-267.
49. Ljung B, Sivertsson R. Inhibition of vascular
    smooth muscle contraction by vibration. Acta
    Physiol Scand (Suppl) 1973; 396, 95 p.
50. Pyykkö I, Hyvärinen J. The physiological basis
    of the traumatic vasospastic disease: A
    sympathetic vasoconstrictor reflex triggered
    by high frequency vibration. Work Environ
    Health 1973; 10: 36-47.
51. Eklund G, Hagbarth K-E. Normal variability of
    tonic vibration reflexes in man. Exp Neurol
    1966; 16: 80-92.
52. Taylor W, Pelmear PL, Person J. Raynaud's
    phenomenon in forestry chain saw operators.
    In: Taylor W, ed. The Vibration Syndrome.
    London: Academic Press, 1974; 121-139.
53. Grounds MD. Raynaud's phenomenon in users of
    chain saw. Med J Aust 1964; 22: 279-272.
54. Juul C, Nielsen SL. Locally induced digital
    vasospasm detected by delayed rewarming in
    Raynaud's phenomenon of occupational origin.
    Br J Ind Med 1981; 38: 87-90.
55. James PB, Galloway RW. Arteriography of the
    hand in men exposed to vibration. In: Taylor
    W, Pelmear PL, eds. Vibration White Finger in
    Industry. London: Academic Press, 1975; 31-41.
56. Zweifler AJ. Detection of occlusive arterial
    disease in the hand and its relevance to
    occupational hand disease. In: Wasserman DE,
    Taylor W, Curry MG, eds. Proc of the Int Occup
    Hand-Arm Vibration Conf. Cincinnati, OH: Dept
    of Health and Human Services, 1977. (NIOSH
    publication no. 77-170): 12-20.
57. Miura T, Kumura K, Toimiaga Y, Kimotsuki KJ.
    On Raynaud's phenomenon of occupational origin
    due to vibrating tools. Jpn J Ind Health 1965;
    42: 725-747. (English abstract).
58. Asanova TP. Vibration disease among workers
    using portable power tools in Finnish ship-
    years. In: Korhonen O, ed. Vibration and
    Work. Helsinki: Inst Occup Health, 1976:
    52-62.
59. Pelmear PL, Taylor W, Pearson CG. Clinical
    objective test for vibration white finger. In:
    Taylor W, Pelmear PL, eds. Vibration White
    Finger in Industry. London: Academic Press,
    1975: 53-82.

DISCUSSION

H. Iwata: Are all 118 subjects in 1972 included among the subjects examined in subsequent years?

Authors' Response: Of 118 forest workers examined in 1972, 72 are still actively working. Because participation in the study was compulsory, we were able to establish the reasons why the forest workers were not available for the survey (retirement, moving to another district, change of occupation or sick leave). In only one case was early retirement due to the Vibration Snydrome. Chronic back pain caused more handicap than the Vibration Syndrome.

What are the prevalence rates of the various symptoms for the same subjects in 1972 and 1979, or 1980?

Authors' Response: The statistical analysis required to answer your question has not yet been completed.

P.V. Pelnar: Pacina and I studied a group of hard rock miners, who operated rock drills, and followed-up those with VWF from 1 to 5 years after the first diagnosis (Pelnar P, Pacina V. Vyvoj professionalni traumaticke vasoneurosy u lamacu rudnych dolu. Proc 8th Cong Occup Health, Czechoslovakia, 1964. (in Czech)). In most of those who had ceased work with vibrating tools, the disease had regressed or disappeared (see Table D1). This is further evidence of the reversibility of VWF. What was surprising, however, were three cases in which the disease regressed or disappeared, even though they had continued exposure to vibration. Would you care to comment on these observations? We speculated that these workers may have become skilled in operating their drills with reduced hand grip, which could have reduced the transfer of vibration into their hands.

Table D1. Results of Re-Examination of 50 Drillers with VWF (Percentages in Parentheses).

	Still Exposed To Vibration (N=8)	No Longer Exposed To Vibration (N=42)
Disease Progressed	3 (37)	3 (7)
Disease Unchanged	2 (25)	8 (19)
Disease Regressed or Disappeared	3 (37)	31 (74)

Authors' Response: The reversibility of VWF seems to be well established in our longitudinal study of lumberjacks, where we found a decrease of VWF from 40% to 7% during the years 1972 to 1981. The average daily exposure time to chain-saw vibration stayed unchanged among the lumberjacks. Since introducing the A/V chain saw in 1969, the prevalence, severity and incidence of VWF have slowly decreased. In very advanced cases, where structural changes probably occur, the extent of reversibility is not yet well established. If reversibility does occur, then the recovery interval will be longer for severe cases.

An important factor in determing the energy entering the hands is the coupling between tool and operator, and this could influence the reversibility of VWF.

Pyykkö et al.: Finnish lumberjacks

Vibration-Induced White Finger Among Chain Sawyers Nine Years After the Introduction of Anti-Vibration Measures

H. F. V. Riddle and W. Taylor

ABSTRACT: A further report on the prospective study, now in its eleventh year, of forest workers using chain saws at Thetford Forest is presented. The data reveal an improvement in the condition of a number of ex-chain sawyers who continue to work in the forest. Improvements are also noted in men continuing to operate saws with vibration-isolated handles (A/V saws), who are known to have suffered from VWF following the use of saws without vibration-isolation systems. However, the hands of some of these men continute to deteriorate. Concern is expressed regarding the occurrence of VWF among men with exposure limited to A/V saws. The relevance of this data to work practice in Forestry Commission forests and current vibration standards is discussed.

RESUME: Il s'agit d'un autre rapport sur l'étude prospective, entreprise il y a maintenant onze ans, sur les bûcherons qui utilisent des tronçonneuses dans la forêt Thetford. Les données révèlent que l'état d'un certain nombre de bûcherons qui n'utilisent plus une tronçonneuse mais qui travaillent toujours en forêt, s'est amélioré. On a aussi noté une amélioration de l'état des hommes qui, ayant souffert de VWF à force d'utiliser des scies non isolées des vibrations, les ont remplacés par des scies munies de poignées avec isolateurs de vibrations (scies A/V). L'état des mains de certains de ces hommes continue toutefois à se détériorer. On s'inquiète des cas de VWF des hommes qui n'utilisent que des scies A/V. On discute de la pertinence de ces données aux techniques de travail dans les forêts de la Forestry Commission et des normes actuelles sur les vibrations.

INTRODUCTION

The prevalence of vibration-induced white finger (VWF) among UK Forestry Commission workers at Thetford, Norfolk was reported in 1975 (1). The current status of a sample of this group of men who continue to work is described in this paper. They include men with experience of work with unprotected chain saws (non-A/V saws) and with saws incorporating anti-vibration devices (A/V saws). Forty-three men have stopped sawing and are employed on other forest work not involving the use of chain saws. Twenty-eight men, having used non-A/V chain saws in the past, continue working using modern A/V saws and there are eighteen men who have work experience limited to the use of A/V saws.

The objectives of the continuing survey of this group are: a) to follow, so far as possible, the natural course of VWF after chain saw use is discontinued, b) to monitor the effects of continuing vibration exposure on those men with past experience using non-A/V chain saws, and c) to assess the effectiveness of current A/V saws.

I METHODS

All available members of the work force with chain sawing experience attended for examination at the time of the survey. Work history, clinical history, clinical assessment of hands and arms, and blood pressure was done by one of us (HFVR). Evaluation of peripheral sensory nerve function was done by the other (WT), and included light touch, two point discrimination and temperature sensitivity. The Stage of VWF was assessed according to the criteria of Taylor and Pelmear (2), and the current Stage was contrasted with the worst recorded Stage, if any, in the past. Separate tables describing the current status of VWF in terms of improvement or deterioration were also prepared. The

Table 1. Prevalence and Stage of VWF Among Ex-Sawyers (N=43).

Year	Number of Sawyers	Mean Age ± SD (Yrs)	Mean Saw Usage ± SD (Yrs)	Never VWF	0	VWF Stage 1	2	3	1+2+3	Prevalence VWF
1981	43	51 ±8	11.7 ±5	15	15	2	10	1	13	30%
*	43			15	0	5	7	16	28	65%

*Worst Stage of VWF recorded for this group.

peripheral neurological findings will be the subject of another paper.

II RESULTS

The workers were analysed in two groups consisting of ex-chain sawyers and active chain sawyers. The active chain sawyers' group was further divided into subjects with non-A/V as well as A/V experience, and subjects with experience limited to A/V saws only.

2.1 Ex-Chain Sawyers

It is perhaps reassuring that among this group of ex-chain sawyers, of whom 65% were affected by VWF, the termination of vibration exposure has resulted in some improvement in their condition (Table 1). This is particularly evident for the 16 (37%) men classified originally as Stage 3, as only one man remains in Stage 3 at the time of this survey. However, the situation is not quite as good as it seems, for when the current status in terms of improvement in the condition of those with VWF is considered, it is found that there are four men who complain that their condition is deteriorating (Table 2).

Table 2. Current Status of the Condition of Ex-Sawyers with VWF (N=28).

Stationary	Improving	Deteriorating
20	4	4

The age, duration of chain saw operation and current Stage VWF (compared with the previous worst Stage) of the four sawyers complaining of deterioration in their condition are, respectively: 46 yrs, 15 yrs, Stage 3 (Stage 3); 56 yrs, 20 yrs, Stage 2 (Stage 3); 46 yrs, 11 yrs, Stage 2 (Stage 3); 35 yrs, 5 yrs, Stage 2 (Stage 1). Among the first three individuals there was no obvious explanation for the deterioration, but the fourth man has recently developed late onset asthma. It is possible that the sympathomimetic drugs being used to manage this condition have acted on vibration-sensitized peripheral vessels or nerves in his hands.

2.2 Active Chain Sawyers

2.2.1 Men with Previous Experience of Non-A/V Saws

The drop in prevalence shown in Table 3 suggests that the introduction of anti-vibration machines together with other measures by the UK Forestry Commission has been of benefit. The fact that thirteen men continue to work despite varying degrees of VWF is perhaps a measure of this. Whether occupational physicians should advise these men to continue to work as chain sawyers, let alone feel any satisfaction with the improvement, is questionable. Certainly whether the three men whose condition is deteriorating should be allowed to continue chain sawing (Table 4) must be considered. It was not possible to distinguish any difference between them and the six men who described an improvement in their symptoms, either in duration of vibration experience or other factors.

Yet another variable has been added to the problems of investigating VWF in the forest situation, following the introduction of the heated handle. This has been generally, though not universally, welcomed by our foresters. One man previously in Stage 2 is currently symptom-free since changing to a saw with heated handles. It should be noted that this saw is also lighter in weight than previous models.

2.2.2 Men with Experience Limited to A/V Saws

The occurrence of VWF in men with experience limited to A/V saws (see Table 5) is a matter of concern, and one of us has similar data from another forest area (HFVR, unpublished).

This raises questions regarding the vibration levels of current A/V saws, though there are other possible explanations. For example, before questioning the A/V characteristics, a review of the three men with symptoms revealed that one man age 42 was being treated for peripheral cramps, which might imply a suspect circulation. Another man, age 27, suffered from chilblains as a child and, concurrent with the onset of his VWF, has developed a trigger finger in the affected hand. The third reported classical symptoms of VWF prior to recruitment, while riding his motorcycle.

Riddle et al.: VWF among chain sawyers

Table 3. Prevalence and Stage of VWF Among Active Sawyers Who Have Operated Non-A/V and A/V saws (N=28).

Years	Number of Sawyers	Mean Age ± SD (Yrs)	Mean Saw Usage ± SD (Yrs)	0	VWF Stage 1	2	3	1+2+3	Prevalence VWF
1981	28	47 ±9	16 ±5	15	2	9	2	13	46%
*	28			11	2	9	6	17	61%

*Worst Stage of VWF recorded for this group.

Table 4. Current Status of VWF During Active Sawyers Who Have Operated Non-A/V and A/V Saws (N=28).

Never VWF	Stationary	Improving	Deteriorating
10	9	6	3

A pre-employment medical examination might have excluded these men from working with chain saws.

III DISCUSSION

The results presented here are open to various interpretations.

Consider first the progress of the ex-chain sawyers. The improvement of workers initially in Stage 3 is striking and confirms observations by Futatsuka (3), and Taylor and Pelmear (2). Earlier studies had suggested that Stage 3 was irreversible and this may still be correct. Jepson went so far as to state that there is no abatement once symptoms occur even after stopping work with vibrating tools (4). The absence of complaint among this group of men may reflect some change in life-style or change in work practice. The men under observation are very aware of VWF as the result of repeated surveys, of the importance of maintaining body temperature and of protecting their hands at work, and at leisure. As Pyykkö states, cold is the provocative factor in VWF (5). Clinical questioning is difficult at the best of times, and care is required in this situation not to lead to the required answer. However, until an adequate measuring technique is developed for use in the field, the current methods of clinical Staging must be applied. Whether or not Stage 3 as defined by Taylor and Pelmear is irreversible, it is a useful guide to the current severity of symptoms.

Turning now to those men with non-A/V and A/V sawing experience, the latest prevalence data suggest that a plateau may have been reached, but it is doubtful whether this situation will continue. Will the prevalence start to increase once more as the years of exposure to the vibration of A/V saws increases? Does the improvement noted over the years imply that the current A/V specifications are satisfactory? The many confounding variables make interpretation of the data difficult. For example, to what extent does the yearly reinforcement of the Forestry Commission's working practices by the survey team's interest affect the health of workers at Thetford? Do the other measures taken by the Forestry Commission mask the presentation of VWF (we refer to the provision of gloves, protective clothing and heated rest shelters)? The latest refinement, heated handles, is a further variable, as is the reduction in weight of these saws. Does the current economic climate in the UK, with some 10% of the work force unemployed, make men complain less? Would prescription of VWF result in more cases being discovered? Whatever the effect of these variables, the complaint by three men of a deterioration in their condition is cause for concern. Two other factors might explain this. First, over the last five years, the extraction rate from the Thetford Forests has increased. Perhaps these men are reaching a danger threshold so far as their vibration exposure is concerned. The second

Table 5. Prevalence and Stage of VWF Among Active Sawyers Who Have Only Operated A/V Saws (N=18).

Years	Number of Sawyers	Mean Age ± SD (Yrs)	Mean Saw Usage ± SD (Yrs)	0	VWF Stage 1	2	3	1+2+3	Prevalence VWF
1981	18	32 ±10	5 ±3	15	2	1	0	3	17%
*	18			16	1	1	0	2	11%

*Worst Stage of VWF previously recorded for this group.

factor is the concern that the vibration characteristics of the chain saw, satisfactory when new, deteriorate with use. Szepesi has reported considerable deterioration in the anti-vibration characteristics of the saws used in the Hungarian Forestry Service (6). A satisfactory method of studying this aspect of the problem is in the process of being designed.

Finally the occurrence of VWF among those men with sawing experience limited to A/V saws must be considered. This suggests that for these men at least the vibration levels are not low enough. What will happen to others after further years of vibration exposure is a matter of concern. There were probable predisposing factors in this group, and it may be possible to eliminate these variables by a rigorous exclusion policy at recruitment. Unfortunately, the specificity and sensitivity of a questionnaire designed with this in mind, and put to the Thetford group during the course of this survey, was not encouraging. So far as the vibration levels are concerned, we can only hope at present to stimulate the design of more stable engineering systems and more satisfactory maintenance procedures. A close watch on these men must be maintained to monitor the development of symptoms. There seems no escape at present from the kind of field study described, though our experience suggests that self-reporting conceals the size of the problem.

ACKNOWLEDGEMENTS

We wish to thank the UK Forestry Commission for encouraging this project, in particular D. Bardy, Safety Officer, the management and staff of the Forestry Commission District Office at Santon Downham, Norfolk, for their help, and finally the forest workers and their union representatives for their continuing co-operation.

REFERENCES

1. Taylor W, Pelmear PL, Pearson JCG. A longitudinal study of Raynaud's phenomenon in chain saw operators. In: Taylor W, Pelmear PL, eds. Vibration White Finger in Industry. London: Academic Press, 1975: 15-20.
2. Taylor W, Pelmear PL. Introduction. In: Taylor W, Pelmear PL, eds. Vibration White Finger in Industry. London: Academic Press, 1975: xxi.
3. Futatsuka M. The change of peripheral circulatory function of the vibrating tool users. Sangyo Igaku 1973; 15: 371-377.
4. Jepson RP. Raynaud's phenomenon in workers with vibrating tools. Br J Ind Med 1954; 11: 180-185.
5. Pyykkö I. Vibration syndrome, a review. In: Korhonen O, ed. Vibration and Work. Helsinki: Inst of Occup Health, 1976: 1-24.
6. Szepesi L. Vibration and Noise Level of Chain Saws. Report to Chain Saw Ergonomics Group FAO/ECE/ILO, 1979. (unpublished).

DISCUSSION

J.R. Barron: Was a medical history taken prior to the study, to detect conditions that may make operators more susceptible to VWF, such as diabetes, vascular conditions and smoking?

Authors' Response: No, but these details were established as part of the routine clinical history which preceded examination.

N. Olsen: What is the reproducibility of your Stage assessments?

Authors' Response: Our impression, having examined this group at frequent intervals over a ten year period, is that the Stage assessments are reproducible and change gradually with improvement or deterioration, as determined from the subject's history.

A. Behar: Are you taking account of vibration exposure that occurs outside the work situation (e.g. riding motorcycles)?

Authors' Response: Yes. We include exposure to other vibration as part of the occupational history.

You presented medical data for workers using A/V saws alone. Do you have results for workers using only non-A/V saws?

Authors' Response: No. Forestry Commission policy has been since 1971 to replace non-A/V saws with A/V saws. All sawyers use saws provided by the Commission.

E. Rivin: What were the differences between the vibration spectra of the conventional and vibration-isolated saws used at Thetford?

Authors' Response: The vibration spectra for A/V and non-A/V saws are to be found in: Taylor W, Pearson JCG, Keighley GD. A longitudinal study of Raynaud's phenomenon in chain saw operators. In: Wasserman DE, Taylor W, Curry MG, eds. Proc of the Int Occup Hand-Arm Vibration Conf. Cincinnati, OH: Dept of Health and Human Services, 1977 (NIOSH publication no. 77-170): 74.

A Pilot Investigation of the Vibration Syndrome in Forestry Workers of Eastern Canada

P. V. Pelnar, G. W. Gibbs and B. P. Pathak

ABSTRACT: In a population of 566 forestry workers from nine lumber camps in Quebec and Ontario, 90 (27.9%) of 323 power saw operators complained of vibration white finger (VWF). The prevalence of reported white fingers was related to the period of work. From this population, 86 workers were selected for an objective clinical study. Modified finger-plethysmography gave the best discrimination between exposure groups. Radiograms of the hands suggested that bone cysts were more common among persons with VWF. The results of nerve conduction studies correlated with the effect of heavy muscular work rather than with the effect of vibration exposure. The octave-band accelerations of saws were measured during the cutting of 50 trees by 16 workers. Differences were found between saws, between sawyers, between cutting operations and between species of trees. The results of the study have implications for establishing standards.

RESUME: Dans une population de 566 travailleurs forestiers provenant de neuf camps de bûcherons au Québec et en Ontario, 90 (27,9%) de 323 opérateurs de tronçonneuses se sont plaints des doigts blancs dûs aux vibrations (VWF). La prévalence des doigts blancs signalés fut mise en relation avec la période de travail; 86 travailleurs furent choisis parmi l'ensemble de cette population pour obtenir une étude clinique objective. Une pléthysmographie modifiée des doigts donna la meilleure discrimination entre les divers groupes d'exposition. Des radiogrammes des mains indiquèrent que des kystes des os étaient plus courants chez les personnes ayant des doigts blancs. Des études de la conduction nerveuse étaient en corrélation avec l'effet de travaux musculaires exigeants plutôt qu'avec l'effet de l'exposition aux vibrations. Les accélérations par bandes d'une octave des tronçonneuses furent mesurées pendant la coupe de 50 arbres par 16 travailleurs. Des variations furent constatées d'une machine à l'autre, d'un scieur à l'autre, d'une opération de coupage à l'autre et d'une espèce à l'autre. Les résultats de l'étude ont des conséquences sur la rédaction de normes.

INTRODUCTION

Raynaud's Phenomenon, an abnormality in the behavior of blood vessels leading to attacks of finger blanching, is known to be associated with long term work with vibrating tools. In this context it is called vibration white finger (VWF). The condition is painless but progressive, often accompanied by paresthesia and other neurological abnormalities, and sometimes by changes in the bones of the affected arms and hands (the Vibration Syndrome or vibration "disease"). Vibration-induced disorders of the hands were first recognized in 1911 and 1918 (1,2). Since that time, an increasing number of vibrating tools have been introduced into industry, mining and construction work. Two international conferences have been devoted to health problems associated with hand-arm vibration in the last decade, (3,4) and the current state of knowledge was summarized recently by Gibbs and Pelnar (5).

In the late 1950's, power saws were introduced into the lumber industry. Unlike most industrial and mining exposures, the effect of this vibrating tool on the hands of workers is combined with the effect of cold, wind and rain, which by themselves may constitute a severe stress on the vessels of the hand, and are believed to influence the development of the Vibration Syndrome (6). The magnitude of the risk of

Table 1. Groups of Forest Workers Selected for Clinical Tests (Total Examined N=86).

Group	Forestry Workers	Reported Symptomatology	N
1	Power saw operators	with VWF	31
2	Power saw operators with injuries to the hands	with VWF	6
3	Not power saw operators	with VWF	10
4	Power saw operators	none	25
5	Not power saw operators	none	14

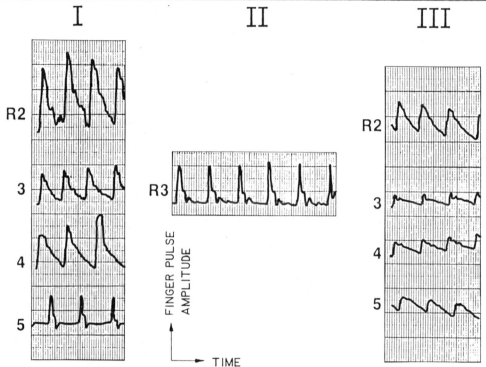

Fig. 1 Finger plethysmograms for a normal hand: I, at room temperature; II, during cooling of the other hand; and III, immediately after cooling the examined hand. R2, 3, 4 and 5, second, third, fourth and fifth fingers of the right hand.

VWF from working with chain saws, and the parameters responsible for the effects, are not known precisely for three important reasons. First, investigations have depended largely on reported symptoms without objective tests. Second, most studies have been cross-sectional in nature, resulting in the possibility of underestimating the risk. Third, measurements of the vibration characteristics of saws have been limited. The occupational-medical concern has been mainly based on the large number of persons at risk, the widespread prevalence of VWF, and on the fact that VWF, although reversible in the first stages, can become an irreversible and disabling disease (6).

In Canada, there is a forestry labour force of approximately 60 000 persons distributed as follows: 26 000 felling,

14 000 skidding and forwarding, 14 000 transporting, and 6000 providing services. At least the 26 000 persons involved in tree felling work regularly with power saws. In order to determine the risk of vibration-induced disorders of the hands in Canadian forestry workers, a pilot study was undertaken, with three main objectives:
1)   To determine the prevalence of signs and symptoms of the Vibration Syndrome disease reported by a sample of forestry workers, and to examine the relationship of the reported signs and symptoms to factors such as age, periods of work with the power saw, and smoking.
2)   To examine the potential of selected, objective clinical tests to distinguish persons reporting signs and symptoms from comparison groups, such tests to be suitable

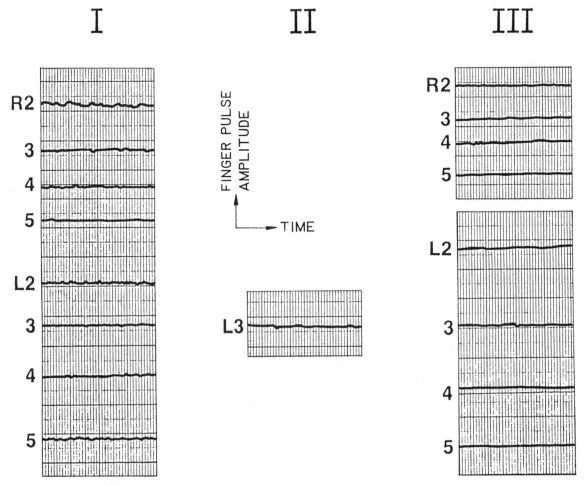

Fig. 2 Finger plethysmograms for a hand with a permanent obstruction (anatomical, spasm ?): L, left hand. (For explanation of other symbols, see caption to Fig. 1).

for use as an objective tool for the diagnosis of vibration-induced disorders.
3)   To examine the vibration characteristics of power saws used at the lumber camps under investigation, and their relation to disease.

I MATERIALS AND METHODS

1.1 Field Survey

All workers present at nine lumber camps (operated by four companies) in the western part of Quebec and the eastern part of Ontario were selected for study. In October and November 1978, two interviewers administered a work history and symptom questionnaire (French and English) to all workers present at the camps. Completed questionnaires were obtained from 566 workers. Of these, 323 were power saw operators. A power saw operator was considered to be a person currently felling with a power saw, or a person with a long history of such work, but currently working at other jobs and so employed for less than two years.

1.2 Clinical Study

From the workers interviewed, five groups were selected for clinical testing, as indicated in Table 1. The tests were performed during a one day visit by the workers to Montreal (in March and April of 1979), during the winter-break in forestry operations, several weeks after the last exposure to the usual working conditions. This timing should have eliminated some acute, transient, health effects.
The clinical study consisted of a neurological examination, a radiogram of the hands and the following vascular tests:
a)   Finger plethysmography in three modes of thermal exposure with three tracings, as introduced to the study of vibration-induced disorders in 1944 by Kadlec and Pelnar (plethysmography K-P) (7);
b)   Finger plethysmography with cooling the opposite hand only, as described by Miday (8);
c)   The Lewis-Prusik test; and
d)   Infrared thermography of the hands. The experimental procedures are described in the following sections.

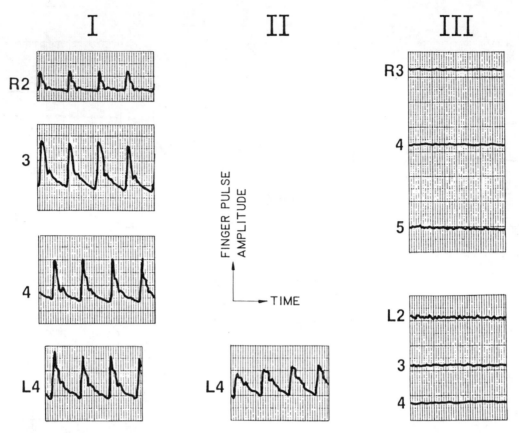

Fig. 3 Finger plethysmograms for a hand with vibration white finger: a spasm occurs only in reaction to local cooling (tracing III). (For explanation of symbols, see captions to Figs. 1 and 2.)

Table 2. Prevalence of Claimed Signs and Symptoms Reported by Persons Exposed and Not Exposed to Chain Saw Vibration (Total Examined N=566: Percentages in Parenthesis).

Signs and Symptoms	Chain Saw Operators*	Other Forestry Workers*	All Persons Interviewed
Finger blanching	90 (27.9)	30 (12.2)	120 (21.2)
Finger numbness	113 (35.2)	58 (23.7)	171 (30.2)
Cyanosis	12 (3.7)	5 (2)	17 (3)
Total	323 (100)	243 (100)	566 (100)

*Not matched for age.

1.2.1 Finger Plethysmography (K-P)

A digital plethysmograph (Hewlett-Packard, model 14301A), was used with a laboratory constructed recording system. The second, third, fourth and fifth fingers of each hand were examined at room temperature (tracing I). Then a finger in which the worker reported symptoms was examined while the other hand was cooled in water at 10°C (tracing II). Finally, the second to the fifth fingers of each hand were examined immediately after the cooling of the one hand (tracing III). Figures 1 to 3 illustrate this procedure, showing plethysmograms for a normal hand, a hand with permanent obstruction of the finger arteries, and a person suffering from VWF. The results were considered positive when there was a total disintegration of the pulse wave in the third tracing, and (±) when there was a clear abnormality but the pulse waves were still discernable. The overall evaluation of the results has been recently discussed in more detail (9).

Pelnar et al.: Forestry workers

Table 3. Prevalence of Claimed Finger Whitening by Age and Period of Work with a Power Saw (Percentages in Parentheses).

Time Operating Chain Saw (yrs)	Age (yrs) <40	>40	All Ages
>5	42/123 (34.1)	28/84 (33.3)	70/207 (33.8)
<5	16/93 (17.2)	4/23 (17.4)	20/116 (17.2)
Total	58/216 (26.9)	32/107 (29.9)	90/323 (27.9)

1.2.2 Finger Plethysmography While Cooling Only the Opposite Hand (8)

In this method, a tracing of the pulse wave in one hand was started at room temperature and then the other hand was cooled in cold water, while the tracing continued. The presence or absence of changes in pulse amplitude while cooling the opposite hand were noted and their size measured. The test was considered positive when the amplitude of the pulse decreased to two-thirds, or less, of its original value.

This procedure was essentially identical to the first and second tracings of Kadlec and Pelnar, but rather than measuring the local reaction typical of VWF, it identifies a general disturbance of the vasomotoric system.

1.2.3 Lewis-Prusik Test

The Lewis-Prusik test is a measure of the time required for the return of normal colour to the nail-bed after compression (10). In a normal person, even after cooling, the blood refills the compressed nail-bed within five seconds. In subjects with VWF, this time may be substantially prolonged.

1.2.4 Infrared Thermography

Infrared thermography of the hands was performed using an AGA Thermovision (type BW-600). An infrared image of both hands was photographed at normal room temperature. A second photograph was taken after cooling each hand. The fingers remaining cold do not appear on the infrared image (displaying "thermal amputation"), in sharp contrast with normally warming fingers and hands.

1.2.5 Radiograms of the Hands

Radiograms were taken of the 86 subjects' hands and evaluated by a collaborator in the study (PJF).

1.2.6 Neurological Examination

A general neurological examination was performed by a collaborator in the study (JS), and tests of motor and sensory nerve conduction were made on the hands and legs of 40 workers. This sample was selected to include men with VWF and comparison groups, and consisted of 18 workers from group 1, and 11 from each of groups 4 and 5 (see Table 1).

1.3 Measurements of Chain Saw Vibration

The vibration characteristics of the chain saws used at four lumber camps were measured at the hand and handle interface, by installing an accelerometer package on both the front and rear handles. Knowles BU-1771 accelerometers containing an FET amplifier stage were used as vibration transducers. The accelerometer package consisted of three accelerometers mounted on a thin rubber sheet, such that the axes of the accelerometers were orthogonal. Data were recorded on a two-channel, FM tape recorder (Bruel & Kjaer 7001).

The vibration characteristics were measured in the X, Y and Z directions specified by the ISO (11), during the felling, limbing (debranching), slashing (bucking), and notching of fifty trees by a total of sixteen professional sawyers.

II RESULTS

2.1 Prevalence of Reported Symptoms of VWF

The prevalence of whitening, numbness and/or cyanosis of the fingers when exposed to cold reported by 566 forestry workers are shown in Table 2. Every fifth forestry worker reported whitening and every third reported numbness.

Whitening, numbness and cyanosis of the fingers are signs and symptoms that are not specific to the Vibration Syndrome, and a certain background prevalence of each of these is acknowledged to exist in the general population. The non-specific background prevalence of whitening of 12.2% in our group of forestry workers was high, but in good agreement with that reported among British forestry workers (3). The background prevalence of numbness was higher, and differed less from the prevalence observed in power saw operators. This is in agreement with the suspected lesser specificity of numbness associated with vibration

Pelnar et al.: Forestry workers

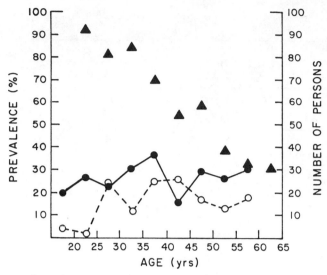

Fig. 4 Prevalence of claimed finger blanching by age and history of hand injury: those with hand injuries reporting VWF are shown by the filled circles, and those without injuries by the open circles. The total number of workers in each age group is shown by the triangles.

Table 4. Results of Plethysmography (K-P) for the Five Groups of Workers Examined (Total Examined N=86: Percentages in Parentheses).

Group*	Positive +++	Positive ±	Total Positive	Total Positive & Negative
1	15 (48.4)	4 (12.9)	19 (61.3)	31 (100)
2	2 (33.3)	1 (16.7)	3 (50)	6 (100)
3	4 (40)	1 (10)	5 (50)	10 (100)
4	0	2 (8)	2 (8)	25 (100)
5	1 (7.1)	1 (7.1)	2 (14.3)	14 (100)
Total	22	9	31	86

*Details of the groups are given in Table 1.

exposure. Cyanosis was rare, but it showed the same trend. Although these signs and symptoms were also claimed by those who had not worked with power saws, the frequency was much greater in the power saw operators. The difference between those working and those not working with chain saws was greatest for finger whitening.

2.2 Relationship Between Symptoms, Age and Period of Work

There was no relationship evident between age and numbness (r=0.19, p=0.3) or cyanosis. There was an increase in the prevalence of whitening of the fingers with age in the youngest age groups (r=0.4, p=0.12), but there was no increase in the prevalence of this sign in the older age groups.

In power saw operators, there was a higher correlation between whitening and age (r=0.59) than in the whole group, but the older age groups showed that this was very likely to be related to the increase in period of work with age (see Table 3). The correlation with period of work was much higher (r=0.83) than the correlation with age, and a t-test indicated that the difference between the two indices was significant. Thus, in the development of vibration-linked finger whitening, the period of work with the vibrating tool is important, but age is relatively unimportant.

The period of work before development of the Vibration Syndrome in power saw operators was examined by analysing the prevalence of symptoms reported each year, during the first ten years of power saw operation. The cumulative frequency of VWF in men with up to seven years of work with a power saw was constant, but increased with a wider spread after more than seven years of exposure. This suggests that the period of work necessary for VWF to develop among our power saw operators was approximately seven years.

2.3 Other Factors Influencing the Prevalence of VWF

The background prevalence of whitening and feeling of numbness (Table 2), although not quite unexpected, was surprisingly high. Although there are several causes of "white fingers" known and mentioned in the literature, such as constitutional Raynaud's Disease, arteriosclerosis, and scleroderma, the main cause of the background prevalence of the symptoms was suspected to be injury to the hands. Opportunities for injury to the hands in forestry work are many. Mechanical injuries, such as cuts to fingers and hands by the saw, lacerations by branches, wood or by tools, and fractures of fingers, are frequent. Significant thermal injury can occur from frost-bite in this outdoor work, and thermal injury is known to change the vasomotorics of the fingers (6).

In our population, 228 (41.8%) of 545 workers had a history of one or more injuries to the hands, and the prevalence of VWF was almost twice as high in those injured than in those without injury. Figure 4 indicates that this was true in almost all age groups. In fact, up to the age of 25, whitening was claimed only by those injured and almost no cases appeared in those who were not injured. The period of work necessary to produce VWF

Table 5. Exposure to Vibration Other than from Occupational Use of Chain Saws Reported by Persons Claiming VWF (Total N=41: Percentages in Parentheses).

	Other Vibration Exposure		
Group*	Yes	No	Total
1	10 (37)	17 (63)	27 (100)
2	2 (40)	3 (60)	5 (100)
3	8 (28.9)	1 (11.1)	9 (100)
Total	20 (48.8)	21 (51.2)	41 (100)

*Details are given in Table 1.

Table 6. Plethysmography While Cooling Only the Other Hand (Total N=85: Percentages in Parentheses).

Group(s)*	Positive	Negative	Total
1†	10 (33.3)	20 (66.7)	30 (100)
2	1 (16.7)	5 (83.3)	6 (100)
3	5 (50)	5 (50)	10 (100)
4	12 (48)	13 (52)	25 (100)
5	4 (28.6)	10 (71.4)	14 (100)
1 + 2 + 3	16 (34.8)	30 (65.2)	46 (100)
4 + 5	16 (41)	23 (59)	39 (100)
Total	32	53	85

*Details are given in Table 1.
†One person was not tested.

had not yet elapsed for most people in these younger age-groups. Thus almost all cases of whitening in these groups were most likely due to injuries to their hands and not related to vibration exposure.

2.4 Clinical Tests

2.4.1 Plethysmography (K-P)

Of the vascular tests, finger plethysmography in three modes of thermal exposure and three tracings, as developed by Kadlec and Pelnar, showed the highest correlation with the subjective history of VWF.

Results for the various groups investigated are shown in Table 4. In all three groups claiming VWF, the proportion of positives was significantly higher than in groups claiming an absence of VWF. Positive (+++) objective signs of VWF were found in 21 of 47 men claiming symptoms, and in one man of the 39 who did not report the whitening of fingers. On the other hand, not all of those claiming the whitening of fingers produced a positive result when tested with this plethysmographic procedure. Either they did have whitening but their

Table 7. Lewis-Prusik Test (N=75).

Group(s)*	Positive	Negative	Total
1	16 (59.3)	11 (40.7)	27 (100)
2	3 (60)	2 (40)	5 (100)
3	6 (60)	4 (40)	10 (100)
4	5 (25)	15 (75)	20 (100)
5	2 (15.4)	11 (84.6)	13 (100)
1 + 2 + 3	25 (59.5)	17 (40.5)	42 (100)
4 + 5	7 (21.2)	26 (78.8)	33 (100)
Total	32	43	75

*Details of the groups are given in Table 1.

VWF has not reached the threshold above which the disease could be revealed by this method, or they incorrectly reported their abnormality.

It should be noted that our control groups of non-power saw workers were not necessarily persons unexposed to vibration. Most of them were operators of skidders and other heavy forestry machinery. Not infrequently, they used power drills and even power saws at home. Thus, some of our background cases may be influenced by exposure to vibration. Table 5 gives support to the suspicion that this may have been the case in group 3 (non-power saw workers claiming VWF).

2.4.2 Plethysmography While Cooling Only the Opposite Hand

The test did not distinguish between persons claiming and not claiming VWF, or between those exposed and not exposed to vibration (Table 6). This result is not surprising. In this test, vasomotoric reaction to a thermal stimulus is registered from the opposite side. The main characteristic of VWF is that it is a local reaction. A reaction mediated by the vasomotoric system of the whole body is not typical of VWF, even if the reaction may be present in some cases.

2.4.3 Lewis-Prusik Test

This test distinguished between those claiming and not claiming VWF almost as well as Kadlec-Pelnar plethysmography (Table 7). It was more often positive among both cases and controls, but the agreement with plethysmography (K-P) was good. The result depends to some extent on the examiner's judgement, and so over-reading or under-reading is possible. Nevertheless, the extreme simplicity of this test has been its major asset in previous field studies (10). This study confirmed its value.

Pelnar et al.: Forestry workers

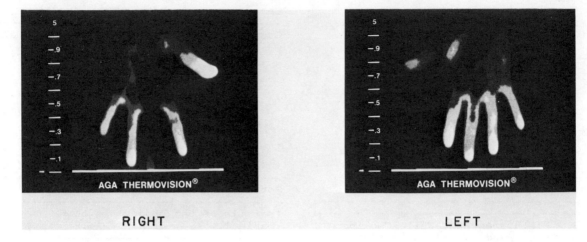

RIGHT   LEFT

Fig. 5 Infrared thermographic photograph of the hands ten minutes after cooling. Note thermal amputation of the third finger of the right hand as a sign of VWF.

Table 8. Radiological Findings in the Hands (N=86) (Fitzgerald PJ, personal communication).

Group*	Cysts	Osteoporosis	Osteoarthritis	Accidental Abnormalities	Tufting	No Abnormalities	Total
1	5	3	8	6	6	12	31
2	1	0	1	1	0	3	6
3	3	1	2	2	1	5	10
4	0	2	0	6	1	14	25
5	0	2	1	1	0	10	14

*Details of the groups are given in Table 1.

2.4.4 Infrared Thermography

The method was very sensitive, and a thermal amputation appeared on infrared photographs after cooling almost every hand. This is probably the reason for the controversy in the literature over the usefulness of thermography. During the course of clinical examinations, it was found necessary to modify the procedure until, finally, heat from the examined hand was not recorded until from 10 to 15 minutes had elapsed after cooling. By that time, a normal hand and fingers should have returned to their normal temperature, and false-positive results should be eliminated. A positive result in the third finger of the right hand is shown in Fig. 5.

If results obtained by the final procedure are compared with plethysmographic results (K-P test), much better agreement between the results of the two methods was observed. Thus, if more subjects were tested, infrared thermography using a strictly defined procedure could prove to be a sensitive method for the diagnosis of VWF, with results well correlated with other objective tests.

2.4.5 Radiography

Small bone cysts have been repeatedly reported and denied in the literature as a phenomenon linked with vibration exposure. The radiological findings in the hands of our workers are summarized in Table 8, and will be published in detail elsewhere (by PJF). All abnormalities, with one exception, were found in persons over 40 years of age. There were only 9 cases with bone cysts, all of them persons claiming VWF. Cysts were also present in those not working with a power saw but claiming VWF. There were no bone cysts in power saw operators who did not have VWF. This apparent link between the cysts and VWF, rather than with work with a power saw, was interesting. A similar relationship was found with osteoarthritis and with tufting of the phalanges.

Confirmation of these links was sought by comparing the radiological results with objective plethysmographic signs of VWF. It was observed that bone cysts alone, cysts combined with signs of osteoarthritis, osteoarthritis of the hand-joints, and tufting occurred more frequently among

Table 9. Average Sensory Action Potentials (Expressed in mV) (Stewart J, personal communication).

| Nerve | Forestry Workers | | | "White Collar" Workers |
	Sawyers Claiming VWF	Sawyers Not Claiming VWF	Others	
Median	20.2	18.9	24.5	33.2*
Ulnar	8.9	8.9	11	18 *
Radial	9.3	9.1	10.4	21.7*
Sural	6.8	6.3	8.4	12.3*

*p < 0.01.

workers with positive plethysmograms. On the other hand, osteoporosis appeared to be equally frequent among those with symptoms and those without symptoms, and among those with positive and negative plethysmograms.

2.4.6 Neurological Examination

In general, the neurological state of health of our forestry workers showed little abnormality, with a weak, if any, relation to VWF. The more sophisticated laboratory testing of nerve conduction revealed no correlation with VWF or with exposure to vibration. Most of the tests and measurements were found to be within normal limits, and there was no significant difference between the right and left hands of any subject. The results will be described in detail elsewhere (by JS).

The important abnormal findings are shown in Table 9. In the nerve conduction study, the sensory action potentials at all sites tested were significantly lower in forestry workers than in "white collar" workers. There was no significant difference between the sawyers and other forestry workers, between persons with and without symptoms of VWF, or between those with and without objective signs of VWF on plethysmograms. Thus, the nerve conduction abnormalities appeared to be associated with the effects of heavy muscular work, and perhaps the effects of past exposure to cold, rather than with vibration exposure.

At the clinical neurological examination, there was slightly more abnormality in sawyers claiming VWF (55.6%) than in those who did not claim disease (45.5%), and even less abnormality in non-sawyers (18.2%). When objective, plethysmographic signs of VWF are considered, there was clearly more abnormality in sawyers with objective signs of disease (77.8%) than in sawyers without such signs (40%) (p=0.05).

2.5 Factors Influencing the Occurrence of Objectively Diagnosed VWF

In most previous studies and in the first part of our study, factors thought

Table 10. Relation Between Smoking and Plethysmography (K-P) (Total N=84: Percentages in Parentheses).

Plethysmogram	Smokers	Non-Smokers	Total
+++	20 (27)	2 (20)	22
±	8 (10.8)	1 (10)	9
-	46 (62.2)	7 (70)	53
Total	74 (100)	10 (100)	84

to be influencing the prevalence of symptoms subjectively claimed by workers were investigated. The factors believed to be the most important, smoking, brand of power saw and the use of anti-vibration (A/V) saws, were examined in relation to objectively diagnosed signs of VWF. The results of previous studies by Kadlec and Pelnar suggested that their finger-plethysmography method was likely to be the most relevant, objective method for the diagnosis of Raynaud's Phenomenon, and thus for the diagnosis of VWF. The present study yielded results consistent with this view, through the good agreement between K-P plethysmography and claimed symptoms, and the minimal occurrence of "false-positive" results. This test was therefore employed for the analysis of potential contributing factors.

Table 10 shows that a somewhat greater proportion of smokers than non-smokers had positive plethysmograms, but the small number of non-smokers makes the observation of limited value. However, among non-power saw workers, there was no objectively diagnosed VWF among non-smokers, and all five positive cases were smokers. It could be that the effect of smoking was masked by the (stronger) effect of vibration in genuine cases of the Vibration Syndrome, while it manifested itself among the "background cases" of Raynaud's Phenomenon. However, our data cannot provide conclusive evidence on this subject.

Table 11 shows significant differences in the prevalence of VWF, depending on the commercial brands of saws used by the

Table 11. Relation Between Plethysmography (K-P) and the Brand of Chain Saw Used During the Last Year (Total N=49: Percentages in Parentheses).

Plethysmogram	Brand of Power Saw 03	04	05	06	07	08	Total
+++	1 (25)	2 (9.5)	6*(54.5)	0 (0)	1 (33.3)	3 (33.3)	13 (26.5)
±	1 (25)	2 (9.5)	2 (18.2)	1 (100)	0 (0)	1 (11.1)	7 (14.3)
−	2 (50)	17*(81)	3 (27.3)	0 (0)	2 (66.7)	5 (55.6)	29 (59.2)
Total	4 (100)	21 (100)	11 (100)	1 (100)	3 (100)	9 (100)	49 (100)

*$p < 0.005$

Table 12. Results of Plethysmography (K-P) for Workers Who Operate Confirmed Anti-Vibration Saws (Total N=19: Percentages in Parentheses).

Group	Finger Blanching	N	Plethysmography (K-P) Positive +++	Positive ±	Negative −	Total Positive & Negative
1 + 2	Yes	17 (89.4) }	6 (31.6)	4 (21.1)	9 (47.4)	19 (100)
4	No	2 (10.6) }				
Total		19 (100)				

sawyers. This difference in health effect (compare "04" and "05") is striking, considering only the brands used in the last year before examination (i.e. presumably the most modern models of each brand), were included in the comparison. The fact that there were 95 models of power saws used by our group of sawyers during the last ten years led to difficulties in trying to establish a link between VWF and particular brands of saw.

The sawyers were also questioned about their use of anti-vibration (A/V) saws. The result was paradoxical: more users of A/V saws claimed symptoms than non-users. To establish that this was not due to the workers' lack of awareness of which saws were truly A/V models, the manufacturers of all brands of saws used by our workers were contacted, to determine which were considered to be A/V saws. The results shown in Table 12 are based on the information received. Of 19 sawyers using confirmed anti-vibration saws for at least one of the last two, or two of the last three, years, 89.4% claimed to have symptoms of VWF. In comparison with the objectively diagnosed prevalence of VWF, only 6 (31.6%) users of A/V saws were positive whereas 9 (47.4%) were negative. The number of men claiming VWF with objective signs of VWF, in spite of their use of A/V saws, was much larger than expected. One possible reason might be that men suffering from VWF preferably chose anti-vibration models to alleviate their symptoms. Hence our study was unable to document any substantial benefit from the use of A/V saws. In fact, one saw, with handle acceleration sometimes in excess of 50 m/s^2 in the octave band with centre frequency at 125 Hz (see Fig. 8), was the latest A/V model from a manufacturer.

2.6 Characteristics of Chain Saw Vibration

The chain saws were observed to produce a complicated vibration pattern, as previously reported by Brammer (12). The rms acceleration measured in each octave frequency band from 16 to 4000 Hz are shown in Fig. 6 for a saw operated by one sawyer. Different ways of cutting the same wood type (yellow birch) produced similar data whether felling, notching, limbing or slashing. The maximum acceleration occurred in the 125 Hz frequency band. Some workers' exposure could easily exceed recommended exposure levels for four to eight hours (12), as many worked almost continuously during their eight hour shift.

The vibration recorded when a sawyer, using the same saw, performed the same operation on different types of wood was examined. In Fig. 7, it can be seen that the acceleration in the 125 Hz octave band when cutting yellow birch was considerably in excess of that when cutting maple. In other measurements, the 125 Hz band acceleration in the Y direction was, in general, greater when cutting maple than when cutting birch. The accelerations along the X, Y and Z axes were essentially the same when cutting beech, but there was less acceleration along the Z axis then along the other two when cutting poplar.

Repeated measurements of handle vibration when one sawyer was cross-cutting the

Pelnar et al.: Forestry workers

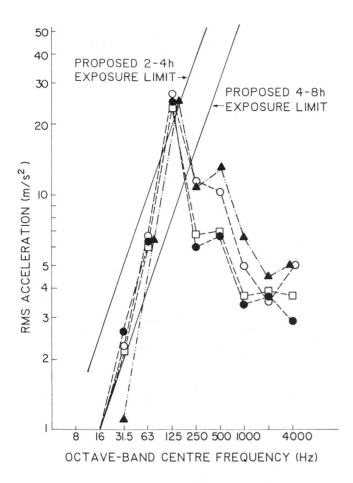

Fig. 6 Octave-band accelerations during various cutting operations (on yellow birch) performed by one sawyer with the same saw: notching, squares; felling, filled circles; limbing, triangles; and slashing, open circles. The exposure limits are from Ref. 12.

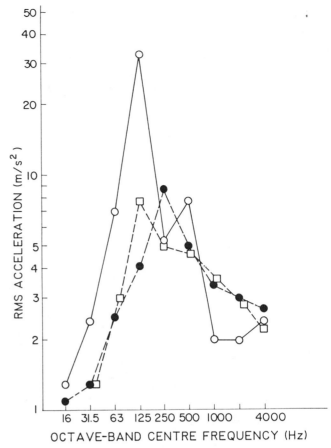

Fig. 7 Octave-band accelerations observed when slashing (cross-cutting) various woods: sugar maple, filled circles; maple, squares; and yellow birch, open circles. Data are for one sawyer using the same saw.

same tree revealed considerable variations in octave band accelerations (Fig. 8). The variation, however, was less than the differences between the accelerations recorded by another operator with another type of saw when cutting yellow birch and sugar maple. A direct comparison of the vibration of the various types of saws when operated by the same person on the same wood was not obtained, as different workers had their own saws, and it was not considered appropriate to ask a worker to cut with a saw other than his own. Substantial differences in vibration were found, however, when two different cutters used the same type of saw on the same type of wood.

III DISCUSSION AND CONCLUSIONS

The Vibration Syndrome has been shown to be associated with the use of power saws by Canadian forestry workers. The prevalence of claimed symptoms increased with the period of work, to a maximum of approximately 50% after 15 years of service. This is not out of proportion with other studies. Direct comparisons are difficult due to the various reported levels of subjective symptoms, and the absence of objective testing in most studies.

The vascular effects of the Vibration Syndrome have been objectively demonstrated by clinical methods at a certain level of abnormality. In our (examined) population, this level was reached by approximately half of those claiming symptoms. The most consistent relationship between reported symptoms and objective tests was obtained for finger-plethysmography (K-P). This method can also distinguish objectively between the reversible stage of arterial spasms and the irreversible, presumably anatomical, obstruction of the arteries.

Pelnar et al.: Forestry workers

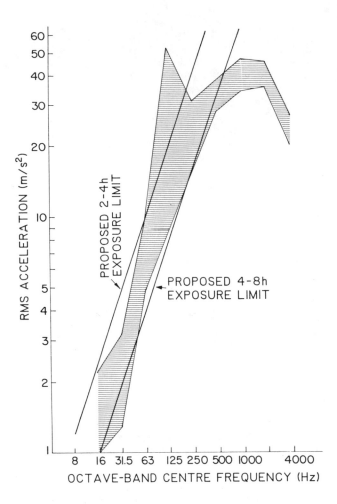

Fig. 8 Range of octave-band accelerations (shaded area) observed during
repeated slashing of maple. Data are
for one sawyer and one saw. The exposure limits are from Ref. 12.

The ability to demonstrate this difference
is important when advising a worker to
cease vibration exposure and change his
job, and for workmen's compensation. Less
consistent, but still potentially useful,
were the Lewis-Prusik test and infrared
thermography. Plethysmography without
cooling the hands, or with only cooling the
opposite hand, did not discriminate between
groups with and without symptoms and/or
vibration exposures, and proved unsuitable
for diagnosing vibration-induced abnormalities.

The results of the neurological
examinations were consistent with the previous conclusions of Pelnar and Pacina that
neurological abnormalities are not necessarily associated with VWF (10), nor are
they a specific effect of vibration exposure. They are often seen in persons with
VWF because neurological impairment may
be the result of strain caused by heavy

muscular work, which is required in many
jobs involving exposure to vibration.

Radiological changes in our examined
population, if present at all, were more
linked with age and/or with heavy, manual
work than with exposure to vibration. The
small number of bone cysts found were present only in persons claiming VWF. Further
study of this relationship is required.

The field investigation of the vibration characteristics of saws operated by
forestry workers indicated that there are
many factors which have to be taken into
account in determining the actual vibration
exposure of workers. The brands of saws,
the models and types of each brand, and also
the age and the state of maintenance of the
saw may change the vibration. In addition,
this study identified other factors influencing the vibration characteristics, such
as the axes of measurement, the position of
the saw relative to the wood, and the
position of the hands on the handles. There
were also variations in vibration associated
with cutting various types of wood with the
same saw. The establishment of a link
between a single index of vibration and
health effects, which would have implications
for setting exposure standards, has not been
possible from our results.

Our study confirmed the general experience that VWF is not a serious clinical
disease. In most cases it was considered
more a nuisance than a disease by the
workers, and it did not cause them much
concern. No gangrene or permanent disability
as reported by Laroche (13), and elsewhere
in the literature was found. Nevertheless,
one half of our men with a positive plethysmogram had to stop working during some (not
all) attacks of VWF, and many reported that
VWF interfered with their leisure activities
and with driving an automobile.

A cross-sectional, retrospective study
such as ours may have underestimated the
risk of VWF by omitting the disabled persons
who might have left the industry. In the
questionnaire, the workers were asked about
other cases of VWF known to them. Only a
few were reported, although the retired
sawyers were unlikely to have moved away
from the lumbering communities. VWF did
not appear to be a major cause for leaving
forestry work. However, the high prevalence
of VWF in an important national industry,
and the possibility of an irreversible disabling disease of the hands in otherwise
able-bodied men (with often limited skills
and job opportunities), makes the Vibration
Syndrome a matter of both medical and social
concern.

ACKNOWLEDGEMENTS

The study was supported by a grant
from Health and Welfare Canada. In planning and carrying out this study we obtained

invaluable help from Mr. D. Myles of the
Canadian Forestry Service, Environment
Canada, from the Canada Department of Labor,
and from Dr. A.J. Brammer of the National
Research Council. We enjoyed the full
support and effective collaboration of
E.B. Eddy Ltd., C.I.P. Company, Consolidated
Bathurst Co. Ltd. and J. Maclaren Co. Ltd.,
and the managing staffs of their lumber
camps. The workers showed great interest
in the study and we are grateful to all who
participated. AGA Infrared Instrument AB
of Lidingö very kindly lent us their
Thermovision-BW-680-Medical equipment.
Mrs. T. Dufresne and Miss C. Ceausu conducted the interviews in the lumber camps
and Miss Ceausu assisted in the clinical
studies. Dr. P.J. Fitzgerald kindly co-
operated in carrying out radiological
examinations, and Dr. J. Stewart in carrying out neurological studies of the workers.
Mr. H. Ghezzo provided statistical advice
and assisted in the data analysis. Measurement of the vibration associated with the
use of saws in the lumber camps were carried
out with the assistance of P. Nicoll,
R. Robb, L. Laferrière and L.A. Monaghan.

REFERENCES

1. Loriga G. Il lavoro con i martelli pneumatici (Work with pneumatic hammers). Bol Ispett Lavoro 1911; 2: 35-60, ibid 1913; 6: 524. (in Italian).
2. Hamilton A. A study of spastic anaemia in the hands of stone cutters. Washington: Government Printing Office, 1918. (Bull US Bureau of Labor Statistics, no. 236 Ind Accidents and Hygiene Series, no. 19) 53-66.
3. Taylor W, ed. The Vibration Syndrome. London: Academic Press, 1974.
4. Wasserman DE, Taylor W, Curry MG, eds. Proc of the Int Occup Hand-Arm Vibration Conf. Cincinnati, OH: Dept of Health and Human Services, 1977 (NIOSH publication no. 77-170).
5. Gibbs GW, Pelnar PV. Occupational exposure of the hands to vibration in Canada. Proc of Seminar on Occup Exposure to Noise and Vibration. Ottawa: National Research Council of Canada, 1982. (to appear).
6. Kadlec K, Pelnar P. Vznik, pruheh a predpoved nemoci poklepavacu (Onset, course and prognosis of the "Pounder's Disease") Cas Lek Cesk 1944; 83: 1251-1259. (in Czech).
7. Kadlec K, Pelnar, P. Prstova plethysmografie jako klinicka vysetrovaci methoda obvodovych cev (Finger plethysmography as a clinical method for examining the peripheral vessels). Cas Lek Cesk 1944; 83: 947-952. (in Czech).
8. Miday R. Cold-induced vasomotor reflexes in early diagnosis of peripheral vascular dis-turbances. JOM 1978; 20: 296.
9. Pelmear PL, Pelnar PV. Vibration white finger. Symptoms, signs and objective tests for diagnosis. Proc of Seminar on Occup Exposure to Noise and Vibration. Ottawa: National Research Council of Canada, 1982. (to appear).
10. Pelnar P, Pacina V. Vyvoj profesionalni traumaticke vasoneurosy u lamacu rudnych dolu (Evolution of the occupational traumatic vaso-neurosis in miners in ore mines). Proc 8th Cong on Occup Health, Marianske Lazne, Czechoslovakia, 1964. (in Czech).
11. International Organization for Standardization. Guide for the Measurement and Evaluation of Human Exposure to Vibration Transmitted to the Hand. ISO/TC 108/SC4/WG3 draft, 1975. (unpublished).
12. Brammer AJ. Chain Saw Vibration: Its Measure-ment, Hazard and Control. Ottawa: National Research Council of Canada, 1978. (Report NRC 18803/APS 599).
13. Laroche GP. Traumatic vasospastic disease in chain saw operators. Can Med Assoc J, 1976; 115: 1217-1251.

DISCUSSION

H. Von Gierke: I assume that workers identified as using anti-vibration saws had previously operated saws without vibration isolated handles. Did you establish how many years they had used "conventional" saws prior to using A/V saws, and whether they reported symptoms of VWF prior to operating A/V saws?

Authors' Response: We have data on the model of saw each man said he had used during the last seven years, but we do not have reliable evidence whether or not symptoms of VWF were present prior to the use of A/V saws. We accept that this could be the case, and suggested that some workers may have chosen an A/V saw in order to alleviate the existing symptoms and signs of VWF.

W. Taylor: It is generally accepted that attacks of finger blanching cannot be provoked at will, that is, a subject does not always respond to a provocative cold test with blanching of the digits. Thus immediately after cold provocation, if the examined hand is cold but not blanched, is the finger pulse plethysmogram abnormal? To my mind, there must be digital blood flow in a pink, but cold, finger, implying the existence of a partially open artery with a pulse wave not equating to that shown in trace III of Fig. 3, even though the subject suffers from VWF.

Authors' Response: According to the classic description of Sir Thomas Lewis, an attack of Raynaud Phenomenon, such as VWF, begins with a complete spasm of the digital arteries. This spasm is demonstrated in Fig. 3. This condition, however, does not immediately produce a change of colour, or blanching of the finger. The change of colour results from secondary spasm of the capillaries, which may or may not occur (along with spasm or dilation of the arterioles) after a short delay, as a consequence of lack of blood supply from the closed digital arteries, and of cold. This secondary reaction of the capillaries usually does not occur at room temperature, and it is usually impossible to produce blanching of the finger in the doctor's office. However, the basic phenomenon is spasm of the arteries and this can occur, and be produced, by local cooling (even at room temperature), and is demonstrated by plethysmography as shown here, even if the fingers are not white. This capability of demonstrating complete arterial spasm in the absence of actual blanching makes plethysmography an important aid for clinical diagnosis in individual persons.

In view of the inability to provoke finger blanching in subjects at will, have you confirmed the repeatability of finger plethysmography on the same subject a) on different days, and b) at different times during the same day (for example, at 09:00 and 16:00 hours)? In other words, is an abnormal plethysmogram always abnormal?

Authors' Response: No, we do not have statistically significant numbers of repeated plethysmographic tests to show that an abnormal plethysmogram is always abnormal. As demonstrated again in this study, one typical positive result should be sufficient for a positive diagnosis of the Syndrome. The negative result may be a sign of either an absence of disease, or of the presence of VWF at a stage that is below a certain level of abnormality detectable by this method. This level of abnormality is probably low because it would be below even the level demonstrated by our ±. VWF at such a stage would probably not require any practical intervention, medical or at work, other than further surveillance.

J.A. Rigby: I believe it is important to clarify the development of osteoarthritis (i.e. the inflammation occurring at the bony surface of a joint). This condition is known to become more common with increasing age, and is often detected on X-rays without the patient being aware of any symptoms in the joint. This is particularly so in heavy manual workers. The diagnosis of the Vibration Syndrome is difficult enough without introducing confounding variables such as osteoarthritis, which have well-established relationships with other non-related factors.

Authors' Response: In our study, we related radiological evidence of osteoarthritis, of bone cysts, of the combination of bone cysts and osteoarthritis, and of osteoporosis (in the hands) to the period of work and to age. Tables D1 and D2 show that osteoarthritis and osteoporosis had a

Table D1. Radiological Findings in the Hands in Relation to Age (Total N=86: Percentages in Parentheses).

Age	Cysts	Osteoarthritis	Cysts and Osteoarthritis	Osteoporosis	Total
<20	0	0	0	0	1
20-25	0	0	0	0	5
25-30	0	0	0	1 (5.9)	17
30-35	0	0	0	0	15
35-40	3 (17.6)	2 (11.7)	1 (5.9)	0	17
40-45	1 (11.1)	1 (11.1)	0	0	9
45-50	2 (20)	2 (20)	2 (20)	4 (40)	10
50-55	1 (14.3)	3 (42.9)	1 (14.3)	3 (42.9)	7
55-60	2 (50)	3 (75)	1 (25)	0	4
60-65	0	1 (100)	0	0	1
Total	9	12	5	8	86

Table D2. Radiological Findings in the Hands in Relation to the Number of Years of Forestry Work (Total N=85: Percentages in Parentheses).

Period of Work (yrs)	Cysts	Osteoarthritis	Cysts and Osteoarthritis	Osteoporosis	Total
0-5	0	0	0	0	5
5-10	1 (3.8)	3 (11.5)	0	2 (7.7)	26
10-15	2 (9.1)	1 (4.5)	1 (4.5)	2 (9.1)	22
15-20	2 (20)	2 (20)	2 (20)	2 (20)	10
20-25	4 (36.3)	3 (27.3)	2 (18.2)	0	11
25-30	0	1 (14.3)	0	0	7
>30	0	2 (50)	0	2	4
Total	9	12	5	8	85

much stronger relation to age than to the period of work. In fact, approximately 80% of the findings were in people over 50 years of age, no matter how long their period of work. This was not the case for the bone cysts. Osteoarthritis or osteoporosis in the hands did not appear to be work related. However, our data provide no information on the large joints and skeleton of the arm and spine.

P.L. Pelmear: Could not the appearance of bone cysts only in power saw operators claiming VWF be due to their being involved in heavy manual work for a longer period of time? In the U.K., James et al. found no significant difference in the prevalence of bone cysts between vibration-exposed workers and controls (James PB, Yates JR, Pearson JCG. An investigation of the prevalence of bone cysts in hands exposed to vibration. In: Taylor W, Pelmear PL, eds. Vibration White Finger in Industry. London: Academic Press, 1974: 43-51.) The latter were manual workers who had never been exposed to vibration. It was concluded that bone cysts in the hand and wrist bones were a consequence of heavy manual activity rather than vibration exposure with vascular impairment. Ischemia of bone tissue leads to the development of sclerosis, e.g. Perthe's Disease, not rarefaction with cyst formation.

Authors' Response: Yes, we agree. Therefore, we found an apparent link to VWF in our study interesting. The number of persons with bone cysts appears to be too small to draw any firm conclusions.

W. Taylor: In setting up this study to determine VWF prevalence and to evaluate VWF objective tests in forestry workers, two populations were selected as controls: a) Group 3, not power saw operators with symptoms of VWF, and b) Group 5, not power saw operators with no symptoms. It is surprising to find that in these control groups there are non-power saw workers, some of whom had used power drills and even power saws at home. It is acknowledged that some of the background cases were influenced by exposure to vibration. From the statistical point of view, in population selection, this is unsatisfactory, particularly in Group 3 (non-power saw workers claiming VWF symptoms) which most likely would have contained cases of Primary Raynaud's Disease and also Secondary Raynaud's Phenomenon from causes other than vibration exposure.

The paper concludes that finger plethysmography (K-P), one of four vascular tests, gave the best discrimination between exposure groups and the best consistency between objective tests and reported symptoms. The results in support of this claim were positive (+++) objective signs of VWF found in 21 out of 47 men claiming symptoms and in 1 man of 39 who did not report finger blanching. From these data, finger plethysmography, whilst statistically separating exposed and non-exposed populations, is no better than other objective tests such as depth sense, two-point discrimination sensory tests, light touch, pain and temperature tests. (See, for example,

Pelmear PL, Taylor W, Pearson JCG. Clinical objective tests for vibration white finger. In: Taylor W, Pelmear PL, eds. Vibration White Finger in Industry. London: Academic Press, 1975: 53-81.) In other words, finger plethysmography cannot be accepted for the diagnosis of VWF in individual subjects, in particular for litigation purposes, when used retrospectively as in this study.

The opinion that VWF is not a serious clinical disease, and is considered more of a nuisance by most workers, is difficult to reconcile with the observation that half of the men with a positive plethysmogram had to stop working during some attacks of VWF, and many reported interference with other activities. The objection to the view that VWF is "trivial" and "a nuisance" is that it can mislead others to believe that all cases of VWF fall into this category. Also, it ignores the mass of epidemiological data pointing to a cumulative relationship in which the signs and symptoms of VWF increase in severity with increasing vibration exposure, leading ultimately to tissue necrosis.

Authors' Response: The selection of a "control group" is always a problem in studies of occupational medicine. Here a comparison is made between professional sawyers and other forestry workers. It would be virtually impossible to find, for comparison, persons exposed to the same environment in life or at work in the woods, farms and country, who had never used a power saw, or a power drill. Cases of Primary Raynaud Disease and of Secondary Raynaud Phenomenon, caused by trivial exposures to vibration or to other causes, form the "background prevalence" of white finger disease. Table 2 shows a comparison of the background frequency of symptoms with their frequency in the professional power saw operators. Tables 4, 6, 7 and 8, on the other hand, show comparisons of the frequency of positive results of the tests in question between those not claiming blanching (groups 4 and 5) and those who report blanching of fingers, whether caused by professional sawing (groups 1 and 2), or possibly by home use of vibrating tools or by other causes (group 3).

We believe that plethysmography (K-P) not only separates groups with and without symptoms for statistical purposes, but also can confirm and even establish a clinical diagnosis of VWF in individual workers. Further, it can distinguish a typical picture of VWF from arterial obstructions and from spasm due to arteriosclerosis, Raynaud's Disease etc., in differential diagnosis.

We agree that in those rare cases, in whom VWF reaches the irreversible stage of permanent obliteration of the finger arteries, it can become a serious clinical condition resulting in gangrene, with subsequent suffering and impairment. It was the opinion of the workers we examined, which we wished to stress, that white fingers were more of a nuisance than a disease. We have never thought of VWF as "trivial" and have always maintained that it is a matter of both medical and social concern.

Vibration White Finger in Motorcycle Speedway Riders

S. Bentley, D. E. O'Connor, P. Lord and O. P. Edmonds

ABSTRACT: Speedway racing is the second most popular spectator sport in the United Kingdom. The motorcycles used are single-cylinder, 500 cc, four-stroke engined machines, with the engines rigidly bolted to the frame: there is no gearbox or brakes and the handlebar is bolted to the steering head. In a recent survey of riders competing in the British League, a very high prevalence of temperature-mediated finger blanching was observed (30/32 riders), with latent interval of approximately five years. Vibration spectrum analysis on a typical speedway machine showed that the vibration was in excess of that associated with the development of vibration-induced white finger (VWF). This condition is demonstrated in a clearly delineated population, with daily exposure to vibration of, typically, from 40 to 50 minutes.

RESUME: Les courses de motos sur piste viennent au deuxième rang des sports les plus courus au Royaume-Uni. Les motos employées sont des monocylindres quatre temps de 500 cc dont le moteur est fixé fermenent au cadre; elles n'ont ni boîte de vitesses ni freins et le guidon est fixé à l'axe de direction. Au cours d'une enquête récente menée auprès des motocyclistes qui participaient aux courses de la British League, on a constaté que l'incidence de blanchissement des doigts d'origine thermique était très élevée (30 pilotes sur 32) et que l'intervalle latent était d'environ cinq ans. Une analyse du spectre des vibrations effectuée sur une moto de compétition typique a révélé que la vibration était supérieure à celle qui entraînait l'apparition des doigts blancs dûs aux vibrations (le VWF). Les auteurs démontrent l'existence de cette affection chez une population bien délimitée, typiquement exposée à des vibrations pendant 40 ou 50 minutes par jour.

INTRODUCTION

The syndrome of finger blanching in workers using vibratory tools was first described in users of pneumatic tools by Loriga in 1911 (1). Since then, several occupations have been observed to cause a high incidence of this condition among workers, and, on occasions, the vibration characteristics of the tools or machinery have also been described. This paper describes a population, composed of professional speedway riders in the British League, which shows a high prevalence of vibration-induced white finger (VWF), as well as a relatively short interval between initial exposure and clinical manifestations.

Speedway racing is the second most popular spectator sport in the United Kingdom. The racing season extends from March until October, and during this period most clubs have two matches every week. In addition, many of the top professional riders compete in world championship events, in grass track and long track meetings in the United Kingdom and Europe, and in various other meetings. The riders surveyed in this study participated in an average of four racing meetings per week. During the average meeting, each rider races approximately seven times.

The motorcycle used in speedway racing is a relatively simple machine, whose construction is regulated by the Federation Internationale de Motorcyclistes (FIM). All machines have a single cylinder, 500 cc four-stroke engine, bolted rigidly to a diamond-shaped frame, and driving the rear wheel directly through a chain. There is no gearbox, but there is a clutch mechanism. The handlebar is bolted rigidly to the steering head, with no damping material interposed. A typical speedway motorcycle is shown in Fig. 1.

I EPIDEMIOLOGY

A preliminary study of speedway riders has been made. Thirty-two professional riders were interviewed in a two week period

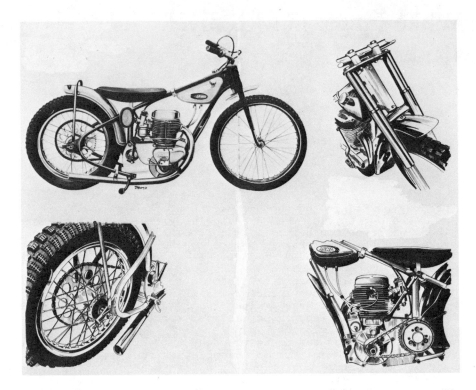

Fig. 1 The air cooled, single cylinder, 500 cc engine motorcycle used in speedway racing (cylinder bore 88 mm and stroke 82 mm; engine power 55 horsepower at 5800 rpm; and weight of 80 kg: note primary chain drive with no gearbox).

during the 1979 racing season. They were selected from an international group competing at the Belle Vue (Manchester) Speedway Stadium. Although some selection was involved due to language limitations, the final sample covering four clubs (Belle Vue, Coventry, Wolverhampton and Ispwich) was considered to be representative of the profession. Each rider was asked about the presence or absence of blanching of the fingers, the anatomical site, the duration of symptoms, the presence of pain, and the length of exposure to vibration during an average week.

Tables 1 and 2 show the reported anatomical distribution (hands and fingers affected) of finger blanching. Only two of the thirty-two respondents were without symptoms. Twelve of the remaining thirty

had symptoms in only one hand. This non-symmetrical condition might be explained by the fact that, during the warm-up period, some riders used only one hand on the throttle.

Table 3 summarizes the average weekly exposure times reported by the riders. In an estimated 28 races per week, the median exposure vibration per race is approximately six minutes, including the warm up. It is clear that these daily exposures (of approximately 45 min) are much shorter than those of workers exposed to vibration in industry.

Table 4 shows the time interval reported between the initial exposure and the onset of symptoms, which, typically, is between four and five years.

Table 1. Numbers of Riders Reporting Anatomical Distribution of Finger Blanching, by Hands Affected.

Symptoms	Number of Riders, N
No Blanching Noted	2
Right Hand Only Affected	10
Left Hand Only Affected	2
Both Hands Affected	18

Table 2. Number of Riders, N, Reporting Finger Blanching, by Fingers Affected.

| Hand Affected | Finger Affected | | | |
	Little N	Ring N	Middle N	Index N
Right Only	10	10	6	1
Left Only	2	2	1	0
Both Right	18	18	10	2
Left	18	14	1	0

Table 3. Average Vibration Exposure Times Per Week During Warm-Up and Racing Reported by Riders.

Exposure Time (h)	Number of Riders, N
1	0
1-2	2
2-3	10
3-4	16
>4	4

Table 4. Time Interval Between Initial Exposure to Vibration and the Onset of Symptoms Reported by Riders.

Years Exposure	Number of Riders, N
1	0
2	0
3	2
4	10
5	12
6	6
6+	2

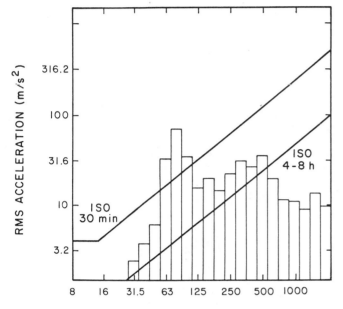

Fig. 2 Frequency spectrum measured at the handlebar of a speedway motorcycle during warm-up, and ISO exposure guidelines for 4 to 8 h and for 30 min (from Ref. 2).

II MEASUREMENT OF VIBRATION AND RESULTS

A general purpose accelerometer (Bruel & Kjaer (B&K) 4369) mounted on a mechanical filter (B&K UA 0559) was attached to the handlebar of the motorcycle by a Jubilee clip (hose clip). The signal was conditioned by a charge amplifier (B&K 2635), and was recorded on a tape recorder (B&K 7003). The one-third octave band frequency spectrum was obtained using true integration with a real time frequency analyser (B&K 2121). The spectrum during engine warm-up is shown in Fig. 2, together with the guidelines recommended by the International Standards Organization for 30 minutes exposure (2).

It is evident that the vibration was in excess of the ISO recommended values,

particularly in the 80 Hz band, which contains the rotational speed of the engine. Note that the rider spends some time before the race warming up the engine, and this operation contributes significantly to the total vibration exposure.

III DISCUSSION AND CONCLUSIONS

In the sample of speedway riders studied, the prevalence of finger blanching was 30/32 or 93%. The latent interval, the period between initial exposure and onset of symptoms, was five years or less. Because high levels of vibration were observed, the incidence of VWF was not unexpected.

This survey was different from most previous surveys of VWF, in that the study group was not industrially exposed, and the daily exposure times were very short. The riders typically are exposed for no more than forty to fifty minutes per day. If the latent period is determined by total exposure time, then a typical industrial exposure of four to five hours per day to this vibration would result in a latent interval of about ten months. Such an interval was found in swaging, and was discussed by Hempstock and O'Connor (3). The vibration spectrum due to swaging was observed to be higher than that of the motorcycles in all but the 80 Hz band. This suggests that frequencies around 80 Hz may be particularly harmful to the hand. It is interesting to note that Agate and Druett suggested that frequencies in the range 40 to 125 Hz were most instrumental in the production of VWF (4); and, more recently, Reynolds has suggested that frequencies in the range 100 to 200 Hz are isolated and dissipated in the fingers (5).

It has been thought that rest periods are helpful in reducing the risk of vibration damage (2). However, speedway riders have very long rest periods between exposure to vibration. Even the daily exposure is not continuous. It appears, therefore, that the vibration to which speedway riders are exposed presents a high risk of vibration damage, despite the long rest periods which are associated with the exposures of speedway riders.

ACKNOWLEDGEMENTS

The authors wish to thank P. Collins, 1976 World Speedway Champion, for his help in providing speedway machines for testing, as well as the staff of the Belle Vue Speedway for their help.

REFERENCES

1. Cited by Teleky L. Occupational and Health Supplement. Geneva: International Labour Office, 1938.
2. International Organization for Standardization. Principles for the Measurement and Evaluation of Human Exposure to Vibration Transmitted to the Hand. Draft International Standard ISO/ DIS 5349, 1979.
3. Hempstock TI, O'Connor DE. Assessment of hand transmitted vibration. Ann Occup Hyg 1978; 21: 57-67.
4. Agate JN, Druett HA. A study of portable vibrating tools in relation to the clinical effects which they produce. Br J Ind Med 1947; 4: 167-174.
5. Reynolds DD. Hand-arm vibration: a review of three years' research. In: Wasserman DE, Taylor W, Curry MG, eds. Proc of the Int Occup Hand-Arm Vibration Conf. Cincinnati, OH: Dept of Health and Human Services, 1977. (NIOSH publication no. 77-170): 99-128.

DISCUSSION

J. Ellen: Is the rapid, and consistent development of VWF due to the riders intense grip on the handlebar when racing?

Authors' Response: Yes. Speedway riders do grip the handle hard during racing.

Is the difference between the VWF statistics for left and right hand caused by the additional stress on the right hand due to holding the motorcycle in a sliding attitude?

Authors' Response: Probably not, as the right hand only is used during the warming-up period.

W. Taylor: With reference to the measurement of vibration carried out with the motorcycle stationary during the warming-up period, would the vibration data be representative when the rider is actually racing around the track? From observation of these riders, they appear to be using additional grip force and are being subjected to additional vibration from the track surface, both adding materially to the vibration dose. Secondly, it is disappointing not to find in the diagnosis of VWF, any reference to other causes of white finger (such as lacerations and fractures of the digits, Primary Reynaud's Disease), which account for 10 to 20% of any VWF survey sample.

Authors' Response: The total vibration dose include contributions from both the warming-up period and the race. Only the levels during the warming-up period were measured because of the difficulties involved in obtaining measurements on a moving motorcycle. It is believed that the handlebar acceleration when racing would be similar. We have not tried to determine accurately the total vibration dose.

Vibration-Induced White Finger— Reversible or Not? A Preliminary Report

H. J. Hursh

ABSTRACT: This paper presents a preliminary report on blood flow and digital temperature measurements on 46 patients who have previously been positively identified as Stage 2 or 3 of vibration white finger (in Taylor and Pelmear's classification). Of the 46 patients studied, 36 (78%) have shown improvement following their removal from vibration exposure.

RÉSUMÉ: Cette communication présente un rapport préliminaire sur des mesures du débit sanguin et de la température des doigts effectuées auprès de 46 malades qui ont atteint le deuxième ou troisème stade des doigts blancs dûs aux vibra- tions (selon la classification établie par Taylor et Pelmear). L'état de 36 (78%) d'entre aux s'est amélioré lorsqu'ils ont cessé d'être exposés aux vibrations.

INTRODUCTION

This study concerns workers using pneumatic hand-held tools for chipping and grinding. The population group has been continuously exposed to vibration until 1980, at which time all members were removed from further vibration exposure.

I SUBJECTS AND METHOD

This is a preliminary report of an on- going study of vibration-induced white finger (VWF), presently involving 46 healthy, young, white males. The subjects had all been exposed to hand-arm vibration, the mean duration being 3.4 years with a range of six months to thirteen years. Latency of onset of white finger was usually 1.7 years, with a range of nine months to five years. At the time of their last evaluation in 1981, all patients had not been exposed to vibration at work for a mean period of 2 years (a range of one month to five years).

All 46 subjects were using vibrating tools at the time of diagnosis of vibration- induced white finger (VWF). All subjects were assessed as either Stage 2 or 3 VWF (1). Any subjects with other illnesses known to cause Raynaud's Phenomenon or diagnosed as possible Primary Raynaud's Disease were excluded from the study. Thirty-one of the subjects (67%) gave a history of being exposed to other types of hand-arm vibration, such as frequent use of chain saws or motorcycles. Twenty-six of the subjects (56%) stated that they smoked from 10 to 30 cigarettes per day.

On each patient, two evaluations of upper extremity blood flow have been per- formed, the first in July 1980, the second approximately nine months later. The tests included: a) history and physical examination; b) Doppler upper extremity pressures (2); and c) digital temperature recovery after 20 seconds cold stimulation. (Note: This test is normal when rewarming occurs within 20 minutes (3).)

II RESULTS AND DISCUSSION

Pressure testing on each upper extrem- ity yielded eight values. The data were converted to a single number pressure ratio. First, the digital pressures were averaged and then were divided by the brachial pres- sure in order to arrive at a (single-number) ratio. By using this ratio, a comparison between the measurements performed in July 1980 and again in April 1981 can be made (see Table 1).

Figure 1 shows changes per patient on the basis of the 1980 and 1981 evaluations. Of the 46 subjects, 31 stated that their symptoms were less frequent, less severe, shorter in duration, involved fewer fingers and occurred more distally on the fingers. Eleven subjects stated that they had no change in symptoms and four subjects com- plained of increased symptoms.

A comparison of the 1980 and 1981 objective tests showed that the pressure ratios tended to follow symptomatic improvement more closely than temperature values. Digital pressure tests showed improvments in 36 subjects, no change in

Table 1. Ratio of Average Digital Blood Pressure
to Brachial Pressure for One Subject.

	Digital Blood Pressure (mm Hg)	Brachial Blood Pressure (mm Hg)	Ratio DBP/BBP
July 1980	154	138	1.12
April 1981	181	132	1.37

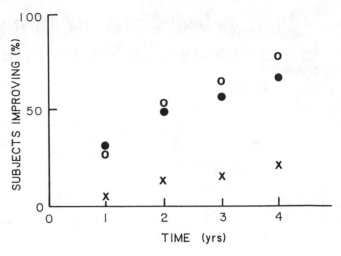

Fig. 2 Percentage of subjects showing
improvements in symptoms (solid circles),
pressure ratio (open circles), and digital temperature (crosses) one to four
years after terminating vibration exposure. Only data for subjects whose
condition improved have been included.

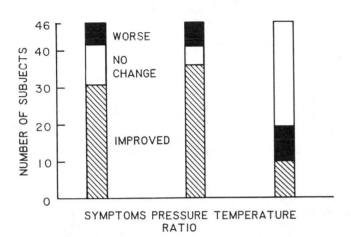

Fig. 1 Results of physical examinations, blood pressure ratios and digital temperatures recorded after an
interval of nine months.

five subjects and decreased pressure in
five subjects. Temperature response tests
were improved in nine subjects, worse in
nine subjects and unchanged in 28.

Vibration white finger assessed at
Stage 3 was previously thought to be an
irreversible injury, though recovery from
this stage has been reported in the literature (4). The data presented here tend
to support reversibility, at least on the
basis of the subjective assessment of
symptoms and the blood pressure ratios.

Figure 2 shows only subjects whose
symptoms, blood pressure ratios and finger
temperatures improved. These comprised 78%
of the population group. The subjects were
separated into four groups according to the
number of years each subject had been away
from vibration exposure. In the group
that had been removed from vibration for
two years, 50% of persons showed an improvement in symptoms and pressure ratio.
Note that pressure tests tended to follow
more closely the subjective symptoms, whereas the results of the temperature tests
lagged behind the assessment of subjective
symptoms.

Additional longitudinal studies of
these subjects are presently in progress.

REFERENCES

1. Taylor W, Pelmear PL, eds. Vibration White
Finger in Industry. London: Academic Press,
1975.
2. Dean RH, Yao JST. Hemodynamic Measurements in
Peripheral Vascular Disease. Chicago, Ill:
Yearbook Medical Publishers, Aug. 1976.
3. Blackburn DR, Peterson LK, Flinn WR, Yao JST.
Non-invasive assessment of occupation-induced
white finger. Third Int Symp on Hand-Arm
Vibration. Ottawa, 1981 (unpublished).
4. Taylor W, Riddle HFV, Bardy DA. Vibration-
Induced White Finger in Chain Saw Operators
in Thetford Chase Forest, Norfolk, England.
Report to the UK Forestry Commission, 1980.
(unpublished).

DISCUSSION

T. Azuma: I would like to suggest that a
reactive hyperemia test may be useful to examine
the reversibility of VWF. The degree of reactive
hyperemia may be greater in reversible cases and
less in irreversible cases.
Author's Response: Good suggestion.

J.R. Barron: It was reported that a large
number of workers removed from the use of vibratory
tools partially recovered from their symptoms. I
wonder if there is a recurrence of these symptoms
in workers who still smoke, or ride motorcycles, or
use lawn mowers, or simply use a hand drill frequently? My experience is that this is so.

Hursh: VWF-reversible or not?

Author's Response: Recovery seems to be noticeably slower in subjects who smoke or live with smokers, and in subjects who continue to be exposed to vibration.

W. Taylor: Were all the 46 subjects taken off the job at an advanced Stage? If not, then if Stage 1 cases did 'reverse', this is an important finding for legal purposes and future litigation.

Author's Response: The cases were not selected according to Stage but I believe that all white finger cases should be removed from further vibration exposure.

If VWF is reversible to the extent of 78%, would you tell us whether the Stage 3 cases take longer to reverse than, say, Stage 1?

Author's Response: The data have not been broken down to differentiate between stages.

E.S. Harris: You appear to be dealing with a relatively young population. Does your data allow you to determine whether the degree of reversibility is related to the age at which the subjects stopped using vibrating tools?

Author's Response: Yes, this could be done in the future. It has not been done as yet.

P.L. Pelmear: How have you been able to remove so many (46) workers from exposure and watch their recovery in the plant? Do you not experience difficulties from workers (e.g. loss of earnings) and management (e.g. finding alternative work)?

Author's Response: Most of these workers were eager to change jobs. Less than five were concerned about decreased income. Management has been very co-operative finding new jobs quickly.

G.I. Renwick: What are these workers doing who have been removed from occupations involving vibration exposure?

Author's Response: These workers have been moved to the machine shop, if they have appropriate skills.

T.P. Oliver: Are all the workers in your study both grinders and chippers?
Author's Response: Yes.

What is the average number of hours daily that the employees actually use these tools?
Author's Response: Approximately 6-7 hours per day - the employees are on piece work.

I. Pyykkö: Different criteria for staging VWF are being used. This seems to be rather confusing because a staging of VWF, which is not the same as a staging of the Vibration Syndrome, seems to be too dependent upon the subjective evaluation of both the investigator and subject. We should limit staging to factors which are not very difficult to interpret, and, if the criteria are subjective, dependent only on the subject. In the index you are using, you are including symptoms like tingling or numbness of finger as a predisposing factor to VWF, which is not necessarily so. Furthermore, the index is composed of factors indicating social handicap. This may be confusing because a factory worker who is indoors can be placed in a wrong Stage compared with a forest worker working continuously outdoors. Furthermore, our work suggests that the limits between Stages 3 and 4 might not be justifiable, because subjects even with extensive VWF can recover.

Author's Response: Good comment. Yes we need a universal method of Staging of VWF based on objective criteria. When we have such objectivity, then we will be able to communicate findings more effectively and make more accurate comparisons.

A. Behar: You are studying a very noisy industry. Have you attempted to relate exposure to noise to the development of white fingers, for example, by comparing the frequency of disorders among workers wearing hearing protectors with those who do not?

Author's Response: All of our workers wear hearing protection.

TOOL AND MACHINE
VIBRATION

Chain Saw Vibration: Effects of Age of the Saw and the Repeatability of Measurements

*J. P. Starck, S. A. Aatola, M. J. Hoikkala,
M. A. Färkkilä, O. S. Korhonen and I. Pyykkö*

ABSTRACT: The vibration of nine A/V chain saws (three samples of three makes) was measured when cutting wood according to the FAO/ECE/ILO hand-held method, both when the saws were new and after every 100 hours of operation. The acceleration levels were found to increase by up to 10 dB, depending on the chain saw make, the direction of vibration and the handle selected. The increase occurred during the first 100 h; thereafter the vibration tended to remain constant. By repeatedly measuring the vibration at the handle and wrist when the same saw was operated by 46 sawyers, it could be shown that the repeatability of field measurements was acceptable. The standard deviation in repeated measurements by one operator was less than 5 dB. Differences in the overall (summed) vibration level between operators were 6 dB at the handle and 8 dB at the wrist.
RESUME: On a mesuré les vibrations produites par 9 tronçonneuses A/V (3 marques différentes) pendant une coupe de bois effectuée selon la méthode manuelle du FAO/CEE/OIT, ceci au début d'utilisation et après chaque 100 heures de travail. On a constaté que l'accélération augmentait d'une valeur pouvant atteindre jusqu'à 10 dB, selon la marque de scie, la direction des vibrations et la poignée utilisée. L'augmentation se produisait durant les 100 premières heures, l'importance des vibrations ayant tendance à demeurer constante par la suite. On a montré que la répétabilité des mesures sur le terrain était acceptable en mesurant à plusieurs reprises les vibrations produites au poignet et à la poignée par une même scie confiée à tour de rôle à 46 ouvriers. L'écart-type de mesures répétées chez un même ouvrier était inférieur à 5 dB. La différence (sommation) entre les niveaux de vibration mesurés chez les différents ouvriers s'élevait à 6 dB pour la poignée et à 8 dB pour le poignet.

INTRODUCTION

The development of chain saws with vibration-isolated handles in the late 1960's has reduced the vibration exposure of lumberjacks by 6 to 14 dB (1,2). In Finland, since 1973, regulations accept only those chain saws that produce oscillating forces in the handles of less than 50 N (3). These regulations concern new saws which have been studied under laboratory conditions. This vibration limit still allows rather high exposure. In addition, vibration exposures may later increase, because of deterioration of the vibration damping capacity owing to use and ageing. In consequence, chain saws need to be tested repeatedly in the field in order that these effects may be controlled. It is simplest to base the measurements on the acceleration recorded at the handles.

This two-part study addresses the questions of: a) whether changes in the vibration of chain saws occur with use, and b) whether field measurements of the vibration of chain-saw handles are repeatable, and correlated with measurements of vibration at the wrist.

I EXPERIMENTS

1.1 Experimental Procedure

Three samples of three makes of the chain saws most commonly used by professional lumberjacks in Finland (total nine saws) were used to study the effect of ageing. The vibration was measured when the chain saws were new and after every 100 hours of use. A normal cutting operation was simulated: for this the log was supported

198

horizontally in order to cut, vertically, thin discs (Fig. 1). All measurements were made with fresh, not frozen, spruce, shaped as stated in the procedure specified by the ECE/FAO/ILO (4).

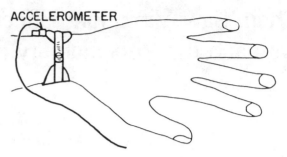

Fig. 3 Method of attaching the accelerometer to the wrist. (From Ref. 6, with permission of Scand J Work Environ Health).

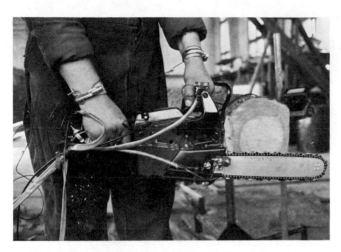

Fig. 1 Photograph of apparatus for vibration experiments.

The same operator was employed for all the measurements. He was instructed to use a normal gripping force, which was measured to be from 24 to 50 N at the front handle and 25 N at the rear handle. The method of measuring grip force has been described in detail elsewhere (5).

For vibration measurements, triaxial transducers were mounted on both handles using hose clamps to which steel studs had been soldered. The orientation of the coordinate system is shown in Fig. 2. The wrist transducers were fastened to acryl plates, which were adjusted to fit against the styloid process of the ulna (Fig. 3).

The signals were recorded during three operational phases: idling, cutting and racing. The engine speed was monitored with a tachometer. Idling measurements were made at the engine speed most appropriate for each chain saw. Cutting measurements were made at the speed corresponding to the maximum power, and racing measurements at an engine speed 133% of the maximum power (4). Details of the saws and the engine speeds are given in Table 1. The vibration measurements were performed six times on each saw with the exception of the Partner type P48 saws, which were only measured four times.

Table 1. The Makes, Weights and Engine Speeds of Anti-Vibration Chain Saws Used in the Measurements.

Type	Weight* kg	Engine Speed (Hz) Idling	Cutting	Racing
Raket 451 EV	6.8	38	150	200
Partner P 48	6.5	42	142	188
Husqvarna 162	7.9	38	142	188

*Contains 0.5 l fuel

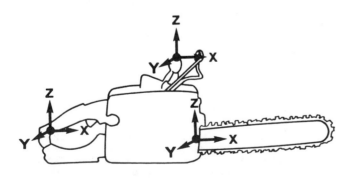

Fig. 2 Location of transducers on the front and rear handles, and on the body of the saw showing the orientation of the X, Y and Z axes.

The second part of the study dealt with the repeatability of field measurements. By repeatability we mean the comparison of results obtained when the same laboratory performs the analyses, and the same operator and apparatus are employed for vibration measurements (7). The measurements for this part of the study were obtained only on the front handle and the corresponding wrist, and used a Partner type R22 chain saw, which weighed 8.7 kg. The normal cutting operation was simulated in the same way as in the first part of the study. Logs were selected from spruce and other species, and were not shaped. The operators were 46 professional lumberjacks and each of them repeated the test five times. There was a break of about half an hour between

Starck et al.: Chain saw vibration

tests, when the accelerometer was not fastened to the wrist.

In all experiments the acceleration signals were simultaneously recorded, using charge amplifiers and FM tape recorders. Each recording, corresponding to a single saw cut, lasted about 30 seconds.

1.2 Measurement and Analysis System

The transducers used were all piezo-electric accelerometers. Bruel and Kjaer (B&K) model 4321 accelerometers were used in the study on the effect of saw age, and B&K model 4366 in the repeatability study. For the wrist, a B&K model 4371 accelerometer weighing 11 g was used. The types of charge amplifiers were B&K 2635 and Wärtsilä VIB 1075. The signals were simultaneously recorded by 4-channel FM-tape recorders, type B&K model 7003. An accelerometer calibrator, type B&K model 4291, was used to generate a calibration signal.

Two different analyzing systems were used. In the study on the effect of age, the analyzing system consisted of a real time 1/3 octave-band frequency analyzer (B&K type 3347), a laboratory built interface, a paper tape punch (Facit type 4070) and a Tektronix 4051 computer. The results obtained were the average octave-band spectra from 6 to 12 1/3 octave-band analyses taken at one second intervals. For comparison purposes, the vibration levels in the 31.5 and 63 Hz octave-bands were summed when the engine was idling, as were the levels in the 125 and 250 Hz bands when the saw was cutting, or the engine racing.

In the repeatability study, the acceleration signals were analyzed by a B&K digital frequency analyzer, model 2131, controlled by a Tektronix computer type 4052. A 1/3 octave-band spectrum was calculated from each tape recording. The result was the average of 20 spectra, which were taken from the recordings at half second intervals. The average spectra obtained from each recording were stored on magnetic discs. The final result for each lumberjack was obtained by forming the average and standard deviation of five stored spectra. The total acceleration levels were also calculated from the 1/3 octave-band spectra for each lumberjack.

II RESULTS

2.1 Effects of Ageing of the Chain Saw

The vibration increased during the first 100 h and then remained nearly unchanged. The most prominent increase was found to be in the X direction at the front handle and in all directions at the rear handle (Figs. 4 and 5). In some cases slight decreases in level were also found, which may be due to a decrease in engine power. A comparison between the different makes of chain saw showed only slight differences in the vibration levels at the front handle: Husqvarna chain saws generally had the lowest levels on the rear handle.

The measurements at the wrists and the handles of the saw showed that more vibration was transmitted to the wrist of the hand grasping the rear handle than the front handle (Fig. 6). This may be due to

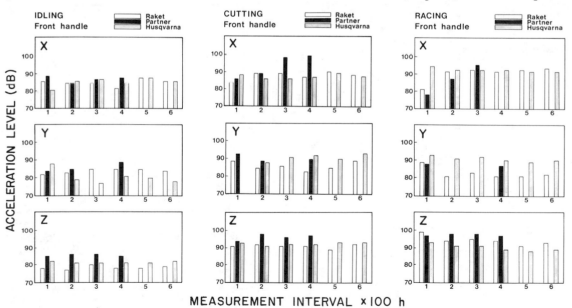

Fig. 4 Overall acceleration levels at the front handle of three makes of chain saws during 500 hours of operation (dB re 4.38×10^{-4} m/s^2). Data for engine idling and racing, and for cross-cutting wood.

Starck et al.: Chain saw vibration

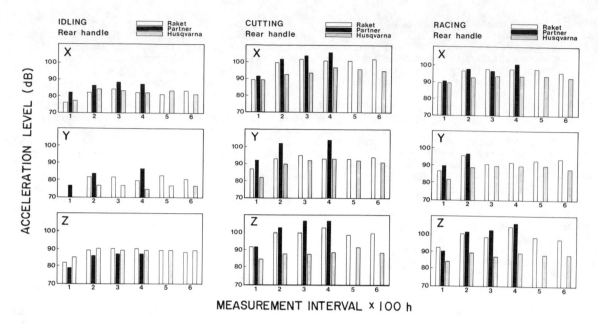

Fig. 5 Overall acceleration levels at the rear handle of three makes of chain saws during 500 hours of operation (dB re 4.38×10^{-4} m/s^2). Data for engine idling, racing, and for cross-cutting wood.

the different grip of the handles (8). Also low frequency vibration was transmitted better than high-frequency vibration.

2.2 Repeatability of the Measurements

The 1/3 octave-band acceleration spectrum obtained for a lumberjack whose overall level corresponds to the mean of the 46 lumberjacks is shown in Fig. 7. For reference purposes, data for the lumberjacks exhibiting the lowest and the highest overall acceleration levels are also shown. As already noted, the measurements were made on the front handle of a Partner type R22 chain saw.

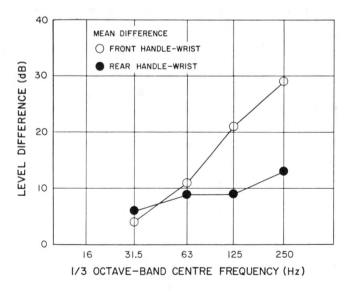

Fig. 6 Hand-transmitted vibration. The mean value recorded between the handle and the wrist: front handle to wrist, data shown by open circles; rear handle to wrist, data shown by closed circles.

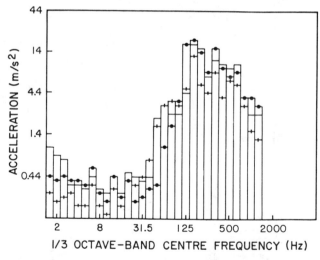

Fig. 7 Average 1/3 octave-band acceleration spectra at the front handle during normal cutting (Partner model R22). Selected data for various overall (summed) levels: mean value, continuous line; maximum value, closed circles; minimum value, +.

The mean value of the overall handle acceleration level in all these measurements was 97 dB (re 4.38×10^{-4} m/s^2); the minimum was 93 dB and the maximum 99 dB. The corresponding standard deviation was 1 dB (see Fig. 8).

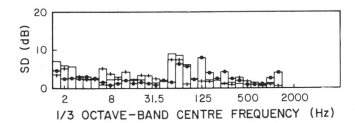

Fig. 8 Standard deviations from repeated measurements of the 1/3 octave-band acceleration spectra at the front handle during normal cutting (Partner model R22). Selected data for various overall (summed) levels: mean value, continuous line; maximum value, closed circles; minimum value, + (dB re 4.38×10^{-4} m/s^2).

When compared to the exposure guidelines proposed by the ISO (9), the most critical frequencies are between 125 and 800 Hz, when slices of wood are being cut. In this frequency range, the standard deviation formed from repeated measurements by a sawyer was less than 5 dB in most cases. The largest standard deviations, of up to 10 dB, were in the 1/3 octave-bands between 50 and 80 Hz.

Results from the wrist vibration measurements showed that the mean value of the overall acceleration levels was 75 dB, with a maximum of 78 dB and minimum of 70 dB (Fig. 9). The standard deviation of these data was 3 dB.

In the 1/3 octave-bands, the standard deviation in most cases was less than 7 dB, and in all cases less than 10 dB (Fig. 10). The values in 1/3 octave-bands with centre frequencies at 63 and 80 Hz generally had the largest standard deviation.

III DISCUSSION

The greatest changes in the vibration level of chain saws occurred during the first 100 hours of use. The levels clearly increased both at the rear and front handles, in the direction of the cutting blade. The application of the proposed ISO draft standard to the results of the first round of measurements shows that the standard would permit these saws to be used for a period of less than four hours a day (9). Presently, this is regularly exceeded in some types of lumbering operations.

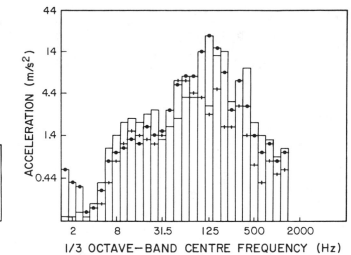

Fig. 9 Average 1/3 octave-band acceleration spectra at the wrist during normal cutting (Partner model R22). Selected data for various overall (summed) levels: mean value, continuous line; maximum value, closed circles; minimum value, +.

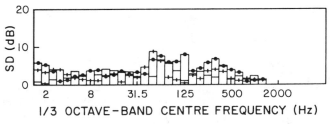

Fig. 10 Standard deviations from repeated measurements of the 1/3 octave-band acceleration spectra at the wrist during normal cutting (Partner model R22). Selected data for various overall (summed) levels: mean value, continuous line; maximum value, closed circles; minimum value, + (dB re 4.38×10^{-4} m/s^2).

The wrist vibration measurements show that the levels of vibration decreased more between the front handle and the wrist than between the rear handle and the wrist. As suggested, the reason for this may be the different hand grips employed (8). Also, the first finger of the right hand controls the throttle trigger and does not support the saw. The angles between the palm and the forearm are different for the two hands, which again may cause variability in the test results (10).

The standard deviation of the wrist measurements was from 1 to 2 dB more than that at the handle. Mounting the accelerometer to the wrist had to be done

resonance fell outside the frequency range
of interest and of the bandpass of the
amplifiers (11,12).

IV CONCLUSIONS

The vibration of A/V chain saws increases with saw age, and with saw use.
The increase in vibration may be as much
as 10 dB. A similar increase in vibration
was also observed at the wrist of the
operators. Therefore, vibration measurements on new saws will not lead to representative estimates of the vibration exposure occurring during the life of a chain
saw. Field measurements are necessary to
monitor the vibration levels and, according to our study, the repeatability of the
field measurements described appeared
satisfactory.

ACKNOWLEDGEMENTS

Some of the work reported in this
paper has appeared in Työterveyslaitoksen
tutkimuksia 175 (1981), and is reproduced
with permission.

REFERENCES

1. Taylor W, Pelmear PL, Pearson JCG. A longitudinal study of Raynaud's phenomen in chain
   saw operators. In: Taylor W, Pelmear PL,
   eds. Vibration White Finger in Industry. New
   York: Academic Press, 1975: 15-20.
2. Pyykkö J, Starck J, Hoikkala M, Korhonen O,
   Nurminen M. Hand-arm vibration in the etiology
   of hearing loss in lumberjacks. Br J Ind Med
   1981; 38: 281-9.
3. Ministry of Social Affairs and Health. Chain
   Saws, Instructions for Manufacturers. Technical Instructions for Safety No. 8. Helsinki:
   Government of Finland, 1971. (in Finnish).
4. Joint Committee on Forest Working Techniques
   and Training of Forest Workers. Hand Operated
   Chain Saws With Internal-Combustion Engine:
   Protection Against Vibration Diseases, Part II.
   Geneva: Economic Commission for Europe/Food &
   Agriculture Organization/Int Labour Organization, 1976.
5. Färkkilä M, Pyykkö I, Korhonen O, Starck J.
   Hand grip forces during chain saw operation
   and vibration white finger in lumberjacks. Br
   J Ind Med 1979; 36: 336-341.
6. Färkkilä M, Starck J, Hyvärinen J, Kurppa K.
   Vasospastic symptoms caused by asymmetrical
   vibration exposure of upper extremities to a
   pneumatic hammer. Scand J Work Environ Health
   1978; 4: 330-335.
7. International Organization for Standardization.
   Acoustics - Statistical Methods for Verifying
   Stated Noise Emission Values of Machinery and
   Equipment. Draft Proposal ISO/DP 7574, 1981: 24.
8. Reynolds DD. Hand-arm vibration: A review of
   3 years' research. In: Wasserman DE, Taylor W,
   Curry MG, eds. Proc of the Int Occup Hand-Arm
   Vibration Conf. Cincinnati, OH: Dept of Health
   and Human Services, 1977. (NIOSH publication
   no. 77-170): 99-123.
9. International Organization for Standardization.
   Principles for the measurements and the evaluation of human exposure to vibration transmitted
   to the Hand. Draft International Standard
   ISO/DIS 5349, 1979.
10. Hoikkala M, Aatola S, Starck J. Chain saw
    vibration test: a long-term follow-up study.
    NAS-80. Proc Abo 10-12 Juni 1980 Helsinki:
    Acoustical Society of Finland, 1980: 185-188.
11. Rasmussen G. Measurement techniques for hand-
    arm vibration. In: Wasserman DE, Taylor W,
    Curry MG, eds. Proc of the Int Occup Hand-Arm
    Vibration Conf. Cincinnati, OH: Dept of Health
    and Human Services, 1977 (NIOSH publication
    no. 77-170): 173-175.
12. Broch JT. Mechanical Vibration and Shock
    Measurements. 2nd ed. Naerum: Bruel & Kjaer,
    1980: 122-129.

DISCUSSION

A.G. Taylor: What was the reason for the
increase in vibration with the age of the saw; could
it be due to imbalance or a lack of sharpness of the
saw teeth?

Authors' Response: It was not engine imbalance.
Sometimes the vibration level decreased. There
seems to have been a reduction in the damping properties of the vibration-isolation system with age.

T. Miwa: The acceleration was measured on the
wrist. On the surface of the human body, the mass
of the accelerometer forms a resonance system with
the elastic properties of the skin. What allowance
was made for this effect?

Authors' Response: An accelerometer with little
mass was used (11 g). It was located on the hard,
boney part of the wrist and a wrist bracelet was
developed.

Why did you measure the vibration acceleration
below 8 Hz?

Authors' Response: We were interested in the
motion of the hand at these frequencies. Of course,
we are not suggesting that these frequencies are
directly related to the incidence of VWF.

N. Olsen: Do the higher acceleration levels on
the rear handle lead to more vibration white fingers
of the hand holding this handle?

Authors' Response: The differences in VWF
between the right and left hand have not been
significant.

Measurement of Chain Saw Handle Vibration

R. Lombard and S. Holt

ABSTRACT: Without control and complete specification of the experimental procedure, substantial differences can occur in the results of handle vibration measurements when a chain saw is hand-held and used to cut wood. At present,
measurements on the same model saw by different laboratories can vary by over
200% in some octave bands, and similar variations can occur between production
samples. Smaller variations, however, have been observed in the ISO frequency-
weighted acceleration sum of the three components. In addition, the handle
vibration of a new saw may not be a good indicator of the vibration exposure of
a worker, owing to changes in vibration with engine speed, chain sharpness, isolator performance, deterioration of the saw with age and work techniques. The
implications of these factors on the development of exposure risk criteria and
regulations are discussed.

RESUME: En l'absence de contrôles et d'une spécification complète de la méthode
expérimentale, les mesures de la vibration du manche peuvent varier considérablement dans le cas d'une tronçonneuse à main servant à la coupe du bois. A
l'heure actuelle, les mesures effectuées pour un même modèle de tronçonneuse
dans différents laboratoires peuvent varier au-delà de 200% dans certains bandes
d'octave et des écarts semblables peuvent exister entre des échantillons de
production. Toutefois, des variations moins importantes ont été observées dans
la somme des trois composantes de l'accélération pondérée en fréquence selon
l'ISO. En outre, la vibration du manche d'une tronçonneuse neuve peut ne pas
constituer un bon indice de l'exposition d'un ouvrier aux vibrations, en raison
de changements dans les vibrations selon la vitesse du moteur, l'état de la
chaîne, le rendement de l'isolateur, l'usure et l'âge de la machine et les techniques de travail. On étudie l'incidence de ces facteurs sur l'établissement
d'exigences et de règlements concernant les risques d'exposition.

INTRODUCTION

Today's chain saw designer faces
numerous challenges in trying to optimize
his product. Not only must power, weight,
efficiency, handling, safety, reliability
and cost elements be carefully balanced to
suit a variety of users, but the designs
must meet a multitude of regulatory requirements. The variety of vibration
standards proposed or adopted in different
countries poses a confusing and somewhat
contradictory situation to the designer.
On occasion, these regulations may force
design compromises that impair utility or
safety in some manner unforeseen by those
imposing the requirements. To complicate
matters further, each regulatory body seems
to have its own procedure for measuring
vibration and processing the data. These
variations can introduce significant discrepancies in results.

We have conducted an extensive handle
vibration measurement programme for several
years, to develop vibration isolation
systems, to verify that chain saws meet
particular standards, and to investigate
the influence of the test procedure on the
results, so as ultimately to improve their
reliability. (More than 750 vibration tests
were conducted during the past year and
over 2500 during the last five years.)
From these measurements, it has become
evident that the results can be sensitive
to seemingly small variations in test conditions and procedure.

The purpose of this paper is to provide
details of our measurement procedure and
to discuss the difficulties inherent in
attempts to characterize the handle vibration of saws with compliant isolating
systems.

I MEASUREMENT PROCEDURE

A block diagram of the apparatus is
shown in Fig. 1. The three signals from a
triaxial accelerometer clamped to the saw
handle (Columbia 610-TX: weight with

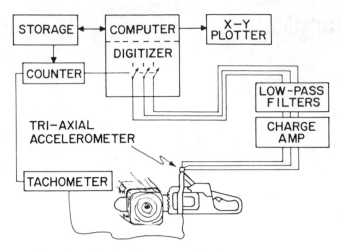

Fig. 1 Block diagram of the apparatus.

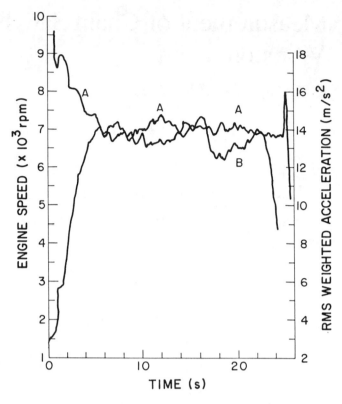

Fig. 2 Variation of engine speed (curve A) and ISO frequency-weighted acceleration sum, WAS, (curve B) recorded during a cut: data for the front handle of a 49 cc chain saw (serial no. 603530457).

mounting pad and clamps, 36.5 g) were fed simultaneously to charge amplifiers (Columbia, model 4102) and low-pass filters, (Hewlett Packard 54440A), to prevent aliasing, and then to a real time analyser (Hewlett Packard 5451B). The filter cutoff frequency and the input overload voltage were controlled by software. Signals were digitized at a rate of 2500 points per second and stored on disc memory. Once data acquisition had been completed, a Fourier analysis was performed and narrow band, 1/3 octave-band or full octave-band frequency spectra plotted. A frequency weighted acceleration sum was also calculated from the three component weighted accelerations a_F, a_V, a_S, as suggested in the ISO Draft Proposal for chain saws (1),

$$WAS = (a_F^2 + a_V^2 + a_S^2)^{\frac{1}{2}} \qquad (1)$$

and at frequencies from 16 to 50 Hz and from 50 to 1000 Hz, as required by the French Norm (2). The component directions are as specified in Ref 1: F-front to rear; V-vertical; and S-side-to-side.

The acquisition of data was controlled by a tachometer signal obtained from the engine ignition, which permits sampling only when the engine speed is within a specified range (usually ±50 Hz). Each sample was of approximately one second duration and the results consisted of the average of ten samples.

Measurements of handle vibration were performed while the saw was hand held by an operator and used to cross cut horizontally-mounted, squared (30×30 cm) red oak logs.

The change in engine speed and in handle vibration during a cut are shown in Fig. 2. In this diagram, the acceleration is expressed in terms of the ISO three component, frequency-weighted sum, WAS,

which was formed by an analogue filter network from the charge amplifier outputs. It can be seen that the weighted acceleration sum changed during the cut at times when the engine speed was essentially constant. As the source of this discrepancy is unclear, the method used to obtain values of the weighted acceleration sum, that is, by means of a filter network or by calculation from average frequency spectra, is identified in the results.

II RESULTS AND DISCUSSION

2.1 Effect of Chain Sharpness

Chain sharpness influences handle vibration. With a properly sharpened chain, a chain saw will almost self-feed during a cut: the operator need only guide the saw, and so needs to apply very little pressure to the handles to maintain control. Under these conditions, a vibration-isolation system employing "soft" (compliant) isolators will lead to low handle vibration levels in laboratory tests. However, if the chain is dull or not well matched to

Lombard et al.: Chain saw vibration

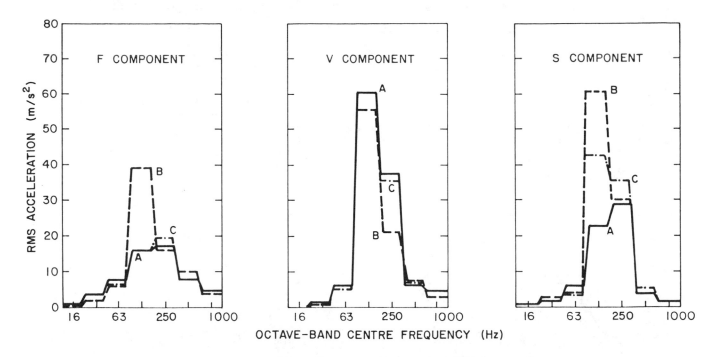

Fig. 3 Component octave-band accelerations observed on the front handle of an A/V chain saw with different chain sharpness: A, saw chain in "factory sharpened" condition (100%); B, 89% sharp; and C, resharpened to give 101% cutting rate.

the wood being cut, the operator may have to apply sufficient pressure for soft isolators to "bottom out" and contact some restraining device at the limit of their deformation, thereby short circuiting the vibration-isolation system. This situation will result in a significant change in the handle vibration.

The results of a three-step experiment on chain sharpness with a 66 cc capacity saw, which possessed vibration isolators that are not considered particularly compliant, are shown in Fig. 3. Curves A show the octave-band component accelerations of the front handle when the chain was in the "factory sharpened" condition. These values correspond to an ISO weighted acceleration sum of 10.1 m/s^2. The saw was then used to cut wood for approximately two hours until the cutting rate was reduced to 89% of the factory sharpened chain. The octave-band frequency spectra under these conditions are given by curves B. Note that the ISO frequency weighted acceleration sum has increased to 13.1 m/s^2 (Table 1), an increase of 23%, and in this experiment the vibration isolators did not "bottom out". The chain was then resharpened and the handle vibration again measured when the same operator cut wood. The results, curves C, are similar to the original spectra (curves A) and the weighted acceleration sum is now 10.9 m/s^2, or within 8% of the initial value.

Table 1. Frequency-Weighted Acceleration Sums Observed on the Front Handle of an A/V Chain Saw for Different Chain Sharpness (engine speed 7000 rpm).

Chain Sharpness*	ISO Sum (m/s^2)	French Norm (m/s^2) 16-50 Hz	French Norm (m/s^2) 50-1000 Hz
100%	10.1	3.07	9.73
89%	13.1	2.68	13.1
101%	10.9	2.64	10.8

*Determined from the rate of cutting wood

We would expect that much larger variations in handle vibration are likely to be experienced by the sawyer who encounters a range of wood sizes and types, who must use his saw in different orientations when cutting, who may not always be able to maintain his saw chain within 10% of factory sharpness and who may be operating a saw with very compliant vibration isolators. Any increase in vibration exposure will, of course, be in addition to that resulting from isolator or saw deterioration with age. It thus appears that the results of saw qualification tests may not be a good indicator of user exposure to vibration, and that designs optimized to provide minimum handle vibration in product tests (by employing very compliant isolators) may

Table 2. Maximum Octave-Band Accelerations and Peak Acceleration Sums on the Handles of a Chain Saw Used by Seven Operators to Cross Cut Squared Timbers.

| Operator Experience | Maximum Octave-Band Acceleration (m/s²) (Band Frequency, Hz) | | | | | | ISO Frequency-Weighted Acceleration Sum, WAS (m/s²) | | $(F^2+V^2+S^2)^{\frac{1}{2}}$ (m/s²) | |
| | Front Handle | | | Rear Handle | | | Front Handle | Rear Handle | Front Handle | Rear Handle |
	F	V	S	F	V	S				
1 h: Non-User of Saws	11.4 (125)	41.2 (125)	16.6 (125)	17.3 (125)	43.2 (125)	23.6 (125)	7.66	13.1	45.9	52.2
10 yrs, 5 h/wk: Professional Pulpwood Cutter*	7.5 (250)	42 (125)	31 (125)	17.5 (125)	39 (125)	25 (125)	9.3	10.5	52.7	49.5
10 h: Non-User of Saws*	8.84 (250)	40.4 (125)	18.1 (125)	10.3 (125)	35.4 (125)	22.4 (125)	8.55	11.6	45.2	43.1
5 yrs, 3 h/wk:	10.3 (250)	48.3 (125)	19.5 (125)	20.5 (125)	51.3 (125)	29.9 (125)	9.51	15.8	53.1	62.8
3 yrs, 2 h/wk	7.5 (125)	35.7 (125)	13 (125)	19 (125)	38.5 (125)	27.5 (125)	7.29	13	38.7	51
15 yrs, 2 h/wk	14.8 (125)	36 (125)	9.8 (250)	10 (125)	33.5 (125)	20.5 (125)	7.51	11.4	40.1	40.5
30 yrs, 10 h/wk: Professional Cutter	8 (250)	39.5 (125)	11.5 (125)	11.5 (125)	37.5 (125)	16.5 (125)	7.12	12.8	41.9	42.6

*Operator left handed.

be more susceptible to increases in vibration during actual use.

The repeatability of our measurements of handle vibration during cutting can also be deduced from the results shown in Fig. 3. When a saw is hand-held, operated by the same sawyer and the chain maintained at factory sharpness, differences in octave band acceleration such as those between curves A and C may occur. The corresponding variation in the ISO frequency weighted acceleration sum is, as already noted, 8%. Changes in vibration in excess of these values may therefore be considered significant.

2.2 Measurements by Different Operators

The potential influence of the operator on the vibration recorded when the saw is hand-held has been recognized by many research workers. The results of a carefully controlled experiment in which seven operators cut wood with the same saw (volumetric capacity 66 cc) are given in Table 2.

It can be seen from the Table that there was considerable variation in handle acceleration between operators, though no pattern could be established for the differences from either the octave band spectra or the ISO frequency weighted sums. However, when the maximum values obtained for the vibration components were combined to form a peak unweighted acceleration sum

for each handle (expressed by the square root of the sum of the squares), it became evident that the manner in which the sawyer's hands controlled the cutting operation influenced the results. An examination of the values for the unweighted sum in Table 2 reveals that the acceleration of the rear handle usually exceeds that of the front, except in two cases. It was subsequently found that the operators in these cases were left handed.

This presumed effect of hand grip and/ or the manner in which the sawyer operates the saw not only influences the results of hand held measurements and qualification tests, but also introduces errors in vibration-exposure risk evaluation.

2.3 Measurements on Production Samples of the Same Chain Saw

An experiment was performed to assess the variations in handle vibration between production samples of the same model of chain saw. Five nominally identical saws were obtained from the warehouse and operated sequentially by one sawyer. The results are shown in Table 3.

It can be seen from the Table that the vibration of the saw handles differed from under 15 to over 200%, depending on the measure selected. It is interesting to note that the smallest standard deviation was recorded during measurement of the ISO frequency-weighted acceleration sum by the

Lombard et al.: Chain saw vibration

Table 3. Maximum 1/3 Octave-Band Accelerations and Acceleration Sums on the Handles of Five Production Samples of a Chain Saw when Cross Cutting Squared Logs.

| Chain Saw Serial No. | Maximum 1/3 Octave-Band Acceleration (m/s²) (Band Frequency, Hz) | | | | | | ISO Frequency-Weighted Acceleration Sum, WAS (m/s²) | | | | Frequency-Weighted Sum (French Norm) (m/s²) | | | |
| | Front Handle | | | Rear Handle | | | Analogue Filter | | Computed Sum | | 16-50 Hz | | 50-1000 Hz | |
	F	V	S	F	V	S	Front Handle	Rear Handle	Front Handle	Rear Handle	Front Handle	Rear Handle	Front Handle	Rear Handle
603530056	15.8 (125)	9.74 (125)	12.7 (125)	13.7 (125)	16.4 (125)	15 (125)	12.5	13.2	8.46	16.1	3.81	6.57	1.06	2.81
603530410	33 (125)	13.9 (315)	21.6 (125)	14.2 (125)	31.4 (125)	18 (125)	11.8	14.2	10.2	14	7.12	11.3	8.31	11.6
603530451	30.1 (125)	13.3 (125)	12.8 (250)	16.6 (125)	34.3 (125)	18.5 (125)	12.5	14.6	10.3	15.8	7.8	13.3	8.58	13.2
603530457	29.7 (125)	11.8 (315)	20.2 (125)	9.3 (125)	12.6 (50)	10.8 (40)	13.5	13	11.1	12.2	8.64	11	8.43	6.95
603530463	25.3 (125)	9.11 (125)	26.1 (125)	22.7 (125)	29.8 (125)	18.7 (125)	-	13.3	8.63	14.8	5.96	12.3	7.58	12
Mean Value							12.6	13.7	9.75	14.6	6.66	10.9	6.79	9.28
SD							0.699	0.698	1.16	1.58	1.87	2.56	3.22	4.32

Note: The 49 cc chain saws were equipped with 40.6 cm (16 in) bars and Oregon type 72DP chains.

analogue filter network. Though there can be no assurance that these samples display variations typical of those found in other production models, the experiment does reveal that substantial differences can occur in hand held measurements of handle vibration by one sawyer, even between saws manufactured on the same production line.

It can be assumed that as these saws are used, normal wear and the ageing of parts, particularly the rubber vibration isolators, will lead to increases in these differences. We have observed, for example, that the elastic modulus of some commonly used isolator elastomers increases with age, a phenomenon sometimes known as the "marching modulus". Also, the replacement isolators offered by manufacturers sometimes possess an elastic stiffness significantly greater than those originally supplied. In both cases, increased vibration on the saw handle will result. In summary, differences in the handle vibration of production saws and changes occurring during the life of the saw can affect the vibration exposure of the operator by more than a factor of two.

2.4 Comparison Between Measurements from Different Laboratories and Vibration Standards

By careful attention to the experimental technique, we have obtained repeatable measurements of handle vibration when the saw is hand-held and used to cut wood.

Unfortunately, the results do not always agree well with measurements on similar saws by other laboratories, though this should not be unexpected in view of the sources of variability discussed in the preceding sections.

Figure 4 illustrates the magnitude of the problem, by comparing the results of measurements on the same model saw by the official testing laboratories in two countries (3,4), and by Homelite. It is evident that the maximum, component octave-band accelerations, which have been determined under operating conditions specified by the National Standards, differ considerably (data for the octave band with the largest acceleration only are available from Finland). In fact, when tested at the official Government Test Laboratories in Japan, Czechoslovakia and Finland (and also when tested by a different method in Sweden), the vibration of this model saw was found to be acceptable (3-6), and the saw was approved according to the pertinent National Standard. However, based on our measurements, this model would only meet the requirements for vibration in Japan. In addition, this model would not satisfy the vibration limits contained in the Canadian Standard for Chain Saws (7), nor those proposed for day-long exposure by the ISO (8), which are also shown in Fig. 4. Thus, it is difficult for a chain saw designer (and manufacturer) to establish prior to the actual certification tests whether a new design will comply with the various national requirements.

Lombard et al.: Chain saw vibration

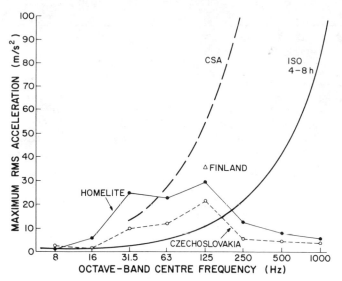

Fig. 4 Maximum, component octave-band accelerations observed on the handles of a small A/V saw in tests performed by official government laboratories and by Homelite. Also shown are the vibration limits proposed in the Canadian Standard for chain saws (CSA) and by the ISO for 4 to 8 h daily exposure (7,8).

2.5 Low-Frequency Performance of Vibration-Isolation Systems

There are design difficulties associated with further reducing the vibration of A/V saws at low frequencies. Non-isolated saw handles typically possess less vibration than the handles of A/V saws at these frequencies, because of resonances in the vibration-isolation systems. It also appears that the consequences of isolators "bottoming out", overloading, or stiffening with age, and environmental factors are most important at low frequencies. Unfortunately, these same frequencies are considered most hazardous by some authorities.

To illustrate the performance of vibration-isolation systems, a series of measurements were made on four pairs of "matched" saws. Each matched pair consisted of two chain saws of approximately the same volumetric displacement, weight and geometry; one with and one without vibration-isolated handles. The saws for this experiment were selected from our laboratory inventory and were not new. However, all were in good working condition. The rubber isolators were also checked to ensure that none had visible signs of failure or deterioration, though some may have become harder with age.

The change in handle vibration for each pair of saws, expressed as an effective transmissibility (i.e. the ratio of the acceleration observed on the A/V saw handle to that observed on the handle of

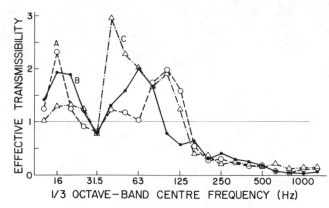

Fig. 5 The effective transmissibility of some isolated saw handles observed as a function of frequency when cutting red oak. Data for selected saws and vibration components: A, V direction, rear handle of a 41 cc capacity saw; B, V direction, rear handle, 57 cc saw; and C, F direction, front handle, 82 cc saw.

the paired non A/V saw), is shown as a function of frequency in Fig. 5. Data are shown for only one vibration component of one handle for each saw pair, but these are sufficient to indicate the magnitude of the effect. In each case, the vibration of the A/V saw handle exceeds that of the comparable non A/V handle at some frequencies below 125 Hz.

In order to reduce the resonance frequency of these vibration isolation systems, the spring rate of the rubber isolators would have to be significantly reduced. This would decouple the handles from the bar and power-head of the saw to such an extent that an operator would have only marginal control over the cutting operation, thereby increasing the risk of accidents. In addition, the soft elastomer compounds often used to achieve low spring rates tend to be less durable and more likely to stiffen with age. Hence, improving vibration isolation at low frequencies by reducing the stiffness of the rubber isolators does not appear to be practicable: in all probability, more complex isolation systems will be required.

III CONCLUSIONS

1. Without control of the experimental procedure, substantial differences can occur in the results of handle-vibration measurements when the saw is hand-held.
2. At present, the results of hand-held vibration tests by different laboratories on the same model chain saw can vary by more than 200% in some octave bands. Much smaller variations, however, were observed

in the ISO frequency-weighted acceleration sum of the three components.

3. The handle vibration measured in current, hand-held laboratory tests on a new saw may not be a good indicator of the vibration exposure of a worker using the saw. The potential for discrepancies should be taken into account by those responsible for developing exposure risk criteria, as well as by those authorities setting regulations.

4. The imposition of requirements for extremely low vibration, particularly at low frequencies, may lead to saw designs "tuned" for the test conditions. If this is done by using "soft" rubber isolators, the operator may have only marginal control of the saw, and may experience increased vibration exposure as the isolators age under actual working conditions.

5. Agencies imposing vibration requirements on chain saws should sponsor research to develop improved test methods for measuring vibration, and ensure that the results are representative of operator exposure and repeatable in different laboratories.

6. Authorities from the various agencies should make a greater effort to adjust their vibration limits and their test procedures to a common, world-wide standard.

7. Authorities should place more emphasis on the control of work practices to reduce vibration exposure, rather than relying on increasingly restrictive regulatory requirements based on potentially misleading tests.

REFERENCES

1. International Organization for Standardization. Chain Saws - Measurement of Hand-Transmitted Vibration. Draft Proposal ISO/DP 7505, 1980.
2. Commission de normalisation des vibrations et chocs mechaniques. Guide pour l'évaluation de l'exposition des individus à des vibrations transmises par les mains. Paris: Association française de normalisation, 1978. (E90K-doc 2).
3. Brno Branch Testing Station. Final Protocol No. 5422 Concerning Approval of Homelite VI Super 2 SL Automatic Oiling One-Man Power Chain Saw. Prague, Czechoslovakia: State Testing Station of Agricultural, Food Processing and Forestry Machines, 1979.
4. Vakola. Information on Chain Saws Available in Finland. Helsinki, Finland: Finnish Research Institute of Engineering in Agriculture and Forestry, 1979. (Test Report 1017).
5. Statens Maskinprovningar. Typogodkända Motorkedjesågar. Uppsala, Sweden: Statens Maskinprovningar, 1979. (Meddelande 2509). (in Swedish).
6. Extract from test report by Government Forest Experimental Station, Tokyo, Japan. (in Japanese).
7. Canadian Standards Association. Chain Saws. Toronto: Canadian Standards Association, 1977. (CAN 3-7621.1-M77).
8. International Organization for Standardization. Principles for the Measurement and the Evaluation of Human Exposure to Vibration Transmitted to the Hand. Draft International Standard ISO/DIS 5349, 1979.

DISCUSSION

A.J. Brammer: The influence of hand grip, that is, the average compressive force exerted by the hand on a handle, on the vibration of an A/V chain saw handle has been discussed in the literature. In controlled experiments, changes in hand grip alone (i.e. no change in instrumentation, engine speed, wood cut, saw chain sharpness, operator, push - or cutting - force, or posture) can produce changes in handle vibration of up to 300% in some octave bands (Brammer AJ. Influence of hand grip on the vibration amplitude of chain-saw handles. In: Wasserman DE, Taylor W, Curry MG, eds. Proc of the Int Occup Hand-Arm Vibration Conf. Cincinnati, OH: Dept of Health and Human Services, 1977. (NIOSH publication no. 77-170): 179-186.) It is also known that different operators employ different grip forces when cutting wood (Färkkilä M, Pyykkö I, Korhonen O, Starck J. Hand grip forces during chain saw operation and vibration white finger in lumberjacks. Br J Ind Med 1979; 36: 336-341). These factors could account for the differences you recorded between sawyers. The changes in handle vibration with grip force apparently result from the coupling of different amounts of flesh to the motion of the handle. In consequence, all forces exerted by the hands on the handle of an A/V saw must be controlled before differences attributable to other sources can be reliably identified.

The implications for compliance testing of chain saws are also clear. For product evaluation, where the primary goal is surely to obtain a measure of handle vibration that is repeatable, reproducible in different laboratories, and consistently ranks saws according to their vibration hazard, the mechanical coupling of the hands to the handles must be explicitly defined. This could be achieved by measurements of grip and push forces, and mechanical impedance on a selected hand, and subsequent control of these and other variables during vibration tests when the saw is hand-held. However, a satisfactory measure of handle vibration is much more likely to be obtained by means of a test machine, with approximate, but consistent, simulation of the dynamical response of the hand, and simultaneous control of other variables.

Mechanical Test Stand for Measuring the Vibration of Chain Saw Handles During Cutting Operations

D. D. Reynolds and F. L. Wilson

ABSTRACT: A mechanical test stand for measuring the vibration of chain saw handles during cutting operations has been developed for the Chain Saw Manufacturers Association. The stand is designed to accommodate saws of all types, and shapes, and uses compliant mechanical coupling devices, which approximate the dynamic characteristics of the hand, to clamp the top and rear handles. The results of hand-held and machine-held measurements of the handle vibration of four chain saws are discussed. The overall correlation between the vibration levels and frequency spectra obtained from the two measurement procedures was good. The variability of the data, the performance of the test stand, and the construction and performance of the mechanical "hands" are examined in detail.

RESUME: Un banc d'essai mécanique pour mesurer les vibrations de poignées de tronçonneuses qui se produisent pendant la coupe a été mis au point pour la Chain Saw Manufacturers Association. Le banc est conçu pour recevoir des scies de tous les types et de toutes les formes; il comporte des dispositifs d'accouplement mécanique souple dont les caractéristiques dynamiques sont presque semblables à celles de la main, pour immobiliser la poignée du haut et celle de l'arrière. On étudie le résultat des mesures des vibrations des poignées de quatre tronçonneuses, tenues à la main et tenues mécaniquement. Il y a eu une bonne corrélation globale entre les niveaux de vibrations et le spectre de fréquence obtenu à partir des deux méthodes de mesure. On examine en détail la variabilité des données, le fonctionnement du banc d'essai, ainsi que la conception et le fonctionnement des "mains" mécaniques.

INTRODUCTION

The vibration of hand tools has long been associated with problems of occupational health and safety, the most important of which is the Vibration Syndrome. For this reason, several countries have established standards for vibration exposure which define the maximum vibration deemed tolerable. In these countries, many of the tools sold must undergo tests to verify that they conform to the vibration limits.

The purpose of this paper is to describe the development of a standardized method for measuring the vibration of chain saw handles. To date, most measurements of chain saw vibration have been performed while simulating actual field conditions. Tests performed when a saw is hand-held usually result in a lack of repeatability between measurements performed by the same operator and between those conducted by different laboratories. This lack of repeatability is usually associated with the different grip forces and methods of operating a saw used by sawyers. As a result, the Chain Saw Manufacturers

Association (CSMA) initiated a programme to develop a mechanical test stand and test procedures for measuring the vibration of chain saw handles. Its objectives were as follows:

a) The design and construction of a machine for holding the handles of a chain saw during vibration measurements.

b) The acceleration measured on the handle of a saw held in the machine must be repeatable and correlate with measurements made when the saw is hand-held.

c) The machine must not introduce any preload on the saw other than that introduced by human hands and arms during normal use; must not develop any resonant interaction with the saw other than that occurring with human hands and arms; must provide for tests whether or not the saw is cutting wood; must be so designed that identical machines may be readily constructed by others; and must include a method for calibration so that machine performance may be frequently checked against a standard and against other machines.

d) The relationship between the machine and hand-held tests is to be established by

a mathematical model and verified experimentally. Variations in grip force, and operational parameters such as mass, stiffness, and damping of the hand-arm system are to be explored.
e)   Establish the required instrumentation.
f)   Determine the useful operating range and the limitations of the machine.
g)   Identify proper operating procedures.

I   THE VIBRATION TEST MACHINE

1.1   General Description

Figures 1 to 3 show a chain saw mounted in the CSMA chain saw vibration test machine. The basic superstructure of the machine was constructed of solid steel, two inch diameter circular shafts and two inch square bars. These were fastened together using Thomson pillow blocks so that the machine is extremly rigid in all directions. The machine is sufficiently massive (around 1000 lb) so that no resonant interactions occur between the test stand and the saw being supported.

The basic support structure for the chain saw is adjustable to accommodate saws of all shapes and sizes. The two supporting "arms" attached to the top circular shaft of the test machine can be moved back and forth, or rotated from side-to-side, to line up

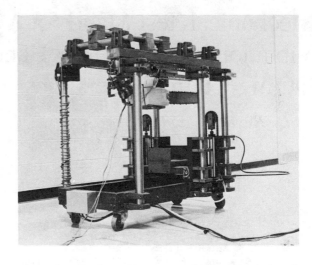

Fig. 2   Chain saw mounted in test stand.

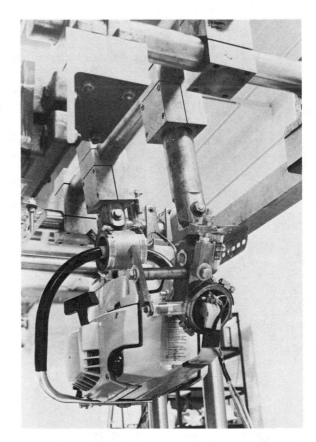

Fig. 3   Chain saw mounted in test stand.

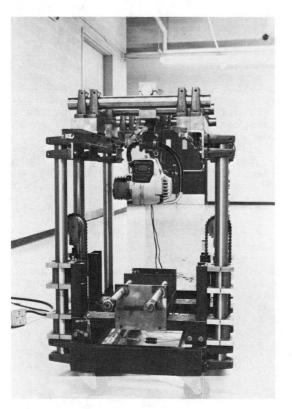

Fig. 1   Chain saw mounted in test stand.

with the top and back handles of different saws. The handle clamps at the lower end of the arms can also be positioned to match the handle configurations of various saws (Fig. 4). The top circular shaft, to which the arms are attached, can be moved from side-to-side to align the saws with the wood during cutting tests (Fig. 5).

Reynolds et al.:   Chain saw test stand

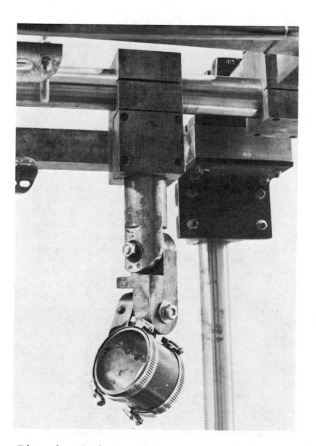

Fig. 4   Chain saw clamping mechanism.

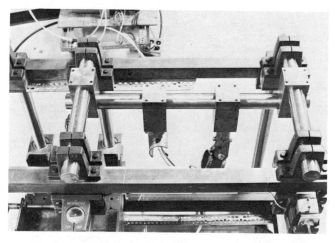

Fig. 5   Adjustable support structure
for chain saw.

The wood is raised on a steel carriage, which is lifted by two hydraulic
cylinders. The carriage rides on eight
self-adjusting linear bearings, which are
adjusted to provide a zero tolerance between the bearings and shafts (Fig. 1).
The bearings are kept clean by commercial

plastic window shades, which are affixed
to the stand so as to move in conjunction
with the carriage. The window shades can
be seen in Fig. 11.

The hydraulic operation is controlled
by an electric switching circuit. This
enables the operator to control the upward
motion of the carriage, or to lower it
immediately, in case of emergency. The
circuit also causes the carriage to reverse
direction automatically when it reaches the
limiting height of its travel.

A chain saw is mounted in the test
stand by means of molded elastomers (Fig. 6)
that are wrapped around the saw handles and
then placed inside rigid circular clamps.
These, in turn, are rigidly attached to the
support structure of the test stand (Figs. 3
and 4). In this manner it is possible to
mount a chain saw in the test stand without
attaching additional mass to the saw handles.

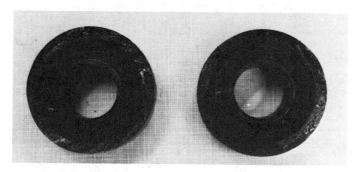

Fig. 6   Elastomer for use in chain saw
test stand.

1.2   The Molded Elastomers

Figure 7 shows a sketch of the elastomer configuration that was used for the
machine-held chain saw vibration tests.
The elastomer was constructed in the

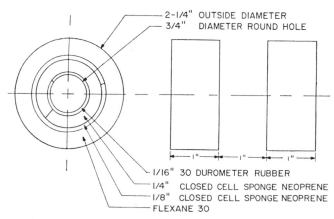

Fig. 7   Final elastomer configuration.

Reynolds et al.:   Chain saw test stand

214

following manner. First, a 0.16 cm (1/16 in) thick by 6.35 cm (2.5 in) wide single layer of 30 durometer neoprene rubber, cut to a length equal to the circumference of the inner core of the elastomer mold, was wrapped around the inner core. The two ends of the 30 durometer neoprene rubber were bonded together with Eastman 910 contact cement. Second, a single layer of closed-cell sponge neoprene measuring 0.64 cm (1/4 in) thick by 6.35 cm (2.5 in) wide was cut to a length equal to the circumference around the 30 durometer rubber. Goodyear Contact Cement (trade name) was applied to the outside of the 30 durometer rubber and to one side and the two ends of the closed-cell sponge neoprene. The cement was allowed to dry for five to ten minutes. The closed-cell sponge neoprene was then wrapped around the 30 durometer rubber. It is important to insure that the ends of the closed-cell sponge neoprene are pressed securely together. Third, a single layer of closed-cell sponge neoprene measuring 0.32 cm (1/8 in) thick by 6.35 cm (2.5 in) wide was cut to a length equal to the circumference around the 0.64 cm (1/4 in) thick layer of closed-cell sponge neoprene. Goodyear Contact Cement was used to attach the 0.32 (1/8 in) thick layer of closed-cell sponge neoprene to the 0.64 cm (1/4 in) layer as was previously described. Fourth, the elastomer assembly was placed in a mold and a 0.64 cm (1/4 in) layer of Flexane 30 (trade name) was poured around the assembly and allowed to cure for a minimum of twenty-four hours. Finally, before being used for a machine-held chain saw test, two 2.54 cm (1 in) sections were cut from the finished elastomer assembly.

The basic elastomer configuration, when attached between the saw handles and the test machine clamps, supported the saw without applying any static compressive pressure on the saw handles. This worked well for light-weight chain saws. However, when this configuration was used with heavier saws, the larger static weight of the saws resulted in the cement bond between the handles and elastomers breaking, or, in excessive static deformation of the elastomers during testing. These problems were solved by using Goodyear contact cement, in the manner already described, to attach a 0.08 cm (1/32 in) thick layer of 50 durometer neoprene rubber to the outside surface of the Flexane 30. This resulted in a compressive static pressure being applied to the handles of heavier saws, eliminating the difficulties just described. The results of the machine-held chain saw tests, when compared to the hand-held tests, indicated that the increased dynamic stiffness of the elastomer associated with the 0.08 cm (1/32 in) thick layer of 50 durometer neoprene rubber had no apparent adverse effects upon the results.

It was decided at the beginning of the project to design a chain saw clamping mechanism that was relatively simple in nature, and easy to construct and use. It was considered neither desirable nor practical to duplicate exactly the dynamic properties of the hand in such a mechanism. Past investigations have shown that the dynamic mass of the hand, when excited by vibration, is small when compared with the mass of a saw handle (1,2). Thus, any elastomer or clamping configuration should add little or no additional rigid mass to a saw handle. The elastomer configuration was designed so that it would roughly approximate the one-degree-of-freedom dynamic stiffness and damping coefficients, K and R respectively, for vibration in each of three mutually orthogonal directions. Referring to Fig. 8, vibration in the X or Z directions will result in the rubber elastomer being loaded or excited in compression, and vibration in the Y direction will result in the elastomer being excited in shear. Acceptable values of K and R for the elastomers excited in compression are $K = 5 \times 10^4$ to 4×10^5 N/m and R = 26 to 263 N-s/m. Acceptable values of K and R for the elastomers excited in shear are about 1/10 to 1/2 the corresponding values for the elastomers excited in compression. These values for K and R resulted in a one-degree-of-freedom displacement mobility that would roughly approximate the actual displacement mobility of the hand at frequencies above 60 to 70 Hz. At lower frequencies, the displacement mobility of the elastomer will be lower than that associated with the hand by up to a factor of ten, or more.

Table 1 shows the K and R values for elastomers with a 2 cm diameter, 2.5 cm diameter and 2.5 cm × 3.5 cm rectangular cross-section hole in the centre, measured in both compression and shear. These values are for the elastomers tested in the configuration indicated in Figs. 6 and 7. If one notes that the one-degree-of-freedom natural frequency is given by $\omega_n = (K/M)^{\frac{1}{2}}$,

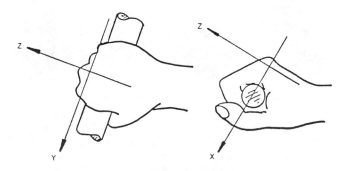

Fig. 8 Coordinate system for the hand-arm system.

Reynolds et al.: Chain saw test stand

Table 1. K and R Values for Elastomers of Various Cross Section.

Elastomer	Compression		Shear	
	K (N/m)	R (N-s/m)	K (N/m)	R (N-s/m)
2 cm Dia. Round Hole	2.1×10^5	35	1.75×10^5	26.25
with 50 Durometer Rubber Added	3.85×10^5	35	1.75×10^5	26.25
2.5 cm Dia. Round Hole	1.4×10^5	40.25	2.1×10^5	35
with 50 Durometer Rubber Added	2.98×10^5	40.25	1.93×10^5	26.25
2.5 cm × 3.5 cm Square Hole	2.63×10^5	52.5	1.58×10^5	43.75
with 50 Durometer Rubber Added	3.5×10^5	52.5	1.49×10^5	40.25

then the maximum variation from lowest to highest natural frequency was less than 15% for the elastomers without the 50 durometer rubber. The maximum variation for the elastomers with the 50 durometer rubber was also less than 15%. There was only, on average, a 20% difference in natural frequencies between the elastomers with and without the 50 durometer rubber. These variations were judged to be acceptable, and the results of the chain saw vibration tests confirmed this belief.

Table 2 shows the K and R values of four identical elastomers constructed on four separate days. These elastomers had a 2.5 cm diameter hole in the centre and a 0.08 cm layer of 50 durometer rubber added to the outside surface. These were the elastomers used on the top handle of chain saw D for the four machine-held vibration tests reported in Figs. 14-19. The results in Table 2 indicate that the maximum variation in the one-degree-of-freedom natural frequency was less than 10%. These elastomers were tested in the configuration indicated in Figs. 6 and 7.

Table 2. K and R Values for Four Elastomers of Identical Cross-Section with Round, 2.5 cm Diameter, Inner Hole and with 50 Durometer Rubber Outer Layer.

Elastomer	Compression		Shear	
	K (N/m)	R (N-s/m)	K (N/m)	R (N-s/m)
No. 1	2.98×10^5	40.25	1.93×10^5	26.25
No. 2	3.15×10^5	52.5	1.84×10^5	26.25
No. 3	2.63×10^5	36.75	1.93×10^5	26.25
No. 4	2.98×10^5	40.25	1.93×10^5	26.25

In general, the values of K and R for the elastomers loaded in compression were within the desired ranges. The stiffness coefficients were always at or near the upper limit of acceptable values, and the damping coefficients were at or near the lower limit of acceptable values. For the case where the elastomers were loaded in shear, the resistances were generally within the range desired, but the shear stiffnesses were always above the desired values. The results of the machine-held chain saw vibration tests indicated that this was not important, so no measures were taken to design an elastomer with lower K values in shear.

All the materials used in the construction of the layered elastomers were readily available off-the-shelf items. They have been referred to here by either their trade or generic names, and we were unable to obtain specific information concerning their physical properties. Static test procedures could, of course, be devised to determine the density, stiffness, etc. However, the static properties of individual components may not be indicative of the dynamic properties of the elastomer configuration used for the machine-held vibration tests. As the results in Tables 1 and 2 indicate, elastomers with similar dynamic properties could be readily constructed. Whether or not significant differences in the dynamic properties will occur when layered elastomers are constructed at different laboratories is not known at present.

The inner core of all the elastomers was shaped to conform to the handles around which they were placed. It was initially thought that all elastomers could be made with circular centre sections, even though they would be placed around handles that had non-circular cross-sections, but this proved to be unsatisfactory.

Elastomer life and deterioration was a concern throughout this project. For any machine-held chain saw test, no chain saw was placed in the machine until just before the cutting tests were to begin. Allowing the dead weight of the saw to hang on the elastomers for a period of over 40 to 60 minutes before testing could result in the elastomer taking a permanent set, which could affect the test results. No set of front and back handle elastomers was ever used for more than one series of tests. The static loads applied to the elastomers during cutting operations usually resulted in some deterioration. The elastomers on the front handle always experienced greater deterioration than those on the back handle. Also, since it was necessary to glue the elastomers to the saw handles and the test machine clamps, they were usually seriously damaged when removing the saw from the stand after a series of tests. The deterioration of the elastomers as a result of exposure to vibration was also considered.

Reynolds et al.: Chain saw test stand

However, because each elastomer was only used for one series of tests that lasted, typically, for between 40 and 60 minutes, vibration deterioration was not found to be a problem. The greatest deterioration was associated with the static forces applied to the elastomer when the saw was cutting or when it was just hanging, being supported by the elastomers.

II EXPERIMENTAL PROCEDURES

2.1 Hand-Held Vibration Measurements

Two triaxial accelerometer modules were mounted on the top and back handles of the saw to be tested. Each accelerometer weighs about 2 grams, and the entire module (including the mounting block) weighs approximately 11 grams. When compared to the weight of an average chain saw (approximately 10 kg), 11 grams is negligible. This small mass will in no way preload the saw enough to alter the results. An accelerometer module was mounted on the top handle just to the right of where the hand clasps the handle, and on the rear handle just to the rear of where the hand clasps that handle. The accelerometers were located such that their principle axes corresponded roughly to the biodynamic coordinate system specified in the ISO Draft International Standard (3) (see Fig. 8). Figure 9 and Table 4 provide the exact position of the accelerometer blocks on the four saws tested.

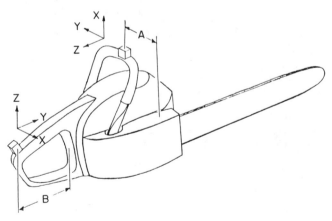

Fig. 9 Location of the accelerometer module on, and the vibration components for, each handle.

During testing, the signals from the Endevco accelerometers (type 2222B) were fed into charge amplifiers and then into a Hewlett-Packard (HP) four-channel FM tape recorder. The engine speed of the saw was monitored using a tachometer. The output of the tachometer was fed into Channel 4 of the tape recorder, and also into an HP

oscillograph, so that the engine speed of the saw could be continuously monitored during the tests. The recorded vibration signals were analysed by a General Radio 1921 1/3 octave-band real-time analyzer and an HP 9820A calculator via an HP A/D converter. The results were then plotted on an HP 9862A plotter.

During each chain saw vibration test, the signals from three accelerometers (one triaxial module) and the tachometer signal were recorded, first for the module on the top saw handle and then for the module on the rear handle. This procedure was continued until there were at least ten recordings for each handle, each of four seconds duration, during which the engine rpm remained within the desired speed range. It was usually necessary to run a minimum of five separate cutting tests for each handle to obtain these data records. Then ten samples of recorded data where the chain saw engine speed remained within the desired range were found for each of the three accelerometers on each handle, and analysed into 1/3 octave bands. After all samples had been stored in the HP 9820A, the average acceleration levels and 90% confidence bands at each centre frequency were calculated for the ten tests.

All vibration tests were conducted with the saws operating at full throttle. The wood was cut with the operator applying sufficient pressure to the saw to keep its engine speed as constant as possible. The desired engine speed for each saw was determined by instructing the operator to cut the log in what he judged to be an optimum manner. Several cuts were made in this manner to establish the engine speed for each saw (Table 3). The operator was

Table 3. Saw Engine Speeds When Cutting Wood (rpm)

Saw A:	7500	Saw C:	8000
Saw B:	7000	Saw D:	9000

also instructed to remember the "sensations" produced by each saw to assist in achieving the desired engine speed. During the chain saw vibration tests, the operator was not allowed to monitor the tachometer. He was instructed to operate each saw so as to produce the same "sensations" that were experienced during the experiment used to determine the engine operating speeds. An instrument technician monitored the tachometer during the cutting tests. He conveyed information to the saw operator by means of hand signals, instructing him to press harder to decrease the engine speed or to press lighter to allow the engine speed to increase. During each hand-held cutting test, efforts were made to maintain the engine speed to within ±400 rpm of the desired engine speed.

Reynolds et al.: Chain saw test stand

The wood used in all the tests was fresh-cut, unseasoned oak. A 30 cm × 30 cm square cross-section log was used for the larger saws. On the smaller saws, the guide bar was not long enough to extend through a 30 cm thick log and so a 30 cm × 20 cm rectangular cross-section was used.

2.2 Machine-Held Vibration Measurements

For the machine-held tests, the instruments were calibrated and operated in the same manner as for the hand-held tests. The accelerometers were attached to the chain saws in the same locations as were used in the hand-held tests.

Reasonable care was exercised when attaching the elastomers to the saw handles. First, a cleaning solvent was used to remove all dirt, oil, grease, etc. from the saw handles and the brass clamps. The rubber hand grips, commonly found on chain saw handles, were not removed. One inch wide 3-M masking tape was placed on the surfaces over which the elastomers were to be attached. The inside of the brass cylinders that were to be in contact with the elastomers were also covered with one inch wide 3-M masking tape. Care was taken to insure that a high quality masking tape with excellent adhesive qualities was used. Two one-inch sections of elastomer, placed approximately one inch apart, were required for each handle (see Figs. 6 and 7). A single slit was made along one side of each elastomer so that it could be wrapped around a handle. Goodyear Contact Cement was applied to the taped handle surfaces, to the inner surface of each elastomer which was to be in contact with a taped handle, and to the two surfaces formed by the slits in the elastomers. The cement was allowed to dry for five to ten minutes. The elastomers were then attached to the handles. Care was taken to ensure that the

elastomers were securely cemented to the complete circumference of each handle, and that the sides of the slits were securely cemented together. Goodyear Contact Cement was then applied to the outer surface of the elastomers and to the inside, tape-covered surfaces of the two brass cylinders. To facilitate assembly, the latter were cut in half lengthwise, along the axis of the cylinders. The cement was allowed to dry and the cylinder half-sections were placed around the top and rear handles (Fig. 10). The cylinder associated with each handle was finally placed in the circular clamp attached to the support structure of the test stand (see Fig. 3).

The test machine was next adjusted to accommodate the saw being tested. It was important to ensure that the clamps were aligned properly with the handles of the saw. The saw was visually aligned so that the wood carriage could be fed into the saw without the cutting chain coming into contact with any metal parts. This ensures that the saw properly cuts the wood. The saw was also aligned so that its static weight was evenly distributed between the elastomers of each handle. It was important that the clamps and elastomers not be twisted or skewed relative to the handles. This part of the saw alignment was also done visually. Finally, the limiting carriage height was adjusted to ensure a complete cut without the cutting chain coming into contact with the carriage base. Note that the saw was not placed in the test stand until after the instruments had been calibrated and the cutting tests were ready to begin, as allowing the saw to hang in the test stand for even up to an hour before the tests commenced could result in the elastomers experiencing a permanent deformation.

It was necessary to attach the nozzle of an air blower to the front of the test

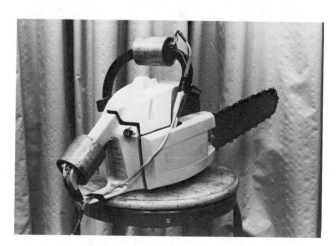

Fig. 10 Chain saw prepared for vibration testing in the CSMA test stand.

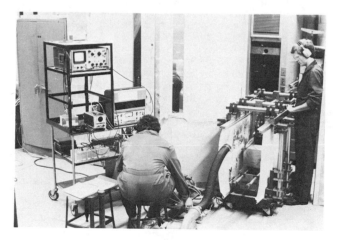

Fig. 11 Machine-held chain saw vibration test in progress.

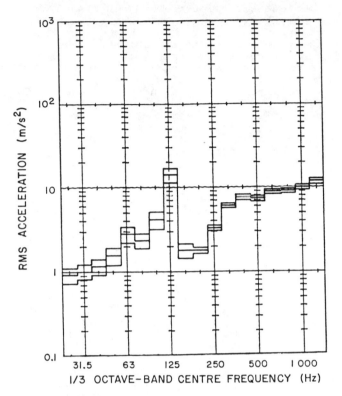

Fig. 12 Typical 1/3 octave-band accelerations for a hand-held saw: average
value and 90% confidence limits for the
X direction, top handle, of saw A.

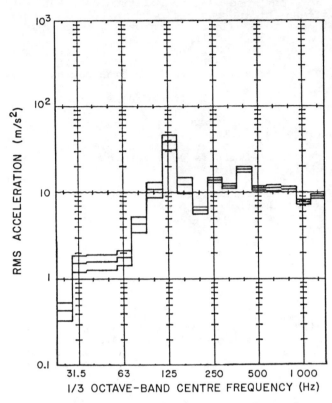

Fig. 13 Typical 1/3 octave-band accelerations for a machine-held saw: average
value and 90% confidence limits for the
X direction, rear handle, of saw C.

stand during cutting tests. The air was
directed such that it flowed over the part
of the saw containing the exposed engine
cooling fins. This prevented the saw from
overheating, as the saw did not receive
enough cool air owing to its confined location. The air flow also carried the
exhaust fumes into a small room, from
where they were removed by means of a fume
hood. The blower can be seen in use in
Fig. 11.

It was discovered when analyzing some
of the preliminary vibration data that
possible vibration resonances occurred on
some of the larger saws at frequencies corresponding to the engine speed and its
second harmonic. For this reason, controlled air dampers were attached to the
triaxial accelerometer blocks when machine
tests were conducted on the larger saws.
These were mounted in two directions on
both the top and back handle.

The tests were conducted with the saws
operating at full throttle. At the beginning of a cut, the wood was raised slowly,
allowing the saw to begin its cut without
binding. The feed rate of the wood was
then increased until the load on the saw
was sufficient to decrease the engine speed

to within the desired speed range, which
was usually within ±200 rpm of the values
shown in Table 3. The machine tests were
conducted exactly as were the hand-held
tests. Since the top handle elastomer sustained more damage, the top handles were
tested first to ensure optimum results.

The vibration measurements were analyzed in the same manner as the data from
the hand-held tests. Figure 11 shows a
machine-held chain saw test in progress.

III RESULTS

The precise location of the accelerometer modules on, and some specifications
of, the four chain saws used in this study
are given in Table 4. Each used an Oregon
Chipper chain to cut unseasoned oak.

Typical results from the hand-held
vibration measurements are given in Fig. 12,
and from the machine-held measurements in
Fig. 13. The data are shown as average 1/3
octave-band accelerations with their corresponding upper and lower 90% confidence
limits. Figures 14 to 19 give results from
both the hand-held and machine-held tests
on a medium sized saw for the six vibration

Reynolds et al.: Chain saw test stand

Table 4. Chain Saw Specifications and Accelerometer Locations (See Also Fig. 9).

Chain Saw	A	B	C	D
Weight (kg)	4.5	4.9	9.7	10
Engine Displacement (cc)	32	32	66	69
Chain Bar Length (cm)	40.6 (16 in)	40.6 (16 in)	48.3 (19 in)	48.3 (19 in)
Chain Pitch (cm)	0.6125 (1/4 in)	0.6125 (1/4 in)	0.9525 (3/8 in)	0.9525 (3/8 in)
Width of Cut (cm)	20 (8 in)	20 (8 in)	30.5 (12 in)	30.5 (12 in)
Dimension A (cm)	3.5	4	3	3
Dimension B (cm)	10	12.5	13	12

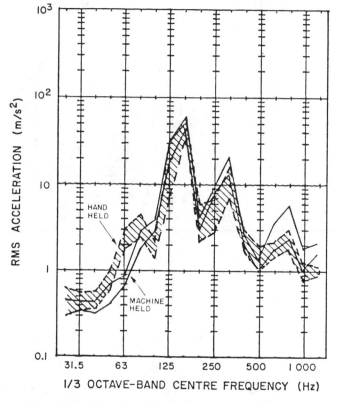

Fig. 14 90% confidence limits obtained from hand-held and machine-held tests: top handle, X direction, of saw D.

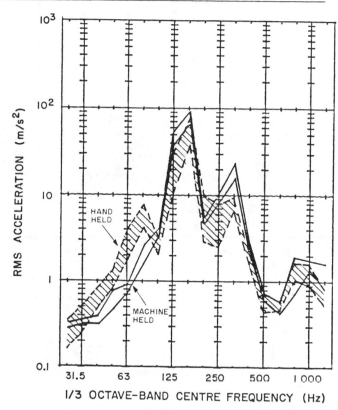

Fig. 15 90% confidence limits obtained from hand-held and machine-held tests: top handle, Y direction, of saw D.

components specified in Fig. 9.

3.1 Hand-Held Vibration Measurements

Two separate sets of hand-held tests were conducted by a single operator on chain saws A, B and C. Two separate sets of hand-held tests were conducted by each of three different operators on chain saw D. Of interest is the variation in the vibration level between different tests on each saw. Table 5 gives extreme values for the ratio of the maximum to the minimum accelerations in each 1/3 octave-band, for all four chain saws. The results for saws A, B and C indicate the typical difference

in vibration between two tests performed by the same operator. The difference in vibration between the two tests conducted by each operator on saw D was similar to that for saws A, B and C. However, as indicated by Table 5, the variation associated with all of the tests on saw D was larger than that for saws A, B and C. Figures 14 to 19 show the maximum and minimum accelerations found in all tests on saw D. Compared with the variation in vibration reported in other measurements on a single chain saw by different sawyers, the results of these hand-held tests are considered very consistent.

The 90% confidence limits shown in Fig. 12 are representative of those found

Reynolds et al.: Chain saw test stand

Table 5. Extreme Values for the Ratio of the Maximum to the Minimum Accelerations in 1/3 Octave-Bands Recorded During Hand-Held Tests.

| Chain Saw | Range of Maximum/Minimum 1/3 Octave-Band Accelerations | | |
	Frequency Bands below Engine Operating Speed	Frequency Band at Engine Operating Speed	Frequency Bands above Engine Operating Speed
A	1.4 - 1.6	1.2 - 1.8	1.2 - 1.5
B	1.7 - 2.5	1.3 - 1.7	1.2 - 1.5
C	1.2 - 2	1.2 - 1.8	1.1 - 1.3
D	1.6 - 3	1.4 - 3	1.4 - 2

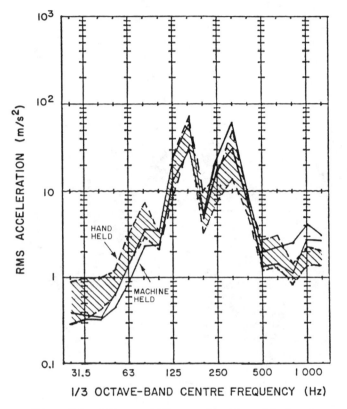

Fig. 16 90% confidence limits obtained from hand-held and machine-held tests: top handle, Z direction, of saw D.

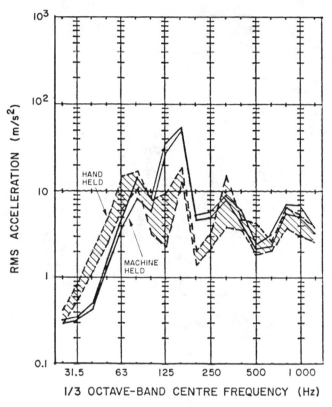

Fig. 17 90% confidence limits obtained from hand-held and machine-held tests: back handle, X direction, of saw D.

in hand-held tests. For each 1/3 octave-band containing frequencies less than the engine firing frequency, the 90% confidence interval was, on average, about 0.23 times the mean acceleration. For the band containing the engine firing frequency, the 90% confidence interval was, on average, about 0.21 times the mean acceleration; at higher frequencies, this ratio was, on average 0.06. Some vibration tests yielded 90% confidence intervals consistently greater than two to three times the above values. This was usually an indication that something was wrong; i.e. the cutting chain was not properly sharpened, the engine was not running efficiently, the section of the wood being cut contained

knots, etc. When this happened, the test results were discarded and the test repeated.

3.2 Machine-Held Vibration Measurements

Chain saws A, B and C were tested twice and saw D was tested four times. Table 6 gives extreme values for the ratio of the maximum to the minimum accelerations in each 1/3 octave band, for all four chain saws. With the exception of the results for saw B at frequencies below the engine firing frequency, the repeatability of all the tests was nearly the same. A comparison of the results in Table 6 with those of Table 5 indicates that the repeatability

Reynolds et al.: Chain saw test stand

Table 6. Extreme Values for the Ratio of the Maximum to the Minimum Accelerations in 1/3 Octave-Bands Recorded During Machine-Held Tests.

Chain Saw	Range of Maximum/Minimum 1/3 Octave-Band Accelerations		
	Frequency Bands below Engine Operating Speed	Frequency Band at Engine Operating Speed	Frequency Bands above Engine Operating Speed
A	1.2 - 1.4	1 - 1.2	1 - 1.3
B	1.2 - 3	1.1 - 1.7	1.1 - 1.3
C	1 - 1.8	1.2 - 2	1 - 1.5
D	1.1 - 1.7	1.2 - 2	1.3 - 1.6

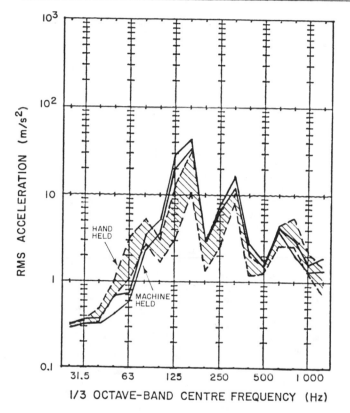

Fig. 18 90% confidence limits obtained from hand-held and machine-held tests: back handle, Y direction, of saw D.

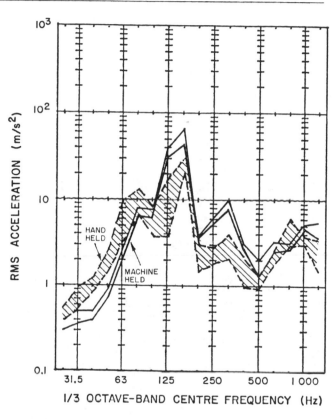

Fig. 19 90% confidence limits obtained from hand-held and machine-held tests: back handle, Z direction, of saw D.

of the machine-held tests on saws A, B and C did not differ much from that found in the hand-held tests on these saws, where only one operator was involved. However, the repeatability of the four machine-held tests on saw D was much better than that found in the six hand-held tests conducted by three different operators.

The confidence bands shown in Fig. 13 are typical of those obtained in all machine-held tests. The average values of the confidence intervals for the machine-held tests were nearly the same as those for the hand-held tests. As in the hand-held tests, excessively large confidence intervals were usually an indication that

the data were unacceptable due to some malfunction in the test procedure.

IV DISCUSSION

The test machine was designed to overcome the variability in vibration measurements associated with hand-held tests. An advantage of the machine is that the engine speed can be maintained more constant than in the hand-held method, thus providing the potential for more consistent results. Figure 20 contains typical records of the engine speed (from the oscillograph) during a machine-held and a hand-held test on the

Reynolds et al.: Chain saw test stand

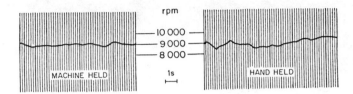

Fig. 20 Records of engine speed as a
function of time during cutting tests:
desired speed 9000 rpm.

same saw. It can be seen that the machine
controlled the engine speed to within ±200
rpm of the desired value. In contrast, it
was only possible to control the engine
speed to within ±400 to 500 rpm of the
desired value during the hand-held test.

One of the major design objectives at
the test machine is to obtain values of
handle vibration that are either the same
as, or well correlated with, the values observed in hand-held tests. In this project,
four saws were tested. Saw A was a small
hobby saw without vibration isolation. Saw
B was a small A/V hobby saw (with vibration-isolated handles), and saws C and D
were medium-weight, professional A/V saws.

For saw A, the machine-held test
results correlated well with the corresponding hand-held data. For the top
handle of saw A, the machine-held results
were consistently a factor of about two, or
more, greater than the hand-held results at
frequencies above 250 Hz. It is not uncommon for broad-band structural resonances
to occur in non-A/V saws at these frequencies. As will be discussed later, the
damping of the elastomers was less than was
needed. Increasing the damping associated
with the machine clamping mechanism can
reduce the differences between the machine-
and hand-held vibration test results for
small saws that are not vibration isolated.

For saw B, the machine- and hand-held
vibration test results usually agreed well
at frequencies above 125 Hz. For frequencies at or below 125 Hz, the machine-held
test results were always consistently less
than the corresponding hand-held results.
Figure 21 indicates the type of relation
that exists between machine- and hand-held
results for saw B. However, more saws of
this size and type need to be tested to
determine the exact form of the relation.

An understanding of the dynamic properties of the elastomer, compared to the
dynamic properties of the hand, is needed
to interpret the differences between the
machine- and hand-held test results on saw
B at low frequencies. The dynamic compliance of the elastomer is substantially
lower than that associated with the hand
at frequencies below 70 Hz. The overall
dynamic stiffness of the elastomer is

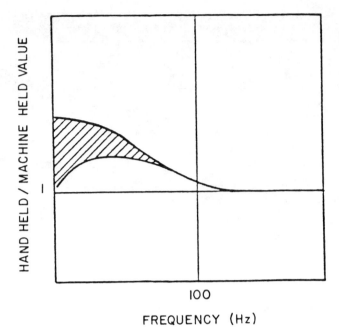

Fig. 21 Probable ratio of the handle
acceleration obtained from hand-held
and machine-held tests on small A/V
hobby saws (upper curve), and on medium
weight, A/V professional saws (lower
curve).

possibly a factor of ten, or more, greater
than that associated with the hand at these
frequencies. In addition, the vibration-
isolation system of saw B may have resonances in the frequency range from 25 Hz to
80 Hz. When this is the case, the vibration level observed will be very sensitive
to the manner in which the saw is clamped
in the machine or hand-held. Due to the
excess stiffness of the elastomer at low
frequencies, it is reasonable to expect
machine-held vibration levels to be less
than the corresponding hand-held results at
these frequencies.

In general, the machine-held test
results for saws C and D compare well with
the corresponding hand-held results. In
some cases, the machine-held test results
were greater than the corresponding hand-
held results at frequencies above 125 Hz,
and somewhat less at frequencies below
125 Hz. The explanations given for the
differences found with saws A and B may
account for these results. Figure 21
indicates the form of the relation between
the machine- and hand-held results at frequencies less than 125 Hz for saws C and D.
More tests involving similar saws are needed
to establish the exact form of this relation. It should be noted that adding more
damping to the clamping mechanism should
reduce the difference between the machine-
and hand-held test results at frequencies
above 125 Hz.

Reynolds et al.: Chain saw test stand

The damping of the elastomer was near the lower acceptable limit. It was initially anticipated that this damping would be sufficient. However, some machine-held test results indicated the presence of substantial saw handle resonances at frequencies above 100 Hz. Sufficient time was not available before completion of the project to investigate this problem fully. As a stop-gap measure, air dampers were purchased and added to the clamping mechanism, as shown in Fig. 3. Some improvement in performance was achieved, but more work is needed to determine the amount of damping required and the type of dampers that can be most effectively used.

During the machine-held tests, it was found that the elastomers must be bonded to both the chain saw handle and the clamp, because when the saw was loaded, unbonded elastomers tended to pull away from the handles. This not only altered the stiffness coefficient of the elastomer, but it also resulted in the saw being poorly constrained by, and aligned in, the test stand. If a saw was not firmly constrained by the test stand, it tended to cut irregularly. The elastomers could also only be used for one set of tests. The jerk when starting, the static forces applied to the elastomers during cutting and the weight of the saw caused the elastomer to deteriorate during the test. The top handle was tested first, as this elastomer always sustained the greater damage. It was also found that proper alignment of the test stand clamps with respect to the chain saw handles was critical. Clamps improperly oriented (i.e. twisted or skewed with respect to the handle) put a preload or prestress on the elastomer, thereby altering the results.

V CONCLUSIONS

5.1 The Elastomer

1. The elastomer configuration is simple and easy to construct, and the components are readily available.
2. The inner core shape of the elastomer must conform to the shape of the handle around which it is wrapped.
3. The variation in K and R obtained from elastomers with different sized and shaped cores did not noticeably affect the chain saw vibration test results. In general, the maximum variation in the natural frequencies so introduced was less than 15%.
4. The variation in K and R obtained by constructing identical elastomers on different days did not noticeably affect the chain saw vibration test results. In general, the maximum variation in the natural frequencies from this source was less than 10%.
5. It is necessary to allow the molded rubber to cure for a minimum of twenty-four

hours before it can be used for a machine-held vibration test.
6. It is necessary to bond the elastomer to both the chain saw handles and to the clamps.
7. The elastomers can only be used for one set of machine-held vibration tests; a new elastomer must be constructed for each series of tests.
8. Test should be done on the top handle first, as this elastomer tends to deteriorate more rapidly.

5.2 The Test Machine

1. The test machine does not introduce any preload on the saw other than that likely to be introduced by human hands and arms in normal use.
2. The test machine is sufficiently massive so that it does not develop any resonant interaction with the saw other than that likely to occur with human hands and arms.
3. The test stand is designed such that tests may be conducted whether or not the saw is cutting wood.
4. The test stand may be reproduced exactly using either off-the-shelf or easily manufactured components.
5. The test stand performs well and is reliable; no fracture or malfunction occurred during approximately one year of testing.

5.3 Comparison Between Hand-Held and Machine-Held Chain Saw Vibration Tests

1. The engine speed of the saw can be maintained within ±200 rpm during machine-held tests compared with ±400-500 rpm during hand-held tests.
2. The repeatability of the vibration measurements on saws A, B and C was approximately the same for both the hand-held and machine-held methods.
3. The variability of results from hand-held tests on saw D was, on average, about 1.5 times that from the corresponding machine-held tests.
4. The range of vibration levels in hand-held tests repeated by a single operator was approximately the same. The range of vibration levels for three sawyers (operating saw D) increased by a factor of, on average, about 1.6.
5. There was insufficient damping in the elastomer. Additional damping in the form of an air damper proved beneficial.
6. For the small saw with vibration-isolated handles, the vibration levels below 80 Hz measured on the test machine were consistently lower than those obtained by the hand-held method. Above 80 Hz, the machine-held test results correlated well with the hand-held results.
7. The small, non A/V chain saw produced vibration levels on the test machine that correlated reasonably well with hand-held

tests throughout the entire frequency range of interest.

8. Generally, the vibration levels measured in hand-held and machine-held tests correlated well for medium-size professional saws with vibration-isolated handles.

9. When machine-held test results differed from hand-held results at frequencies below 125 Hz, the machine-held results were consistently less than the hand-held results. This was due to the fact that the dynamic stiffness of the elastomers is more than the dynamic stiffness of the hands at these frequencies. When these differences occur, correction factors similar to those indicated in Fig. 21 must be used to transform machine-held test results to correspond to hand-held test results.

10. When machine-held test results differed from hand-held results at frequencies above 125 Hz, the machine-held results were consistently greater than the hand-held results. This was possibly caused by the damping in the saw clamping mechanisms being less than necessary, as the discrepancy can be reduced by increasing the damping.

11. In both hand- and machine-held vibration tests, the 90% confidence intervals were, on average, about 0.23 times the mean acceleration at frequencies less than the engine firing frequency; about 0.21 times the mean acceleration in the band containing the firing frequency; and about 0.06 times the mean accelerations at higher frequencies.

12. To optimize the repeatability and reliability of the test procedure, the saw must always be in the best operational condition. This includes proper carburettor tuning, a clean spark plug, and a sharp chain.

ACKNOWLEDGEMENTS

The research reported in this paper was carried out under a contract funded by the Chain Saw Manufacturers Association of the United States while D.D. Reynolds was an Associate Professor in the Dept. of Mechanical Engineering at the Univ. of Pittsburgh.

REFERENCES

1. Reynolds DD, Soedel W. Dynamic response of the hand-arm system to a sinusoidal input. J Sound Vib 1972; 21: 339-353.
2. Reynolds DD, Keith RH. Hand-arm vibration part I: analytical model of the vibration response characteristics of the hand. J Sound Vib 1977; 51: 237-253.
3. International Organization for Standardization. Principles for the Measurment and the Evaluation of Human Exposure to Vibration Transmitted to the Hand. Draft International Standard ISO/DIS 5349, 1979.

DISCUSSION

M.R. Noble: Do you consider the test stand to be fully developed for measuring chain saw vibration?

Authors' Response: We consider the test stand to be 90% developed. Its completion has been shelved because of more pressing problems in the industry (e.g. kickback).

Has the test stand been adopted as the preferred method for vibration measurement by the CSMA or an organization concerned with standardization? If it has not yet been adopted, is it likely to be adopted for the purposes of standardization in the future?

Authors' Response: The test stand has not yet been adopted for the measurement of chain saw vibration, though it may be in the future.

Vibration Acceleration Measured on Pneumatic Tools Used in Chipping and Grinding Operations

D. D. Reynolds, D. E. Wasserman, R. Basel,
W. Taylor, T. E. Doyle and W. Asburry

ABSTRACT: This paper presents the acceleration measurements and data analysis aspects of a comprehensive multidisciplined field study of several hundred chipper and grinder workers using pneumatic hand-held tools. Measurements indicate that acceleration levels are approximately 2400 G(rms) on the chisel and 30 G(rms) on the handles of impact chipping hammers in the frequency range from 6.3 to 1000 Hz. Grinder acceleration levels are approximately 0.5 to 2 G(rms) over the same frequency range. The results are compared with guidelines for vibration exposure proposed by the ISO/DIS 5349. It is found that chipping hammers generally possess acceleration levels in excess of the guidelines, and grinders possess levels that fall between the guidelines for thirty minutes' and eight hours' exposure.

RESUME: La présente communication contient les mesures d'accélération et les résultats de l'analyse des données fournies par une étude multidisciplinaire approfondie effectuée in situ, portant sur plusieurs centaines d'opérateurs de marteaux-piqueurs et de broyeurs utilisant des outils manuels pneumatiques. D'après les mesures, les niveaux d'accélération dans la gamme de fréquences de 6,3 à 1000 Hz sont de 2400 G environ (valeur efficace) sur les poignées du marteau-piqueur. Dans le cas du broyeur, les niveaux d'accélération s'élèvent de 0,5 à 2 G (valeur efficace) pour la même gamme de fréquences. On compare les résultats aux limites proposées par l'ISO/DIS 5349 pour une exposition à des vibrations. On a trouvé que les marteaux-piqueurs présentent généralement des niveaux d'accélération supérieurs aux limites proposées, et que dans le cas des broyeurs ces niveaux sont compris entre les limites correspondant à une exposition d'une durée de trente minutes et de huit heures.

INTRODUCTION

In October 1975, the National Institute for Occupational Safety and Health (NIOSH) organized a one week international conference where the epidemiological, medical, clinical, physiological, and engineering aspects of VWF and vibration measurements were discussed in detail. The conference summary and recommendations comprised ten points, two of which applied to the engineering aspects of the problem:
a)   there were extreme difficulties in performing vibration measurements on percussive pneumatic tools (because the attendant acceleration levels were very high and resulted in destruction of the transducers); and
b)   there was a need to validate an engineering model (i.e. simulation of the hand and arm) to assist the designer in producing a vibration-free tool.

The 1975 conference became the catalyst for a multidisciplinary field study of pneumatic tool chipper and grinder workers. This paper will address the vibration measurements of the chipper and grinder study. Other aspects of this study are reported elsewhere in this volume (2-4). Complete details of the engineering study are given in Ref. 5.

I   WORK SITES, WORK PRACTICES, AND TOOLS

A total of 415 males from four work sites were medically investigated in the chipper and grinder study, including workers from two grey-iron foundries, a shipyard, and the stone-workers of Bedford,

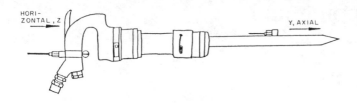

Fig. 1 Pneumatic chipping hammer showing location of transducers and coordinate system.

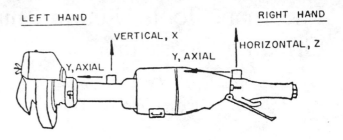

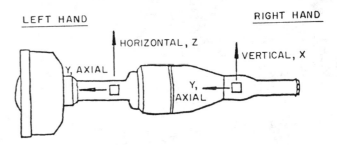

Fig. 2 Horizontal grinder showing location of transducers and coordinate system.

Indiana. The pneumatic tools used by foundry and shipyard workers in this study were: Type 2 chipping hammers or impact hammers (Fig. 1); vertical grinders (Fig. 2); and horizontal grinders (Fig. 3). These same tool types are made by various manufacturers. The limestone workers used a smaller, lightweight chipping hammer similar to the Type 2, except the unit is purely barrel-shaped and without a handle.

The Type 2 chipping tool generally produces 2100 blows/minute (corresponding to a 35 Hz repetition rate). It weighs about 12 pounds and its length can vary from 12 to 15 inches (depending on the manufacturer). The diameter of the rear handle is approximately 1.5 inches. The diameter of the chisels used with these hammers is approximately 0.75 inches, and the length can vary from a few inches to two feet. Characteristics of the working end of the chisels differ somewhat depending on the chisel application. Most important, the chisel is inserted freely into the bore of the chipping hammer, so that the worker can change chisels quickly. It is not usually restrained while in use (i.e., the chisel, if not guided by the operator's hand and not working against resistance, is free to shoot out of the chipping tool). This is why the operator must place one hand around the chisel.

The foundries studied used pneumatic horizontal grinders accommodating six or eight inch diameter grinding wheels. These units rotate from 4500 to 6000 rpm (corresponding to 75 to 100 Hz). They weigh about 14 pounds and their length is from 20 to 25

inches. The vertical grinders used in the shipyard accommodated similar grinding wheels, ran at about the same speed as the horizontal grinders, and weighed about eight pounds.

For all these pneumatic tools, the usable air pressure was in the range of 90 to 110 psi. Each of the three work sites studied had a central tool crib and repair/maintenance station for the tools. A detailed description of the work practices at each of the foundries and the shipyard is given in the Appendix. Table 1 summarizes estimates of the time spent chipping, grinding and in non-vibratory activity, for each of these work sites. The estimates are given both for an eight hour workday, and for a year's exposure, assuming no overtime and a two-week vacation period.

There are two types of limestone workers who use pneumatic tools: a) cutters and carvers; and b) drillers. Cutters and carvers are true artisans, who use a

Table 1. Duration of Vibration Exposure for Foundry Workers

Activity	Foundry #1 hours/day	Foundry #1 hours/year	Foundry #2 hours/day	Foundry #2 hours/year	Shipyard hours/day	Shipyard hours/year
Chipping	3.5	840	3	720	3	720
Grinding	2.5	600	4	960	3	720
No vibration	2	480	1	240	2	480

*Assuming an 8 hour day (40 hours/week) and a yearly work schedule of 50 weeks/year (2 week vacation period).

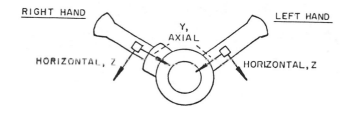

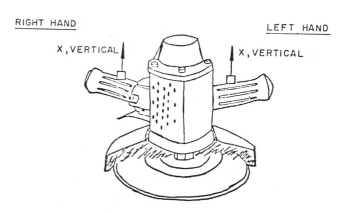

Fig. 3 Vertical grinder showing location of transducers and coordinate system.

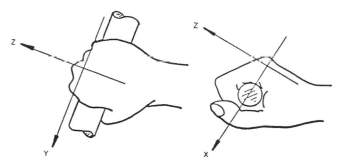

Fig. 4 Coordinate system for the hand-arm system.

myriad of chipping chisels, most not longer than six inches, with the smaller impact hammer. These workers frequently change chisels, and grip the chisel and barrel of the chipping tool very tightly. The tool is usually operated at full throttle without the benefit of a trigger-grip throttle control. The thumb of the dominant hand (barrel hand) controls the tool throttle by pressing on a small exhaust hole. An operator uses the tool for 5 to 6 hours/day, or a total of 1500 hours/year vibration exposure.

Unlike carvers and cutters who perform the finishing operations, drillers work in the quarry. They use an impact hammer type of tool with a pointed chisel from 2 to 3 feet long. After the face of the lime-stone block to be quarried is exposed, the drillers then drill a line of holes (spaced a few feet apart) across and down the sides of this face. They use the tool from 2 to 2.5 hours/day or 600 hours/year.

II MEASUREMENT METHODS

2.1 Accelerometers

Acceleration was used as the primary measure in this study because of: a) the ability to obtain three parameters (acceleration, velocity, and displacement) from one measurement (by electronic integration of the signal observed); and b) the large variety of accelerometers available.

Because of the large acceleration levels expected from pneumatic tools, as well as the frequency range anticipated (approximately 6 Hz to 2 kHz), piezoelectric accelerometers were used exclusively in this study.

Many investigators have attempted to measure the vibration from percussive pneumatic tools and have experienced numerous problems (6-9). These stem from the very high impulse vibration levels that may destroy the accelerometers, as well as problems of spectrum accuracy at low frequencies (referred to as "DC shift"). The methods of tackling these measurement problems have been two-fold: a) using a mechanical low-pass filter between the tool and accelerometer; and/or b) modifying the design of the accelerometer itself.

Using a mechanical filter prevents destruction of the accelerometer, but the acceleration recorded by an accelerometer in series with a mechanical filter is modified by the characteristics of the filter. Thus, the combination may not provide a true measure of the source's vibration. It seemed therefore that modifications should be made to the accelerometers, so as to eliminate the need for mechanical filters. A Bruel and Kjaer (B&K) compression-type piezoelectric accelerometer model 8309 was chosen as the best device for this application (1 Hz to 60 kHz range, sensitivity 0.3 mv/G or 0.04 pC/G, weight 3 grams), knowing, in advance, that it might require factory modification.

2.2 Chipping Hammer Mount

Acceleration levels were obtained from four (Type 2) pneumatic chipping hammers (from various manufacturers), and two different pneumatic grinders. The Type 2 chipping hammers are shown in Fig. 1. (The grinders used are shown in Figs. 2 and 3.) The measurement coordinate system is shown in these diagrams and is consistent with that proposed in the Draft International Standard ISO/DIS 5349, as can be seen from

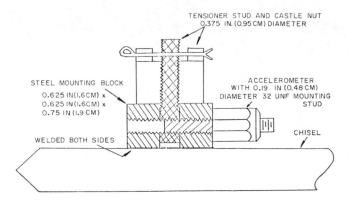

Fig. 5 Accelerometer mounting block for chipping hammer chisels.

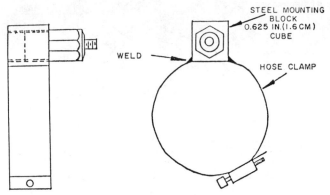

Fig. 6 Accelerometer mounting for chipping hammer handles.

Fig. 4 (10). Chipping hammers A, B, and C and the horizontal grinder are used in the engine foundry. Chipping hammer D and the vertical grinder are used by the shipyard workers. The small limestone chipping hammer (not shown) is used for decorative carving and finishing limestone blocks and monuments.

One of the operations performed in the foundry is the chipping and grinding of flash from slots in the cast iron castings. The chipping hammer is operated at full throttle, with the chisel directed into a corner of the casting. Slot chipping data were taken for chipping hammers A, B, C, and D, so that a comparison could be made between the various types of chipping hammers. To indicate the influence of work material on the acceleration levels produced by the tool, data were also taken for hammer D chipping nickel-aluminum bronze (Ni-Al bronze) and mild steel. For these tests, chipping hammer D was operated at 1/2 to 3/4 throttle, to cut a groove in the material 0.76 inch wide and 0.1 inch deep. Acceleration levels were also measured for the small limestone chipping hammer chipping on limestone at full throttle.

Chipping hammers B, C, and D were all of roughly the same size and weight. Chipping hammer A was somewhat larger and heavier, whereas the limestone chipping hammer was much smaller and lighter than any of the chippers. The chisels used with chipping hammers A, B, and C were 10 to 12 inches long. The chisels used with the limestone chipping hammer and chipping hammer D were three to five inches long.

For the chipping hammer measurements, two Bruel and Kjaer type 8309 accelerometers were used, one at the chisel end of the tool, the other at the rear handle of the tool. At the chisel end, a steel block was welded directly to the chisel and positioned where the worker would normally

hold his chisel. The mounting block (Fig. 5) had a tapped hole with the accelerometer screwed into it and held by a tension stud and castle nut. The accelerometer sensed vibration in the axial direction parallel to the axis of the chisel. It was recognized that vibration might appear in other directions (especially transverse), but because of the extreme difficulty in making these measurements and the high cost of damaging accelerometers, measurements were made only in the axial direction. Welding the block to the chisel was necessary due to the extremely high acceleration levels generated on the chisel end of the chipping hammer. A steel mounting block welded to a stainless steel hose clamp (jubilee clip) as shown in Fig. 6 was found to be effective on the handle. The accelerometer was equipped with a mounting stud for attachment to the mounting block. The hose clamp was securely tightened around the handle of the chipping hammer, as close as possible to the hand. In the case of the small limestone chipper, the accelerometer was mounted on the barrel of the tool.

Initially, hose clamps were attached to the chisel. However, they broke or slipped while on the chisel. As a solution, the steel mounting blocks were then welded directly to the various chisels. Several accelerometer failures also occurred. These were believed to be caused by fatigue, resulting in the shearing of studs or stripping of threads, and the loosening of welds of the "top hat" structure that protects the crystal element. The actual crystal element did not fail. Damaged accelerometers were sent back to the manufacturer who in turn supplied modified model 8309 accelerometers, which eventually worked reasonably well for up to 30 minutes continuous chipping.

It is important to note that the accelerometers must be screwed tightly into

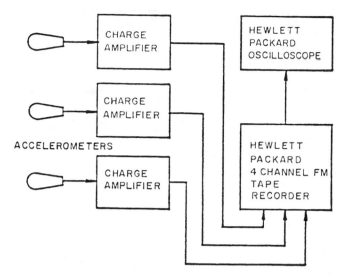

Fig. 7 Block diagram of measurement system.

CHARGE AMPLIFIER

CHARGE AMPLIFIER

ACCELEROMETERS

CHARGE AMPLIFIER

HEWLETT PACKARD OSCILLOSCOPE

HEWLETT PACKARD 4 CHANNEL FM TAPE RECORDER

the mounting holes, in order to avoid spurious signals in the measurement system and to reduce accelerometer fatigue. Tension in the mounting stud, however, should not be excessive. The mounting arrangement shown in Fig. 5 was found to be effective and was used to obtain acceleration data on the chisel. A hole was drilled into the mounting block at right angles to the accelerometer mounting hole. A stud loading pin was inserted into the hole, then drilled and tapped to accept the accelerometer mounting stud. The pin was threaded at its outer end to accept a castle nut. After the accelerometer was screwed with moderate tightness into the mounting block, the tensioning pin was pulled tightly against the accelerometer mounting stud. The resulting shear load on the mounting stud proved more effective in reducing fatigue failure than did increasing the stud tension.

Failures also occurred in the electrical connectors, both in the attachment threads and by shearing of the centre contact pins, after several minutes of testing. The lifetimes of the electrical connectors were finally extended by changing cable manufacturers (to Endevco), and by carefully strain relieving and taping the leads to the chisel.

Professional chipper, grinder, and stonecutter workers operated the tools during the tests and were asked to work normally. Most chipping tools were operated at full throttle (with 100 psi supply air pressure); a few were tested at 1/2 to 3/4 throttle. Data were obtained for three operators in the field.

2.3 Grinding Tool Mount

Grinder acceleration levels were measured while grinding cast grey-iron. The vertical grinder was operated with a sanding pad and medium grit paper. Data were obtained for the horizontal grinder with three grinding wheels: a coarse radial wheel, a fine radial wheel and a coarse flared cup wheel.

A triaxial accelerometer block was mounted on each grinder handle as shown in Figs. 2 and 3. Each block consisted of three Columbia Research model 6063 crystal accelerometers mounted on three perpendicular faces of the steel cube. These steel cubes were glued to the grinders using epoxy cement. The accelerometer leads were strain relieved, bundled, and taped to the handles, to avoid electrical noise from vibration of the leads.

The grinders were operated at full throttle (with 100 psi supply air pressure). Data were obtained for two operators.

2.4 Data Acquisition System, Calibration Procedure and Data Analysis

A block diagram of the instrumentation used to obtain and record acceleration levels of both the pneumatic chipping hammers and the grinders is shown in Fig. 7. The charge output from the accelerometers is converted to voltage signals by charge amplifiers and recorded on a multichannel FM tape recorder. In order to avoid overloading the electronic circuits, the charge amplifier signals and tape recorder outputs were observed on an oscilloscope. A Fourier spectrum analyzer was also used to observe spectra as the measurements were taken.

All crystal accelerometers were calibrated before use in a field mobile unit (11), by means of a minishaker (B&K model 4809) driven by an amplifier (B&K model 2706) from an oscillator Spectral Dynamics model SD104. These crystal accelerometers were calibrated against a known piezoresistive accelerometer (Entran, EGAL 125).

Before data were recorded, trial data were played through the tape recorder to establish the maximum signal levels. No DC shift was observed from the accelerometers. The tape recorder input gain was adjusted to give recorded levels large enough to be easily read, but small enough to avoid overloading the tape-recorder input amplifiers. During testing, charge amplifiers and the tape recorder were constantly monitored for possible overloading. Static and dynamic calibration signals were later used to scale the data during digitization.

Most measurements were made while professional and experienced chippers and grinders worked under normal working conditions, using metal castings taken directly from the given work place. Tool operators

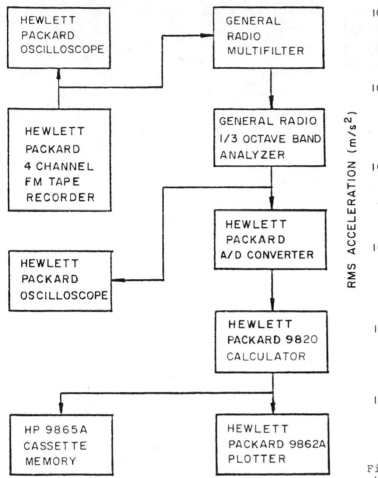

Fig. 8 Block diagram of the spectrum analysis and digitization system.

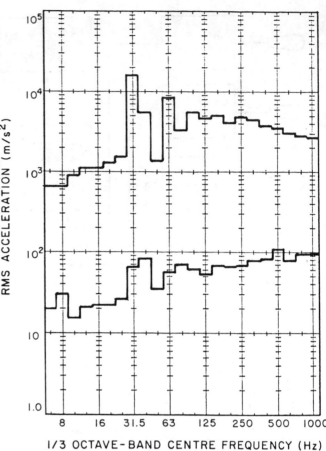

Fig. 9 RMS acceleration levels for chipping hammer A cleaning castings at full throttle: slot chipping on nodular cast iron - chisel, top; handle, bottom.

were instructed to begin chipping or grinding before the tape recorder was started. Approximately one minute runs of data were then recorded. Handle and chisel data were taken simultaneously during chipping hammer tests. As vibration measurements were taken, the subjects' hand motions were simultaneously video-taped for later observation.

Data analyses were performed in the laboratory. Third-octave band acceleration levels for the grinder and chipping hammer data were obtained using the system shown in Fig. 8. The FM tape recording of the analogue acceleration data for the various tools was played into a General Radio model 1921 1/3 octave-band real-time analyzer. The 1/3-octave-band frequency spectrum output from the frequency analyzer was digitized using the Hewlett-Packard analogue/digital converter and the model 9820A calculator. The digital data was stored on cassette tapes.

In those few instances where insufficient and/or inadequate acceleration data

were obtained in the field, supplemental data were obtained in the laboratory using the same pneumatic tool types and similar conditions as that found in the field.

III RESULTS

3.1 Chipping Hammer Acceleration

The chipping hammer is an impact type tool. Third octave-band acceleration spectrum plots for typical Type 2 pneumatic chipping hammers are given in Figs. 9 and 10; spectra for the smaller limestone chipping hammer are given in Fig. 11. Both chisel and rear handle acceleration levels are given in the diagrams. A summary of the overall acceleration levels from 6.3 to 1000 Hz for all of the chipping hammers investigated is given in Table 2.

The spectra for the Type 2 chipping hammers have peaks at 31.5 and 63 Hz; those for the small limestone chipper have peaks at 80 and 160 Hz. The first peaks, at 31.5

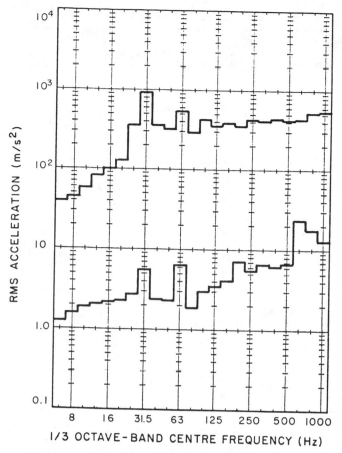

Fig. 10 RMS acceleration levels for chipping hammer D when shaping propeller blades at 1/2 to 3/4 throttle: chipping on Ni-Al bronze - chisel, top; handle, bottom.

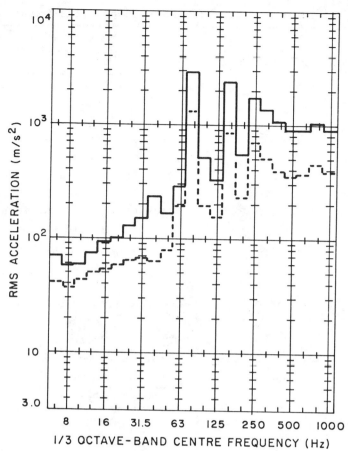

Fig. 11 RMS acceleration levels of small chipping hammer when carving limestone at full throttle - chisel, top; barrel, bottom.

and 80 Hz, are the fundamental excitation frequency for each tool.

Of the Type 2 chipping hammers, hammer A exhibits the highest chisel acceleration levels. The chisel acceleration levels for chipping hammer D and the small limestone chipper are comparable to each other, and considerably less than chipping hammer A. Data were taken for hammer D during slot chipping on cast iron and chipping on mild B steel and Ni-Al bronze, to assess the influence of material and operating conditions on acceleration levels. The levels for mild B steel and Ni-Al bronze are generally the same. The levels for slot chipping are approximately ten times higher than those for other chipping operations. This is generally a more severe operation, since the chisel is operated at full throttle. Shipyard workers operated the chipping hammers at 1/2 to 3/4 throttle on Ni-Al bronze or mild steel.

The acceleration levels for the chipper handles are considerably lower than those for the chisels. The attenuation

of the vibration transmitted from the chisel to the handle depends on the chipper. Chipping hammer A shows an attenuation of 1/150 for the peaks and 1/65 for the general acceleration level. Chipping hammer D shows an attenuation of 1/150 for the peaks and 1/60 for the general level. The small limestone chipper, which is the smallest of the five chipping hammers, shows the least attenuation of all: 1/3 for the peaks and 1/2 for the general level.

It is interesting to note the attenuation from chisel to handle of the small limestone chipper. The chisel acceleration levels for the small limestone chipping hammer are the smallest measured, comparable to those for hammer D and much less than for hammer A; the handle accelerations are the largest, approximately four times the levels for the hand of hammer A. This situation is probably associated with the relative magnitude of the masses of the handles and the chisels. The larger hammers have more mass in their handles than the limestone chipper. The larger the mass of the chipping hammer handle, the less the acceleration

Reynolds et al.: Vibration levels

Table 2. Overall RMS Accelerations for Chipping Hammers (6.3 to 1000 Hz).

Chipping Tool	Operation and Transducer Location Type 2	Direction	Throttle	Overall Acceleration m/s^2	G*
Hammer A	Slot Chipping (cast iron)				
	Handle	Z	Full	2.99×10^2	30.5
	Chisel	Y	Full	2.34×10^4	2390
Hammer B	Slot Chipping (cast iron)				
	Handle	Z	Full	3.52×10^2	35.8
Hammer C	Slot Chipping (cast iron)				
	Handle	Z	Full	1.20×10^2	12.3
Hammer D	Slot Chipping (cast iron)				
	Handle	Z	Full	6.47×10^2	66
Hammer D	Chipping (Ni-Al bronze)				
	Handle	Z	1/2-3/4	3.71×10^1	3.78
	Chisel	Y	1/2-3/4	1.91×10^3	194
Hammer D	Chipping (Mild B Steel)				
	Handle	Z	1/2-3/4	3.97×10^1	4.05
	Chisel	Y	1/2-3/4	1.99×10^3	203
Small (Limestone) Hammer	Slot Chipping				
	Handle	Y	Full	2.01×10^3	205
	Chisel	Y	Full	4.85×10^3	494

*1 G = 9.81 m/s^2

of the handle required to absorb the force transmitted from the chisel. It appears that it is not necessarily true that smaller chipping hammers, by virtue of delivering lighter chisel blows, expose both the operator's hands to lower acceleration levels.

It is possible that the handle acceleration levels are far more significant to the operator than are the chisel levels. Perhaps only a small part of the chisel acceleration is transmitted to the hand, since the chisel is usually guided by resting it on the open palm, or by cradling it between the thumb and index finger. The handle, on the other hand, must be grasped firmly, which results in good mechanical coupling and good energy transfer from the handle to the hand-arm system.

3.2 Grinder Acceleration

The pneumatic grinder is not an impact tool. Its rotary action results in continuous vibration. Typical grinder acceleration levels are shown in Figs. 12 to 15. The grinder acceleration levels are very much less than those measured on the chipping hammer chisels and on most of the handles. The grinder acceleration levels

vary between 0.03 m/s^2 and 10 m/s^2 (approximately 0.003 to 1 G, respectively). Chipping hammer handle accelerations generally range between 10 m/s^2 and 100 m/s^2 (approximately 1 to 10 G). A summary of the overall grinder acceleration levels from 6.3 to 1000 Hz are given in Table 3.

Peaks occur in many of the horizontal grinder spectra at 63, 250 and 1000 Hz. These may be the operating frequencies of mechanical parts within the tools. Peaks occur frequently at 40, 80, and 250 Hz in the vertical grinder spectra, but these are difficult to characterize.

It is interesting to note that the accelerations during some of the coarse radial wheel and flared cup measurements are comparable to the handle acceleration of hammer D chipping on mild B steel and Ni-Al bronze. Between 63 and 250 Hz, the left handle of the horizontal grinder with the coarse flared cup wheel attached has acceleration levels which are lower, but close to, those for the handle of hammer D chipping on Ni-Al bronze. In fact, for discrete frequency ranges, workers using chipping hammer D and the horizontal grinder with the coarse wheels experience similar acceleration levels.

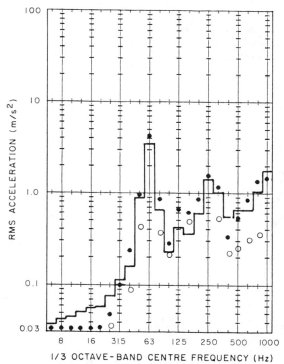

Fig. 12 RMS acceleration levels for horizontal grinder with coarse radial wheel: right hand - X direction, continuous line; Y direction, open circles; Z direction, closed circles.

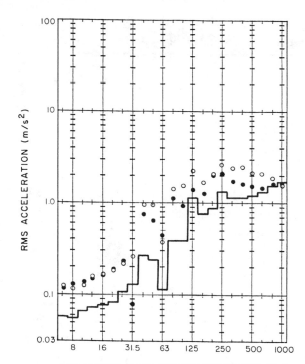

Fig. 14 RMS acceleration levels for vertical grinder with sanding pad, medium paper: right hand - X direction, continuous line; Y direction, open circles; Z direction, closed circles.

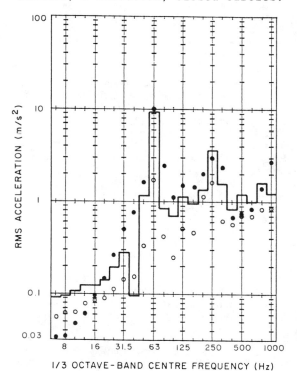

Fig. 13 RMS acceleration levels for horizontal grinder with coarse radial wheel: left hand - X direction, continuous line; Y direction, open circles; Z direction, closed circles.

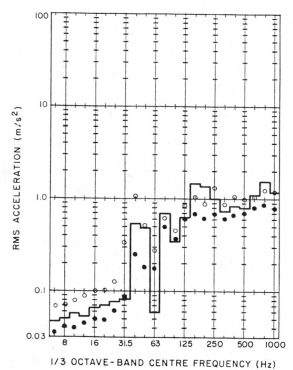

Fig. 15 RMS acceleration levels for vertical grinder with sanding pad, medium paper: left hand - X direction, continuous line; Y direction, open circles; Z direction, closed circles.

Reynolds et al.: Vibration levels

Table 3. Overall RMS Accelerations for Grinders (6.3 to 1000 Hz).

Tool	Handle	Direction	Component Acceleration (m/s^2)	Total Acceleration, A_T* m/s^2	G
Horizontal Grinder with Coarse Radial Wheel	Right	X	4.54	7.3	0.74
		Y	2.49		
		Z	5.2		
	Left	X	10.5	15.8	1.61
		Y	3.17		
		Z	11.4		
Horizontal Grinder with Fine Radial Wheel	Right	X	4.21	6.36	0.64
		Y	2.46		
		Z	4.08		
	Left	X	3.73	7.75	0.79
		Y	2.3		
		Z	6.4		
Horizontal Grinder with Flared Cup Wheel	Right	X	6.7	16.7	1.71
		Y	7.77		
		Z	13.2		
	Left	X	9.29	20.5	2.09
		Y	8.54		
		Z	16.2		
Vertical Grinder with Sanding Pad	Right	X	3.81	9.56	0.97
		Y	6.96		
		Z	5.34		
	Left	X	3.51	5.51	0.56
		Y	3.58		
		Z	2.29		

Note: *1 G = 9.81 m/s^2 and $A_T = (A_x^2 + A_y^2 + A_z^2)^{\frac{1}{2}}$

IV COMPARISON OF TOOL ACCELERATIONS WITH GUIDELINES PROPOSED BY THE ISO

Some years ago, an ISO subcommittee on human vibration was formed to determine tolerable levels for persons exposed to vibration. The data used to generate the proposed hand-arm vibration standard (ISO/DIS 5349) were based, for the most part, on subjective studies and some chain saw data, and not on medical data (12). The standard has yet to be universally adopted. However, since it represents the only international attempt to develop a standard in this area, it is useful to compare the acceleration levels obtained in this study with the ISO guidelines (10).

4.1 Chipping Hammer Acceleration

The data indicate that all chipping hammer chisel accelerations measured are in excess of the ISO levels for thirty minutes exposure. In fact, one peak at 31.5 Hz for the chisel of chipping hammer A is 1500 times the exposure limit. None of the chisel acceleration levels fall below the thirty minute exposure limit within the 6.3 to 1000 Hz frequency range.

Since accelerometers were not placed on the subject's hands or arms, it is difficult to determine how much vibration is transmitted from the chisel to the open palm of an operator, but the levels can be estimated. The chisel acceleration levels transmitted to the hand from chipping hammer D and the small limestone chipper may be reduced by a factor of 50 or 100, depending on the worker/tool hand grip force and the work practices employed. However, it is unreasonable to expect a reduction of 1500 for chipping hammer A. Even so, reductions of 50 or 100 for chipping hammer D and the small limestone chipper would almost reduce the levels to the ISO guideline for thirty minutes exposure.

For handle acceleration levels, chipping hammers A, B and C substantially exceed the thirty minute guideline in the low and middle frequency ranges. For hammer A, Fig. 9 shows that acceleration levels for all frequencies below 300 Hz are in excess of the thirty minute guideline. For hammers B and C, the minimum frequency with vibration less than the thirty minute exposure guideline occurs at 80 Hz. It should be noted that for hammer B, the acceleration levels for 80, 125 and 160 Hz are all near the thirty minute exposure guideline.

235

According to the ISO guidelines, the worst chipping hammer for handle vibration is the small limestone chipper, which exceeds the proposed thirty minute exposure over the entire 6.3 to 1000 Hz frequency range. The acceleration levels are 1.5 times to 65 times the guideline with most of the range being more than ten times the level proposed.

On the other hand, the handle acceleration levels for hammer D chipping on Ni-Al bronze at 1/2 to 3/4 full throttle (shown in Fig. 10) lie entirely within the suggested ISO exposure for thirty minutes. According to the ISO proposal, the acceleration level at 31.5 Hz would restrict continuous exposure to approximately 1.5 hours per day. For hammer D chipping on mild B steel, only the peak at 31.5 Hz exceeds the thirty minute exposure guideline. For slot chipping on cast iron at full throttle, all acceleration levels below 1000 Hz are in excess of the thirty minute guideline. This demonstrates the severity of the slot chipping operation, together with the work practice of operating the tool at full throttle in order to get the work completed in a reasonable time.

4.2 Grinder Acceleration

The grinder acceleration levels are all below the thirty minute exposure guideline. The horizontal grinder with the fine radial wheel has acceleration levels on both handles, in all directions and at all frequencies, that are lower than the levels proposed for eight hour exposures. The horizontal grinder with the coarse radial wheel is limited by the left hand X and Z directions: these acceleration levels fall approximately at the two hour exposure guideline. The right X and Z directions also exceed the eight hour guideline, but are within the four hour guideline. The ISO proposal would restrict operation of the horizontal grinder with the coarse flared cup wheel to four hours exposure per day (by the left hand Y direction). The left hand Z direction and the right hand Y direction barely exceed the eight hour exposure guideline. These data appear to agree with grinder studies performed by other investigators (13,14).

V CONCLUSIONS

Vibration acceleration measurements were obtained on four large Type 2 chipping hammers and a small stone chipper during actual work conditions. The results indicate that when these Type 2 hammers are operated at full throttle chipping grey-iron, Ni-Al bronze or mild steel castings, acceleration levels on the chisel were approximately 2400 G(rms) and 30 G(rms) on the rear handle, at points where workers grip these tools. In the case of one chipping hammer (A), the ratio of chisel to rear handle acceleration was approximately 78/1. When the throttle was reduced from full to 1/2 or 3/4, the chisel acceleration levels were reduced by a factor of approximately 12 (2400 to 200 G rms). Correspondingly, rear handle accelerations decreased from 30 G(rms) to approximately 4 G(rms). The ratio of chisel to rear handle acceleration at 1/2 to 3/4 throttle was reduced to 50/1, as compared to 78/1 at full throttle.

The levels measured on the small stone chippers were approximately 500 G(rms) on the chisel and 200 G(rms) on the rear handle (a factor of 2.5/1). These levels are quite high, especially on the rear handle. This is apparently due to the very little mass damping associated with the light weight of the tool. Thus, the attenuation of vibration transmitted from the chisels to the handles is larger for large chipping hammers than for small chipping hammers. At the same operating conditions, substantially more energy is transmitted to the hand-arm system from the handles of small chipping hammers than from the handles of large chipping hammers. Spectra for each tool extended from approximately 6.3 Hz to 1 kHz.

For comparative purposes only, the acceleration measurements were compared with the maximum levels for daily exposure contained in the proposed ISO hand-arm vibration standard. In no case did the chipping hammer chisel acceleration measurements fall within an acceptable ISO exposure guideline. Under some conditions, such as operating at 1/2 to 3/4 throttle, some chipping handle acceleration levels did fall within acceptable exposure levels.

Similarly, triaxial acceleration measurements were obtained on pneumatic horizontal and vertical grinders when using a variety of grinding wheels. All grinders were operated at full throttle. The vector summed acceleration levels ranged from a low of 0.56 G(rms) on the vertical grinder, to a high of 2.09 G(rms) on the horizontal grinder. These levels are considerably lower than the chipping hammer levels, and are distributed within the range of exposures recommended by the ISO for durations of between thirty minutes and eight hours per day.

ACKNOWLEDGEMENTS

The research reported in this paper was carried out under NIOSH Contract No. 210-77-0165, while Dr. D.D. Reynolds was an Associate Professor in the Dept. of Mechanical Engineering at the Univ. of Pittsburgh.

Reynolds et al.: Vibration levels

DISCLAIMER

Mention of commercially available services, apparatus, instrumentation, devices, products, or proposed standards does not constitute endorsement by the National Institute for Occupational Safety and Health.

REFERENCES

1. In: Wasserman DE, Taylor W, Curry MG, eds. Proc of the Int Occup Hand-Arm Vibration Conf. Cincinnati, OH: Dept Health and Human Services, 1977. (NIOSH publication no. 77-170).
2. Reynolds DD, Wasserman DE, Basel R, Taylor W. Energy entering the hand of operators of pneumatic tools used in chipping and grinding. In: Brammer AJ, Taylor W, eds. Vibration Effects on the Hand and Arm in Industry. New York: Wiley, 1982.
3. Reynolds DD. Three- and four-degrees-of-freedom models of the vibration response of the human hand. In: Brammer AJ, Taylor W, eds. Vibration Effects on the Hand and Arm in Industry. New York: Wiley, 1982.
4. Behrens V, Taylor W, Wasserman D. Vibration syndrome in workers using pneumatic chipping and grinding tools. In: Brammer AJ, Taylor W, eds. Vibration Effects on the Hand and Arm in Industry. New York: Wiley, 1982.
5. Wasserman D, Reynolds D, Behrens V, Taylor W, Samueloff S, Basel R. Vol II-Engineering Testing - Vibration White Finger Disease in U.S. Workers Using Pneumatic Chipping and Grinding Hand Tools. Cincinnati, OH: Dept Health and Human Services, 1981. (NIOSH publication no. 82-101).
6. Hemstock TI, O'Connor DE. Evaluation of human exposure to hand-transmitted vibration. In: Wasserman DE, Taylor W, Curry MG, eds. Proc of the Int Hand-Arm Vibration Conf. Cincinnati, OH: Dept Health and Human Services, 1977 (NIOSH publication no. 77-170): 129-135.
7. Frood ADM. Testing methods and some of the problems involved in measuring the vibration of hand-held pneumatic tools. In: Wasserman DE, Taylor W, Curry MG, eds. Proc of the Int Hand-Arm Vibration Conf. Cincinnati, OH: Dept Health and Human Services, 1977. (NIOSH publication no. 77-170): 146-152.
8. Kitchener R. The measurement of hand-arm vibration in industry. In: Wasserman DE, Taylor W, Curry MG, eds. Proc of the Int Hand-Arm Vibration Conf. Cincinnati, OH: Dept Health and Human Services, 1977. (NIOSH publication no. 77-170): 153-159.
9. Rasmussen G. Measurement techniques for hand-arm vibration. In: Wasserman DE, Taylor W, Curry MG, eds. Proc of the Int Hand-Arm Vibration Conf. Cincinnati, OH: Dept Health and Human Services, 1977. (NIOSH publication no. 77-170): 173-178.
10. International Organization for Standardization. Principles for the Measurement and the Evaluation of Human Exposure to Vibration Transmitted to the Hand. Draft International Standard ISO/DIS 5349, 1979.
11. Wasserman DE, Doyle TE, Asburry W. Whole-body Vibration Exposure of Workers During Heavy Equipment Operation. Cincinnati, OH: Dept Health and Human Services, 1978. (NIOSH publication no. 78-153).
12. Taylor W, Wasserman D. Relationship between occupational vibration and morbidity. J Envir Path Tox 1979, 2: 67.
13. Glass SW. Vibration analysis of high cycle hand grinders. Arbete Och Malsa, 1979: 32.
14. European Committee of Manufacturers of Compressors, Vacuum Pumps and Pneumatic Tools. Vibrations in pneumatic hand tools: investigations on hand held percussive tools. (Copies available from British Compressed Air Society, 8 Leicester Street, London WC2H 7BL, England.)

APPENDIX: WORK PRACTICES IN THE FOUNDRIES AND SHIPYARD

A1. Foundry #1

Foundry #1 was a large, high-volume production, grey-iron foundry manufacturing large castings weighing more than 100 pounds, such as motor-vehicle engine blocks, transmission cases, etc. The casting method in use falls under the Class 30 Grey Iron designation. This type of metal is a perlitic (nodular iron having a minimum of 30 000 psi tensile strength with a general hardness range of 187 to 255 BHN (Brinell Hardness Number).

We observed several workers using pneumatic chipping and grinding tools, and discussed with various department supervisors and foremen how a worker uses both chipping and grinding tools interchangeably.

The men worked in teams of two and each team's work station consisted of a semi-enclosed cubicle (approximately ten feet long and five feet wide). Approximately 20 of these stations were side-by-side. Compressed air (90 psi) was brought to each work station to power two Type 2 chipping hammers with assorted chisels (each from one to three feet long) and two vertical grinders (with six and eight inch diameter grinding wheels). Each cubicle had a waist-high steel table. Above this table was an electric hoist used to manipulate large castings. In operation, large castings were brought to each of these work stations via a continuous overhead moving chain conveyor or by a forklift truck carrying pallets of castings.

The men on these teams were paid on a piece-work basis and worked very quickly. After they received a casting, one man immediately began chipping the burrs off the visible faces of the casting, and the other man followed grinding the area just chipped. After doing one to three surfaces, they would interchange tools. Sometimes both chipped simultaneously (e.g., one on the surface metal and the other in the deep cyclinder cavities of an engine block). After all visible surfaces were chipped and ground, they then hoisted the casting onto the table to work on the remaining surfaces. A team could completely chip and grind an 800 pound transmission case, for example, in an average of 54 minutes. On occasion, some castings were "burnt" - sand from the mold had impregnated itself on the casting. These were extremely difficult castings to chip and grind and were, as a rule, sent back to a single "reclaim/salvage chipper/grinder" (paid as an hourly employee, not as a pieceworker) who spent all the necessary time it took to do this difficult job. The ratio of two-man teams to reclaim/salvage chipper/grinders was ten teams to one reclaim man.

These two-man teams worked very hard and very fast, operating their chipping and grinding tools virtually all of the time at full tool throttle. They clasped the chipping tool (both at the chisel and rear end) with a tightly coupled wrap-around palm grip (grip strength approximately 6 pounds of force for each hand). The hand holding the chisel was always gloved (to reduce the heat reaching the hand). The hand holding the rear handle was occasionally gloved, depending on operator preference. The method of clasping the pneumatic grinder was essentially the same as that for the chipping tool. Since the same operator interchangeably used both chipping and grinding tools, operator preference with regard to gloves did not change.

The gloves were of medium-weight leather or similar man-made materials and, we believe, did very little to attenuate the vibration except at the very high frequencies (above 500 Hz), where some absorption in the material undoubtedly took place. All chippers and grinders wore hearing protection, and each wore a ventilated hood connected to a filtered, compressed-air supply line. The hood also prevented flying metal and dirt particles from striking the eyes.

Based on our observations and discussions with supervisors, we estimate that in a normal eight hour shift each chipper and grinder spent an average of 3.5 hours chipping, 2.5 hours grinding, 1.5 hours manipulating and moving castings, and 0.5 hours break time. The reclaim/salvage chipper/grinder (hourly) worker averaged about the same time as the piece-workers (except that he worked longer on much fewer castings). In this plant, there were about five or six different types of castings.

A2. Foundry #2

Foundry #2 is another large, high-volume production, grey-iron foundry manufacturing small (less than 100 pounds) motor-vehicular castings (oil pans, manifolds, etc.). The casting metal was the same type as that used in Foundry #1. Here we examined 66 chippers and grinders, and 79 machine shop set-up men who were not exposed to either hand-arm or whole-body vibration. In this plant, the chippers and grinders were not teamed. Each man was paid on a piecework basis, and the foundry operation was composed of many such workers. Castings were brought to the work station via forklift truck and pallet. A variety of types of small castings were handled with more grinding than chipping taking place. The same types of tools used in Foundry #1 were used here. Chisel lengths varied from 3 to 12 inches and were not, as a rule, as long as those in Foundry #1.

The men in Foundry #2 were also incentive workers and worked very quickly. Chipping and

grinding time varied depending on the casting type, e.g., an 85 pound oil pan took about ten minutes to complete, whereas a 44 pound manifold took about 1.5 minutes to complete. Here, again, there were a few hourly paid reclaim/salvage chipper/grinder operators (ten pieceworkers for each reclaim/salvage operator).

Each man wore hearing protection as well as a ventilated hood. As a rule, at least one glove was worn and, at times, both hands were gloved, depending on operator preference. The estimated work time was 4 hours grinding, 3 hours chipping, 0.5 hour casting manipulation, and 0.5 hours break time.

We discussed with supervisors in both foundries the training given to their workers. It appears that they developed skills naturally. This was accomplished by placing a new worker on the midnight to 8:00 a.m. shift, when the workload is lighter than on the other two shifts. As his skill level increased, the trainee was eventually transferred to another shift. There appeared to be little specific training as to a preferred or a more appropriate method of working with the vibrating tools. Thus, each operator chose a working method that seemed to suit him.

A3. Shipyard

The large shipyard operation investigated employed about 10 000 workers. Large ships and ship propellers of all descriptions were built, repaired, modified, etc., at this location. These workers used the same chipping hammer as the foundry workers (Type 2 chipping hammers), and a rotary type vertical grinder.

We observed workers using pneumatic chipping and grinding tools, and talked with supervisors in two departments to determine how the workers used these tools. Department X included men who worked in the holds of ships. Department Y included workers who chipped and ground propellers. All worked on a single daily work shift. The metals chipped by workers in both departments were nickel-aluminum-bronze alloy and mild steel.

A3.1 Department X

The men in this department worked in the holds of ships and used both pneumatic chippers and grinders. An average eight hour workday consisted of four hours of chipping, two hours of grinding, and two hours of performing other non-vibratory activities. On occasion, the chipping could extend to 5.5 hours per day. The workers were under continuous pressure to complete the work quickly and accurately.

One man trained all of the men in this department on the use of pneumatic chipping hammers. All chippers were instructed to use their body for leverage, and thereby absorb some of the vibration energy from the chipping hammer. Their arms were to be held close to the body, with the arm braced by the body, knee, etc., for extra leverage. Generally, the chipping hammer chisel was guided with the first finger and thumb, or the flat palm of the hand. The chisel was rarely in complete contact with the fingers. The chippers were trained to work holding the chipping hammer in either the right or left hand according to preference. The workers always wore leather gloves on both hands, to reduce the heat reaching the hands. Generally, they operated the chipping hammers for 15 to 29 minutes without resting. They also sharpened their own chisels, altering them to suit themselves. The length of the chisel was from 3 to 5 inches.

The men in this department basically performed two types of chipping operations: tamp and cut. The tamping operation included tamping and packing metal, and other caulking compounds, into holes. Welders initially welded metal into a hole and the chippers finished the job, by tamping the metal down to even it out and form a smooth surface. The chisel was held and guided by the flat part of the palm of the hand. The back handle was loosely clasped by the fingers. The workers leaned into the chipping hammer, pushing on the back handle with the palm of their hand, using their bodies as leverage. They interchanged hands frequently while holding the chipping hammer and chisel.

Using the chipping hammer for cutting involved removing metal, cleaning welds, etc. Sometimes workers used chisels to cut through bulkheads. For these operations, the workers guided the chisel with the flat part of the palm of the hand, and gripped the back handle fairly tightly. They also used their body for leverage, and interchanged hands frequently while holding the hammer and chisel. Frequently, they had to hold the chipping hammer over their head to perform some cutting operations. During nearly all of the chipping operations, the worker used the chipper at full throttle. Both horizontal and vertical grinders were used for the finishing work.

A3.2   Department Y

The men in this department cleaned and formed ship propellers. The workers spent about three hours of their time chipping, three hours grinding, and two hours on other activities. Because of the high precision required for finishing propellers, the work proceeded very slowly. It was not unusual for a worker to work from 40 to 50 weeks on a newly-cast propeller. Normally, a worker worked on one side of a propeller, first chipping the entire surface of the propeller and then grinding the surface. When these operations were completed on one side, the propeller was turned over and the operations were repeated on the other side. These chipping and grinding operations generally occurred continuously over a several-week period before changing to another operation.

Chipping a propeller is very demanding and tiring work. The worker leaned into the chipping hammer with his body, pushing on the back handle of the hammer with the palm of his hand. He then guided the 3 to 5 inch long chisel with the flat part of the palm of his hand. Thus, his fingers never contacted the surface of the chisel and rarely contacted the back handle. In many cases, the worker rested the hand that guided the chisel on the front end of the chipping hammer. Thus, no part of his hand came in contact with the chisel. Each worker wore a glove only on the one hand that was used to guide the chisel. The hand that pushed against the back handle remained ungloved, so that the worker's hand was free to control the throttle trigger of the hammer. The workers mostly operated this tool at 1/2 to 3/4 throttle and chipped in 15 to 30 second bursts, with a two to three minute rest period between bursts.

Workers reported that the general maintenance of the tools (obtained from a central supply tool crib) was poor. They claimed that this, along with bent chisels, usually resulted in higher vibration levels.

DISCUSSION

D.E. O'Connor: You measured accelerations on the chisel of over 10^4 m/s^2 in the third octave band centred on 31.5 Hz (Fig. 9). If this level were generated from a sinusoidal signal, a reasonable assumption for a signal with a third octave bandwidth, then the corresponding displacement is of the order of a metre. Clearly this is incorrect. How can you explain the excessive displacements associated with some of your acceleration measurements?

Authors' Response: Your statement appears to be correct. The accelerations measured on chisels during slot-chipping operations are known to be very large because of the measurement problems experienced (see Section 2.2). Because of the various sources of measurement error, the actual accelerations may not be exactly as reported, but we do believe that they are of the correct order of magnitude. During slot-chipping operations, plastic deformation occurs at the cutting edge of the chisel and in the work piece. This may influence significantly the nature of the acceleration pulses, and it may not be possible to construct the corresponding displacements from linear combinations of the Fourier components.

Motorcycle Handlebar Vibration

R. T. Harrison and W. A. Murphy

ABSTRACT: Concern for the health of Forest Service motorcycle riders has led to an investigation of handlebar vibration. Ten different motorcycles were instrumented and data were obtained from stationary tests, during which engine speeds were quickly increased to their maximum safe value (with transmissions in neutral) and then allowed to return to idle. One machine was also ridden over a 3/4 mile course in two different modes - "hard" and "easy." The results indicate that hand-arm vibration would not significantly affect a Forest Service operator who rides at work for no more than two hours per day. However, those who ride for eight (or more) hours per workday experience vibration exposure that could exceed the limits proposed in ISO/DIS 5349.

RESUME: Des inquiétudes concernant la santé des motocyclistes au service du Service des forêts ont mené à une enquête sur les vibrations des guidons. Des instruments furent installés sur dix motocyclettes différentes, et des données furent obtenues de tests stationnaires, pendant lesquels la vitesse des moteurs fut rapidement augmentée jusqu'à leur plein régime (les transmissions étant en position neutre) puis retournée normalement au régime ralenti. Une moto fut également conduite sur un parcours de 3/4 de mille de deux façons différentes: à fond de train et doucement. Les résultats indiquent que les vibrations du système main-bras n'auraient pas d'effet significatif sur un opérateur du Service des forêts qui conduit sa moto pour un maximum de deux heures par jour. Cependant, ceux qui roulent pendant huit heures ou plus par jour subissent une exposition aux vibrations qui pourrait dépasser les limites proposées dans ISO/DIS 5349.

INTRODUCTION

The Forest Service, U.S. Department of Agriculture, is responsible for the multiple-use management of nearly 188 million acres of National Forests and Grasslands in the United States. Its employees are making increasing use of motorcycles for transportation at work. In addition, motorcycling is a popular recreational activity on forest roads and trails. A very practical way for Forest Service personnel to patrol designated motorcycle recreation areas is on motorcycles.

While motorcycles are cost-effective and relatively safe vehicles, they do present some concerns for the health of their operators. One of the more interesting health questions, raised by several Forest Service field units, pertains to handlebar vibration. To establish and evaluate the hand-arm vibration experienced by our motorcycle-riding employees, we instrumented ten different motorcycles to obtain data during a series of tests.

I HAND-ARM VIBRATION TEST PROGRAMME

1.1 Test Motorcycles

Until recently, Forest Service employees mostly used off-road 90 cc step-through frame trailbikes. These have now generally been supplanted by 125-175 cc dual-purpose enduro motorcycles, which can be used as both off-road and on-highway vehicles. This not only eliminates the need for pickup trucks to transport trailbikes to their point of use, but also allows many field tasks to be accomplished with a very energy-efficient vehicle. Patrol personnel who enforce off-road vehicle regulations use performance-oriented "serious" enduro competition motorcycles, such as the Can-Am 175 Qualifier or the Kawasaki KDX175.

A 1980 Can-Am 175 Qualifier was chosen to be the most extensively investigated motorcycle, since it is typical of both the dual-purpose transportation motorcycles and the true enduro off-road patrol machine. The following nine motorcycles were also tested while stationary, with the engine revving: two-stroke, dual-purpose - a 1981 Kawasaki KE125, a 1981 Suzuki TS185, and a 1980 Yamaha DT125; four-stroke, dual-purpose - a 1981 Honda XL185S, a 1981 Suzuki SP500 and a Kawasaki KL250; competition, off-road - a 1981 Kawasaki KDX175 (enduro) and a 1981 Suzuki RM250 (motocross); and a 1981 Yamaha Special 400 (an on-highway twin cylinder motorcycle equipped with rubber-isolated handlebars). The primary test motorcycle - a two-stroke, single-cylinder, six-speed Can Am 175 Qualifier (see Fig. 1) - is built in Canada; it has an Austrian engine.

1.2 Instrumentation

The instrumentation used was a Bruel and Kjaer model 4338 uniaxial piezoelectric accelerometer and an Ivie Electronics

IE-30A real-time spectrum analyzer (Fig. 1). These instruments were configured to provide an accumulated maximum spectrum, i.e., a "worst case" spectrum. The accelerometer was mounted on a thin piece of aluminum (see Fig. 2), as described in the Draft International Standard ISO/DIS 5349 (1). Since we could not mount the accelerometer beneath the operator's hand, it was placed as seen in Figs. 2, 3, and 4. These are, respectively, the X, Z, and Y axes, as specified in ISO/DIS 5349.

The handgrip attached to the handlebar is an important part of the vibration-absorbing system. We therefore mounted the accelerometer outside the handgrip. We also realized the firmness with which the thin aluminum plate is attached to the handgrip affects the grip-to-accelerometer coupling. Therefore, tape was applied loosely - just tight enough to hold the accelerometer in

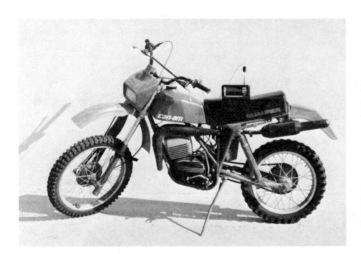

Fig. 2 Photograph showing accelerometer mounted in the X direction.

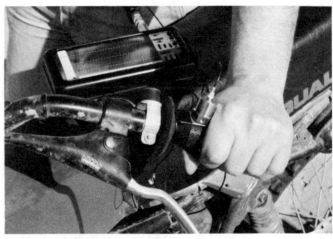

Fig. 1 Primary test motorcycle (Can-Am 175 Qualifier) with test instrumentation.

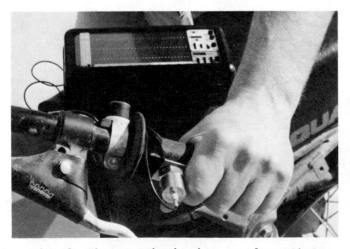

Fig. 3 Photograph showing accelerometer mounted in the Z direction.

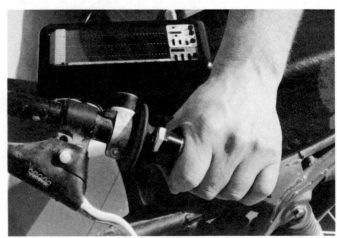

Fig. 4 Photograph showing accelerometer mounted in the Y direction.

Harrison et al.: Motorcycle vibration

place; the "clamping force" was provided by the operator's hand in all X and Z direction tests.

Because of the twist-grip throttle design, the accelerometer could not be mounted in a fixed position in the Z-X plane. It was mounted so that it was roughly aligned with the Z axis at rest and with the X axis when the throttle was opened. In some cases, data were obtained while the motorcycle was moving. Since mounting instrumentation tape recorders on off-road motorcycles has not always provided reliable measurements, we decided to accumulate data by using the Ivie analyzer in the accumulate mode. Thus, the highest vibration level in each third octave was recorded during each run. This accumulated maximum spectrum is probably approximately 3 dB higher than the instantaneous spectrum. The precision of the results depends on the smallest increment that the analyzer can display. In the mode we used, it was 1.5 dB.

1.3 Test Methods

All ten motorcycles underwent stationary tests. The Can-Am was also ridden over a 3/4 mile test course, which consisted of 1/4 mile of asphalt, 1/4 mile of rutted dirt road, and 1/4 mile of unimproved surface covered with weeds and low brush. The stationary tests were run with the transmissions in neutral while the engine speeds were quickly increased to their maximum safe rpm; they were then allowed to return to idling speeds (often referred to as a "revving" test).

Two modes were used to ride the Can-Am over the 3/4-mile course: "easy," an average 15 mph pace that a recreational motorcyclist would probably consider sensible; and "hard," an average 30 to 35 mph pace that might seem reckless to the recreational rider, but which was, in fact, significantly slower than a skilled competition rider would use to negotiate the course. There were no jumps in the test course; the few jumps that were tried overloaded the instrumentation.

II RESULTS AND DISCUSSION

The test results are summarized in Figs. 5 through 11.

Figure 5 shows the vibration, in metres per second squared, at the left handlebar in each of three directions, X, Y, and Z, for the Can-Am. These data indicate that the vibration in the Y direction (along the cylindrical axis of the handlebar) is not significant. The peaks in both the X and Z direction (up and down, and fore and aft, respectively) are roughly equivalent. However, there are two significant peaks in the X direction and only one in the Z direction. This is not surprising, given

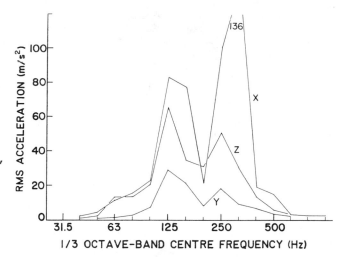

Fig. 5 X, Y, and Z components of the left handlebar vibration: Can-Am stationary test.

that the main forcing function (the engine) is closely aligned to the X direction. Based on these data, a decision was made to evaluate different operating modes only in the X direction.

Figure 6 shows the vibration in the X direction at the left handlebar when riding "hard" and "easy." The data indicate that the manner in which the motorcycle is operated is of primary importance in the amount of vibration transmitted to the operator's hands. Also apparent is that the band corresponding to the maximum power engine speed (7500 rpm) of the motorcycle greatly exceeds the selected safety standard (the small circles on Fig. 6 are the levels given in ISO/DIS 5349 with a correction

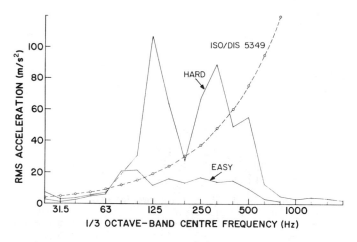

Fig. 6 X component of the left handlebar vibration: Can-Am riding "hard" and "easy" tests.

Harrison et al.: Motorcycle vibration

factor of three). The reasons for selecting this safety standard will be discussed later. All data in Fig. 6 were obtained with the same rider, who attempted to compress the handgrip the same amount during each test. The higher values seen in Fig. 6 when riding hard are unlikely to result from the firm grip naturally employed when riding fast on an off-road motorcycle. It is also apparent that the most damaging vibration comes from the engine and not from some other source.

Figure 7 shows data similar to those in Fig. 6 for the right handgrip. This cannot properly be called acceleration in the X direction, because, as mentioned before, the most sensitive axis of the accelerometer is aligned with the X axis during only a portion of the test ride. These data were taken with the accelerometer aligned with the X axis under wide-open throttle conditions. The spectrum observed during the stationary test shows the same peaks at 125 Hz and 320 Hz as that recorded on the left handgrip, but the 320 Hz peak is about 5 dB lower. The right handgrip, which contains the throttle, is not firmly affixed to the handlebar itself, but is mounted on a concentric tube that operates the throttle, which in turn is slipped over the handlebar. There is necessarily some clearance between the two concentric tubes, allowing for more movement and more damping than occurs in the left handgrip. This could explain the difference.

14 dB down at 125 Hz, and 20 dB down at 320 Hz.

In Fig. 7, the peaks at 125 Hz and 320 Hz are roughly 3 dB less in the stationary test compared with the riding "hard" test. Again, the vibration levels during the riding "easy" test are much lower. From these observations, it can be concluded that the most severe vibration will be encountered at the left hand when riding hard, and that a stationary engine "revving" test gives a fair indication of the maximum vibration that the rider will experience. For the riding "easy" condition, the operator is likely to experience much less vibration at either hand than would be measured during a stationary engine "revving" test, with the accelerometer located at the left handlebar.

A short series of tests were run over the test course with two different riders. No significant difference in vibration levels occurred during the slow runs. Slightly lower peak accelerations were recorded with rider 2 during the fast runs, but since rider 1 is a much more experienced operator and traversed the course considerably quicker, this might have been expected.

The nine other motorcycles were tested in the stationary engine "revving" mode, with the accelerometer attached to the left handlebar, oriented to record the X component. The test results are shown in Figs. 8 through 11. Figure 8 shows results obtained on three small, dual-purpose motorcycles, the kind most commonly used by the Forest Service for transportation purposes. All of the spectra are somewhat lower than that of the Can-Am. These motorcycles would probably not exceed the selected permissible vibration limits under any but the hardest riding conditions. All of the motorcycles referred to in Fig. 8 have two-stroke engines.

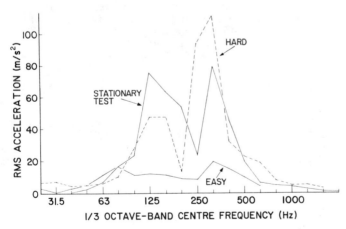

Fig. 7 Right handlebar vibration: Can-Am riding "hard" and "easy" tests and stationary test.

For the left hand, comparing Figs. 5 and 6, the 125 Hz peak is slightly higher during the riding "hard" test than during the stationary test. However, the stationary test yielded a 320 Hz band level roughly 5 dB greater than the riding "hard" test. The riding "easy" test peaks are roughly

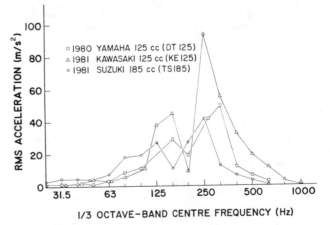

Fig. 8 X component of the left handlebar vibration: Two-stroke, dual-purpose motorcycles; stationary test.

Harrison et al.: Motorcyle vibration

Eight identical Yamahas were tested. The differences in the spectra from motorcycle to motorcycle were found to be of the same order of magnitude as the differences observed in repeated runs with the same motorcycle. Therefore, we conclude that the differences among motorcycles of the same model are negligible, at least for new motorcycles.

Figure 9 shows the handlebar vibration of two four-stroke, dual-purpose motorcycles - a Suzuki SP500 cc motorcycle and a Honda XL185S 185 cc motorcycle. The Honda incorporates weights in the handlebars, probably to reduce the handlebar vibration. The subjective impression of most who have ridden this motorcycle is that it is very vibration-free. The measurements substantiate that the levels are indeed comparatively low.

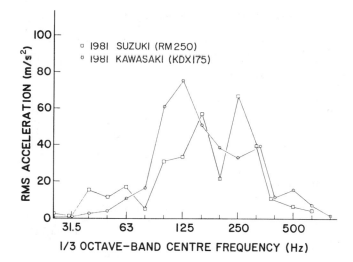

Fig. 10 X component of the left handlebar vibration: Competition, off-road motorcycles; stationary test.

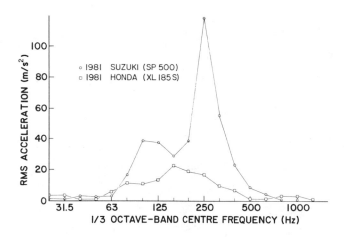

Fig. 9 X component of the left handlebar vibration: Four-stroke, dual-purpose motorcycles; stationary test.

Figure 10 shows vibration spectra obtained at the left handlebar, in the X direction, of an all-out competition motocross motorcycle (Suzuki RM250) and a serious enduro motorcycle (Kawasaki KDX175). The spectra reveal that serious competition motorcycles are not likely to present a significantly greater hazard than dual-purpose motorcycles.

Finally, Fig. 11 shows the vibration spectra obtained on (Kawasaki KL250), a four-stroke dual-purpose motorcycle, and an on-highway motorcycle with rubber-isolated handlebars (Yamaha Special 400). The rubber isolation is apparently effective, as the Yamaha spectrum is quite low throughout the frequency range.

A literature review reveals that there are no universally accepted vibration limits. The limits proposed in ISO/DIS 5349 were selected because they probably represent the broadest consensus available. A tentative

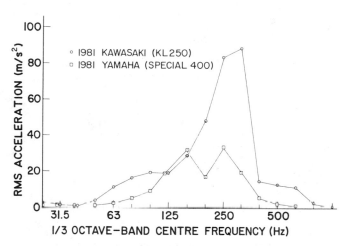

Fig. 11 X component of the left handlebar vibration: "Other" motorcycles; stationary test.

correction factor of three from Table 2 of ISO/DIS 5349 was chosen, as this was representative of a "typical" Forest Service trailbike workcycle. Normally, an employee will ride for under an hour from station to work site. The employee may then perform his required duties, move to another work site 15 to 20 minutes away, and then return to the station, for a total of about two hours riding per day. Normally, when the employee is riding, the ride will not be interrupted. Consequently, a factor of three is appropriate and this was employed in Fig. 6. This assessment does not take into consideration those employees who might be exposed to other hand-arm vibration during the day; e.g., those who use chain saws.

Harrison et al.: Motorcycle vibration

III CONCLUSIONS AND A RECOMMENDATION

We performed extensive tests only on one motorcycle. Firm conclusions must await tests on additional models. However, there is a similarity in the design of popular makes of motorcycle for the same application. We would be surprised if test results on similar motorcycles were greatly different. Thus, based on our limited test programme, we tentatively conclude that:

1. The most severe axis of hand-arm motorcycle vibration is the X direction.

2. The vibration measured in the X direction while the rpm of the engine is increased to its maximum safe speed is a good indication of the maximum vibration that would be transmitted to the hands while riding the motorcycle hard, and is considerably more than the hands would receive during easy riding.

3. Operator aggressiveness determines the maximum vibration received by the hands. Other variables, including differences intrinsic to different operators, are less important.

4. Dual-purpose motorcycles produce handlebar vibration spectra that are very similar to each other and are probably not dangerous to the operator under most field conditions.

5. True enduro and motocross competition motorcycles present only a slightly greater hazard to the operator from hand-arm vibration than do dual-purpose motorcycles.

6. Weights in the handlebars, and rubber isolation of the handlebars from the rest of the motorcycle, are effective in damping operator hand-arm vibration.

Based on these six conclusions, we believe that hand-arm vibration is probably not a problem for Forest Service motorcycle operators. However, there are some Forest Service workers who ride motorcycles as part of their official duties. They should be made aware of the possibility of hand-arm vibration damage and be alerted to its symptoms, so they can recognize any problem before it becomes serious. These employees either patrol on motorcycles for a full eight hour (or longer) workday, or they encounter other sources of hand-arm vibration in addition to motorcycle riding during their workday.

DISCLAIMER

The Forest Service, U.S. Department of Agriculture has developed this information for the guidance of its employees, its contractors, and its co-operating Federal and State agencies, and is not responsible for the interpretation or use of this information by anyone except its own employees. The use of trade, firm, or corporation names in this publication is for the information and convenience of the reader, and does not constitute an endorsement by the U.S. Department of Agriculture of any product or service to the exclusion of others that may be suitable.

REFERENCES

1. International Organization for Standardization. Principles for the Measurement and the Evaluation of Human Exposure to Vibration Transmitted to the Hand. Draft International Standard ISO/DIS 5349, 1979.

DISCUSSION

C.H. Grace: To what extent were the higher acceleration levels obtained with the experienced driver due to: a) greater engine speed, and b) tighter grip of the handlebars by the rider?

Authors' Response: We did not assess this directly. However, comparison of Figs. 5 and 6, and inspection of Fig. 7, may provide some information. The stationary tests were done with a moderate grip and maximum engine revolutions. The riding "hard" tests were done with a tight grip and maximum engine revolutions. The spectra are at least qualitatively similar. Thus one can tentatively conclude that engine speed is more important than grip strength.

Harrison et al.: Motorcycle vibration

Vibration of Power Tool Handles

C. W. Suggs, J. M. Hanks and G. T. Roberson

ABSTRACT: Measurements of the handle vibration of a selection of power tools revealed that many violate hand-arm vibration guidelines after only 0.5 hours of use. Reciprocating tools, such as sabre saws and pad sanders, generated significant vibration at the operating frequency. A gasoline-powered chain saw produced intense vibration at the engine rotational frequency due to the reciprocating engine parts. In well balanced rotating tools, such as drills, routers and circular saws, most of the vibration was traced to the interaction of the cutter with the work piece. The vibration levels observed on some of the electric tools suggest that it may be desirable to develop vibration-isolation systems for a range of tool handles.

RESUME: La mesure des vibrations présentes aux poignées de certains outils mécaniques a révélé qu'un grand nombre excède le niveau de vibration tolérable pour le système main-bras après seulement 0,5 heure d'utilisation. Les outils à mouvements alternatifs, comme les scies à chantourner et les ponceuses à tampon, ont engendré des vibrations importantes à leur régime normal de fonctionnement. Une tronçonneuse à essence a produit d'intenses vibrations à la fréquence de rotation du moteur causées par les pièces du moteur à mouvement alternatif. Dans le cas des outils portatifs bien équilibrés, comme les perceuses, les toupies et les scies circulaires, les vibrations sont surtout attribuables à l'interaction du couteau et de la pièce. L'importance des vibrations que produisent certains des outils électriques rend souhaitable la mise au point d'éléments amortisseurs pour toute une gamme de poignées d'outil.

INTRODUCTION

Vibration is inherent in reciprocating power sources, and is usually present at lower levels in the rotary power sources used to drive hand tools. Vibration is also generated at the tool-work piece interface by the cutting, grinding, drilling or other action taking place. The power tool industry is well aware of these problems and has found some ingenious methods of reducing the sources of vibration. In addition, if the vibration of a tool is excessive and cannot be adequately attenuated at the source, it has been found beneficial to place vibration isolators between the tool handle(s) and body, or to provide resilient handgrips which further reduce transmission of vibration into the hands. The use of resilient handgrips has technical and intuitive appeal, in part because of their simplicity, and is discussed elsewhere (1).

The use of power tools has increased dramatically since the Second World War and is now not limited to professional users. During this period, the risks of vibration-induced disorders of the hands and arms have been widely recognized, and have been responsible, in part, for the development of exposure guidelines. The International Organization for Standardization has proposed exposure boundaries in a Draft International Standard (2). In this paper, the letters CF (correction factor) identify the number by which the four to eight hour exposure values are multiplied to compensate for short duration or intermittent exposure. A hand-held power tool might be considered to violate these guidelines if its frequency spectrum exceeded the appropriate exposure duration curve at any frequency. One could speculate, however, that a tool which exceeded the allowable limit in only one frequency band and had low vibration levels in all other bands might be less damaging than a tool which approached, but did not exceed, the limits in all frequency bands.

This paper reports the vibration characteristics of several hand-held power tools and relates them to levels and durations that are considered acceptable according to the proposed Standard ISO/DIS 5349 (1979). The group of tools selected were chosen on the basis of availability and usage.

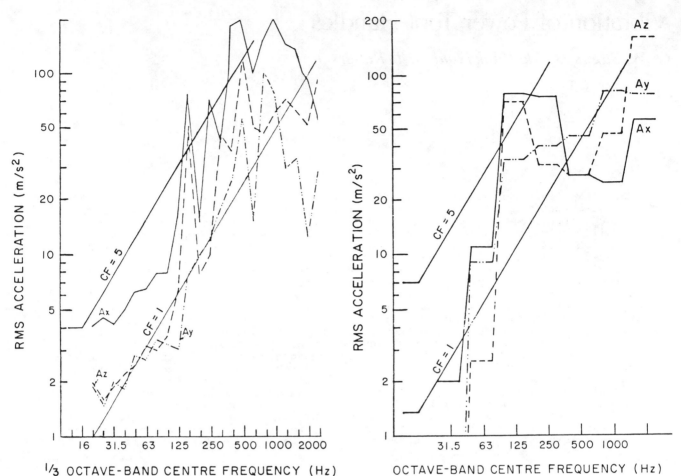

Fig. 1 Front handle vibration of a 33 cc gasoline powered chain saw, when cross cutting wood. (Overall component accelerations: A_x = 500 m/s^2; A_y = 400 m/s^2; and A_z = 360 m/s^2.)

Fig. 2 Rear handle vibration of a medium size, 54 cc, gasoline powered chain saw without handle isolation, when cross cutting wood (engine speed 7000 rpm).

I METHODS

Vibration was measured by attaching an accelerometer to the tool handle near the hand. Because tool handles vibrate in more than one direction, it was necessary to make a sequence of observations, one for each of three orthogonal axes. In accordance with the ISO proposal (2), these were designated A_x, A_y and A_z for acceleration normal to the plane formed by the palm, across the palm (in the direction required for orthogonality) and parallel to the third metacarpal bone, respectively. The vibration signals were obtained from a small accelerometer (Bruel & Kjaer, type 4344) attached to a special mount, which was shaped to fit between the hand and the handgrip as recommended in the Draft International Standard. The accelerometer

signals were amplified (Bruel & Kjaer, type 2635) and fed into a frequency analyzer (Nicolet, type 446A - some of the graphs shown were drawn by a companion recorder directly from the analyzer output). Data are reported as root mean square (rms) accelerations, in units of metres per second square (m/s^2).

The results are presented as octave- or 1/3 octave-band frequency spectra. In each diagram, the ISO guidelines for 0.5 hours and from four to eight hours of exposure are included for comparison. Table 1 gives the factors which may be applied to the four to eight hours exposure curve to compensate for shorter exposure durations or for interruptions in vibration exposure (intermittent tool operation).

The tools were operated by experienced operators who were instructed to operate the tools in a normal manner while the

Suggs et al.: Power tool vibration

Table 1. Correction Factors by Which the 4 to 8 h Exposure Guideline May be Multiplied for Shorter Exposures or When Various Rest Schedules are Employed (from Ref. 2).

Exposure Time Per 8 h Day	Interruptions in Vibration Exposure Minutes Per Working Hour				
	<10	10-20	20-30	30-40	>40
up to 30 min	5	-	-	-	-
30 min to 1 h	4	-	-	-	-
1 h to 2 h	3	3	4	5	5
2 h to 4 h	2	2	3	4	5
4 h to 8 h	1	1	2	3	4

Table 2. Listing of Tools Tested and Tabulation of Vibration Guideline Violations.

Tool	Frequency and Allowable Exposure Duration					
	Low*		Medium*		High*	
	8 h	0.5 h	8 h	0.5 h	8 h	0.5 h
0.95 cm (3/8 in) air wrench	x	-	-	-	-	-
1.27 cm (1/2 in) drill, rear handle	-	-	x	-	A_y only	-
1.27 cm (1/2 in) drill, side handle	x	A_x only	-	-	-	-
Reciprocating sander	x	x	x	-	-	-
Sabre saw	-	-	x	A_y only	x	x
Circular saw	-	-	x	-	-	-
Router	-	-	-	-	x	x
Disk grinder, side handle	-	-	x	-	-	-
Disk grinder, rear handle	x	-	-	-	x	-
Electric chain saw, control handle	-	-	-	-	x	-
Electric chain saw, guide handle	-	-	-	-	x	-
0.64 cm (1/4 in) drill	-	-	A_z only	A_z only	-	-
0.95 cm (3/8 in) drill	x	-	A_x only	-	-	-
Cordless shrub trimmer	-	-	-	-	-	-
Gasoline chain saw, rear handle	-	-	x	A_y only	-	-
Gasoline chain saw, front handle	-	-	x	x	x	-
Cordless string trimmer	-	-	-	-	-	-
Belt sander	-	-	-	-	A_y only	-

x - indicates that all vibration components are in excess of the guideline.
* - low, below 30 Hz; medium, from 30 to 250 Hz; and high, above 250 Hz.

measurements were being made. The tools investigated are listed and briefly described in the first column of Table 2. Brand names are not given because the purpose of the study was to evaluate hazard potential rather than to show that one brand is better than another. Also vibration measurements of hand tools precise enough for brand comparisons are difficult to make, because small changes in operating conditions can significantly change the results in some cases.

II RESULTS AND DISCUSSION

2.1 Chain Saws

Chain saws, especially units powered by internal-combustion engines, were found to have very high levels of vibration, as can be seen from Figs. 1 to 3, and exceed the 4 to 8 h exposure guideline over much of the spectrum; in several cases, the saw vibration exceeds the 0.5 h exposure guideline.

Suggs et al.: Power tool vibration

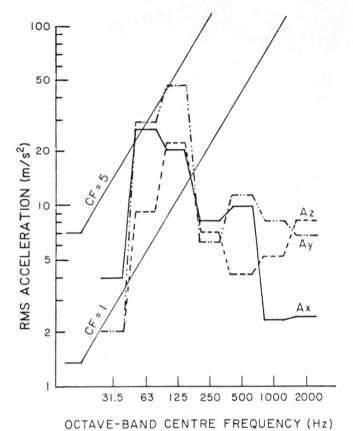

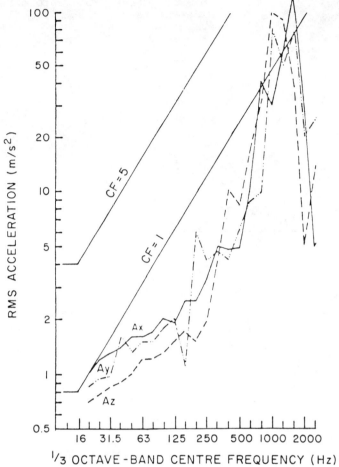

Fig. 3 Rear handle vibration of the saw used to obtain the data shown in Fig. 4 after the addition of handle isolation, when operating under the same conditions.

A small saw, with volumetric capacity of approximately 33 cm^3 and a 36 cm (14 in) bar was found to have more handle vibration than larger commercial saws. The small saw violated the 0.5 h daily exposure curve at several frequencies (see Fig. 1). Its use would need to be limited to short periods, followed by intervals without vibration exposure. The relatively high vibration levels can be tolerated because these tools are designed for the casual user and are seldom operated for more than a few hours per week, during weekends or evenings. They do not usually possess vibration-isolated handles.

A saw with larger volumetric capacity (54 cm^3) produced less vibration than the smaller saw just discussed (see Fig. 2). However, it did violate the 0.5 h exposure guideline in one octave band. The effect of handle isolation can be clearly seen by comparing Figs. 2 and 3: there is a dramatic decrease in vibration at frequencies above about 125 Hz. The engine firing frequency occurs at an engine speed of 7000 rpm (about 117 Hz) and is

Fig. 4 Front handle vibration of an electric powered chain saw, when cross cutting wood. (Overall component accelerations: A_x = 210 m/s^2; A_y = 300 m/s^2; and A_z = 360 m/s^2.)

responsible for the peak acceleration in the 125 Hz band. Higher frequencies are mainly harmonics of the engine speed and handle responses.

While the vibration of an electric chain saw will not peak at the motor frequency, unless it is unbalanced, there will probably be significant vibration at higher frequencies (Fig. 4). These peaks can usually be associated with the sprocket tooth passage frequency or with impacts between the cutting teeth and the wood, which occur at three to ten times the motor frequency. Handle isolation is difficult, on many of these tools, as the handle is an integral part of the motor housing in most current designs. The high frequencies could readily be reduced by handle isolation.

Suggs et al.: Power tool vibration

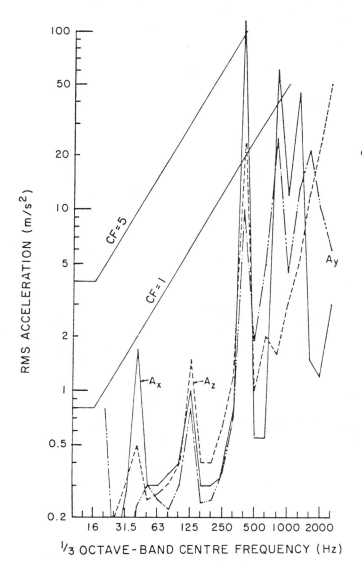

Fig. 5 One-third octave-band accelerations at the handle of a router when cutting wood.

2.2 Other Hand-Held Power Tools

The vibration characteristics of a selection of electric tools and some gas or pneumatic tools are summarized in Table 2. The vibration of each tool was evaluated at "low", "medium" and "high" frequencies, and violations of the 8 h or 0.5 h exposure guidelines are marked with an X. The frequency ranges are as follows: "low" frequencies, below 30 Hz; "medium" frequencies, from 30 to 250 Hz, and "high" frequencies, above 250 Hz.

In addition, one-third octave band accelerations at the handles of some of the tools are shown in Figs. 5 to 9, which also include the 8 h and 0.5 h ISO exposure guidelines for comparison purposes.

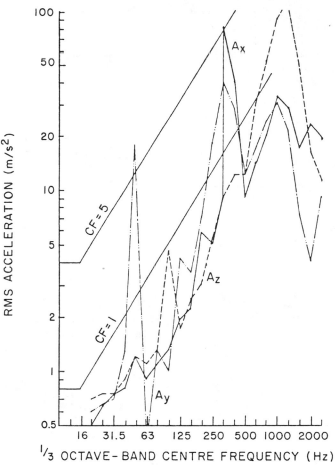

Fig. 6 One-third octave-band accelerations of a reciprocating sabre saw when cutting wood.

A router, with shaft rotating at about 25 000 rpm (417 Hz), produced intense vibration in the 400 Hz frequency band (which contains 417 Hz) and lower levels at harmonics of the fundamental, as can be seen from Fig. 5. This vibration appeared to be due primarily to the impact of the two lobed cutting bit against the wood. Some peaks at lower frequencies were attributed to vibration of the work piece and supporting table.

A reciprocating electric sabre saw generated intense vibration at frequencies around 50 and 300 Hz (Fig. 6). The peaks appear to be at the reciprocating frequency of the saw and at the tooth passage frequency of the saw blade, respectively. Both of these peaks violate the 0.5 h guideline. While vibration at high frequencies could be isolated from the handle by resilient mounts, isolation of the lower frequencies would be difficult. A reciprocating counterweight might reduce the low frequency vibration, particularly in the 50 Hz band.

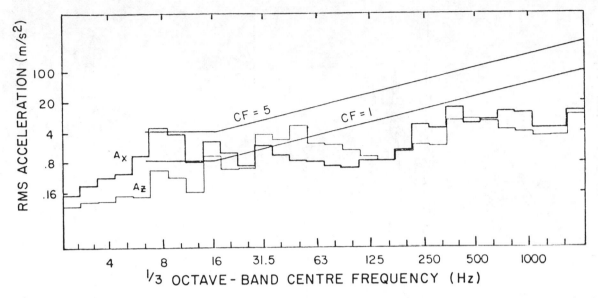

Fig. 7 One-third octave-band accelerations at the side handle of a 1.27 cm (1/2 in) electric drill with a 1.27 cm diameter bit, when drilling mild steel plate.

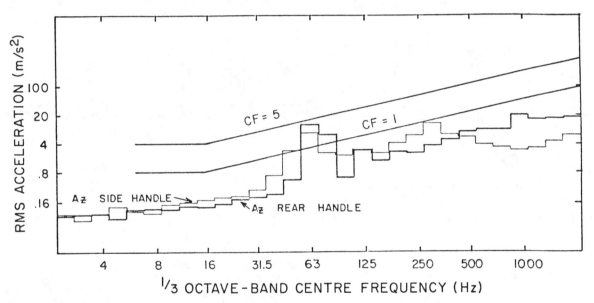

Fig. 8 One-third octave-band accelerations at the side and rear handles of a 23 cm (9 in) disk grinder.

The side handle of a large electric drill vibrated excessively in the X and Z directions, as can be seen from Fig. 7. Changes in rotational speed were found to excite vibrations in the X direction, and acceleration parallel to the long axis of the drill bit would excite motion in the Z direction. The rotational speed of the drill was about 500 rpm (8 Hz), which corresponds to the band in which most vibration was observed.

The handles of a disk grinder with a 23 cm (9 in) carborundum wheel vibrated most at frequencies in the 63 Hz band (see Fig. 8). The no-load rotation speed of the grinder was about 4200 rpm (70 Hz), which is within the 1/3 octave band centred at 63 Hz. The peak was attributed to imbalance in the grinding wheel and was most pronounced in the Z direction, on both handles. There was some higher frequency vibration which could possibly be associated with contact between the grit and the work piece or handle resonances. Gullander and Peterson have also found intense vibration on the handles of disk grinders (3).

The handle vibration of a 19 cm (7.5 in) wood-cutting circular saw violated the

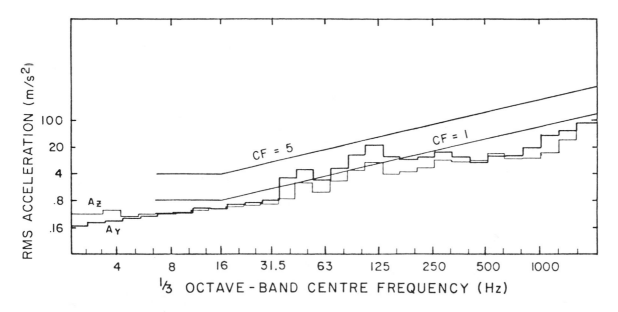

Fig. 9 One-third octave-band accelerations at the handle of a 19 cm (7.5 in) circular saw, when cutting wood.

8 h guideline but did not quite violate the 0.5 h guideline, as can be seen from Fig. 9. Vibration isolation of the handle could reduce the acceleration at the frequencies of concern.

III CONCLUSIONS

While chain saws are well known to produce intense vibration, it is not generally recognized that many electric tools also produce unpleasant, often harmful, vibrations. Efforts to reduce the vibration of chain saws and its transmission to the handles have been successful in most cases. However, the vibration of many small saws intended for limited duration usage is poorly isolated from the handles. Some of these saws exceed the ISO vibration guidelines for exposures lasting as little as 30 minutes. Larger saws, while they may exceed the guidelines, tend to be fitted with vibration isolators which attenuate the transmission of vibration to the hands.

When electric tools were found to possess significant vibration, it could usually be traced to impacts between the tool and work piece or to the reciprocating nature of the tool. A high speed router and a reciprocating saw were examples of two vibration sources that generated sufficient vibration to restrict safe exposures to 30 minutes' duration.

ACKNOWLEDGEMENTS

The permission of the Standards Council of Canada, under authority of the International Organization for Standardization, to reproduce Table 2 from Draft International Standard ISO/DIS 5349 (1979) is gratefully acknowledged.

DISCLAIMER

The use of trade names in this publication does not imply endorsement by the North Carolina Agricultural Research Service of the products named, nor criticism of similar ones not mentioned.

REFERENCES

1. Suggs CW, Hank JM. Resilient hand grips. In: Brammer AJ, Taylor W, eds. Vibration Effects on the Hand and Arm in Industry. New York: Wiley, 1982.
2. International Organization for Standardization. Principles for the Measurement and the Evaluation of Human Exposure to Vibration Transmitted to the Hand. Draft International Standard ISO/DIS 5349, 1979.
3. Gullander A, Peterson NF. Arbetsbelastning Samt Buller- och Vibrationsexponering vid Arbete med Handslipmaskiner (Physical Strain, Noise and Vibration from Work with Hand Sanding Machines). Stockholm: Arbetarskyddsstyrelsen, Arbetsfysiologiska enheten, 1976. (in Swedish).

Vibration of Manual Tool Handles

C. W. Suggs

ABSTRACT: The handle vibration of traditional impact hand-held tools, such as axes, hammers, mauls, adzes and hoes, has been measured by means of an accelerometer placed between the hand and the handle. A large transient oscillation occurs, with a peak acceleration of as much as 14 000 m/s^2 in some cases, which usually decays within 8 ms. A high frequency (>1000 Hz) ringing was observed with some combinations of workpiece and handle material. Long-handled, two-handed tools exhibited less intense but longer lasting vibration. The short duration, intermittent nature and high frequency of the exposure can be expected to result in less damage to the hand than from comparable continuous vibration.

RESUME: La vibration du manche des outils manuels à impact traditionnels, comme les haches, marteaux, masses, herminettes et houes, a été mesurée au moyen d'un accéléromètre placé entre la main et le manche. Une oscillation transitoire importante se produit, avec une amplitude de pointe atteignant 14 000 m/s^2 dans certains cas, qui décroît généralement en 8 ms. Une résonance à haute fréquence (>1000 Hz) fut observée avec certaines combinaisons de pièces de travail et de matériaux de manche. Les outils à manche long à double poigne ont révélé une vibration moins intense mais de durée plus longue. On peut prévoir que la courte durée, l'intermittence et la haute fréquence de l'exposition peuvent provoquer moins de dommages à la main qu'une vibration continue comparable.

INTRODUCTION

Hammers, axes, mauls and other impact tools operate by storing energy in the kinetic form during a muscle input stroke and rapidly releasing this energy during impact with the workpiece. During impact, high working forces are generated by the rapid deceleration of the tool head. Depending on the hardness of the materials being worked, the impact time is often less than a millisecond, and the acceleration often exceeds several thousand meters per second squared. Fortunately, the tool handle serves as an attenuator so that most of this vibration does not reach the hand.

Tool mass has apparently been optimized by an evolutionary process, which tends to select tool size so that muscles are loaded for maximum power output, consistent with stroke control and other requirements of the job. Also, good design requires that the centre of percussion be located in the tool head near the centre of resistance, so that generation of moments in the handle during impact (handle "sting") will be minimized. This relationship was not fully understood by ancient tool designers, and only in fairly recent history was a poll or head added to a blade to form the present axe.

I   EXPERIMENTAL METHOD

Handle vibration was measured by means of a small piezoelectric accelerometer located at the hand-handle interface. Acceleration values were measured in three mutually orthogonal directions by orienting the sensitive axis of the accelerometer along the axis of the handle, perpendicular or parallel to the plane of motion. Signals were fed into a charge amplifier before being displayed on an oscilloscope. Selected signals were recorded from the oscilloscope by a digital plotter.

Efforts to obtain frequency spectra were unsuccessful because the sampling time of the real time analyzer was, for the desired frequency range, longer than the duration of the signal. Spectra recorded under these conditions would contain an input from the signal combined with a much smaller input after the signal had essentially disappeared. Because of these problems, the results are presented in the time domain rather than in the frequency domain.

The hand tools evaluated were all impact devices and, except where noted, were fitted with wooden handles. All were being used in a normal manner during collection of the data. Some, like small

254

hammers, were designed for one-handed operation; others, like axes and large sledge hammers, were designed for two-handed, over the shoulder strokes.

No effort was made to evaluate the effect on handle vibration of the different size or strength of subjects. Also, no effort was made to investigate a wide range of operating conditions.

II RESULTS AND DISCUSSION

2.1 One-Handed Tools

Peak acceleration values of about 14 000 m/s^2 were observed at the handgrip position of a 0.88 kg ball pein hammer with a 37 cm wooden handle when striking a 10 cm thick steel block (Fig. 1). The

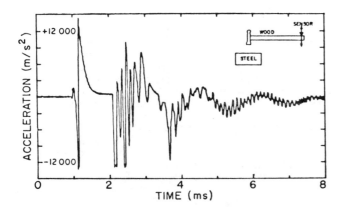

Fig. 1 Vertical component acceleration of the wooden handle of a 0.88 kg ball pein hammer striking a steel block.

manner in which the signal passes through the storage buffer allowed the instrumentation system to display the signal for about 1 ms before the blow occurred. At the moment the blow occurred, there was a large, rapid, downward and upward excursion of the acceleration signal followed in about 1 ms by a general oscillatory response. Most of the response occurred in 3 to 4 ms and consisted of a low level, high frequency signal superimposed on a low frequency wave. Striking a wooden block gave similar peak values (Fig. 2), but did not show the high frequency ringing as when striking the steel block. Substitution of a steel handle for the wooden handles caused the ringing to reappear (Fig. 3). The results in Figs. 1, 2 and 3 were observed with the sensitive axis of the accelerometer parallel to a tangent of the arc of swing (hereafter referred to as the vertical component).

The handle of a carpenter's claw hammer was observed to ring for several milliseconds (Fig. 4), after striking a 16 penny nail protruding from a wooden

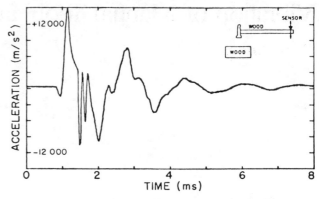

Fig. 2 Vertical component acceleration of the wooden handle of a 0.88 kg ball pein hammer striking a wood block.

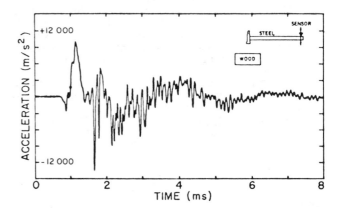

Fig. 3 Vertical component acceleration of the steel handle of a 0.88 kg ball pein hammer striking a wood block.

block. The vibration of the side of the handle, perpendicular to the plane of swing (referred to as the horizontal component), was appreciably less (Fig. 5). The acceleration along the handle (referred to as the axial component) was in turn smaller than on the side of the handle (Fig. 6 - note the change in the vertical scale). Driving a smaller six-penny nail resulted in lower levels of acceleration (Fig. 7). Compare Fig. 7 with Fig. 4 to observe the effect of nail size on the vibration of the handle.

The vertical component acceleration of the handle of a machete with a 46 cm blade was only about 1200 m/s^2 (Fig. 8), and the horizontal component about 1800 m/s^2 (Fig. 9). In both of these signals, there was a large high-frequency component.

2.2 Two-Handed Tools

In general, two-handed tools had lower vibration levels than one-handed tools.

Suggs: Vibration of manual tool handles

255

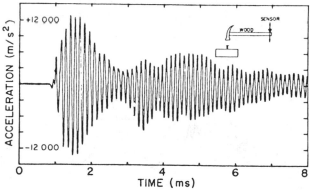

Fig. 4 Vertical component acceleration
of the wooden handle of a claw hammer
striking a 16 penny nail.

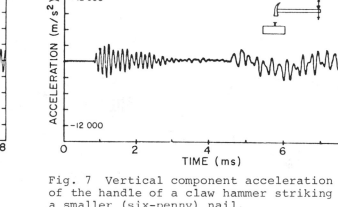

Fig. 7 Vertical component acceleration
of the handle of a claw hammer striking
a smaller (six-penny) nail.

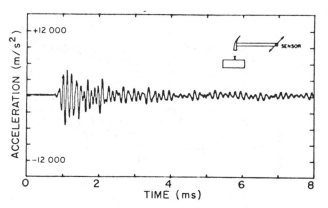

Fig. 5 Horizontal component acceleration
of the wooden handle of a claw hammer
striking a 16 penny nail.

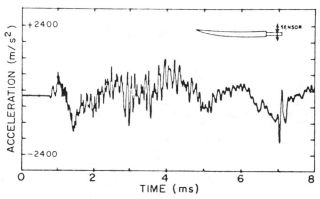

Fig. 8 Vertical component acceleration
of the handle of a machete handle striking a small tree trunk.

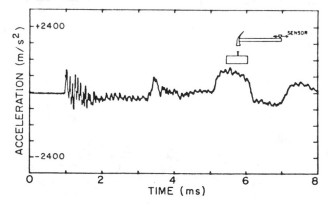

Fig. 6 Axial component acceleration
along the handle of a claw hammer
striking a 16 penny nail. (Note change
in scale.)

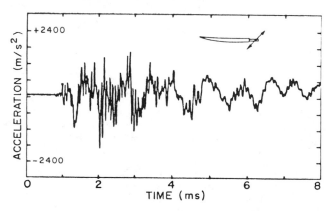

Fig. 9 Horizontal component acceleration
of a machete handle striking a small tree
trunk.

Suggs: Vibration of manual tool handles

Part of the reduction is probably associated with the longer handle, and with the fact that the two-handed tools usually engage a softer workpiece, e.g., soil or wood.

A single bit axe with a 76 cm handle had a vertical component acceleration of about 3000 m/s^2 (Fig. 10). The other two components were about one half this value.

An adz, a wood cutting tool with similar size and configuration as the mattock, had a peak handle acceleration of about 1200 m/s^2 (Fig. 12), or twice the amplitude of the mattock. This may be due to the fact that wood is harder than soil.

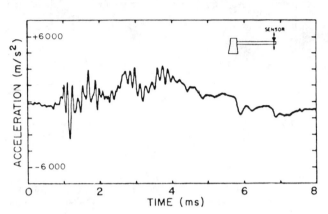

Fig. 10 Vertical component acceleration of the handle of a single bit axe striking a pine log.

The vertical component acceleration of a 5 kg sledge hammer with an 81 cm handle was about 9000 m/s^2 when driving a 6 cm diameter tube into the ground, as can be seen from Fig. 11. The horizontal and axial components were much lower. A

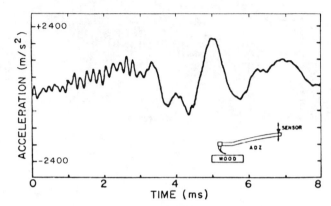

Fig. 12 Vertical component acceleration of the handle of an adz.

The peak axial acceleration of a light-weight garden hoe with a 122 cm handle was about 900 to 1200 m/s^2. The high frequency content was small and the vibration was damped out rapidly (Fig. 13). The acceleration varied with direction and hand position, but ranged between 600 and 1200 m/s^2, except for a few large excursions of the signal that occurred in the axial direction at the upper hand position.

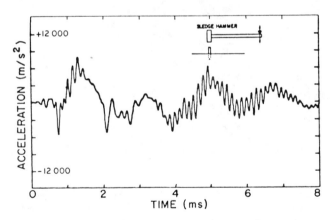

Fig. 11 Vertical component acceleration of the handle of a 5 kg two-handed, sledge hammer driving a metal stake into the ground.

mattock, which had about the same weight, handle length and configuration as the sledge hammer, had a peak acceleration of about 600 m/s^2, or 15 times smaller than the sledge hammer. The difference is believed to be due to the fact that the mattock engaged the soil rather than the metal tube struck by the sledge hammer.

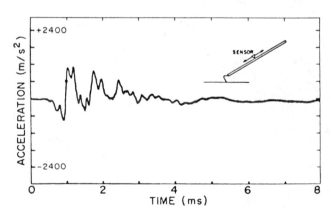

Fig. 13 Axial component acceleration of the handle of a garden hoe.

All the tools discussed so far are swung in an arc. In contrast, a post hole digger is operated vertically, in a straight line. Figure 14 shows the vibration present in the side-to-side direction at the hand-grip position, near the end of the handle, which is about 130 cm from the ground-engaging component. The ground-engaging edges are offset from the point of support,

Suggs: Vibration of manual tool handles

so that upon impact, a moment is generated in the handles in the side-to-side direction.

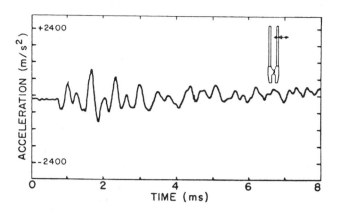

Fig. 14 Horizontal component acceleration of the handle of a post hole digger.

The impacts observed in this study were all high-intensity, short-duration events. In essentially all cases, the duration of the impact was 8 ms or less, and usually it was about 4 ms. In most cases, there was a high amplitude vibration at several thousand hertz and, in some cases, a lower frequency can also be identified. It would appear that the high frequencies could easily be isolated by means of resilient covering material on the handles. This subject will be treated elsewhere (1).

III SUMMARY AND CONCLUSIONS

Traditional hand tools such as axes, hammers, mattocks, adzes and hoes were found to generate high levels of short-duration acceleration during normal operation. Levels as high as 14 000 m/s^2 were measured and levels over 1000 m/s^2 were common. Many of these tools appear to violate the ISO hand-arm exposure guidelines for the shortest exposure duration listed, 0.5 hours (2). While much of the high-frequency component occurs at frequencies greater than 1000 Hz, which are beyond the upper frequency limit of the hand-arm vibration guideline, there is often a component at several hundred hertz sufficiently large to exceed the guidelines. The fact that the duration of each impact is only several milliseconds would, of course, allow a period of rest before the next exposure. Therefore the duration of exposure per hour of work would be small.

DISCLAIMER

The use of trade names in this publication does not imply endorsement by the North Carolina Agricultural Research Service of the products named, nor criticism of similar ones not mentioned.

REFERENCES

1. Suggs CW, Hanks JM. Resilient hand grips. In: Brammer AJ, Taylor W, eds. Vibration Effects on the Hand and Arm in Industry. New York: Wiley, 1982.
2. International Organization for Standardization. Principles for the Measurement and the Evaluation of Human Exposure to Vibration Transmitted to the Hand. Draft International Standard ISO/DIS 5349, 1979.

DISCUSSION

E.I. Auerbach: The response of the tool handle to an impact has been measured, but not the force input. Has any consideration been given to the effect of the force input on the handle vibration?
Author's Response: The author recognizes the desirability of having force measurements. However, due to the sensing devices required, force measurements were not made.

A.J. Brammer: Many workers have discussed the difficulties inherent in measuring impulsive vibrations. The problems encountered are mostly related to exciting the normal modes of vibration of the system, including those of the transducer; this can lead to overloading and non-linearities in the measurement system. I notice that Fig. 1 contains three negative peaks of equal amplitude. Could the author provide details of the transducer and its method of attachment to the handles, and comment on the possibility of overloading occurring in Fig. 1?
Author's Response: Acceleration was sensed by a Bruel & Kjaer (B&K) type 4344 piezoelectric accelerometer, amplified by a B&K charge amplifier, type 2635, and displayed by a Nicolet analyzer, model 446A. While overloading of the instrumentation was not indicated or recognized, it may have occurred. If overloading did take place, then actual acceleration levels may differ from those measured.

P.V. Pelnar: There is a machine in the shoe-making industry which hammers clamps attaching an under-sole to a mold held by the worker. The blows of 3 to 4 kg are transferred directly to the hand of the worker by the wooden mold, approximately 4000 times during each shift. In one worker, we found an aneurysm of the superficial arterial palm arch, in which a total disruption of the elastic layer of the arterial wall was demonstrated histologically. Another worker developed varices of the dorsum of the exposed hand after operating a similar machine with 10 000 blows per shift. He also had bone changes in the thumb. We considered both cases to be due to repeated impacts attacking the larger vessels and structures (Pelnar PV. Arterial aneurysma and venous varices due to occupation. Ces Lek Ces 1943, 82: 634-638 (in Czech)).

DOSE–EFFECT RELATIONS, EXPOSURE LIMITS AND STANDARDS

Hand–Arm Vibration Standards and Dose–Effect Relationships

M. J. Griffin

ABSTRACT: Existing hand-arm vibration standards are compared and objectives of a new vibration standard are proposed. It is advocated that standards should concentrate primarily on the definition of measurement methods, and on reporting the factors causing injury and the injuries that occur. The need for improved definition of the parameters describing exposure to vibration and appearance of vibration white finger (VWF) are discussed. Data on the prevalence of VWF reported in many studies of workers occupationally exposed to vibration are then compared. The vibration levels, frequencies and exposure durations causing injury are shown. A dose-effect relationship between frequency-weighted acceleration and the probability of VWF symptoms is defined. It is concluded that standards could usefully define dose-effect relationships but should not normally specify vibration limits.

RESUME: On compare les normes existantes de vibration du système main-bras et on propose les objectifs d'une nouvelle norme sur les vibrations. Il est recommandé que la norme définisse d'abord des méthodes de mesure et de consignation des facteurs responsables des lésions, puis les lésions qui se produisent. On étudie le besoin d'améliorer la définition des paramètres qui décrivent l'exposition aux vibrations et l'apparition des doigts blancs dus à ces dernières. On compare ensuite les données sur la fréquence de cette maladie signalée dans de nombreuses études chez les personnes qui sont exposées aux vibrations au cours de leur travail. On montre les niveaux, les fréquences et les durées des vibrations qui causent des lésions. On définit une relation effet-dosage entre l'accélération pondérée en fréquence et la probabilité de l'apparition des doigts blancs dus aux vibrations. On conclut que les normes pourraient définir utilement les rapports effet-dosage, mais qu'elles ne devraient pas normalement spécifier des limites de vibrations.

INTRODUCTION

Several past, current and proposed standards present limits for vibration of the hand and arm. Although vibration limits have received most attention, they are probably neither the simplest nor the most useful objective of a standard. The specification of a limit presumes knowledge of:
a) a reliable means of measuring the vibration "dose";
b) a reliable means of measuring the "effect";
c) the relationship between "dose" and "effect"; and
d) the threshold level of an unacceptable effect.
Few standards provide adequate definitions of any of these matters.

In this paper, the possible objectives and forms of vibration standards are considered. An alternative approach is defined such that standardization is primarily applied to the measurement of vibration dose. Existing data are then used to determine a dose-effect relation that might be used to set limits for particular situations.

I VIBRATION STANDARDS

1.1 Objectives

A standard is primarily intended to encourage the use of standardized methods. The specific objectives of a standard concerned with the development of vibration injuries could involve:
a) standardized vibration measurement, analysis and vibration exposure reporting procedures;
b) standardized vibration testing procedures for specific tools;
c) standardized measurement and reporting of the effects of vibration;
d) standardized dose-effect relationships; and
e) standardized vibration limits.
These objectives could result in five types of standard that are interdependent - for

example, the optimum measurement procedure cannot be specified without knowledge of the relationship between vibration parameters and injury, and a vibration limit is not meaningful without a vibration measurement and test procedure. The fundamental barrier to a good standard is the lack of knowledge of the relationship between the complex vibration-related parameters and the effects they produce. Although a standard may help highlight the uncertainty, this alone is not a sufficient objective for a standard.

The desire to prevent vibration injuries has generally led to emphasis on the specification of a vibration limit. In order to avoid the implication of certain knowledge of the dose-effect relationships, it has then been necessary to define vague or ambiguous methods of assessing the vibration exposure. This unfortunate combination fails to achieve any of the five objectives specified above.

A vibration standard may be used by a variety of different groups (Table 1), all of which may require a physical method of quantifying vibration exposures. Dose-effect relationships are also desired by most, but they are meaningless without the definition of the dose measurement procedure.

Table 1. Potential Users of Vibration Standards.

Tool manufacturers

Tool users (employers and employees)

Works' Medical Officers

Health and Safety Inspectors

Legislators

Courts of Law

Epidemiological researchers

Other academic researchers

Manufacturers of vibration measurement instruments

Other Standards Committees

Vibration limits are primarily the responsibility of legislators. They require dose-effect data upon which to frame legislation indicating measures to be taken under different circumstances. Vibration limits are of limited value to any group unless they are supported by a satisfactory measurement procedure, contain a definition of the limit, and allow trade-offs between various parameters such as vibration level and exposure duration.

Not only will the standardization of vibration measurement procedures prove useful to most groups, they are a prerequisite for the provision of the other types of data. Great care, however, is required to ensure that the measurement procedure is

not entirely dependent on false assumptions about the dose-effect relationship. The following sections attempt to define the variables, compare existing vibration standards, and establish a relationship between the physical variables and the prevalence of vibration white finger.

1.2 Variables Whose Effects Should be Specified in a Vibration Measurement Standard

There are four principal groups of variables that require consideration:
a) vibration exposure variables (level, frequency etc.);
b) exposure-related variables (grip, push forces, tool weight, temperature etc.);
c) worker-related variables (health, smoking etc.); and
d) other factors that may assist injury prevention.
The vibration exposure variables are those whose effects must be specified in order to define the vibration measurement procedure. The exposure-related variables may either affect the magnitude of the measured vibration or influence the severity of its effects. The standard should state preferred ranges for these variables. The worker-related variables are those that may alter the susceptibility of an individual. The worker-related variables and those factors that may assist injury prevention will not necessarily be included in a standard solely concerned with vibration measurement.

All practical vibration measurement procedures involve averaging. The vibration standard must specify how this averaging is to be performed. If all exposures were of constant intensity, single frequency and in one direction, it might be sufficient merely to specify the relative effects of different vibration levels, frequencies, directions, and exposure durations. These effects could be specified in one or two equations or graphs. The vibration levels, frequencies, directions and exposure durations for different tools could then be simply weighted to produce an equivalent weighted level. This weighted level would be used to compare different exposures and relate the incidence of VWF to its cause.

In practice, most hand-arm vibration exposures are intermittent and vary in intensity during each exposure period. They are rarely single frequency or single axis. Therefore the standard must also specify methods for averaging different vibration levels, frequencies, directions, and exposure durations. If the standard is to provide a measurement procedure useful for those evaluating the effects of an exposure, it may also be necessary to define a procedure for averaging exposures during a working day to form a vibration "dose". Guidance on a method of accumulating exposures over a complete period of tool use (months or years) may also be valuable. Table 2 lists the variables whose effects should be made clear in a document designed to encourage standardized methods of measurement.

Table 2. Variables Whose Effects Should be Made Clear in a Standard.

Vibration level

Vibration level combinations

Vibration frequency

Vibration frequency combinations

Vibration bandwidth

Vibration direction

Vibration direction combinations

Intermittency

Vibration duration

Duration combinations

Rest periods

Daily dose

Total dose

Grip and push force

Tool weight

Temperature

1.3 Discussion

1.3.1 Comparison of Standards Presenting Vibration Limits

The evolution of various standards has been previously reviewed (1). Figure 1 shows a comparison of the limits proposed in nine different publications (2-10). (This graphical comparison should be interpreted with great care, since the standards allow different methods of assessing complex vibration and exposure duration. The levels shown are usually those applicable to single frequency vibration.) Other standards not shown in Fig. 1 have been evolved for specific tools (see, for example, Refs. 11 and 12), and in Sweden a maximum permissible vibration level (expressed in force) has been defined for chain saws (13).

A detailed consideration of the formulation of each standard in relation to the variables in Table 2 shows that none provides a complete and unambiguous measurement procedure. All of the standards presented in Fig. 1 have, in effect, defined vibration limits. In some cases, there is little or no guidance on what vibration parameter should be considered, or how it should be analysed prior to comparison with the limit. It is evident that most standards are in

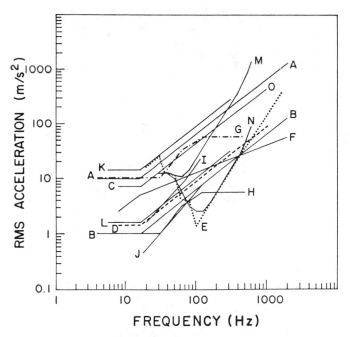

Fig. 1 Comparison of proposed vibration limits: A - BSI DD43 (1975) 150 min; B - BSI DD43 (1975) 400 min; C - ISO/DIS 5349 (1979) <30 min; D - ISO/DIS 5349 (1979) 240-480 min; E - USSR 191-55 (1955); F - USSR 626-66 (1966) & 17770-72 (1972); G - CSSR Hygiene Reg. 33 <30 min (1967); H - CSSR Hygiene Reg. 33 <120 min (1967); I - Miura (1957) 50% slight complaint; J - Miura (1957) no complaint; K - Japan Assoc. Ind. Health (1970) 10 min; L - Japan Assoc. Ind. Health (1970) 480 min; M - Axelsson (1968) occup. injury limit; N - Axelsson (1968) injury risk limit; and O - Canadian Standards Assoc. (1977) chain saws.

agreement that higher acceleration levels are permissible at higher frequencies. However, as explained elsewhere (1), this is because several are based on the same data and assumptions.

1.3.2 Alternative Formulation of Standards

The principal, current need is for the specification of a complete, and unambiguous, vibration measurement standard. This should state the principles of how to make vibration measurements at typical hand/tool interfaces. It should also define how the measures should be analysed so as to produce comparable data from different studies.

The basic standard should not present any vibration limits, since it is reasonable that these may vary with different tools, in different countries or at different times. Vibration measuring equipment manufacturers should therefore neither be required nor encouraged to construct instruments to

Griffin: Vibration standards

262

determine vibration in relation to a limit. It should be clearly recognized that the definition of a vibration limit requires both knowledge of the "dose-effect relationship" and a decision on an "acceptable" effect.

The standard must use such knowledge of dose-effect relationships as exists, in order to define the effects of the variables specified in Table 2 and the methods for averaging the variables. Clearly, knowledge is not currently sufficient to define all these effects with any precision. However, this must not lead to ambiguity in defining the measurement procedure. The uncertainty should be documented, but a clear unambiguous procedure should be defined. If both the uncertainty surrounding the method of assessing any variable is great and the consequent error is likely to be very large, the physical conditions may need to be specified in some detail.

The measurement and analysis procedure should lead to one (or a small number) of parameters which specify the vibration "dose". The desirability of additional and more detailed data about exposures should be made clear and a procedure for reporting all the principal data should be defined. This would be based on the variables specified in Table 2.

II DOSE-EFFECT DATA FOR VIBRATION WHITE FINGER

Although several hundred studies of workers with vibration-induced white finger symptoms have been reported, only in remarkably few have both the vibration conditions and their effects been documented. This section attempts to relate vibration level, and frequency, to the prevalence of VWF and the duration of vibration exposure before the onset of VWF symptoms (i.e. latency).

2.1 Vibration Level and Frequency

Figure 2 is an updated version of a graph which shows the accelerations and frequencies at which VWF has been reported (1). The compilation of this graph is impeded because few studies report the required data, and several processes produce broadband vibration which cannot be easily presented in this format. Any uncertainty in vibration level or frequency reported by the investigators responsible for the studies is marked by a rectangle. The studies concerned are listed in Table 3 (14-29).

Also shown in Fig. 2 are the 1/3 octave-band vibration limits defined in the Draft International Standard (Ref. 3). Although the data presented in Fig. 2 are not sufficient to support the limits in the Draft International Standard, they may be

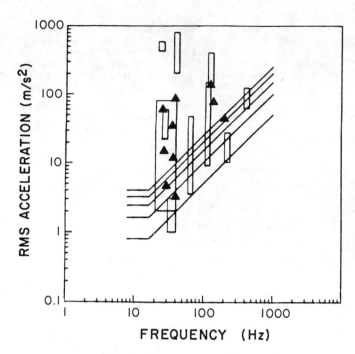

Fig. 2 Conditions causing VWF, and ISO/DIS 5349 (1979) limits.

considered to be broadly compatible. The data are not sufficient to establish whether the frequency dependence in the proposed Standard is correct and it is notable that only one report is for a frequency above 250 Hz. Similarly, the data do not allow any conclusions on the validity of the effect of exposure duration proposed in the Draft Standard.

The presentation in Fig. 2 conceals any effect of exposure duration, latent interval, tool type, and of other factors. Further, the data points come from situations where the prevalence of VWF ranged from about 5% to about 79%.

2.2 Vibration Level, Prevalence of VWF, and Latency

It has previously been suggested that there is a relation between a frequency-weighted acceleration and the latent interval before the onset of vibration white finger (30,31). Although more severe vibration may reasonably be expected to produce early onset of injury, this will only be apparent in the data if other conditions (e.g. the incidence of symptoms and method of defining latent interval) are uniform.

Figure 3 shows the weighted accelerations and latent intervals reported in thirteen studies. The frequency weighting used for the vibration levels is that from the Draft International Standard, which is shown in Fig. 4. The data in Fig. 3 are not the same as those used in Fig. 2, since the latent interval has not been reported

Griffin: Vibration standards

Table 3. Sources of Epidemiological Data.

Ref.	Author	Date	Tool/Process	VWF Prevalence	2	3	5	6	7	8
14	Peters	1946	Air Polisher	11.6%	x	x	–	x	x	x
15	Dart	1946	Rotary Burring Tool	68% (pain)	x	–	–	–	–	–
16	Miura et al.	1956	Pneumatic Drilling	5%	x	–	–	–	x	x
16	Miura et al.	1956	Pneumatic Chipping	25%	x	–	–	–	x	x
16	Miura et al.	1956	Pneumatic Drilling	10%	x	–	–	–	x	x
17	Williams & Riegert	1961	Jack-Leg Drill	11 cases	x	x	–	–	–	–
18	Malinskaya et al.	1964	Perforator Drill	24%	x	–	–	–	x	x
18	Malinskaya et al.	1964	Press & Saws	59%	x	–	–	–	x	x
18	Malinskaya et al.	1964	Electric Saws	23%	x	–	–	–	x	x
18	Malinskaya et al.	1964	Grinding	70%	x	–	–	–	x	x
19	Kakosy et al.	1970	Grinding	79%	x	–	–	–	x	x*
20	Kakosy & Szepesi	1973	Chain Saws	30%	x	–	–	–	x	x
21	Crosetti et al.	1974	Pneumatic Hammers	Unknown	x	–	–	–	–	–
22	Turtiainen	1974	Chain Saws	49%	x	x	x	x	x	x
23	Taylor & Pelmear	1975	Chain Saws	73%	x	–	–	–	x	–
23	Taylor & Pelmear	1975	Pedestal Grinding	52%	–	–	–	–	x	–
23	Taylor & Pelmear	1975	Swaging	2 cases	–	x	–	–	–	–
23	Taylor & Pelmear	1975	Pedestal Grinding	96%	–	x	x	x	–	x
23	Taylor & Pelmear	1975	Pedestal Grinding	100%	–	x	x	x	–	x
23	Taylor & Pelmear	1975	Hand Grinding	35%	–	x	x	x	–	x
23	Taylor & Pelmear	1975	Chain Saws	68%	–	–	–	x	–	–
23	Taylor & Pelmear	1975	Chain Saws	89%	–	x	x	x	–	x
23	Taylor & Pelmear	1975	Chain Saws	48%	–	x	x	x	–	x
23	Taylor & Pelmear	1975	Nobblers	46%	–	x	–	x	x	x*
23	Taylor & Pelmear	1975	Pedestal Grinding	11%	–	x	–	x	–	x
24	Koradecka	1975	Pneumatic Drill	24%	x	–	–	–	x	x
25	Jayat et al.	1977	Hammer Drills	70%	x	–	–	–	x	x
26	Robert et al.	1977	Pneumatic Drill	73%	x	x	x	x	x	x
27	Chatterjee et al.	1978	Pneumatic Drills	50%	x	x	x	x	x	x
28	Färkkilä et al.	1978	Pneumatic Hammer	87%	–	–	–	–	x	–
29	Lie	1980	Pneumatic Hammers	40%	x	–	–	–	x	x

*Not included in the regression between weighted acceleration and VWF prevalence.

in many studies, and weighted levels are known for some studies in which the dominant vibration frequency has not been reported (see Table 3). Where a range of levels has been specified, the average has been used.

It is evident from Fig. 3 that the data are very scattered. However, three points might be eliminated: those at 19 weeks and 3.5 m/s², and at 14 years and 15 m/s² both correspond to a low VWF prevalence of about 11%; that at 16.5 years and 55 m/s² rms is from a group who are known to have only used tools intermittently. For the remaining ten points, a regression between the logarithm of the weighted acceleration, V, and the logarithm of the latent interval, L, produced:

$$L = 9.34\ V^{-0.36} \qquad (1)$$

with a correlation coefficient of 0.529. The regression line shown in Fig. 3 is the more simple relation:

$$L \simeq 10/\sqrt{V} \qquad (2)$$

Considering the large scatter of the data, and the poor definition of latency, it would not be wise to attach great significance to this relation.

Figure 5 shows how the percentage prevalence of VWF varies with the latent interval and weighted acceleration. The three doubtful points mentioned previously, and two for which the percentage prevalence of VWF was not recorded, are not shown. The trend to higher weighed rms acceleration being responsible for short latent periods is no more apparent than the relation between acceleration and prevalence of VWF.

Griffin: Vibration standards

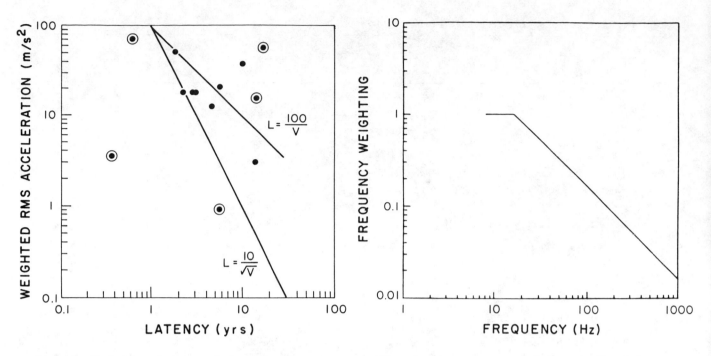

Fig. 3 Relation between latency and
weighted acceleration.

Fig. 4 Frequency weighting defined in
ISO/DIS 5349 (1979).

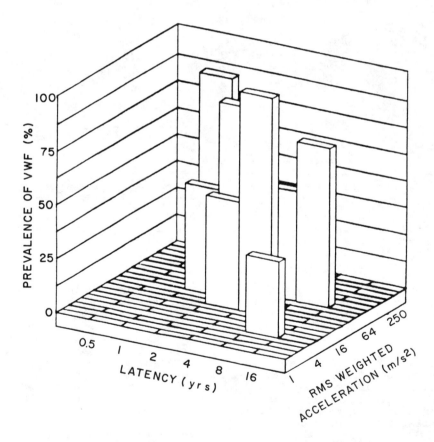

Fig. 5 Relation between weighted acceleration, latency and VWF prevalence.

Griffin: Vibration standards

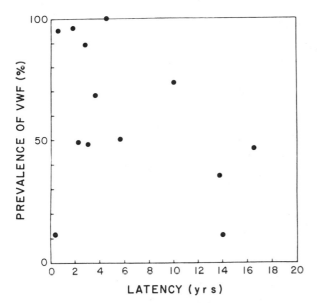

Fig. 6 Relation between latency and
prevalence of VWF.

Figure 6 shows, for more conditions, that
there is a trend in the reports towards a
reduced prevalence of VWF at longer latent
periods. The use of the term latent period
without consideration of the percentage
prevalence of VWF in the exposed group is
therefore likely to bias conclusions.

It is concluded that high weighted
vibration levels produce a high prevalence
of VWF in a short period which might be
called the latent period. Lower levels produce a lower prevalence in a longer period
which may also be called the latent interval. A more precise definition of the
latent interval is desirable.

It would be convenient to specify a
latent period corrected for the prevalence of VWF. However, this requires knowledge of the interacting relationship
between latency, prevalence of VWF and
vibration amplitude, which may be expected
to be an ogive. In the absence of sufficient data to form this relationship, it is
suggested that studies should attempt to
document prevalence as a function of exposure period, and determine the latent
interval for, say, 25%, 50% and 75% prevalence, or at least clearly specify the
percentage prevalence corresponding to the
quoted latency. (A standard means of
reporting latent intervals could encourage
the provision of adequate information, for
example, L_{50}^{1} could signify the period, in
years, before 50% develop Stage 1 symptoms.
However, in view of the widely scattered

nature of the data, it would be more beneficial to provide more complete guidance
on the reporting of latent periods.)

2.3 Vibration Level, Frequency, and
     Prevalence of VWF

Figure 7 shows the percentage prevalence of VWF corresponding to the vibration
amplitudes and frequencies of data from
twenty studies. (Figure 7 is restricted to
those studies in which sufficient information was provided for a percentage prevalence to be determined.) Again, it may be
seen that greater vibration levels produce
a higher prevalence of VWF and that data
are restricted to the vibration frequency
range from about 25 to 250 Hz. For constant
acceleration, there is some evidence of
reduced prevalence of VWF with increasing
vibration frequency. This is in general
agreement with the use of a frequency weighting which attenuates higher frequencies.

Figure 8 shows the percentage prevalence of VWF as a function of the weighted
acceleration. The curve shown was obtained
from a regression between the mean weighted
acceleration and the corresponding prevalence of VWF, using logarithmic and arcsine
transformations. The correlation coefficient of the regression for the twenty-one
data points was 0.56. The probability, P,
of VWF (in the range 0 to 1) is given by:

$$P = 0.5 (1+\sin\{22 \ln(V)-55\}) , \quad (3)$$

where V is, again, the mean weighted
acceleration.

It might be concluded from Fig. 8 that
there is a trend for pneumatic chipping-type
tools to fall below the regression line.
Any such discrepancy may be partially a
consequence of the frequency weighting, but
is more likely to be associated with either
the daily or total period of use of the
tools, or factors such as the tool grip;
rarely have these been reported.

2.4 Discussion

There are some data upon which to base
a dose-effect relationship. Vibration level,
frequency and the cumulative exposure period
are the principal factors which determine
the dose. These factors should be combined
to produce a uniform dose measurement procedure, so as to assist the collection of
additional data and subsequently improve
the definition of the dose-effect relationship. One of the principal difficulties in
the formulation of a measure of vibration
dose is the inadequate information on the
effects of daily exposure times, intermittent tool use and rest periods. This is
almost certainly one of the reasons for the
scatter apparent in the preceding figures.

All vibration measurements involve
averaging over time. Different applications

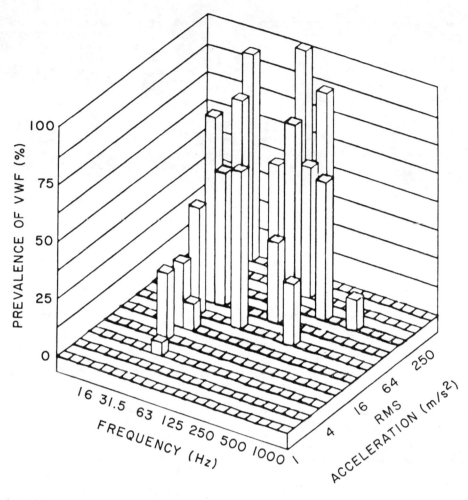

Fig. 7 Relation between acceleration, dominant vibration frequency and prevalence of VWF.

of common averaging methods can yield very different results with the intermittent operation of some tools. It is clearly desirable to encourage the collection of data and this may be assisted by the specification of a standard method of quantifying the periods of tool use and occurrence of rest periods in a vibration standard. Meanwhile, a good standard cannot be formulated without the definition of a method of time-averaging the vibration. The principal convenient method of integrating both short and long periods of vibration exposure is by means of true integration of the square of the frequency-weighted acceleration. This integrated value may then be divided by the exposure period to produce a value which, after taking the square root, might be considered to be the magnitude of the continuous acceleration that would have the same effect. For this method to be useful, it must be likely that, for example, with a halving of vibration magnitude, a four-fold increase in exposure duration will be

required to produce the same effect. It is also to be assumed that the location of rest periods is relatively unimportant, and that their benefit is also predicted by this relation between rms acceleration and time.

The preceding dose relation ($V^2 t =$ constant, where t is the time) provides for a fourfold reduction in weighted acceleration with a sixteenfold increase in exposure duration, from, say, 1/2 hour to 8 hours. In contrast, for much longer periods of time, one of the regression lines shown in Fig. 3 suggests a relationship in which a four-fold reduction in weighted acceleration results in only a doubling of the time before the onset of VWF symptoms (i.e. $L^2 V =$ constant). This relation places great emphasis on the benefits of reduced exposure time. For example, if a weighted level of 10 m/s^2 rms caused a 50% incidence after 100 days, this relation would imply the same incidence after 316 days exposure to 1 m/s^2 rms. The use of this relation for daily exposures would allow accelerations for 30 minutes

Griffin: Vibration standards

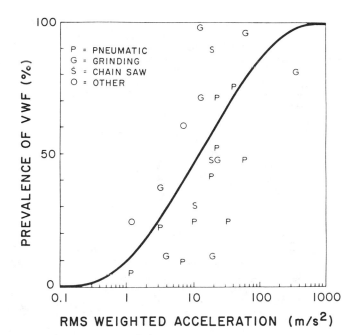

Fig. 8 Relation between weighted
acceleration and prevalence of VWF.

that are 64 times greater than those
allowed for 8 hours. Although the vibration exposure period must be important,
it seems unlikely that the vibration level
is of such low relative importance.

It thus seems doubtful whether a common
procedure can be used for accumulating doses
both during the day and over many days. It
would appear both reasonable and beneficial
to define a standard procedure for accumulating the daily dose, for example:

$$\text{equivalent daily level} = \left(T^{-1}\int_0^T a^2(t)dt\right)^{\frac{1}{2}} \quad (4)$$

where a(t) is the frequency-weighted acceleration time function and T is the daily
period during which vibration exposure may
occur. This should be accompanied by a
standard procedure for quantifying daily
exposure periods, rest periods and work
intermittency.

It will usually be necessary to assume
that the equivalent daily level is approximately similar for the same job on separate
days. There is therefore little to be
gained by standardizing the definition of a
procedure for integrating different levels
on different days. It would appear to be
sufficient to standardize separately the
method of reporting daily equivalent levels
and the method of reporting the number of
days' exposure.

III CONCLUSIONS

During the formulation of a vibration
standard, its objectives, potential users
and applications should be precisely
defined. In the absence of precise information for the formulation of a standard, it
is important to distinguish between approximation and ambiguity.

Standardization could be beneficial to
several aspects of the development of
vibration-induced white finger. Some uniformity is desirable in the measurement of
both the vibration and its effects. Guidance on the method of reporting additional
detailed information is also very desirable.
Knowledge of the dose-effect relation between
standardized measures of vibration and VWF
could be provided to assist in the formulation of limits for specific circumstances.
Without standardizing the means of measuring
vibration, quantifying the effects of vibration, and defining the dose-effect relation,
the standardization of a vibration limit is
meaningless.

REFERENCES

1. Griffin MJ. Vibration Injuries of the Hand and
    Arm: Their Occurrence and the Evolution of
    Standards and Limits. London: Her Majesty's
    Stationery Office, 1980. (Health and Safety
    Executive Research Paper 9.)
2. British Standards Institution. Draft for
    Development: Guide to the Evaluation of Expo-
    sure of the Human Hand-Arm System to Vibration.
    London: British Standards Institution, 1975.
    (publication no. DD43).
3. International Organization for Standardization.
    Principles for the Measurement and the Evalu-
    ation of Human Exposure to Vibration Transmitted
    to the Hand. Draft International Standard
    ISO/DIS 5349, 1979.
4. USSR Ministry of Health. Hygiene Regulation
    No. 191-55, 1955.
5. USSR Ministry of Health. Hygiene Regulation
    No. 626-66, 1966.
6. CSSR Ministry of Health. Health Regulation
    No. 33, 1967.
7. Miura T, Morioka M, Kimura K, Isida N. On the
    Occupational Hazards by Vibrating Tools (Report
    III). Tokyo: The Inst for Science of Labour,
    1957. Report of the Inst for Science of Labour
    no. 52-12-23).
8. Subcommittee on hazards from local vibration.
    Jpn J Ind Health 1970; 12: 198-203.
9. Axelsson SA. Analysis of Vibrations in Power
    Saws. Stockholm: Royal College of Forestry,
    1968. (Studia Forestalia Suecica no. 59).
10. Canadian Standards Association. Chain Saws.
    Toronto: Canadian Standards Association, 1977.
    (CAN 3-Z62.1-M77).
11. Bulgarian Standard. Pneumatic Equipment. Hand
    Tools Norms of Vibration. BDS 11141-73; 1974.
12. International Organization for Standardization.
    Chain Saws - Measurement of Hand-Transmitted
    Vibration. Draft Proposal ISO/DP 7505, 1980.

13. Axelsson SA. Progress in solving the problems of hand-arm vibration for chain saw operators in Sweden, 1967 to date. In: Wasserman DE, Taylor W, Curry MG, eds. Proc of the Int Occup Hand-Arm Vibration Conf. Cincinnati, OH: Dept of Health and Human Services, 1977. (NIOSH publication no. 77-170): 218-224.

14. Peters FM. A disease resulting from the use of pneumatic tools. Occup Med 1946; 1: 55-66.

15. Dart EE. Effects of high speed vibrating tools on operators engaged in the airplane industry. Occup Med 1946; 1: 515-550.

16. Miura T, Morioka M, Kimura K. On the Occupational Hazards by Vibrating Tools. Tokyo: The Inst for Science of Labour, 1956. (Report of the Inst of Science of Labour no. 50-7-10).

17. Williams N, Rieqert AL. Raynaud's phenomenon of occupational origin in uranium miners. Occup Health Rev 1961; 13: 3-8.

18. Malinskaya NN, Filin AP, Shkarinov LN. Problems of occupational hygiene in operating mechanized tools. Vestnik Academy of Medical Science (USSR) 1964; 19: 31-36.

19. Kakosy T, Roazsahegyi I, Soos G. Occupational vasoneurosis in medical instrument grinders. Int Arch Arbeitsmed 1970; 26: 145-156.

20. Kakosy T, Szepesi L. Effects of vibration exposure on the localization of Raynaud's phenomenon in chain saw operators. Work Environ Health 1973; 10: 134-139.

21. Crosetti L, Casalone E, Meda E. An Ergonomic Evaluation of Several Modified Pneumatic Hammers. Brussels: European Coal and Steel Community, 1974. (Technical Report no. 16. Community Ergonomic Research Doc. no. 1522/74 e RCE).

22. Turtiainen K. Chain saw operators' opinions of chain saw vibration. A questionnaire study. Work Environ Health 1974; 11: 132-135.

23. In: Taylor W, Pelmear PL, eds. Vibration White Finger in Industry. London: Academic Press, 1975.

24. Koradecka D. Peripheral blood circulation under the influence of occupational exposure to hand-arm transmitted vibration. In: Wasserman DE, Taylor W, Curry MG, eds. Proc of the Int Occup Hand-Arm Vibration Conf. Cincinnati, OH: Dept of Health and Human Services, 1977. (NIOSH publication no. 77-170): 21-36.

25. Jayat R, Roure L, Bitsch J, Robert J, Mereau P, Cavelier C, Chameaud J. Vascular and nervous disorders caused by the vibration of hammer drills. Paris: Institut National de Recherche et de Sécurité, 1977. (Cahiers de notes Documentaries no. 87 2e Trimestre, Note 1059-87-77): 205-218. (in French).

26. Robert J, Mereau P, Cavelier C, Chameaud J, Albi M, Vera J-C, Toamain J-P. Occupational angio-neurotic disorders induced by the vibrations of manual tools. Survey in miners using pneumatic drills. Arch Mal Prof 1977; 38: 437-455. (in French).

27. Chatterjee DS, Petrie A, Taylor W. Prevalence of vibration induced white finger in fluorspar mines in Weardale. Br J Ind Med 1978; 35; 208-218.

28. Färkkilä M, Starck J, Hyvarinen J, Kurppa K. Vasospastic symptoms caused by asymmetrical vibration exposure of the upper extremities to a pneumatic hammer. Scand J Work Environ Health 1978; 4: 330-335.

29. Lie A. Articular Changes in Construction Workers. Oslo: Yrkeshygienisk Institut Arbeidsforskningsinstituttene, 1980. (Report HD 815/791220).

30. Taylor W, Pelmear PL, Hempstock TI, Kitchener R. Correlation of epidemiological data and measured vibration. In: Taylor W, Pelmear PL, eds. Vibration White Finger in Industry. London: Academic Press, 1975: 123-134.

31. Brammer AJ. Chain Saw Vibration: Its Measurement, Hazard and Control. Ottawa: National Research Council of Canada, 1978. (Report NRC 18803/APS-599).

DISCUSSION

T. Miwa: To determine the vibration "dose", it is desirable to measure both the vibration entering the hand and the grip and/or push forces rather than the vibration of the machine. Could you comment on the method of measurement you consider preferable for the purposes of standardization?

Author's Response: It appears that both grip and push forces are important factors and that they should therefore be controlled during standardized vibration measurements. However it may be inappropriate to specify either the maximum or the minimum grip force for this purpose. Although various means of measuring the grip during tool use are possible, none is very convenient and further development is desirable.

W. Taylor: It is difficult to base a standard, or dose-effect relationship, on the prevalence of VWF, as this can vary from 50 to 100% in the same population working with the same tool for the same working hours. For given working conditions, the prevalence depends on the vibration exposure time. Thus, workers only recently exposed to a particular process will initially present a low prevalence of VWF, but an old population with, say, 30 years exposure to the same stimulus will exhibit close to 100% prevalence. The measure which relates dose and effect in these circumstances is the latent interval for the population.

Author's Response: The prevalence of VWF and the time before onset of symptoms are not alternative measures: they are both necessary. However their measurment is rarely simple - partly because one affects the other. Ideally, a numerical relation is required between the vibration dose and its effects. The duration (e.g. years) of vibration exposure may be incorporated into the measure of dose while both the severity of symptoms and their percentage incidence should be the measure of the effects of the vibration. It has been common to obtain the mean of this time for these persons and call this the latent interval of all the vibration exposed. Unfortunately this convenient measure is necessarily dependent on the rate of incidence of symptoms among the population. Like a simple measure of prevalence of symptoms, mean latency is also dependent on the rate at which new persons join and leave the vibration-exposed population.

Griffin: Vibration standards

Development of the Vibration Syndrome Among Chain Sawyers in Relation to Their Total Operating Time

K. Miyashita, S. Shiomi, N. Itoh,
T. Kasamatsu and H. Iwata

ABSTRACT: A dose-response relationship for the Vibration Syndrome has been established for chain sawyers, by correlating various symptoms with the total saw operating time (TOT). A population of 266 sawyers was classified into four groups according to their TOT, as determined from a questionnaire. A group of 46 forestry workers not using chain saws was used as controls. Sawyers with less than 2000 h TOT generally possessed symptoms confined to tingling, numbness or pain. Those with exposures of from 2000 to 5000 h experienced not only peripheral nerve and/or circulatory disturbances but also muscle, bone and joint symptoms. Sawyers with vibration exposures from 5000 to 8000 h showed a further progression of the Syndrome. Those with TOT in excess of 8000 h suffered functional and organic changes caused by vibration. The prevalence of Raynaud's Phenomenon had increased to 50% and there was damage to bones and joints.

RESUME: Une relation réaction-dosage a été établie en ce qui concerne le syndrome des vibrations, pour les utilisateurs de tronçonneuses. Cette relation fait un lien entre les divers symptômes et le temps total d'utilisation de la scie (TOT). Deux-cents soixante-six (266) utilisateurs de tronçonneuses ont été classés en quatre groupes selon leur TOT, lequel a été déterminé à l'aide d'un questionnaire. Quarante-six (46) travailleurs forestiers n'utilisant pas de tronçonneuses faisaient office de groupe témoin. Les scieurs comptant moins de 2000 h de TOT présentaient généralement des symptômes qui se limitaient à des fourmillements, à un engourdissement ou à une douleur. Pour des TOT variant de 2000 à 5000 h, il y avait des cas de troubles nerveux ou circulatoires périphériques avec également des symptômes frappant les muscles, les os et les articulations. Le syndrome était plus avancé chez les scieurs exposés aux vibrations de 5000 à 8000 h. Les scieurs ayant des TOT supérieurs à 8000 h souffraient de modifications fonctionnelles ou organiques dues aux vibrations. La prévalence du Phénomène de Raynaud avait augmenté à 50% et il y avait également dommage aux os et articulations.

INTRODUCTION

Several papers investigating the frequency and severity of the Vibration Syndrome in population groups whose members operate vibrating tools have been published by, among others, Taylor (1,2) and Pyykkö et al. (3), who have proposed criteria for the diagnosis of vibration-induced white finger (VWF). These epidemiological and clinical investigations indicated increasing severity of VWF with increasing vibration exposure times. Apart from this early work, there is little evidence of a dose-response relationship for the Vibration Syndrome (2-4). In an attempt to establish a correlation between the severity of the Vibration Syndrome and the hand-tool operating time, we have studied the Syndrome in a population of chain saw workers.

I SUBJECTS AND METHODS

Over 2000 forestry workers in the South Kinki area near Osaka, Japan, were contacted by questionnaire concerning symptoms of the Vibration Syndrome. From these, 266 subjects occupationally exposed to chain saw vibration were selected, together with 46 controls who were forestry workers, never exposed to vibration. All subjects were male and ranged from 40 to 59 years of age. The field study was carried out from 1975 to 1979.

The vibration exposure time for each individual was determined by calculating the total chain saw operating time (TOT) from each occupational history, using the following product: chain saw operating hours per day × days per year × years. The TOT was considered to be a better parameter for the assessment of vibration exposure time than the number of years of saw usage or the time of employment, because the duration of saw operation per day and the number of days of operation per year varied among the sawyers.

Subjects were classified according to the TOT into five groups as follows: Group A: control group never exposed to vibration (N=46); Group B: operators with less than 2000 h exposure (N=39); Group C: operators with 2000 to 5000 h exposure (N=76); Group D: operators with 5000 to 8000 h exposure (N=51); and Group E: operators with 8000 h exposure (N=100). Table 1 summarizes the mean age and mean chain saw usage in years for each group. Figure 1 shows the correlation between chain saw usage expressed in years and TOT, which was found to be significant (r=0.627, p<0.005).

Table 1. Age and Chain Saw Usage, Expressed in Years, of the Subjects Classified into Groups According to the Total Operating Time of Chain Saws (TOT) (Mean ± SD).

Group	N	TOT (h)	Chain Saw Usage (yrs)		Age (yrs)	
A	46	0	0		49.8 ±	5.3
B	39	0-2000	5.8	3.2	47.9 ±	8.9
C	76	2000-5000	8.6	3.5	47.6 ±	7.2
D	51	5000-8000	9.4	4.8	45.4 ±	11.7
E	100	8000-	12.6	5.5	47.5 ±	8.1

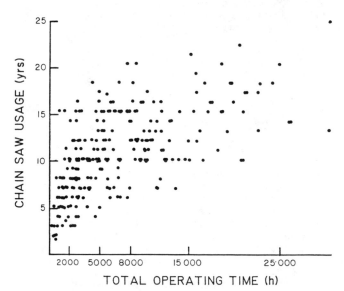

Fig. 1 Relation between the number of years using chain saws and the total operating time reported by 266 subjects.

The relationship between the severity of the Vibration Syndrome and the TOT was determined by calculating the prevalence of subjective symptoms and abnormal findings in each group at the time of the medical examination. The signs and symptoms included circulatory and sensory disturbances of the fingers, damage to muscles and joints, and symptoms of mental and physical exhaustion. The prevalence of symptoms and findings in each group were then statistically compared.

II RESULTS

2.1 Circulatory Disturbances of Fingers

Figure 2 shows the prevalence of subjective symptoms and abnormal findings in the peripheral circulation function tests. Raynaud's Phenomenon, one of the most typical symptoms found in the Vibration

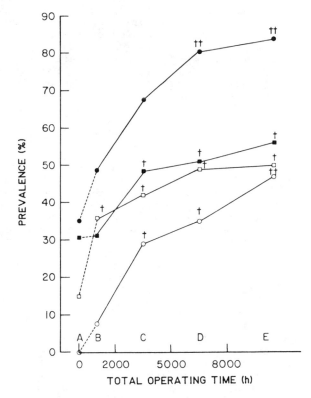

Fig. 2 Prevalence of subjective symptoms of, and clinical findings on, circulatory disturbances of the fingers, expressed in terms of the total operating time: solid circles, numbness or tingling of the hand; open circles, Raynaud's Phenomenon; solid squares, delayed recovery of finger skin temperature (below 45%); and open squares, prolonged reactive hyperemia time of the nail (over 3 s). Prevalences significantly different from those of Group A are shown by †, and from those of Group C by †† (p<0.05).

Miyashita et al.: Chain saw use time

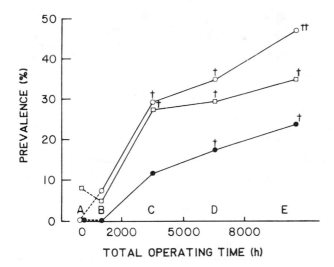

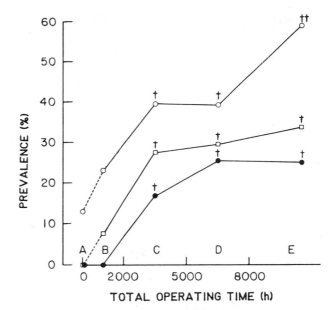

Fig. 3 Prevalence of Raynaud's Phenomenon and abnormal findings in two circulatory function tests, expressed in
terms of the total operating time:
open circles, Raynaud's Phenomenon; open
squares, delayed recovery of finger skin
temperature with prolonged reactive
hyperemia time of the nail; and solid
circles, Raynaud's Phenomenon with delayed recovery of finger skin temperature and prolonged reactive hyperemia
time of the nail. Prevalences significantly different from those of Group A
are shown by †, and from those of Group
C by †† (p<0.05).

Fig. 4 Prevalence of loss of vibratory
sense and loss of pain, expressed in
terms of the total operating time:
open circles, loss of vibratory sense
(over 10 dB at 125Hz); open squares,
loss of pain sense (over 3 g); and
closed circles, loss of both vibratory
and pain sense. Prevalences significantly different from those of Group A
are shown by †, and from those of Group
C by †† (p<0.05).

Syndrome, was more frequently observed with
increased TOT. There were significant
differences in the prevalence of Raynaud's
Phenomenon between Groups A and C, and between Groups C and E (p<0.05). An increase
in prevalence occurred at 2000 h exposure
time, with a marked increase over 8000 h
(to 47%). Numbness or tingling of the
hand and arm occurred among 34.8% of subjects in Group A; the complaints increased
to 48.7% in Group B, to 66.9% in Group C,
to 80.3% in Group D and to 84% in Group
E. The prevalence of numbness or tingling
was significantly elevated after a total
operating time of about 2000 h.

The finger skin temperature, recovery
rate, and reactive hyperemia time after
pressing the nail, were measured to assess
peripheral circulatory function before and
after immersing the hand in cold water
(10°C) for ten minutes. The recovery rate
(in %) of the skin temperature (T_s) is
given by the equation: $100 \times T_s$ (ten minutes after immersion)$/T_s$ (before immersion).
The lower limit of normality was set at 45%,
as determined from experiments on controls.
A delayed recovery of skin temperature
(below 45%) was observed in 30.4% of

subjects in Group A, but a significant increase to 48.7 to 56% occurred in Groups C
to E (p<0.05). The reactive hyperemia time
was determined from the time required for
colour to return after pressing the subject's fingernail between the tester's
thumb and index finger for ten seconds,
immediately after cold water immersion. It
became significantly longer in all groups
compared with the controls (p<0.05).

The prevalence of abnormal findings
among chain saw operators in these two circulatory function tests was 27.6% in Group
C, 29.4% in Group D, and 35% in Group E,
all significantly different from those
found in the control group (see Fig. 3). As
is also evident from this diagram, the
prevalence of Raynaud's Phenomenon accompanied by these peripheral circulatory
abnormalities increased with TOT, by 11.8%,
17.6%, and 24% in Groups C to E, respectively. These results established a strong
correlation between the prevalence of
Raynaud's Phenomenon and the vibration exposure time.

2.2 Sensory Disturbances of Hands

Sensory disturbances due to vibration
exposure include clinical loss of vibratory

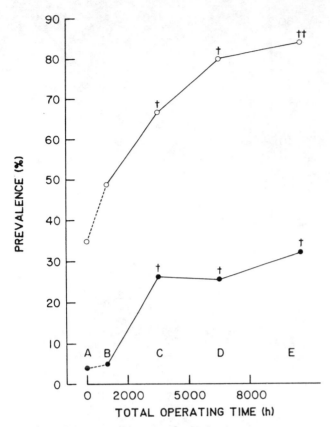

Fig. 5 Prevalence of numbness or tingling of hand (open circles) and hypesthesia of hand and arm (closed circles), expressed in terms of the total operating time. Prevalences significantly different from those of Group A are shown by †, and from those of Group C by †† (p<0.05).

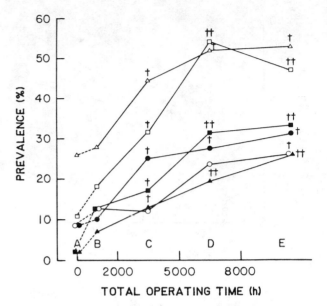

Fig. 6 Prevalence of pain in the muscles and joints of the hand and arm expressed in terms of the total operating time: solid circles, hand; open circles, wrist; solid squares, forearm; open squares, elbow; solid triangles, upper arm; and open triangles, shoulder. Prevalences significantly different from those of Group A are shown by †, and from those of Group C by †† (p<0.05).

or pain sense, and subjective numbness or hypoesthesia of hand and arm.

The vibration sense threshold was measured at 125 Hz by a vibration sensation meter (Rion, AU-02). The upper limit of normality was considered to be 10 dB, from experiments on healthy subjects. The percentage of each group with vibration sense threshold level greater than 10 dB rose significantly with TOT in all groups with more than 2000 h exposure. Differences between Group E (over 8000 h) and Group C (over 2000 h) were significant (p<0.05), as can be seen from Fig. 4.

Pain sensitivity was measured by pricking the back of the finger tip with successively graded, weighted needles (weighing from one to ten grams). The subject was asked to signify when he felt pain and the threshold was then quantitatively assessed by the weight of the needle. Loss of pain sense (over three grams) was observed more frequently in Groups C to E (TOT>2000 h) than in Groups A and B (TOT< 2000 h). The prevalence of loss of both

vibratory and pain sense was markedly increased in all groups with more than 2000 h TOT (Fig. 4).

Clinically manifest hypoesthesia of the hand and arm was observed to occur in groups with less than 2000 h exposure, but was observed more frequently in those with prolonged exposure times (Fig. 5).

2.3 Damage to Muscles and Joints

Damage to muscles and joints was determined from subjective symptoms of pain in the hand and arm, and from clinical evaluations of grip strength, disturbance of joint mobility, or muscle atrophy of the hand. Many operators subjectively complained of muscle and joint pain in the upper extremities. The prevalences of these subjective symptoms are shown in Fig. 6. The prevalences of pain in the hand, forearm, elbow, upper arm, and shoulder were significantly higher after more than 2000 h exposure to vibration (p<0.05). The prevalences of pain in the wrist, forearm, and elbow also increased significantly from 2000 h to over 5000 h exposure time (p<0.05).

A reduction in grip strength is one of the first clinical signs of muscle and joint changes, and is therefore a good parameter for evaluating muscle damage in the Vibration Syndrome. We examined not only

Table 2. Grip Strength and Sarcoplasmic Enzymes in Groups Selected According to the Total Operating Time (Mean Values ± SD).

TOT (h)	N	Grip Strength (kg)	Sarcoplasmic Enzymes		
			ALD (IU)	CPK (IU)	LDH (IU)
Controls	36	52.5 ± 6.9	3.3 ± 1	58.2 ± 14.4	287 ± 51
0-2500	28	46.5 ± 9.1*	3.5 ± 1	71.7 ± 25.6*	331 ± 47*
2500-5000	40	43.6 ± 9.6*	3.8 ± 1.5	70.2 ± 23.4*	324 ± 79*
5000-7500	25	41.8 ± 7.5*	4 ± 1.5*	75.2 ± 34.5*	339 ± 63*
7500-	41	40.1 ± 9.9*	4.3 ± 1.7*	69.6 ± 29.9*	324 ± 60*

*Compared with the controls, differences are significant at the 5% level.

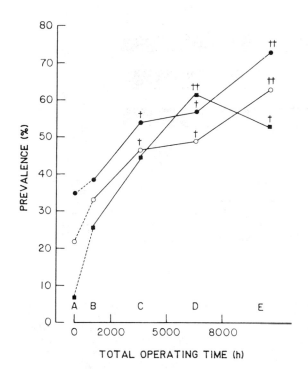

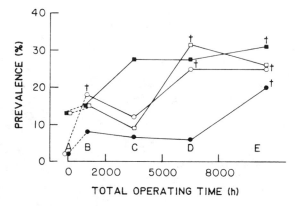

Fig. 8 Prevalence of symptoms due to autonomic nerve disorders expressed in terms of the total operating time: solid circles, vertigo; open circles, irritability; solid squares, sleeplessness; and open squares, palmar sweating. Prevalences significantly different from those of Group A are shown by † (p<0.05).

Fig. 7 Prevalence of symptoms due to physical exhaustion expressed in terms of the total operating time: solid circles, general fatigue; open circles, tiredness in the arm; and solid squares, pain in the back. Prevalences significantly different from those of Group A are shown by †, and from those of Group C by †† (p<0.05).

grip strength, but also in another field study, the sarcoplasmic enzymes of muscles including aldolase (ALD), creatine phosphokinase (CPK) and lactic dehydrogenase (LDH) (5,6). The mean values and standard deviation of these three enzymes in serum, and the grip strength are listed in Table 2 for groups defined according to the TOT. The value for ALD, CPK and LDH showed a tendency to increase with saw usage time, while the grip strength decreased. There

was a significant difference in serum enzymes of CPK and LDH between the control group and each operator group, and of ALD between the control and each group with more than 5000 h exposure. These results suggest that the muscles of the upper extremities are subclinically affected by vibration exposure of around 2000 to 2500 h.

Muscle atrophy of the hand and restriction of joint mobility in the upper extremities are not very common among chain saw operators. These signs are important, however, as they indicate organic changes due to the use of vibrating tools. The prevalence of muscle atrophy, commonly observed in the dorsal interosseous muscles, increased gradually to 7% in groups with more than 8000 h exposure time. Disturbances of the mobility of joints, more commonly observed in the elbow than other joints and affecting one third of the range of motion, occurred in about 10% of subjects in Groups B and C, from 16 to 18% in Groups D and E, and about 9% in the control group.

Miyashita et al.: Chain saw use time

Table 3. Concentrations of Urinary Catecholamines in Groups Selected According to the Total Operating Time (Mean Values ± SD).

TOT (h)	N	Age (yrs)	Adrenaline (ng/mg creatinine)	Noradrenaline (ng/mg creatinine)
Controls	21	39.2 ± 10.2	7.9 ± 3.3	33.9 ± 11.3
0- 4000	27	48 ± 5.9	20.6 ± 9.9**	40.5 ± 11.9
4000- 8000	30	47.4 ± 7.5	21.1 ± 12.5**	45.3 ± 23.1*
8000-12 000	20	45.6 ± 7	21.3 ± 10.2**	43.8 ± 16.4*
12 000-	21	45.5 ± 5.1	21.2 ± 13.7**	45.2 ± 14.7*

Compared with the controls, differences are significant:
*at the 5% level; and
**at the 0.5% level.

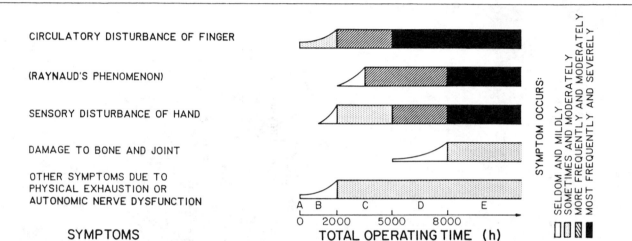

Fig. 9 Frequency and severity of each symptom of the Vibration Syndrome in chain sawyers expressed as a function of the total operating time (TOT).

2.4 General Symptoms Due to Physical and Mental Exhaustion

Chain saw operators suffering from the Vibration Syndrome complain of other subjective symptoms, which are due not only to vibration exposure but also to the working environment, such as their posture, cold weather, or the noise of the chain saw. Figure 7 shows the prevalence of subjective symptoms resulting from physical exhaustion, including general fatigue, tiredness in the arm and pain in the back. These increased significantly with the increase of TOT (p<0.05). More than 50% of operators with over 8000 h experience complained of all three symptoms. The prevalence of vertigo, irritability, sleeplessness or palmar sweating, considered to be autonomic nerve disturbances due to stress, cold weather, or noise are shown in Fig. 8. The prevalences of these symptoms were significantly higher in groups with over 5000 or 8000 h than in the control group (p<0.05).

To evaluate the effects of vibration during stress, we measured, in another field study, the hormones secreted by the adrenal medulla which is said to be a target organ of stress in the human body. Table 3 shows the average concentrations of catecholamines (adrenaline and noradrenaline) in urine, excreted at the noon hour, in relation to the TOT. The differences in urinary excretion of catecholamines between each operator group and the controls were significant (p<0.05), suggesting that increased sympatheco-adrenomedullary activity may result from use of vibrating tools (7).

III DISCUSSION AND CONCLUSIONS

It is generally recognized that the Vibration Syndrome is a disease of the bones, joints, muscles, blood vessels and nerves of the hand, arm or shoulder, and includes Raynaud's Phenomenon (1). From the evidence accumulated during the study of these symptoms for five years, we have found that they may be divided broadly into four categories: a) circulatory disturbances of the fingers; b) sensory disturbances of the hands; c) damage to muscles and joints; and d) subjective symptoms due to mental and physical exhaustion, or autonomic nerve dysfunction (4). We have investigated the prevalence of various symptoms in each of four groups, classified by total chain saw operating time, and have attempted to construct an exposure time-response relationship for the Vibration Syndrome among chain saw operators (Fig. 9). We believe that this will constitute a dose-response relationship for persons operating this power tool.

In the group operating the chain saw for less than 2000 h (Group B), the findings were characteristic of the early stage of the Syndrome and were, clinically, confined to peripheral function disorders. Symptomatology in this group was reported as tingling, numbness and pain. In a few cases, early functional peripheral circulation changes were noted, as shown by the delayed recovery rate (below 45%) of finger skin temperature ten minutes after cold water immersion (ten minutes at 10°C). There was overlap in the results of this test, however, between this vibration exposed group and the controls.

With vibration exposures of 2000 to 5000 h (Group C), the prevalence of Raynaud's Phenomenon reached 29%, compared with 7.9% in Group B. A delayed recovery rate of finger skin temperature, and/or prolonged reactive hyperemia time after pressing the nail, were observed more frequently. At the same time, peripheral nerve disturbances were observed clinically by loss of either vibratory or pain senses, or by hypoesthesia of the hands. Subjective symptoms of pain in the muscles and joints of the hand and arm increased among operators after 2000 h exposure. Not only were the peripheral circulation and nerve systems affected, but muscles, bones and joints (general body condition) were involved to some degree. Specifically, a weakness of grip strength appeared in this group, as well as an elevation of sarcoplasmic enzymes in serum (6). It might be suggested that most workers suffered from disturbance of the autonomic nervous system, from the increased prevalence of the subjective symptoms of vertigo, irritability, sleeplessness, or palmar sweating (7).

With longer exposure times of from 5000 to 8000 h (Group D), there was a steady progression of symptoms compared with those associated with exposures of from 2000 to 5000 h. Raynaud's Phenomenon occurred more frequently and more severely. Both circulatory and nerve functions were observed to deteriorate in repeated objective testing, and the prevalence of muscle disturbance, and pain in the joints and bones increased. The majority of symptoms in this group were considered to be functional changes although, in some cases, organic changes were involved, such as the

limitation of movement in the elbow or shoulders, or muscle atrophy of the hand.

In the group with operating time in excess of 8000 h (Group E), 50% of chain saw operators suffered from questionable functional or organic changes caused by vibration. The prevalence of Raynaud's Phenomenon was 50%, and the area of finger blanching now extended to the base of the finger in this group, whereas, in Group B, it was generally confined to a finger tip. Circulatory disturbances as well as nerve disturbances progressed, to give rise to a typical pathological condition seen in a severe stage of the Vibration Syndrome. Occasionally, this severe stage was combined with damage to bones and joints, evidence of further organic change. Effects on the autonomic nervous system, judged by subjective symptoms, were also evident in this group. With increasing vibration exposure time, almost 100% of chain saw operators can ultimately be expected to be affected.

REFERENCES

1. In: Taylor W, ed. The Vibration Syndrome. London: Academic Press, 1974.
2. Taylor W, Pearson J, Kell RL, Keighley GD. Vibration Syndrome in forestry commission chain saw operators. Br J Ind Med 1971; 28: 83-89.
3. Pyykkö I. The prevalence and symptoms of traumatic vasospastic disease among lumberjacks in Finland - a field study. Work Environ Health 1974; 11: 118-131.
4. Matsumoto K, Itoh N, Kasamatsu T, Iwata H. A study on subjective symptoms based on total operator time of chain saw. Jpn J Ind Health 1977; 19: 22-28. (in Japanese).
5. Kasamatsu T, Itoh N, Iwata H. Biochemical changes in serum constituents in workers operating chain saws. Wakayama Med Rep 1979; 22: 53-60.
6. Kasamatsu K, Miyashita K, Shiomi S, Itoh N, Iwata H. Relationships among sarcoplasmic enzymes in serum, muscular strength and subjective symptoms in chain saw operators. Wakayama Med Rep 1979; 22: 95-102.
7. Makarenko NA. State of the sympatho-adrenal system in patients with vibration disease. Vrach Delo 1968; 1: 94-97. (in Russian).

DISCUSSION

D.E. O'Connor: Do you know the vibration levels of the saws, which can then be correlated with your total chain saw operating time (TOT)?
Authors' Response: No.

I. Pyykkö: We have, for several years, measured vibration detection threshold values from vibration-exposed and non-exposed lumberjacks. We have not been able to show any significant differences between subjects with VWF, and control subjects, or subjects with other components of the Vibration

Syndrome. In your paper, you mentioned that during exposure to vibration, the vibration threshold deteriorated. Could this deterioration be dependent upon ageing of the subjects, or from thickening of the skin of the fingerpad? How did you control these factors and who served as your control subjects?

Authors' Response: Public service workers served as control subjects. They were engaged in the maintenance of roads but did not operate any power-driven vibrating tools. In order to eliminate the effect of ageing, we used all subjects (controls and operators) in one age group from 40 to 59 years of age in this study. The skin of the fingerpad was observed, both in controls and saw operators. There was no difference found in skin thickness.

We suspect that the deterioration of the vibration threshold of the finger in the operator group may be caused by the effects of vibration exposure.

M.A. Färkkilä: What was the time interval of the blood sample taken for the CPK enzyme? This enzyme is quickly lost from the circulation and is elevated by all kinds of mechanical trauma.

Authors' Response: The blood sample was obtained from workers before work (about 09:00 h). We considered that elevated CPK values reflect the muscle changes at that sampling time, but the time-course of CPK activity has not been investigated. However, we excluded the subjects with trauma (e.g. fractures).

Dose–Response Relation for the Vibration Syndrome

Y. Tominaga

ABSTRACT: The dose-response relation for vibration-induced diseases was studied in groups of workers using tools with similar vibration spectra. The development of symptoms was expressed by an index and studied as a function of the total operating time of the tool. The most severe effects were found in workers using air hammers and rock drills. Sand rammers, though considered equally hazardous when evaluated according to the guidelines in the proposed international standard ISO/DIS 5349, were less frequently associated with symptoms of the Vibration Syndrome. It is suggested that the ISO guidelines may overestimate the hazardous effects of exposure at low frequencies.

RESUME: On a étudié la relation dose-réaction, dans le contexte des syndromes dues aux vibrations, chez des groupes d'ouvriers dont les outils produisent une gamme de vibrations semblable. L'apparition des symptômes, exprimée par un indice, a été étudiée en fonction du temps d'utilisation de l'outil. Les effets les plus graves ont été notés chez les ouvriers qui utilisaient un marteau pneumatique ou une perforatrice. Chez les utilisateurs de compacteurs de sable, les symptômes étaient moins fréquents, bien que cet outil soit considéré comme aussi dangereux que les deux premiers dans les directives du projet de norme internationale ISO/DIS 5349. On pense que les effets nocifs des basses fréquences sont surestimés dans cette norme.

INTRODUCTION

In the term "dose-response", "dose" includes many factors: the waveform, the vibration spectrum, the total exposure time (TOT) and the work cycle. At present, we do not have enough knowledge or information to evaluate properly the above factors. But for the same kind of hand tools, the vibration waveforms and frequency spectra are similar, and the variations occur within a certain range depending on the operation. The similarities among waveforms and frequency spectra may be an effective way in which to group vibrating tools, and to establish the relationship between exposure time and the effects on operators from each group. An attempt has been made to obtain this relationship by testing each kind of tool. Epidemological information was obtained from health examinations of about 500 workers who have used vibrating hand tools.

I METHOD

Two concepts were used in the evaluation: 1) total exposure time and 2) an index of symptoms.

By checking each operator's work history and by employing a time and motion study method along with personal monitors to measure noise and vibration, it was possible to determine the total exposure time. For example, an operator said that he had been using a vibrating tool for about one hour a day for five years, but it was found that his actual operating time was about thirty minutes per day. Generally the real exposure time was taken to be half the stated operating time, corrected where necessary by the results of the time study. These results were then compared with an index of symptoms.

After a health examination, workers were placed in one of three categories: A - not affected, B - somewhat affected, such as complaints of numbness in fingers and arms, etc., and C - greatly affected, with injury requiring medical attention. Another method of classification was to assign an index number to each operator. The index number was determined by multivariate analysis.

Figure 1 shows the relationship between the index numbers and the three categories. The graph shows that this index appears to provide an accurate picture of the operator's condition. A number over 30 was given to a subject having VWF, numbness, pain, motor disturbance in the upper limbs and reduced physiological functions. The threshold number between healthy and injured workers was about ten. This point is also the midpoint of category B.

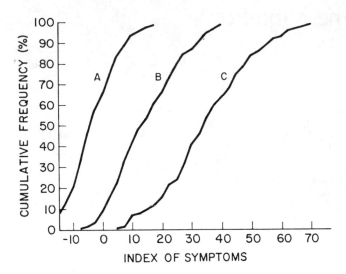

Fig. 1 Cumulative frequency of index.

II   RESULTS AND DISCUSSION

Figure 2 shows the relationship between the total exposure time and the index number in workers who have used rock drills in a mine, chipping hammers to cut stone out-of-doors or to chip metal in two

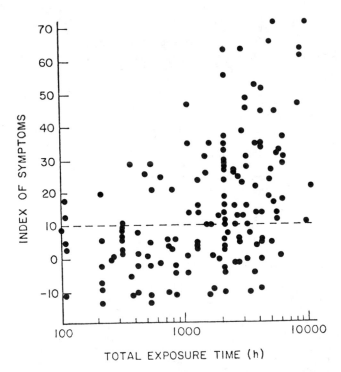

Fig. 2 Relation between total operating time and an index of symptoms for operators of rock drills, and chipping and rivetting hammers.

foundries, or rivetting hammers in a factory. After several hundred hours exposure, they reached the threshold number. The prevalence of VWF was found to be 20% of these workers at about 1000 h exposure, and 35% at about 4000 hrs.

Figure 3 shows the frequency spectrum of the vibration acceleration which was measured during actual operation at the work sites. These tools had similar vibration waveforms and frequency spectra. They possessed components from 0 to 20 dB greater than the levels proposed by the ISO for from 4 to 8 hours exposure in the middle frequency range, and from 10 to 30 dB above the line in the low frequency range (1).

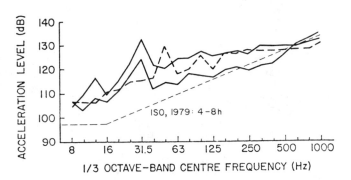

Fig. 3 Vibration spectra of tools used by workers whose symptoms are given in Fig. 2 (levels in dB re 10^{-5} m/s^2).

Figure 4 shows results for the impact wrenches. The operators tested had used wrenches and occasionally grinders. The wrenches were mostly of the small pistol type. Only one type was larger and similar to electric drills used in the home; only two workers had used this type. Each operation was of very short duration, lasting only a few seconds.

The vibration levels of these tools were from 0 to 10 dB greater than the ISO proposal in the mid-frequency range (Fig. 5). The larger type had comparatively more vibration. Two operators who had used this type of tool frequently suffered vibration damage. Larger wrenches or prolonged use of smaller impact wrenches could lead to vibration injuries.

Figure 6 shows results for hand grinders. The vibration levels, shown in Fig. 7, are from 0 to 10 dB greater than the ISO proposal in the mid-frequency range and the average operating time to reach the threshold number was 5000 hours or more.

Figures 8 and 9 show results for sand rammers in foundries. The vibration levels are high at low frequencies, being 30 dB above the ISO proposal. These levels were greater than from other kinds of tool, but the effects of vibration exposure appear to

Tominaga: Dose-response relation

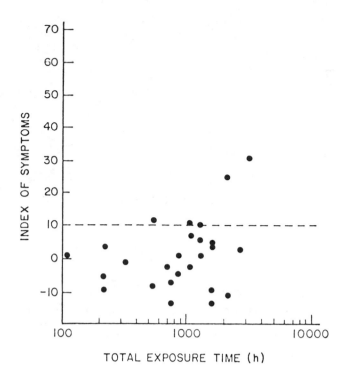

Fig. 4 Relation between total operating time and an index of symptoms for operators of impact wrenches.

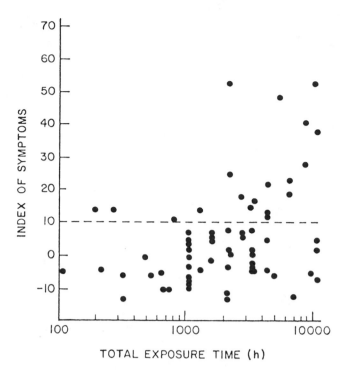

Fig. 6 Relation between total operating time and an index of symptoms for operators of hand grinders.

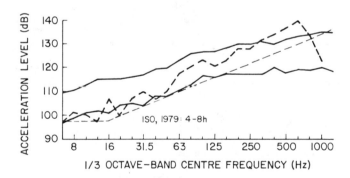

Fig. 5 Vibration spectra of tools used by workers whose symptoms are given in Fig. 4 (levels in dB re 10^{-5} m/s^2).

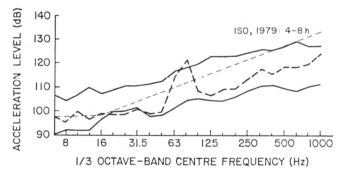

Fig. 7 Vibration spectra of tools used by workers whose symptoms are given in Fig. 6 (levels in dB re 10^{-5} m/s^2).

be less, although few workers had operated these tools for more than 1000 hours.

Epidemiological data from groups of vibrating tool operators with about 1000 h (500 to 2000 h) exposure are compared in Table 1. It can be seen that air hammers and rock drills were the most damaging tools. The percentage prevalence of VWF and motor disturbance in this group was significantly greater than for other groups. In the sand rammer group, significant effects of vibration were not found until after 2000 hrs exposure, although the

vibration of these tools was considered most harmful according to the ISO curves. In the mid-frequency range, (100 to 500 Hz) the vibration levels were smaller than those of the other tools.

In this report the conclusions are limited because the number of subjects was too small. Further investigation of the ISO recommendations is necessary to obtain a better estimate of the effects of vibration exposure, especially in the low frequency range.

Tominaga: Dose-response relation

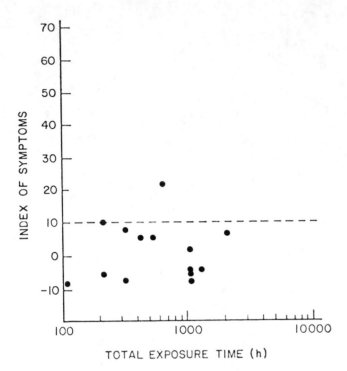

Fig. 8 Relation between total operating time and an index of symptoms
for operators of sand rammers.

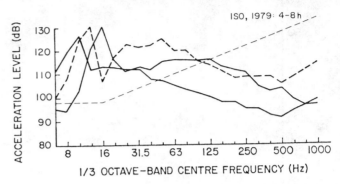

Fig. 9 Vibration spectra of tools used
by workers whose symptoms are given in
Fig. 8 (levels in dB re 10^{-5} m/s^2).

REFERENCES

1. International Organization for Standardization.
    Principles for the Measurement and the Evalu-
    ation of Human Exposure to Vibration Trans-
    mitted to the Hand. Draft International
    Standard ISO/DIS 5349, 1979.

DISCUSSION

A.J. Brammer: Could you describe in more
detail how an index number was established for each
worker?
Authors' Response: The index number gives a
weighted summation of scores for a number of symptoms
and physiological tests. The weighting coefficients
were obtained by means of discriminant analysis,
principal component analysis, and by the multivariate clustering method. The index thus represents
the severity of symptoms. This aspect of the work is
unpublished.

Could you also provide information on the
method of vibration measurement, in particular the
type of transducer, its location, the method of
mounting and the orientation of the vibration components measured?
Authors' Response: Triaxial piezoelectric
ceramic transducers (made of PZT and weighing 6 or
20 g), fixed to a small metal plate, were attached
at points near to a worker's hands by a hose clamp.
The axes were oriented according to each tool. In
most cases, one of the acceleration axes of the
transducer was oriented to the longitudinal axis of
the tool in question. In the diagrams the vibration
spectrum for the axis giving the maximum level for
the tool is shown.

D.E. O'Connor: I noticed that accelerations
of the order of 20 m/s^2 occurred at 8 Hz in the
vibration data presented. This corresponds to a
peak-to-peak displacement of about 3 cm. This
displacement seems unlikely, and suggests that the
measuring system may have gone non-linear. Did
you mount the accelerometer on a mechanical filter?

Tominaga: Dose-response relation

Table 1. Symptoms in the Upper Limbs of Operators
of Various Power Tools After 500 to 2000 Hours
Total Operating Time (expressed as a percentage of
number of subjects in each group)

	Rock Drill Chipping Hammer	Impact Wrench	Hand Grinder	Sand Rammer
White Finger Attack	17.5	0	3	0
Numbness	33.6	42.9	21.2	11.1
Pain	20	9.5	15.2	11.1
Motor Disturbance	47.5	14.3	3	0
Peripheral Circulation	17.5	9.5	12.1	0
Pain Sense	16.3	14.3	18.2	44.4
Vibro-Tactile Sense	23.8	19	18.2	22.2
Two Point Discrimination	22.5	9.5	15.2	11.2
No. of Subjects	80	21	33	9

Author's Response: The data you mentioned refer only to sand rammers which were used to pack sand in foundries. These tools are unique, having peak-to-peak displacements of from 2 to 4 cm in the frequency bands from 8 to 16 Hz. I did not use a mechanical filter during vibration measurements. The waveform did not show any pedestal effects, presumably due to the vibration being without impact. Similar values have been reported for sand rammers by other researchers.

Relations Between Vibration Exposure and the Development of the Vibration Syndrome

A. J. Brammer

ABSTRACT: Three functional relations between vibration exposure of the hand and the development of vibration-induced white finger have been derived. They are based on signs and symptoms reported by members of 40 population groups. Each group consisted of workers whose full-time occupation involved operation of a particular type of vibratory power tool or industrial process. The dose-effect relations suggest that, in these and similar population groups, the average rate of appearance of white fingers, the range of times for them to appear in individual members of a group, and their progression can all be related to the frequency-weighted, rms, component acceleration of a surface in contact with the hand.

RESUME: Trois relations fonctionnelles entre l'exposition de la main aux vibrations et l'apparition des doigts blancs dûs aux vibrations ont été dégagées. Elles sont basées sur les symptômes signalés par les membres de 40 groupes de populations. Chacun de ces groupes était composé de travailleurs à plein temps dont le travail consistait à utiliser un type quelconque d'outil électrique ou de procédé industriel vibrants. Les relations entre les doses et les effets indiquent que dans ces groupes et dans d'autres semblables, la vitesse moyenne d'apparition des doigts blancs, la gamme des durées des périodes écoulées avant l'apparition des doigts blancs chez les membres individuels d'un groupe et la progression des doigts blancs peuvent toutes être reliées à la composante de l'accélération efficace pondérée en fréquence d'une surface en contact avec la main.

INTRODUCTION

Although symptoms of the Vibration Syndrome have been documented in many occupations, particularly during the last forty years (1-3), little information has appeared on the relationship between disorders in workers and their vibration exposures. A link between the repetition rate of percussive pneumatic tools and the incidence of vibration-induced white finger (VWF) was first reported, by Hunter (4), and others. Agate and Druett, after developing a method for measuring the vibration transmitted to the hand from power tools, next suggested the range of frequencies and vibration amplitudes most likely to cause finger blanching (5). This conclusion was reached by comparing their results with those of occupational surveys performed independently by others, where power tools with similar vibration levels were presumed to have been used. The first direct link between epidemiological data and vibration exposure was provided by Miura and co-workers (6), who explored the connection between the dominant frequency of tool vibration, the corresponding vibration amplitude, and symptoms of VWF. A tentative threshold for the onset of the disorders was proposed, based on the experiences of fifty-six population groups from many industries in Japan.

Attempts to establish a threshold limit value for vibration entering the hands, though of considerable interest for establishing limits for vibration exposure, offer little information on the factors controlling the development of the disorders. A correlation between a frequency-weighted measure of vibration amplitude and the latency for finger blanching has been reported for five population groups by Taylor and co-workers (7), but the rationale for the groups selected is unclear. The possibility that the prevalence of VWF is related to the vibrational energy entering the hands has also been suggested by Lidström (8). However, data from only three population groups are available to test this hypothesis.

The purpose of the present paper is to propose functional relations between habitual exposure of the hands to vibration and the development of the early stages of the Vibration Syndrome. The analysis is wholly based on published reports of workers whose full-time occupations involved operation of vibratory power tools or industrial processes that transmitted vibration to the hands.

The general lack of data, particularly concerning the vibration exposure of population groups, and the lack of an objective test for quantifying the onset and severity of the initial disorders dictated the form of the analysis. The latter necessitated the identification of subjective reports of signs and symptoms that appeared to characterize the progression of the Syndrome. The use of retrospective, cross-sectional occupational surveys introduced the need to ensure that data from small population groups, or groups with a low prevalence of symptoms, be representative of a large population group with little influx or efflux of members. This requirement imposed the need to select data. The development of the method is described in more detail elsewhere (9).

I SELECTION OF SIGNS AND SYMPTOMS

The first signs and symptoms consistently reported in the literature are episodes of numbness, or numbness and blanching affecting part of a digit, the former preceding the latter in most, but apparently not all, occupations (10). There are comparatively few epidemiological studies linking the initial neurological symptoms in population groups to the vibration exposure. In consequence, it appears appropriate to examine the development of finger blanching.

1.1 Latent Interval for Finger Blanching

It is first necessary to establish that some sign subjectively reported by workers can be reliably related to some measure of vibration exposure. As the initial appearance of a white fingertip is remembered by most persons, the duration of employment prior to this event, that is the latent interval, has been examined for groups performing the same work with essentially the same power tool. Data for the average latent intervals reported independently by groups of forestry workers using chain saws are given in Table 1 (2,11-23). This tool was selected for study as there were many reports from lumberjacks published at about the same time, and the population groups fulfilled the requirements described above.

It is evident from Table 1 that the average latent interval reported by populations of lumberjacks is generally in the range of 4 ± 2 yrs. There is, however, one exception, the data from Norway, where the forest workers apparently did not operate power saws all day (22).

The consistency of these data has been examined using common, parametric statistical tests, as the probability of individual members of a population group developing white fingers can be expressed by a normal

Table 1. Average Latent Interval Reported in Studies of Chain Saw Operators (Data from Refs. 11-23 & 2).

Location of Population Studied	Exposure Occurred Before	Latent Interval Mean ± SD (yrs)
Australia	1969	< 6.3
Czechoslovakia	1969	> 2
Czechoslovakia	1971	∿ 5
England (Kielder)	1971	3.6
England (Thetford)	1971	2.9 ± 1.1
Finland	1969	2.2
Finland (North)	1971	3
Japan	1967	4.7 ± 1.8
Japan	1968	4.7 ± 1.8
Japan (Kyushu)	1969	3.8 ± 1.7
Japan	1970	4.2 ± 2.5
New Zealand	1971	4.5
Norway	1970	8 ± 3.9*
Scotland (Dumfries)	1971	3
Sweden	1970	> 2

*Chain saws were used for only a few hours per day and usually with long vibration-free interruptions.

distribution (9). The tests indicate that the average latent intervals listed in Table 1 do not differ significantly from each other, with the exception of data from Thetford and Norway.

It thus appears that the duration of employment involving full-time operation of a power tool is generally an acceptable measure of the rate of appearance of white fingers in population groups using essentially the same tool. The detailed nature of each operation, including the pattern of work and interruptions, and epidemiological factors, such as ethnic group, age, lifestyle and climate, appear only to modify slightly the average latent interval. Gross deviations from regular, day-long work involving exposure to vibration can be expected to modify this conclusion.

1.2 Progression of VWF

To establish whether the average duration of employment may also be used as a measure of the progression of the disorders, it is first necessary to select a classification of signs and symptoms that attempts to grade them according to severity. The classification of VWF by Stages proposed by Taylor and Pelmear appears most likely to fulfill this requirement (24). Examples of its use in studies of various population groups are shown in Fig. 1 (2,25).

Brammer: Relations

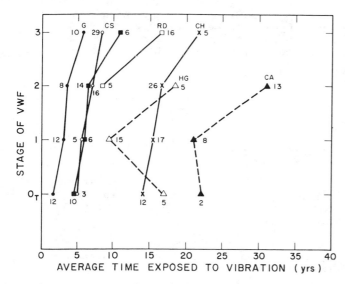

Fig. 1 Examples of the progression of VWF in population groups operating pedestal grinders (G), chain saws (CS), rock drills (RD), chipping hammers (CH), rotary hand grinders (HG) and pneumatic caulking guns (CA) (data from Ref. 2,25). The Stage of VWF is expressed by Taylor and Pelmear's classification, and is shown as a function of the average duration of exposure for the subgroup. The number of persons in the subgroup is indicated adjacent to each symbol. (The latent interval for finger blanching occurs between Stage 0_T and 1.)

It can be seen from this diagram that increasing the duration of exposure to vibration does not always result in an increased Stage of VWF (data shown by the dashed lines). The ability of the classification to separate population groups into distinct Stage-related subgroups was therefore examined statistically (9). It was found that the average time of exposure reported by persons in the Stage 3 subgroup differed from the average time reported for Stage 1, and from the latent interval for finger blanching. Accordingly, the progression of the Syndrome in population groups exposed to vibration will be analysed using two of these measures, the latent interval and Stage 3.

II DOSE-EFFECT RELATIONS

2.1 Progression of VWF in Groups Exposed to a Given Vibration Level

The rate of progression of VWF in a population group operating a particular type of power tool or industrial process can be established from the ratio of the

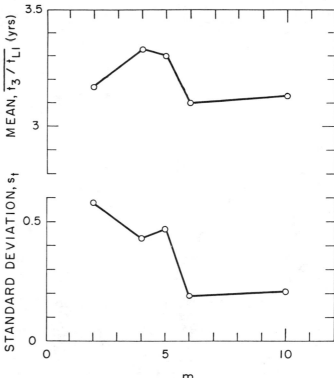

Fig. 2 Repeated calculation of the mean value of the ratios t_3/t_{LI} and its standard deviation, s_t, for all studies in which the Stage 3 subgroups consist of m, or more, persons (data from Refs. 2,25-27).

average time of exposure for persons in Stage 3 to the average latent interval, t_3/t_{LI}. This ratio can be formed without measuring the vibration entering the hands, and so can include data from epidemiological studies that omit this information. Even so, there are only eight reports published in the literature from which this ratio can be derived (2,25-27). The values range from 1.7 to 4.1, but in several studies both the numbers of people in the population group and the Stage 3 subgroup were very small, consisting in the extreme cases of eighteen and two persons, respectively.

Data from small population groups or subgroups are unlikely to be representative of a large population group exposed to vibration. It thus appears that selection rules must be devised to reject data from studies containing unrepresentative samples of vibration-exposed populations.

An example of the procedure used to determine acceptable group and subgroup sizes is shown in Fig. 2. The effect of the number of persons in the Stage 3 subgroup, N_3, on

286

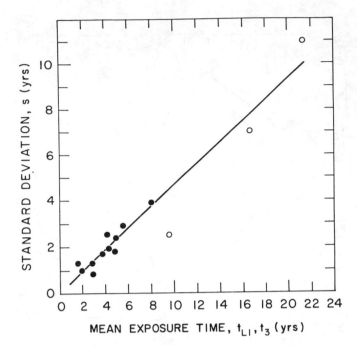

STANDARD DEVIATION, s (yrs)

MEAN EXPOSURE TIME, t_{LI}, t_3 (yrs)

Fig. 3 Range of exposure durations for the onset of selected disorders in members of a population group, expressed by the standard deviation, s, shown as a function of the average latent interval for finger blanching (closed circles), and time for Stage 3 to develop (open circles) (data from Refs. 18-20,22,25-31).

the value of t_3/t_{LI} can be found by calculating repeatedly the mean value of the ratios, $\overline{t_3/t_{LI}}$, and their standard deviation, s_t, for all studies with $N_3 > m$. The arithmetic mean gives equal weight to the value of t_3/t_{LI} from each study, and so tends to emphasize the influence of small samples. Although the changes in $\overline{t_3/t_{LI}}$ are comparatively small, the initial reduction in the standard deviation as the subgroup size (m) increases indicates that the exclusion of subgroups containing less than six persons will minimize the deviations attributable to small subgroups.

By first applying this procedure to determine the effect of group size on the consistency of the ratio t_3/t_{LI}, two selection rules can be devised:
1) All population groups must consist of at least 30 persons whose full-time occupation involves operation of a particular type of power tool or industrial process.
2) The Stage 3 subgroup must consist of at least six persons.

By applying these selection rules, it is found that:

$$\overline{t_3/t_{LI}} = 3.2 . \qquad (1)$$

The duration of exposure for Stage 3 VWF to develop in a segment of a population group thus appears to be 3.2 ± 0.2 times the average latent interval for finger blanching reported by the group. The magnitude of this ratio, which forms the first relation between exposure to vibration and the development of the Vibration Syndrome, is independent of the vibration level, and so depends only on continued operation of a particular power tool or industrial process.

2.2 Range of Latent Intervals for Persons Exposed to a Given Vibration Level

It has already been noted that the range of exposure durations prior to the first reports of a white finger tip by members of a population group follows a normal distribution. This distribution can be completely specified by its mean value, t, and standard deviation, s, so that a relation between s and t_{LI} (and/or t_3), applicable to all population groups, would express the range of times for persons with differing "susceptibility" to develop VWF. In this paper, "susceptibility" is taken to include all factors causing deviations from the mean value, and most probably involves biological differences between individuals as well as differences in hand grip, posture, tool or process operation, and productivity.

Fourteen studies have been identified that comply with the selection rules devised so far, and contain values of s and t (14, 18-20,22,25-31). These are shown in Fig. 3, where it is evident that the standard deviation increases with increasing values of t_{LI} and t_3. A least-squares straight line fit to these data gives:

$$s = 0.01 + 0.46 t , \qquad (2)$$

which implies that the rate at which signs and symptoms appear in members of a population group depends on the magnitude of the average latent interval experienced by the group. Equation 2 forms the second relation between exposure to vibration and the development of the Vibration Syndrome. Like eqn. 1, it also does not depend explicitly on the vibration level, requiring only continued operation of a given power tool or industrial process.

The gradual increase in the range of times for white fingers to appear with increasing t_{LI} (see Fig. 3) also quantifies the errors introduced by population groups in which the prevalence of finger blanching is low. To restrict the magnitude of errors from this source, it is necessary to devise selection rules for the minimum acceptable prevalence of signs and symptoms. As the membership of most population groups changes with time, it is also necessary to ensure that the duration of exposure of those members available for study is sufficient

Brammer: Relations

287

Table 2. Rules for Selecting Epidemiological Data.

For each population group:

1. The group must consist of at least 30 persons whose occupation involves full-time operation of a particular type of vibrating power tool or industrial process, at least 20 of whom must experience finger blanching.

2. The minimum prevalence of finger blanching within the group must be 50% if the latent interval is less than 6 years, and 75% if the latent interval is greater than 6 years.

3. On average, the duration of vibration exposure for group members must exceed the latent interval reported by those affected.

4. Stage 3 data must include results from at least 6 persons, and the prevalence of this Stage within the population group must be at least 15%.

5. A recognized experimental technique must be used to measure the vibration entering the hands of group members.

to provide data representative of the operation.

The complete set of rules devised for selecting data from epidemiological studies is given in Table 2 (9), and includes a provision requiring that a recognized experimental technique be used for measuring the vibration entering the hands of group members (see, for example, Ref. 32).

2.3 Relation Between Frequency-Weighted, RMS, Component Acceleration and the Latent Interval for Finger Blanching

A quantitative relation is required between the vibration transmitted to the hand by a power tool or industrial process and the rate of development of the Vibration Syndrome. As the vibration entering the hand is usually broad-band in nature, it is desirable first to reduce all vibration spectra to a single number measure corresponding to the magnitude of the stimulus. This is most readily achieved by frequency-weighting each vibration component with a function based on a contour of equinoxious frequencies - that is, a contour formed by combinations of vibration amplitudes and frequencies that represent equal risks of causing VWF.

The information from which such a contour may be derived is shown in Fig. 4. It consists of thresholds for the detection of vibration by the fingers (33); combinations of vibration amplitude and frequency judged to produce equal sensations (34); thresholds for inducing pulseless vasospasms in persons suffering from VWF (35); and a contour derived from occupational surveys, corresponding to the vibration amplitudes and frequencies at which 50% of persons

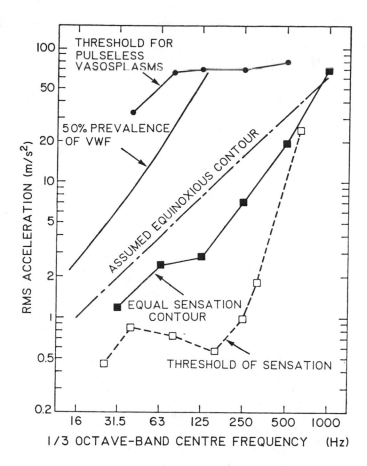

Fig. 4 Information from which to estimate vibration amplitudes at different frequencies that are equally hazardous.

reported "numbness, paleness, stiffness and chill of the fingers" (6).

Only the shape of these functions is relevant to the selection of an equinoxious contour, which, as a compromise between these alternatives, is chosen to be the dash-dot line in the frequency range shown. This is equivalent to a direct measure of the overall vibration velocity, and is identical to the contour proposed in an ISO Draft Standard (32).

There is little information on the shape of an equinoxious contour at lower frequencies, other than the equal sensation contours of Miwa (36). These suggest that the equinoxious contour corresponds to equal acceleration amplitudes rather than equal velocity amplitudes at frequencies of 16 Hz and below. As this transition is also proposed in the Draft Standard, the composite contour has been adopted for the purposes of the present work. It has been applied to the vibration component tending to cause compression rather than shear motion of flesh in contact with the stimulus entering the hand.

Brammer: Relations

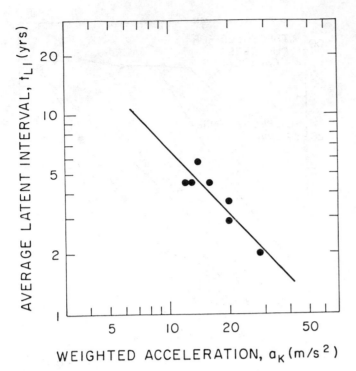

Fig. 5 Relation between the average latent interval and the frequency-weighted, rms, component acceleration for population groups whose members' full-time employment involves operating a particular power tool or industrial process (data from Refs. 2,8,21,25,28,29, 37-42).

If the selection rules in Table 2 are now applied to the thirteen epidemiological studies containing sufficient information to obtain the frequency-weighted, rms, component acceleration, a_K, and the average latent interval, only data from seven studies can effectively satisfy all the requirements. These are shown in Fig. 5 (2,8,21, 25,28,29,37-42). A simple power curve forms the least-squares best fit to these data ($r^2 = 0.82$):

$$t_{LI} = 78.7/a_K^{1.07} \quad . \qquad (3)$$

It thus appears that the average rate of appearance of white fingers in a population group whose members operate a particular type of power tool or industrial process is approximately inversely proportional to the frequency-weighted acceleration entering the hands. Equation 3 forms the third relation between exposing the hands to vibration and the development of the Vibration Syndrome.

III   DISCUSSION

The dose-effect relations derived in Section 2 are based on data from workers in various full-time occupations. In each occupation, the work involved operation of a power tool or industrial process that resulted in vibration entering the hands throughout the workday. By the very nature of every operation, however, the normal pattern of work involved intermittent exposure to vibration. (For example, power saw operators, even if they run the engine between cuts, periodically stop the engine to refuel, and to sharpen and adjust the saw chain.) Hence the dose-effect relations can be expected to apply directly to workers so exposed, that is, to persons who, near daily, nominally operate a power tool or industrial process all day long.

The exposure of each worker to vibration will change from day to day and so cannot be specified precisely. To reduce the effect of these variations, the present work has attempted to establish the average rate of appearance of white fingers in population groups from measurements of typical vibration levels entering the hands of group members (usually the X component of vibration in the coordinate system specified by the ISO). This information is contained in eqn. 3. Among the members of a group, differences in work methods, in the work performed, in holding the tool or workpiece, and in the biological susceptibility to vibration may all cause changes in the time for disorders to appear. These differences are included in the analysis through the standard deviation, s, and are expressed by eqn. 2. It is thus possible to predict the range of times for white fingers to appear in members of a population group from the vibration entering the hand, by first using eqn. 3 to estimate t_{LI} and then eqn. 2 to estimate s.

The progression of VWF within a population group to Stage 3 may now be predicted from eqn. 1. This relation, however, is unavoidably based on studies in which the prevalence of VWF differed considerably. In fact the prevalence of Stage 3 within the population groups included in the analysis ranged from 15 to 45%. It thus appears that eqn. 1 will strictly apply only to that segment of each population group most susceptible to VWF. Even so, eqn. 1 may be employed for estimates of the average rate of progression of the Syndrome, provided it is recognized that the ratio for population means may be somewhat greater than 3.2.

In addition to predicting the consequences of operating an existing vibratory power tool or industrial process, the dose-effect relations may be used to define design goals for new and improved tools and processes. The application of eqns. 1 to 3 to the prediction of tolerable exposures of the hand to vibration is reported elsewhere in this volume (43).

IV CONCLUSIONS

Three functional relations between exposing the hands to vibration and the development of VWF have been derived for members of population groups who use the same tools, or processes, to perform nominally identical work. These suggest that the average rate of appearance of common signs and symptoms, the range of times for them to appear in individual members of a group, and their progression can all be related to the frequency-weighted, rms, component acceleration of a surface in contact with the hand.

REFERENCES

1. Miura T. On the vibration syndrome in Japan due to handheld vibrating tools. J Sci Labour 1975; 51: 771-787.

2. Taylor W, Pelmear PL, Pearson JCG. Vibration-induced white finger epidemiology. In: Taylor W, Pelmear PL, eds. Vibration White Finger in Industry. London: Academic Press, 1975: 1-13.

3. Griffin MJ. Vibration Injuries of the Hand and Arm: Their Occurrence and the Evolution of Standards and Limits. London: Her Majesty's Stationery Office, 1980. (Health and Safety Executive Research Paper 9).

4. Hunter D, McLaughlin AIG, Perry KMA. Clinical effects of the use of pneumatic tools. Br J Ind Med 1945; 2: 10-16.

5. Agate JN, Druett HA. A study of portable vibrating tools in relation to the clinical effects which they produce. Br J Ind Med 1947; 4: 141-163.

6. Miura T, Morioka M, Kimura K, Akutu A. On the occupational hazards by vibrating tools: report IV. J Sci Labour 1959; 35: 760-767.

7. Taylor W, Pelmear PL, Hempstock TI, O'Connor DE, Kitchener R. Correlation of epidemiological data and the measured vibration. In: Taylor W, Pelmear PL, eds. Vibration White Finger in Industry. London: Academic Press, 1975: 123-133.

8. Lidström I-M. Vibration injury in rock drillers, chisellers, and grinders. In: Wasserman DE, Taylor W, Curry MG, eds. Proc of the Int Occup Hand-Arm Vibration Conf. Cincinnati, OH: Dept of Health and Human Services, 1977. (NIOSH publication no. 77-170): 77-83.

9. Brammer AJ. Method for predicting the development of vibration-induced white finger. J Acoust Soc Am (to appear).

10. Matsumoto T, Yamada S, Harada N. A comparative study of vibration hazards among operators of vibrating tools in certain industries. Arh Hig Rada Toksikol 1979; 30: 701-707.

11. Barnes R, Longley EO, Smith ARB, Allen JG. Vibration disease. Med J Aust 1969; 1: 901-905.

12. Huzl F, Stolarik R, Mainerova J, Jankova J, Sykora J. Damage due to vibrations when felling timber by power saws. Pracov Lek 1971; 23: 7-15. (in Czech).

13. Sevcik M, Runstukova J, Hanak L. Damage from vibrations and noise in forestry workers in the region of South Moravia. Pracov Lek 1973; 25: 244-248. (in Czech).

14. Taylor W, Kell R, Pearson J, Thomson CB. The Vibration Syndrome in a Population of Forestry Commission Chain Saw Operators in the Forest of Thetford. Dundee: Dept Social and Occup Med, Univ of Dundee, 1970. (unpublished report).

15. Turtiainen K. Chain saw operators' opinion of chain saw vibration: A questionnaire study. Work Environ Health 1974; 11: 132-135.

16. Laitinen J, Puranen J, Vuorinen P. Vibration syndrome in lumbermen (working with chain saws). JOM 1974; 16: 552-556.

17. Miura T. Historical review of vibration syndrome due to vibrating tools in Japan from 1950's to 1960's. J Sci Labour 1975; 51: 459-478.

18. Takagi S. Raynaud's phenomenon due to chain saw and chipping machine. Jpn Circ J 1968; 32: 99-110.

19. Futatsuka M. Studies on vibration hazards due to chain saw. Kumamota Med J 1969; 43: 467-524. (in Japanese)

20. Wakisaka I, Nakano A, Ando M. Raynaud's phenomenon in chain saw operators. Acta Med Kagoshima 1975; 17: 1-6.

21. Allingham PM, Firth RD. Vibration syndrome. NZ Med J 1972; 76: 317-321.

22. Hellstrom B, Lange Anderson K. Vibration injuries in Norwegian forest workers. Br J Ind Med 1972; 29: 255-263.

23. Kylin B, Lidström I-M. Vibration Disorders in Forestry Workers. Stockholm: Nat Inst of Occup Health, 1970. (Report MF 103/70).

24. Taylor W, Pelmear PL. Introduction. In: Taylor W, Pelmear PL. Vibration White Finger in Industry. London: Academic Press, 1975. XVII-XXII.

25. Chatterjee DS, Petrie A, Taylor W. Prevalence of vibration-induced white finger in fluorspar mines in Weardale. Br J Ind Med 1978; 35: 208-218.

26. Taylor W, Pelmear PL, Pearson J. Raynaud's phenomenon in forestry chain saw operators. In: Taylor W, ed. The Vibration Syndrome. London: Academic Press, 1974: 121-139.

27. Olsen N, Nielsen SL. Diagnosis of Raynaud's phenomenon in quarryman's traumatic vasospastic disease. Scand J Work Environ Health 1979; 5: 249-256.

28. Agate JN. An outbreak of cases of Raynaud's phenomenon of occupational origin. Br J Ind Med 1949; 6: 144-163.

29. Agate JN, Druett HA, Tombleson JBL. Raynaud's phenomenon in grinders of small metal castings. Br J Ind Med 1946; 3: 167-174.

30. Pyykkö I. The prevalence and symptoms of traumatic vasospastic disease among lumberjacks in Finland: a field study. Work Environ Health 1974; 11: 118-131.

31. Pyykkö I, Sairanen E, Korhonen O, Färkkilä M, Hyvärinen J. A decrease in the prevalence and severity of vibration-induced white fingers among lumberjacks in Finland. Scand J Work Environ Health 1978; 4: 246-254.

32. International Organization for Standardization. Principles for the Measurement and the Evaluation of Human Exposure to Vibration Transmitted to the Hand. Draft International Standard ISO/DIS 5349, 1979.

33. Verrillo RT. Investigation of some parameters of the cutaneous threshold for vibration. J Acoust Soc Am 1962; 34: 1768-1773.

34. Mishoe JW, Suggs CW. Hand-arm vibration, part 1: subjective response to single and multi-directional sinusoidal and non-sinusoidal excitation. J Sound Vib 1974; 35: 479-488.

35. Hyvärinen J, Pyykkö I, Sundberg S. Vibration frequencies and amplitudes in the aetiology of traumatic vasospastic disease. Lancet 1973; I: 791-794.

36. Miwa T. Evaluation methods for vibration effect, part 3: measurement of threshold and equal sensation contours on hand for vertical and horizontal sinusoidal vibrations. Ind Health (Japan) 1967; 5: 213-220.

37. Williams N, Riegert AL. Raynaud's phenomenon of occupational origin in uranium miners. U.S. Exec Committee of 13th Int Cong Occup Health, 1961 (Proc): 819-825.

38. Ashe WF, Williams N. Occupational Raynaud's II: further studies of this disorder in uranium mine workers. Arch Environ Health 1964; 9: 425-433.

39. Taylor W, Pearson JCG, Keighley GD. A longitudinal study of Raynaud's phenomenon in chain saw operators. In: Wasserman DE, Taylor W, Curry MG, eds. Proc of the Int Occup Hand-Arm Vibration Conf. Cincinnati, OH: Dept of Health and Human Services, 1977 (NIOSH publication no. 77-170): 74.

40. Hempstock TI, O'Connor DE. The measurement of hand-arm vibration. In: Taylor W, Pelmear PL, eds. Vibration White Finger in Industry. London: Academic Press, 1975: 111-122.

41. Hempstock TI, O'Connor DE. Evaluation of human exposure to hand-transmitted vibration. Appl Acoustics 1975; 8: 87-99.

42. Brammer AJ, Olson N, Piercy JE, Toole FE. Noise and vibration of chain saws. J Acoust Soc Am 1972; 51: 142.

43. Brammer AJ. Threshold limit for hand-arm vibration exposure throughout the workday. In: Brammer AJ, Taylor W, eds. Vibration Effects on the Hand and Arm in Industry. New York: Wiley, 1982.

DISCUSSION

E. Rivin: How sensitive is the correlation between weighted acceleration and latent interval to the function used to weight the vibration spectra; for example, to functions from existing national standards?

Author's Response: The sensitivity of the curve shown in Fig. 5 to the frequency-weighting function applied to vibration spectra is under investigation. The results so far have been inconclusive, partly because not all studies used in the analysis have published vibration spectra. Also, attempting to maximize the correlation coefficient using arbitrary weighting functions assumes that all deviations arise from this source, which is most unlikely. Furthermore, it ignores the information on the nature of an equinoxious contour. The frequency-weighting function adopted in many national standards is identical to that proposed by the ISO in the important mid-frequency range (from 16 to 250 Hz).

I. Pyykkö: We are generally interested in dose-response relationships for the Vibration Syndrome. Actually you, as most of us, have only considered dose-response relationships between vibration and VWF. It has not been shown that all the other components of the Syndrome, such as paresthesias of the hands and arms, and muscle fatigue, have the same dose-response relationship as VWF. It might be unsatisfactory, therefore, to develop standards based only on VWF. However, it seems likely that muscle fatigue and paresthesias of the hands and arms display much the same dose-response relationship as VWF, at least for lumberjacks operating chain saws. In view of this, should we not examine the other components of the Vibration Syndrome when determining the dose-response relationship?

Author's Response: It is indeed desirable to include all common signs and symptoms when establishing relations between exposure to vibration and the development of the Vibration Syndrome. As was mentioned in the paper, the availability of data dictated the form of the analysis. The dose-response relations do indirectly involve some other symptoms, partly through the selection of the equinoxious contour, and through Matsumoto and co-workers observations on the time of exposure prior to the onset of vascular and neurological disorders (Ref. 10). Also, the Taylor-Pelmear classification of VWF considers both neurological and vascular disorders and the effect on task performance in the later Stages.

Threshold Limit for Hand–Arm Vibration Exposure Throughout the Workday

A. J. Brammer

ABSTRACT: The dose-effect relations reported elsewhere (in: Brammer AJ, Taylor W, eds. Vibration Effects on the Hand and Arm in Industry. New York: Wiley, 1982) are extrapolated to predict the vibration level at which the duration of exposure prior to the onset of finger blanching corresponds to a working lifetime. Results are presented for selected percentiles of a cohort exposed to a given vibration level. The vibration threshold so obtained is compared with those derived from other cross-sectional and prospective studies of workers habitually exposed to hand-arm vibration. The agreement between the results suggests that the threshold limit for persons whose hands are exposed to vibration throughout the workday is in the range $1 < a_K < 2$ m/s^2, where a_K is a frequency-weighted, rms, component acceleration specified according to ISO/DIS 5349, 1979.

RESUME: Les relations dose-effet citées dans d'autres documents (dans: Brammer AJ, Taylor W, eds. Vibration Effects on the Hand and Arm in Industry. New York: Wiley, 1982) sont extrapolées pour prédire le niveau de vibration pour lequel la durée de l'exposition avant l'apparition de la maladie des doigts blancs correspond à une durée de vie de travail. Les résultats sont présentés pour des percentiles choisis d'une cohorte exposée à un niveau donné de vibrations. Le seuil de vibration ainsi obtenu est comparé à ceux dérivés d'autres analyses transversales et prospectives effectuées avec des travailleurs habituellement exposés à des vibrations du système main-bras. L'accord entre les résultats suggère que, pour les personnes dont les mains sont exposées aux vibrations pendant leur journée de travail, le seuil se situe dans la fourchette $1 < a_K < 2$ m/s^2, où a_K est une composante efficace de l'accélération pondérée en fréquence et spécifiée selon la norme ISO/DIS 5349, 1979.

INTRODUCTION

In many occupations, the transmission of vibration into the hands from a power tool or machine results in a complex of neurological, vascular and musculo-skeletal disorders known collectively as the Vibration Syndrome (1). Although these disorders have been associated with the operation of certain power tools for over sixty years (2,3), the determination of a vibration threshold below which symptoms do not occur, even after prolonged, near-daily exposure, has proved elusive. The existence of a vibration threshold was first suggested by Miura and co-workers in 1959 (4), but there have been few attempts to establish its value from epidemiological data (5).

Information concerning a vibration threshold is required, however, for the specification of design goals for power tools and industrial processes, and for the formulation of occupational health standards.

In some countries, exposure standards have already been developed for all sources of vibration transmitted to the hand (e.g. Britain, Czechoslovakia, Japan, Romania and the USSR); in others, only the vibration of selected sources, such as chain saws and pneumatic hand tools, is controlled. The vibration limits specified in these standards range in magnitude by approximately a factor of five, and, of equal importance, differ substantially as a function of frequency and duration of exposure (6).

The purpose of the present paper is to establish a tolerable vibration limit for persons whose hands are exposed to vibration throughout each workday. This limit will be defined as the vibration threshold, which, in turn, can be derived from epidemiological studies of workers whose full-time occupations involve habitual operation of a vibratory power tool or machine. A quantitative estimate of the threshold can be obtained from two types of epidemiological data:

a)   prospective studies of selected cohorts of workers; and
b)   cross-sectional, retrospective studies of population groups (of workers) who continue to perform essentially the same task with nominally identical tools or machines. In either case, the development of the initial disorders, often known as vibration-induced white finger (VWF), must have been linked in some way to the vibration exposure.

Few prospective studies satisfy this requirement, and the results of retrospective studies appear to be contradictory unless analysed by a consistent procedure. However, the dose-effect relations reported elsewhere in this volume (8) can be extrapolated to long latent intervals, that is to long durations of exposure before the first appearance of a white finger tip, in order to predict the vibration level required to delay sufficiently the onset of finger blanching. This is discussed in Section 1. The vibration threshold so derived is compared with those deduced from a comparative, retrospective survey of population groups from many occupations (4), and from a prospective study of cohorts of forest workers (7). A limit for habitual exposure of the hand to vibration is then established from the three vibration thresholds.

I   DOSE-EFFECT RELATIONS FOR LONG LATENT INTERVALS

Dose-effect relations, describing the development of VWF, have been derived from retrospective, cross-sectional studies of workers whose hands are habitually exposed to vibration during the course of their occupations (8). Two of these are applicable to the prediction of the onset of disorders. The first relates a representative, single-number measure of the vibration at a surface in contact with the hand to the mean latent interval for a population group (8):

$$t_{LI} = 78.7/a_K^{1.07} \quad . \qquad (1)$$

In this equation, a_K is a frequency-weighted, rms component of the source acceleration, measured in the coordinate system for the hand proposed by the ISO (usually the X component) (9). The second relation links the range of exposure times for the onset of episodes of finger blanching in individual members of a population group to the mean latent interval for the group. As the appearance of VWF in members of a population group appears to follow a normal distribution when expressed as a function of exposure duration, this range of exposure times is conveniently expressed by the standard deviation, s (8):

$$s = 0.01 + 0.46 \, t_{LI} \quad . \qquad (2)$$

The concept of vibration threshold in this paper implies delaying the onset of the Syndrome until after the completion of a working lifetime, as the effects of vibration exposure are cumulative (10). In terms of the dose-effect relations, this is equivalent to predicting the frequency-weighted, rms, component acceleration corresponding to a latent interval in excess of, say, 25 years. However, the relations derived in Ref. 8 are based on epidemiological studies in which the mean latent interval ranged from 2 to 5.7 years (eqn. 1) and from 1.6 to 21.5 years (eqn. 2). Extrapolation of the former to latent intervals of the order of 25 years requires confidence in the accuracy and functional form of the equation, which is dependent, in part, on the errors inherent in the epidemiological data used in its derivation. As these uncertainties are difficult to quantify, it is appropriate to extend the method for predicting the development of VWF, to include additional epidemiological data from population groups in which long latent intervals have been reported.

1.1 Method

The derivation of functional relations between exposure of the hands to vibration and the development of white fingers in Ref. 8 was dependent on the selection of

---

Table 1. Rules for Selecting Epidemiological Data.

For each population group:

1. The group must consist of at least 30 persons whose full-time occupation involves habitual operation of a particular type of vibrating power tool or industrial process, at least 20 of whom must experience episodes of finger blanching.

2. The minimum prevalence of finger blanching within the group must be 50% if the latent interval is less than six years, and 75% if the latent interval is greater than six years*.

3. On average, the duration of vibration exposure for group members must exceed the latent interval reported by those affected.

4. Stage 3 data must include results from at least six persons, and the prevalence of this Stage within the population group must be at least 15%.

5. A recognized experimental technique must be used to measure the vibration entering the hands of group members.

---

*The prevalence required when the latent interval is in excess of six years is reduced in this paper to examine the consequences of long-term vibration exposure.

Brammer: Vibration limit

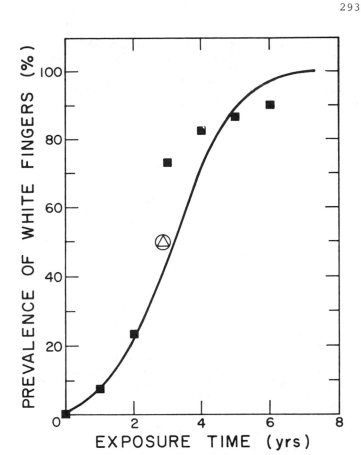

Fig. 1 Cumulative reports of the
latent interval for finger blanching
in a population group expressed as a
function of exposure duration (closed
squares), and the mean value for the
group (triangle within a circle).
Onset of finger blanching predicted
from the tool vibration is shown by
the continuous line.

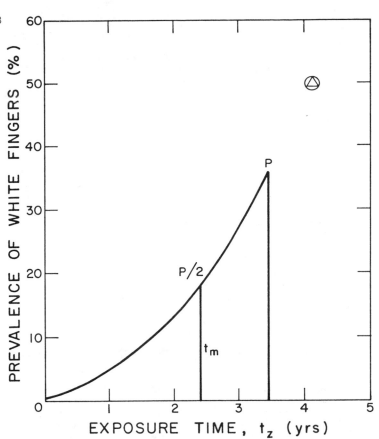

Fig. 2 Onset of white fingers predicted
as a function of exposure duration, t_z,
for a cohort with prevalence P. The
median exposure time, t_m, corresponds to
a prevalence of P/2.

epidemiological data according to the conditions listed in Table 1. These were
designed to ensure that data included in
the analyses were representative of the
effects of vibration on man. Thus, the
requirement that the prevalence of white
fingers in a population group be 75% when
the mean latent interval is in excess of
six years (Rule 2), while appropriate to
establishing the average development of VWF
in groups subject to changing personnel,
needs to be relaxed to examine the consequences of long-term exposure. This single
change to the selection rules permits data
from population groups in which the onset
of disorders commenced only after many
years exposure to be included in the
analyses, provided the tool or machine
vibration is known. The initial low prevalence of VWF in a population group exposed
to vibration is evident from Fig. 1, where
cumulative reports of the latent interval
for finger blanching (the closed squares)

are shown as a function of the duration of
exposure (11).

If it is further assumed that, with
prolonged exposure to vibration of sufficient intensity, the prevalence of VWF in a
cohort of workers ultimately reaches 100%,
then it is possible to predict the "average"
latent interval reported by a cohort with a
low prevalence of white fingers. In this
way, epidemiological data from population
groups with long latent intervals and low
prevalences of symptoms may be compared with
the extrapolated dose-effect relations.

It is first necessary to calculate the
prevalence of finger blanching in a cohort
as a function of the duration of exposure.
This is obtained from the component acceleration, by calculating the duration of exposure prior to the onset of finger blanching
in selected percentiles of the cohort, t_z,
by means of the corresponding values for the
standard normal variable, z (12):

$$t_z = t_{LI} + sz , \qquad (3)$$

with values of t_{LI} and s derived from eqns.
1 and 2. For a group in which the prevalence

Brammer: Vibration limit

Table 2. Latent Interval, Prevalence of White Fingers and Frequency-Weighted, RMS, Component Acceleration for Population Groups Rejected by Selection Rule 2 (See Table 1).

Tool/Process	Prevalence (%)	Latent Interval (yrs)	Component Acceleration a_K (m/s²)	Source (Ref.)
Hand Grinding	37	13.7	3	13,14

of white fingers is P, say, the "average" latent interval experienced by those persons affected can be most simply approximated by the median value of the predicted (truncated) prevalence curve. Thus the predicted "average" latent interval is that exposure time corresponding to a prevalence of P/2.

The calculation is illustrated in Fig. 2, where the curve shown by the continuous line was generated from the predicted mean latent interval (the triangle inside the circle) and eqns. 2 and 3. The estimated latent interval for this low-prevalence cohort is t_m, where m is the value of the normal variable corresponding to a prevalence of P/2.

1.2 Results

There are no cohort data to which the method of the preceding section can be applied. In these circumstances, there is little alternative but to consider epidemiological data from cross-sectional studies, even though persons entering and those leaving a population group during the course of exposure may significantly influence the prevalence of disorders observed. Consequently, agreement between the values reported in and predicted for cross-sectional studies can provide some confidence in the extrapolated dose-effect relations; however, disagreement between them suggests only that either a significant change in group membership occurred during the exposure, or that the method described in Section 1.1 is in error, or both.

An example of the application of the method to data from a cross-sectional study that satisfies the selection rules (Table 1), and so is believed to be representative of the development of VWF, is shown in Fig. 1. The continuous curve shows the prevalence of white fingers as a function of exposure time predicted from the observed component acceleration. The latent intervals reported by group members (the closed squares) and the mean value derived from these data (the triangle within a circle) can be seen to be in reasonable agreement with the predictions.

Epidemiological data from published cross-sectional studies rejected by the selection rules solely because of the low prevalence of white fingers (and so up to now excluded from the analyses) are listed in Table 2 (13,14). There is only one study in this category, which does contain information on the onset of disorders in a

population group with a long latent interval.

A comparison between the calculated and reported latent intervals for this population group is shown in Fig. 3. It is evident that the value of t_m predicted by the method of Section 1.1 (shown by the dashed line for P=37%) is in good agreement with the low prevalence epidemiological data (the open circle). To obtain this prediction, the relation between t_{LI} and a_K had to be extended to a component acceleration of 3 m/s², and a mean latent interval in excess of 24 years. Extrapolation of the dose-effect relations to latent intervals of this magnitude and to population segments other than 50%, without revision to their functional form, thus appears justified on the basis of the available epidemiological data.

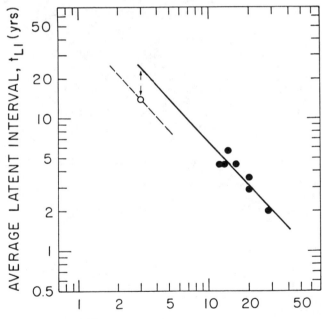

Fig. 3 Extrapolation of the dose-effect relations to predict the median latent interval for a population group with a prevalence of 37% (dashed line) compared with data from Table 2 (open circle). The data shown as filled circles were used in the derivation of eqn. 1 (continuous line) (From Ref. 8).

Table 3. Duration of Exposure Prior to the First Episode of Finger Blanching for Selected Percentiles of a Cohort Exposed to a Given Frequency-Weighted, RMS, Component Acceleration Throughout Each Workday.

Frequency-Weighted Component Acceleration a_K (m/s²)	Exposure Duration* (yrs) Population Percentile				
	10	20	30	40	50
25	-	-	-	2.2	2.5
20	-	2	2.4	2.8	3.2
15	-	2.7	3.3	3.8	4.3
12	2.3	3.4	4.2	4.9	5.5
10	2.7	4.1	5.1	5.9	6.7
8	3.5	5.2	6.5	7.5	8.5
6	4.7	7.1	8.8	10	12
5	5.8	8.6	11	12	14
4	7.3	11	14	16	18
3	10	15	18	21	24
2	15	23	28	33	-
1	32	-	-	-	-

*Durations of less than 2 yrs or in excess of 35 yrs are shown by -.

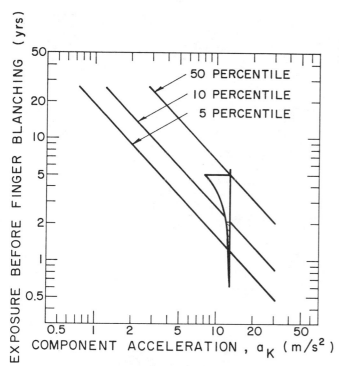

Fig. 4 Predicted duration of exposure prior to the first episode of finger blanching for selected percentiles of a cohort exposed to a given frequency-weighted, rms, component acceleration, a_K, throughout each workday.

The duration of exposure prior to the onset of episodes of finger blanching in selected percentiles of a cohort may thus be calculated with some confidence from the tool or machine vibration. Results are given in Table 3 for frequency-weighted, rms, component accelerations of from 1 to 25 m/s², and for population percentiles of from 10 to 50%. Predictions for persons with an average response to vibration corresponding to the 50 percentile, and for the 5 and 10% of persons within a cohort most susceptible to vibration are shown in Fig. 4.

It should be noted that the extreme percentiles of a distribution are most sensitive to the exact shape of the distribution curve, and so will be most influenced by errors in this function.

II ONSET OF DISORDERS

2.1 Prediction from Dose-Effect Relations

The derivation of a vibration threshold from the dose-effect relations of Section 1 is equivalent to establishing the frequency-weighted component acceleration necessary to delay the onset of finger blanching for the duration of a working lifetime. The predictions applicable to selected percentiles of a cohort, whose members' full-time employment involves habitual operation of a vibrating power tool or machine, are listed in Table 3. It is evident from these results that, at small values of the component acceleration, small changes in a_K correspond to large changes in exposure time prior to the

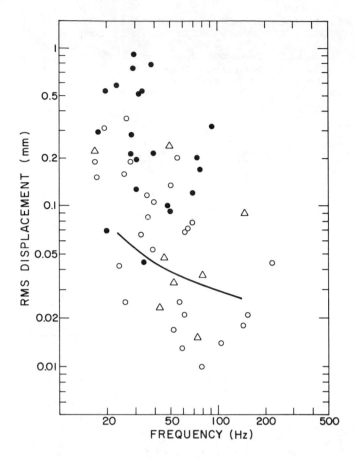

Fig. 5   RMS displacements (mm) of a range of hand-held power tools and machines, expressed as a function of the fundamental vibration frequency. Data shown by closed circles are for rock drills, air hammers, rivetting hammers, chipping hammers, a concrete breaker and a sand rammer; data shown by open circles are for hand grinders, swing grinders, hand sanders, hand drills, a chain saw and an impact wrench; data shown by triangles are for stand-mounted metal polishers and grinders. (Data from Tables 1-3 of Ref. 4).

onset of finger blanching, for all population percentiles. Hence there is little need to specify the duration of a working lifetime with great precision.

Reference to Table 3 and Fig. 4 therefore suggests that the vibration threshold lies in the range $1 < a_K < 2.9$ m/s². The upper extreme of this range corresponds to the component acceleration predicted to delay the appearance of white fingers, on average, for 25 years. The lower extreme corresponds to the component acceleration predicted to delay the appearance of white fingers for over 30 years in the 10% of the population susceptible to VWF.

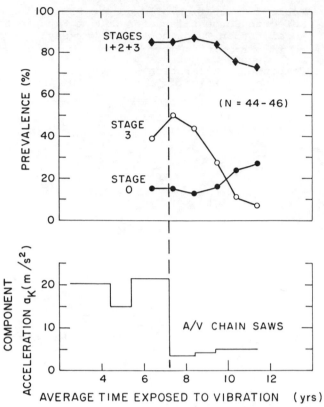

Fig. 6   Prevalence of selected VWF Stages in a prospective study of a cohort of chain saw operators (upper diagram), in which the frequency-weighted, rms, component acceleration entering the hands decreased significantly with the introduction of A/V saws (lower diagram). (Data from Ref. 7).

In the absence of a definitive relation between the development of neurological and of vascular disorders, this range will be taken to define the threshold for the onset of the Vibration Syndrome. It should be noted, however, that users of most, but apparently not all, power tools report that episodes of numbness occur prior to the first episode of finger blanching (15).

2.2   Prediction from Comparative Occupational Surveys

An extensive comparative survey of the onset of the Vibration Syndrome in working populations has been conducted in Japan (4). The prevalences of signs and symptoms reported by workers from a range of occupations were first obtained from a cross-sectional, retrospective study. The epidemiological data were then compared with measurements of the dominant vibration frequency and the corresponding displacement of each source of vibration. The results are summarized in Fig. 5, where the sources have been separated into three groups: piston-operated pneumatic tools (closed circles), portable rotary tools (open circles), and fixed rotary machines, where the operator holds the work piece (triangles). Some impression of the range of power tools, machines and occupations studied may be derived from the figure caption.

Based on these data and a knowledge of the disorders associated with prolonged operation of each tool or machine, it is possible to deduce a contour linking vibration amplitudes and frequencies with the same prevalence of symptoms. According to Miura and co-workers, the line in Fig. 5 corresponds to the vibration threshold below which no workers complained of "numbness, paleness or chill of the fingers". This contour is equivalent to values of the frequency-weighted, rms, component acceleration in the range $1 < a_K < 2.1$ m/s^2, depending on the frequency.

2.3 Prediction from Prospective Studies

There has been only one prospective study of cohorts of workers in which both the development of vibration-induced disorders and the vibration exposure have been repeatedly evaluated (7). In this annual survey of a group of forest workers, the prevalence of signs and symptoms was determined in 46 sawyers, each of whom operated the same model chain saw. The vibration of the saw model used each year was also measured. The results are shown in Fig. 6 for Stage 0 (no signs or symptoms), Stage 3 and Stages 1+2+3 VWF, in Taylor and Pelmear's classification (16). The frequency-weighted component acceleration of the saws used is shown in the lower part of the diagram.

It is evident from Fig. 6 that a significant reduction in vibration occurred after approximately seven years exposure, coincident with the introduction of saws with vibration-isolated handles. Reference to the upper part of the diagram reveals that the reduction in vibration was followed by a gradual decline in the overall prevalence of VWF (Stages 1+2+3), and a marked decline in the prevalence of Stage 3. It can thus be deduced that the vibration threshold must be below $a_K = 20$ m/s^2, though whether it lies above or below the vibration level of the A/V saws ($a_K \sim 4.7$ m/s^2) cannot be established from these data. However, a more recent survey of a second cohort from this population, whose members have only operated saws with vibration-isolated handles, has identified some cases of VWF (Taylor W, personal communication). Hence it appears that the vibration threshold must lie below a frequency-weighted component acceleration of 4.7 m/s^2.

Table 4. Threshold for the Onset of Disorders Derived by Three Methods (Expressed as a Frequency-Weighted, RMS, Component Acceleration in m/s^2).

This Study[1]	Miura and co-workers (Ref. 4)[2]	Taylor and co-workers (Ref. 7)
1 - 2.9	1 - 2.1	<4.7

[1] Onset of episodes of finger blanching delayed for the duration of a working lifetime.

[2] Value depends on the dominant vibration frequency.

III DISCUSSION

3.1 Vibration Threshold

Three methods for establishing a threshold for the onset of the Vibration Syndrome in persons whose full-time employment involves exposure of the hand to vibration throughout the workday have been described. The predictions are summarized in Table 4. Although each method has limitations, each provides an important contribution to the specification of a vibration threshold.

The dose-effect relations provide the only functional expressions linking vibration exposure to the development of VWF. These permit the frequency-weighted component acceleration, necessary to delay sufficiently the onset of finger blanching, to be calculated for any percentile of a cohort of workers performing the same task. To obtain these results, however, the dose-effect relations must be extrapolated to long latent intervals and low prevalences of symptoms. Also, the relation between the appearance of the first white finger tip and other early symptoms of the Vibration Syndrome cannot be specified precisely at the present time.

The results of the comparative, retrospective survey (column 2, Table 4) are not strictly comparable with those of other methods, as the values correspond only to the contribution to the frequency-weighted component acceleration at the dominant vibration frequency. The inclusion of contributions from other components of the vibration spectrum could increase these values somewhat, perhaps by as much as 50%. Also, it would not have been possible to obtain information pertaining to the completion of a working lifetime from active workers, and so the levels reported could well permit the onset of disorders within this period. In addition, cross-sectional studies tend to underestimate the prevalence of disorders, owing to the tendency for those suffering from VWF to withdraw from vibration exposure (i.e change employment). A correction for these two underestimates of the potential hazard of vibration exposure would lead to a reduction of the threshold given in column 2. In the absence of further information on the magnitude of these (opposing) systematic errors, no adjustment to the levels in column 2 is considered appropriate. Nevertheless, despite uncertainty concerning the precise value of the vibration threshold obtained by this method, it alone can provide a confirmed lower boundary for the onset of disorders, by including data from population groups not suffering from any symptoms of the Syndrome.

The prospective study, in contrast, provides information on the progression of disorders in a controlled population exposed to a known source of vibration. As such, it is the only method to avoid explicitly errors arising from the efflux and influx of group members during the course of exposure. Although the population is completely defined and the vibration at the hand is measured repeatedly throughout the exposure, the method can confirm only the progression or appearance of symptoms resulting from this stimulus. Hence a vibration threshold cannot be specified precisely, though the data indicate that it must lie below a_K = 4.7 m/s^2.

When considered together, the three methods provide complementary evidence for the magnitude of the vibration threshold. Thus, the possibility that the extrapolated dose-response relations are significantly in error is to a large extent eliminated by their prediction of a threshold range similar to that deduced from the comparative occupational survey. The possibility that both these methods are systematically in error by the same amount is limited for the upper boundary of the threshold by the results of the prospective study (and for the lower boundary by the comparative survey data from 15 occupations in which no symptoms were observed). It thus appears that the vibration threshold lies in the range 1 < a_K < 3.2 m/s^2, where the upper extreme

is the arithmetic mean of the results in Table 4. As both the dose-effect relations predict, and the low-prevalence data from workers using hand grinders confirm (see Table 2), long-term exposure to a component acceleration of 3 m/s^2 will lead to a substantial prevalence of VWF. A conservative estimate for the upper boundary of the vibration threshold, consistent with all the epidemiological data, would therefore be considerably less than this value.

3.2 Vibration Limit

From the preceding discussion, a vibration limit in the range 1 < a_K < 2 m/s^2 would appear to be necessary to prevent the

Table 5. Limits for Four to Eight Hours Daily Exposure to Vibration Specified in Recent ISO Proposals (Expressed as a Frequency-Weighted, RMS, Component Acceleration in m/s^2).

T* (min/h)	ISO/DIS 5349, 1979 (Ref. 9)	ISO/TC 108/SC 4 Draft 1980 (Ref. 19)
0	1.4	
< 10	1.4	
10 < T < 20	1.4	2-4
20 < T < 30	2.8	
30 < T < 40	4.2	
> 40	5.6	

*T is the recurrent time interval without vibration exposure.

onset of disorders in persons whose full-time employment involves an operation whereby vibration enters the hands throughout the workday. More precise specification of a vibration limit from the results of Section 2 is probably not justified, owing to the potential for error in each method. Even so, the limit can be defined with sufficient precision to serve as a goal for the design of new, and improved, power tools and machines. It should be noted that the vibration of many power tools and industrial processes currently exceed these values (17,18,5).

In addition to information concerning the onset of disorders, the specification of a vibration limit for the purposes of regulating occupational exposure to vibration involves socio-economic considerations beyond the scope of this paper. Vibration limits based solely on the expected adverse health effects have been developed, however, by a committee of the International Organization for Standardization. The limits were apparently derived from subjective assessments of "unpleasant" vibrations, equal sensation contours, and the transmission of vibration into the hand-arm system (6). The two most recent proposals applicable to daily exposures of from four to eight hours duration are listed in Table 5 (9,19). The presumed ameliorative effect of exposure interruptions is included in the Draft International Standard, ISO/DIS 5349, through relaxation of the limit with increased duration of the vibration-free time period per hour, T. In this proposal, the maximum relaxation of the vibration limit for intermittent exposure is a factor of five. In contrast, no adjustment for interruptions is contained in the latest ISO draft (19), which instead proposes for the vibration limit a frequency-weighted, rms, component acceleration in the range 2 < a_K < 4 m/s^2.

It is evident that only the lower extremes of the limits contained in Table 5 are compatible with the vibration limit obtained here from epidemiological studies (in which vibration entered the hands intermittently). From the discussion of Section 3.1, there is considerable evidence that habitual exposure to a component acceleration of 3 m/s^2, or more, will lead to the onset of vibration-induced disorders during the course of a working lifetime.

IV CONCLUSIONS

Three methods have been used to determine a threshold for the onset of the Vibration Syndrome from epidemiological studies of workers occupationally exposed to vibration. The broad base of data, the different methods of analysis, and the general agreement between the results suggest that the vibration threshold can be specified with some confidence to be within the range $1 < a_K < 3.2$ m/s^2, where a_K is the frequency-weighted, rms, component acceleration of a surface in contact with the hands. A conservative estimate of the threshold limit for persons whose hands are exposed to vibration throughout each workday lies in the range $1 < a_K < 2$ m/s^2. Vibration-induced disorders are not expected to result from full-time operation of a power tool or industrial process in which the hands are exposed to frequency-weighted, rms, component accelerations of these magnitudes or less.

REFERENCES

1. Pyykkö I. Vibration Syndrome: a review. In: Korhonen O, ed. Vibration and Work. Helsinki: Inst of Occup Health, 1976: 1-24.
2. Hamilton A. A study of spastic anemia in the hands of stonecutters. Washington: Government Printing Office, 1918. (Bull US Bureau of Labor Statistics, no. 236: Ind Accidents and Hygiene Series, no. 19): 53-66.
3. Rothstein T. Report of the physical findings in eight stonecutters from the limestone region of Indiana. Washington: Government Printing Office, 1918. (Bull US Bureau of Labor Statistics, no.236: Ind Accidents and Hygiene Series, no. 19): 67-96.
4. Miura T, Morioka M, Kimura K, Akutu A. On the occupational hazards by vibrating tools: report 4. J Sci Labour 1959; 35: 760-767.
5. Brammer AJ. Chain Saw Vibration: Its Measurement, Hazard and Control. Ottawa: National Research Council of Canada, 1978. (Report NRC 18803/APS-599).
6. Griffin MJ. Vibration Injuries of the Hand and Arm: Their Occurrence and the Evolution of Standards and Limits. London: Her Majesty's Stationery Office, 1980. (Health and Safety Executive Research Paper 9).
7. Taylor W, Pearson JCG, Keighley GD. A longitudinal study of Raynaud's phenomenon in chain saw operators. In: Wasserman DE, Taylor W, Curry MG, eds. Proc of the Int Occup Hand-Arm Vibration Conf. Cincinnati, OH: Dept of Health and Human Services, 1977 (NIOSH publication no. 77-170): 69-76.
8. Brammer AJ. Relations between vibration exposure and the development of the vibration syndrome. In: Brammer AJ, Taylor W, eds. Vibration Effects on the Hand and Arm in Industry. New York: Wiley, 1982.
9. International Organization for Standardization. Principles for the Measurement and the Evaluation of Human Exposure to Vibration Transmitted to the Hand. Draft International Standard ISO/DIS 5349, 1979.
10. Brammer AJ. Method for predicting the development of vibration-induced white finger. J Acoust Soc Am (to appear).
11. Taylor W, Kell R, Pearson J, Thomson CB. The Vibration Syndrome in a Population of Forestry Commission Chain Saw Operators in the Forest of Thetford. Dundee: Dept Social and Occup Medicine, Univ of Dundee, 1970. (unpublished).
12. See, for example, Wonnacott TH, Wonnacott RJ. Introductory Statistics. 2nd ed. New York: Wiley, 1972.
13. Taylor W, Pelmear PL, Hempstock TI, O'Connor DE, Kitchener R. Correlation of epidemiological data and the measured vibration. In: Taylor W, Pelmear PL, eds. Vibration White Finger in Industry. London: Academic Press, 1975: 123-133.
14. Taylor W, Pelmear PL, Pearson JCG. Vibration-induced white finger epidemiology. In: Taylor W, Pelmear PL, eds. Vibration White Finger in Industry. London: Academic Press, 1975: 1-13.
15. Matsumoto T, Yamada S, Harada N. A comparative study of vibration hazards among operators of vibrating tools in certain industries. Arh Hig Rada Toksikol 1979; 30: 701-707.
16. Taylor W, Pelmear PL. Introduction. In: Taylor W, Pelmear PL, eds. Vibration White Finger in Industry. London: Academic Press, 1975. XVII-XXII.
17. Hempstock TI, O'Connor DE. The measurement of hand-arm vibration. In: Taylor W, Pelmear PL, eds. Vibration White Finger in Industry. London: Academic Press, 1975: 111-122.
18. Miwa T, Yonekawa Y. Measurement of vibrations generated from portable vibrating tools. Ind Health (Japan) 1974; 12: 1-21.
19. International Organization for Standardization. Guide for the Measurement and the Assessment of Human Exposure to Vibration Transmitted to the Hand. Committee document ISO/TC 108/SC 4 N95, 1980. (unpublished).

DISCUSSION

H.F.V. Riddle: In terms of the limits suggested by this paper, what reduction in the vibration of power tools is practicable? Is the only alternative to limit the duration of exposure?

Brammer: Vibration limit

Author's Response: The ability to reduce the vibration of existing power tools to the vibration threshold depends to a large extent on the principle of operation, and the design of each tool. The use of operating principles that minimize vibration at surfaces in contact with the hands is evidently desirable. Many current designs of power tools would benefit from the addition of sophisticated vibration-isolation systems (see, for example, Miwa T. Design of a vibration isolator for portable vibrating tools. J Acoust Soc Jpn (E) 1980; 1: 201-208). However, the performance of any vibration-isolation system must be carefully tailored to the source of vibration and to the coupling of vibration into the hands (see Ref. 5). Failure to recognize these constraints can result in the handle vibration of a tool with a vibration-isolation system exceeding that of a power tool without such a system.

Thus, provided appropriate operating principles and/or vibration-isolation systems are developed, there is no reason why the vibration coupled into the hands from many power tools should not be less than, or equal to, the vibration threshold. However, there will always be some tools with vibration that exceeds the threshold, and for these the daily exposure should be of short duration. Job rotation, whenever practicable, should be employed to reduce the vibration exposure to, perhaps, one day in two, or preferably one week in two. Ideally, such operations should ultimately be automated to eliminate exposure to vibration.

G. Landwehr: I would like to make the following comments concerning the vibration of chain saws:
1) The ISO weighted acceleration sum (defined in: International Organization for Standardization. Chain Saws - Measurement of Hand-Transmitted Vibration. Draft Proposal ISO/DP 7505, 1980), measured on the rear handle of modern A/V chain saws when cutting wood, is mostly between 10 and 15 m/s^2 (see Fig. D1).

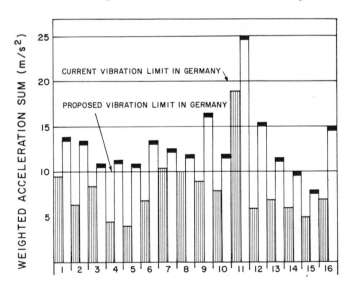

Fig. D1 ISO weighted acceleration sums measured at the front (shaded bars) and rear (unshaded bars) handles of 16 different vibration-isolated chain saw models when cutting beech at 8000 rpm (Stihl and competitors' saws).

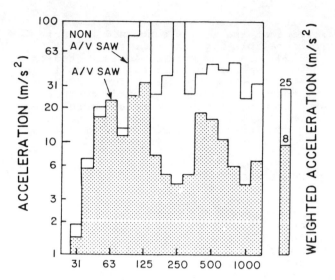

1/3 OCTAVE-BAND CENTRE FREQUENCY (Hz)

Fig. D2 Typical 1/3 octave-band accelerations, and ISO frequency-weighted accelerations, for a chain saw with and without a vibration-isolation system, measured when cutting beech at 8000 rpm. Note that vibration reduction occurs only at frequencies greater than 100 Hz.

The vibration of the front handle is generally less than that of the rear handle.
2) The weighted acceleration observed on the handles of non A/V saws during cutting is between 25 and 30 m/s^2 (see Figs. D2 and D3). Note that there are A/V saws on the market with vibration levels as high as those of non A/V saws (compare the vibration of saw #11 in Fig. D1 with that of the non A/V saw in Fig. D3). Also, the vibration level when the engine is "idling" is higher for A/V saws than for non A/V saws (see Fig. D3).
3) The cutting process itself appears to cause a high level of vibration, especially at low frequencies (see Figs. D4 and D5). The vibration level becomes much higher with a dull and poorly maintained chain.
4) The use of electrically powered or Wankel type (rotary engine) chain saws is not the solution to chain saw vibration. Considering that even these saws produce ISO weighted acceleration sums of approximately 10 m/s^2 while cutting (see Fig. D3), lowering the vibration to 1 to 2 m/s^2, as proposed in this paper, seems to be impossible.

Author's Response: The magnitude of the weighted acceleration sum, WAS, defined by:

$$WAS = (a_{KX}^2 + a_{KY}^2 + a_{KZ}^2)^{\frac{1}{2}} \qquad (D1)$$

should not be confused with that of the frequency-weighted, rms, component accelerations in the X, Y and Z directions (a_{KX}, a_{KY} and a_{KZ}, respectively). Only the latter are used in the paper: they have been consistently written in the abbreviated form a_K, since the discussion is not restricted to a particular direction.

As the vibration of A/V saws tends to be of similar magnitude in the three directions, X, Y,

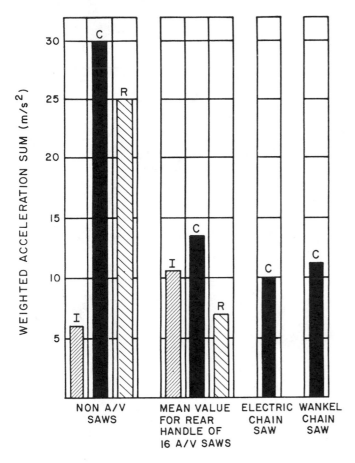

Fig. D3 ISO weighted acceleration sums for
different types of chain saws measured with
the engine "idling" (I) and "racing" (R), and
when cutting wood (C).

and Z (see, for example, Ref. 5), it is evident
from eqn. D1 that the magnitude of each frequency-
weighted, rms, component acceleration will be substantially less than the WAS (by approximately a
factor of 1.7). In fact, a typical value of a_{KX},
a_{KY} and a_{KZ} for the handles of professional A/V saws,
measured when cross-cutting hardwood, is 7 m/s^2 (see
Ref. 5). This value indicates that the frequency-
weighted, rms, component acceleration of a typical
A/V saw needs to be reduced by a factor of approximately three to comply with the vibration threshold.
That maximum, frequency-weighted, rms, component
accelerations of 3 m/s^2, or less, have already
been obtained on the handles of some production
A/V saws during cutting operations can be seen from
the measurements in Fig. 6, and from those of
Politschuk et al. (Politschuk AP, Oblivin VN.
Methods of reducing the effects of noise and vibra-
tion on power saw operators. In: Wasserman DE,
Taylor W, Curry MG, eds. Proc of the Int Occup
Hand-Arm Vibration Conf. Cincinnati, OH: Dept of
Health and Human Services, 1977 (NIOSH publication
no. 77-170): 230-232).

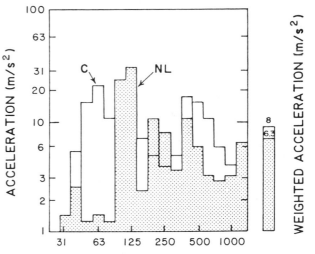

Fig. D4 Typical 1/3 octave-band accelerations,
and ISO frequency-weighted accelerations, for an
A/V chain saw operating at 8000 rpm with no load
(NL) and when cutting wood (C).

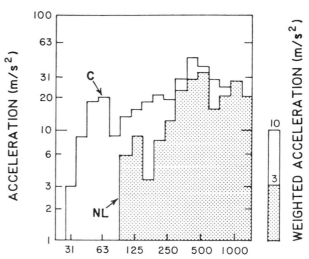

Fig. D5 Typical 1/3 octave-band accelerations,
and ISO frequency-weighted accelerations, for an
electric chain saw operating at 8000 rpm with no
load (NL) and when cutting wood (C).

Brammer: Vibration limit

METHODS FOR REDUCING VIBRATION EXPOSURE

Vibration-Isolation Systems for Hand-Held Vibrating Tools

T. Miwa

ABSTRACT: Vibration-isolating handles have been developed for several hand-held vibrating power tools. An attenuation of about 10 dB was obtained for all vibration directions, even at low frequencies, by attaching compound Nighthart isolators to a jack-leg rock drill and a pneumatic grinder, and air cushions to a small rivetting hammer. The isolation systems were designed by simulation, using equivalent electrical circuits for the mechanical impedance of the tool and the human hand, to establish the spring constant of the isolator from the equivalent low-pass filter.

RESUME: Des poignées antivibrations ont été mises au point pour plusieurs outils mécaniques vibrants tenus à la main. On a obtenu une atténuation d'environ 10 dB pour les vibrations dans toutes les directions, même aux basses fréquences, en fixant des amortisseurs Nighthart sur un marteau perforateur à support réglable et sur une meuleuse pneumatique, et des coussins d'air sur un petit matoir. Ces éléments ont été conçus par simulation, à l'aide de circuits électriques équivalents pour l'impédance mécanique de l'outil et de la main afin de déterminer la constante d'élasticité de l'isolant à partir du filtre passe-bas équivalent.

I BACKGROUND AND METHOD

The principle of vibration isolation can be understood from the motion of a simple (one-degree-of-freedom) mechanical system consisting of a mass connected to one end of a spring (1,2). If an oscillatory motion is applied to the free end of the spring, the motion of the mass will follow that of the source at very low frequencies. As the source frequency increases, the mass-spring system passes through a condition where the oscillation of the mass may exceed that of the source (resonance) to one where its movement becomes progressively less than that of the source. The attenuation characteristic is that of a simple low-pass (mechanical) filter.

It is instructive to analyse an equivalent electrical circuit during the design of vibration-isolation systems (3). Of the two alternative electrical analogies for lumped mechanical systems, the mass-capacitance correspondence proved to be more convenient. Force is then equivalent to an electric current and vibration velocity to a voltage. Hand-held vibrating tools may also be classified into two types of vibrating sources: constant force (e.g. a hand-held rotary grinder) and constant velocity (e.g. a jack-leg rock drill).

Measurements of the mechanical impedance of the human hand have shown that it may be approximately simulated by three lumped elements, one spring and two masses, for both compressional and shearing motion (4). The values of each parameter depend, of course, on the vibration direction relative to the hand. The apparatus used for these experiments and an example of the results obtained are shown in Fig. 1. At very low frequencies, the dynamic model of the hand in Fig. 1 can be further simplified to a single mass.

The electrical analogue of the proposed low-pass mechanical filter may now be inserted between the equivalent circuit of the human hand and that of the power tool, the latter being simulated by a mass and a mechanical resistance. The complete system may then be analysed by transmission circuit theory using matrix methods (4). For multi-dimensional analysis, the transfer matrix method and the finite element method are more powerful tools for determining the natural frequencies of the system (5,6).

A suitable vibration-isolation system for a hand-held vibrating tool must satisfy the following conditions: it must simultaneously reduce vibration in different directions, not influence the operation of the power tool nor increase significantly its weight or cost.

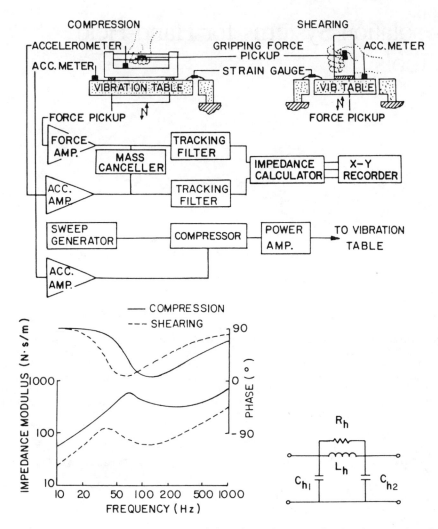

Fig. 1 Apparatus for measuring the mechanical impedance of the human hand during compression and shear vibration. Also shown is an example of the results and the analogous electrical circuit for the hand. (After Ref. 4).

II RESULTS AND DISCUSSION

2.1 Jack-Leg Rock Drill (7)

A jack-leg drill is well known to produce intense noise and vibration. The handle vibration during excavation of granite was measured simultaneously in three orthogonal directions (shown in Fig. 2) by a triaxial accelerometer (Rion PV93) weighing 28 g and a three-channel vibration level meter (Rion VM19A) conforming to the Japanese Standard JIS-1511-C.

Overall rms acceleration levels, AL, rms acceleration levels frequency-weighted according to the Draft International Standard (8), VL, and one-third octave-band levels are shown in Fig. 2 for the three vibration components of the rock drill handle. For industrial health purposes, the most important frequencies of these

spectra occur from 40 to about 125 Hz. The level at 40 Hz is derived from the chisel impact frequency (i.e. the fundamental repetition rate of the tool), and that at 125 Hz from the third harmonic. The components at frequencies above 300 Hz, although their acceleration levels are greater than those at lower frequencies, are partially isolated by a handle cover made of sponge rubber.

The lever principle was used in the design of a vibration-isolation system for this tool. Thus, by incorporating a Nighthart isolator into the hinge of the handle shown in Fig. 3, the static push force exerted by the hand on the handle may be amplified by the lever, while the vibration transmitted in the opposite direction is attenuated. As this system is, in effect, a floating lever, vibration normal to the base of the handle, in the

Miwa: Vibration isolators

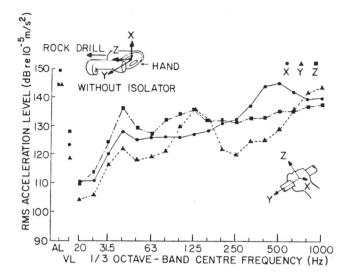

Fig. 2 Overall acceleration level, AL, frequency-weighted level, VL, and one-third octave-band levels at the handle of a jack-leg rock drill excavating granite. Data for the X, Y and Z directions indicated. (After Ref. 7).

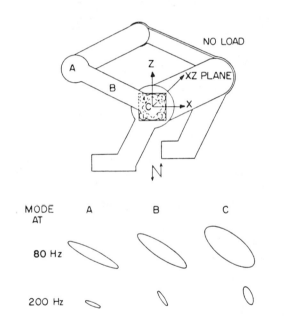

Fig. 3 A Nighthart isolator, showing the two coupled modes of vibration in the XZ plane when driven in the Z direction on a vibration table. (After Ref. 7).

Z direction (see Fig. 2), will be coupled into the X direction leading to motion in the XZ plane (see Fig. 3). The displacements in this plane of the two lowest frequency modes of vibration, occurring at 80 and 200 Hz when the handle was mounted

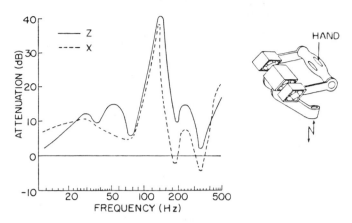

Fig. 4 Attenuation of the type A vibration-isolating handle (see sketch) measured in the X and Z directions as a function of frequency. (After Ref. 7).

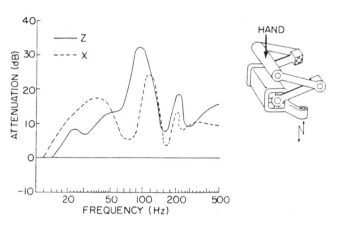

Fig. 5 Attenuation of the type B vibration-isolating handle (see sketch) measured in the X and Z directions as a function of frequency. (After Ref. 7).

on a vibration table and not hand-held, are also shown in the diagram.

The attenuation of this isolating system was found to be less than 6 dB on the vibration table. In order to improve the attenuation characteristics of the Nighthart lever, two Nighthart elements were connected in series and the attenuation of the system again determined on the vibration table. Figure 4 shows the attenuation between the vibration table and the hand grip in the Z and X directions as a function of frequency for the compound isolator sketched (type A). Note that there is significant attenuation in both directions, even at the frequency corresponding to the lowest order mode of the single element isolator (80 Hz), while vibration in the X direction is amplified

Miwa: Vibration isolators

Table 1. Vibration Levels on the Handle of a Jack-Leg Rock Drill With and Without Vibration Isolators.

| | Vibration Component | Acceleration Level (dB re 10^{-5} m/s^2) | | |
		AL[1]	VL[2]	1/3 Octave Band at 40 Hz
Rock drill without isolators	X	152	125	128
	Y	139	118	118
	Z	146	132	137
Rock drill with Type A isolator	X	136	122	124
	Y	127	119	126
	Z	130	120	120
Rock drill with Type B isolator	X	128	121	124
	Y	130	116	117
	Z	129	120	122

[1]AL – overall acceleration level.
[2]VL – overall level, frequency-weighted according to Ref. 8.

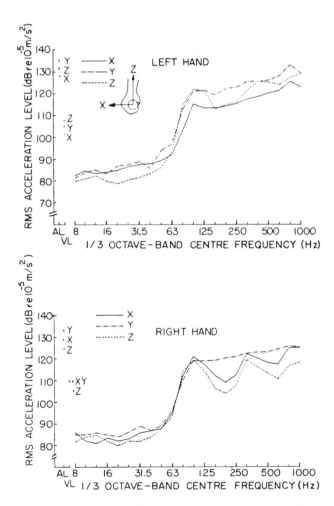

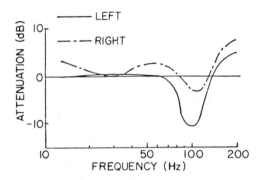

Fig. 7 Attenuation as a function of frequency at the handles, when the grinder is pressed onto the vibration table by both hands. Measurements were made separately at the position of each hand. (After Ref. 9).

Fig. 6 Overall acceleration level, AL, frequency-weighted level, VL, and one-third octave-band levels at the left and right handles of a grinder, when grinding a large iron disk. Data for X, Y and Z directions. (After Ref. 9)

at 180 and 340 Hz. Figure 5 reveals the superior performance of the type B compound isolator (see sketch) for both vibration components. In this design, improved attenuation is obtained in the X direction, except at the resonance frequencies of 80 and 170 Hz.

The vibration levels on the handle of a jack-leg rock drill, with the isolating systems attached, were observed during the excavation of granite. Table 1 gives the overall acceleration and frequency-weighted acceleration levels, and the level for the one-third octave-band dominating the vibration spectrum (40 Hz), for the three vibration components shown in Fig. 2. It can be seen that the vibration-isolating handles provide good attenuation in the Z direction but insufficient attenuation in the other two directions. Note, however, that the frequency-weighted vibration level can be reduced to about 120 dB(VL) by installing a compound Nighthart handle.

Miwa: Vibration isolators

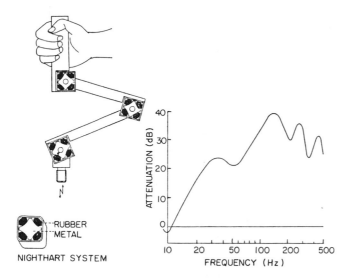

Fig. 8 Attenuation of the three element
Nighthart isolator (see sketch) measured
as a function of frequency. (After Ref. 9).

2.2 Pneumatic Grinder (9)

Operators of a seven inch pneumatic
grinder have a high incidence of the Vibration Syndrome. We considered the design of
a vibration-isolation system for this power
tool.

Vibration spectra in the X, Y and Z
directions were measured at the left and
right hands during the grinding of a large
iron disk (50 cm diameter, 3 cm thick).
Figure 6 shows that the overall frequency-
weighted acceleration levels are between
100 and 110 dB(VL), less than those of the
rock drill, and that the one-third octave-
band spectra contain low levels at frequencies below 100 Hz. Vibration isolation
is somewhat easier for the grinder than for
the jack-leg drill, with dominant vibration
components at frequencies of about 40 Hz:
for the former, both left and right handles
require isolation at 100 Hz and higher
frequencies.

The attenuation of the grinder itself
was first measured on the vibration table
in the Z direction as a function of frequency. The grinder was held in both hands
and the grinding stone was pressed onto the
table to avoid chattering. The attenuation
was measured by the difference between the
vibration levels of the table and the handle
(in the vicinity of the hand) (see Fig. 7).
A resonance can be seen at 100 Hz, which
occurs within the mechanical structure of
the grinder and results in increased vibration of the left handle.

Next, our approach to vibration-isolating handles was reviewed. The measurements during the grinding of the iron plate

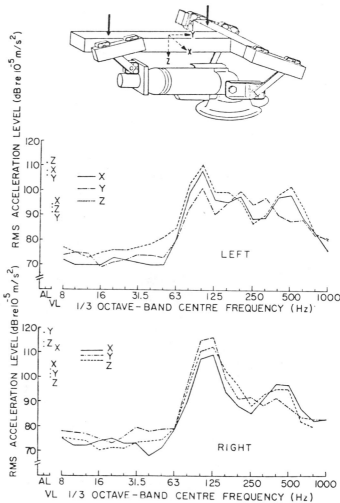

Fig. 9 Overall acceleration level, AL,
frequency-weighted level, VL, and one-
third octave-band levels at the handles
of the grinder when three-element Nighthart isolators (see sketch) were attached.
The tool was again grinding a large iron
disk. Data are for the X, Y and Z
directions. (After Ref. 9).

revealed that the attenuation of the compound isolator was not sufficient. The
vibration in one or two directions can be
effectively reduced, but not in all three
directions simultaneously. It was decided
to separate the grinding function from the
holding function by a system of Nighthart
isolators, in the form of three hinges,
as shown in Fig. 8. The attenuation of
the three element isolator was measured on
the vibration table as a function of frequency (Fig. 8). When hand-held, the
minimum attenuation occurred at a resonance (10 Hz): other minor resonances

Miwa: Vibration isolators

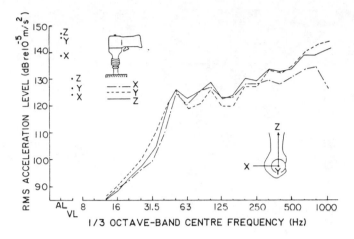

Fig. 10 Overall acceleration level, AL, frequency-weighted level, VL, and one-third octave-band levels at the handle of a baby rivetter with flat-topped hammer (plate snap), when used on a wooden block. Data for the X, Y and Z directions indicated. (After Ref. 10).

were observed but these did not significantly reduce the attenuation. As can be seen from the diagram, an attenuation of more than 20 dB can be expected at frequencies above 30 Hz.

A prototype three-stage isolation system was constructed and attached to the grinder, and the vibration spectra at the handles observed when the same grinding operation was performed (see Fig. 9). For the left hand, the original vibration level in the three directions of, typically, about 105 dB(VL) was reduced by the isolation system to 93 dB(VL), an attenuation of about 12 dB. For the right hand, an attenuation of about 8 dB was obtained.

These results demonstrate the effectiveness of the separation of the holding and grinding functions for the purposes of vibration isolation. The three-stage isolation system was designed by the simulation method described, using the equivalent electrical circuit elements for low-pass filters inserted between the circuits for the tool and the human hand.

A further improved three-stage vibration-isolation system for the grinder was also constructed. The vibration spectra were again measured at the handles during the same grinding operation and an attenuation of about 10 dB was obtained in all directions. The additional weight of this isolating system was less than 1.5 kg.

2.3 Pneumatic Rivetting Hammer (10)

A baby pneumatic rivetting hammer, though its size is small, possesses high vibration levels of between 120 and 130 dB(VL). A vibration-isolation system was

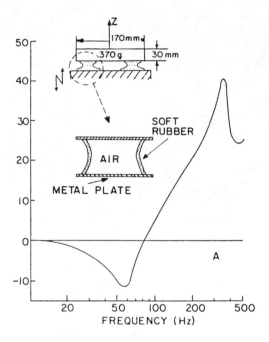

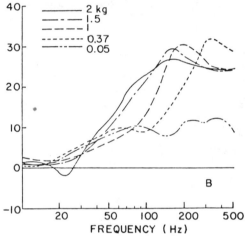

Fig. 11 Attenuation of the isolator (see sketch) as a function of frequency, measured on the vibration table: A, when the bar was not hand-held; and B, for bars of various weights pressed by the hand towards the table. (After Ref. 10)

designed for this power tool using air cushions.

The vibration spectra of the tool were measured in the X, Y and Z directions when a flat-topped hammer was used on a wooden block (see Fig. 10). The fundamental frequency of the hammer was about 50 Hz, below which the tool produced little vibration. It was also evident that the tool vibrates almost equally in all directions.

A vibration-isolating handle was designed around two air cushions (Bridgestone

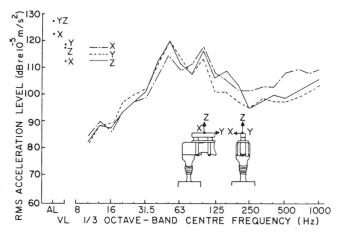

Fig. 12 Overall acceleration level, AL, frequency-weighted level, VL, and one-third octave-band levels on the isolator attached to the baby rivetter with flat-topped hammer, when used on a wooden block. (After Ref. 10).

WF-15, 40 mm top diameter, height 24 mm), which were sandwiched between a rectangular bar (dimensions 3×3×1.7 cm) and a plate (dimensions 18×6×0.5 cm), both made from aluminium. The attenuation of this system as a function of frequency was measured at the centre of the bar when the plate was attached to the vibration table.

Figure 11 A shows the results obtained when the (upper) bar was not hand-held. The natural frequency observed is in agreement with that calculated from the mass of the bar and the spring constant of the air cushion. Figure 11 B shows the attenuation of the system when the bar was varied from 50 g to 2 kg and pressed by the hand with a force of 100 N. The attenuation curves for the bars are generally similar, with the exception of the bar weighing 50 g. The bar weighing 0.37 kg was selected for use in the isolator, as this increase in weight of the tool was considered the most acceptable.

The vibration spectra on the handle of the tool when the isolation system was attached are shown in Fig. 12. To obtain these results, the baby rivetter with a flat-topped hammer was again used on a wooden block. It can be seen from Fig. 12 that peaks occur in all spectra at frequencies of 50 and 100 Hz. The attenuation obtained from the difference between the levels observed with and without the vibration-isolation system, in actual use of the tool, also agrees well with that found in the handle test on the vibration table. An attenuation of more than 10 dB occurs in all directions throughout the frequency range.

III CONCLUSIONS

Vibration-isolating handles have been developed for hand-held power tools as a means of protecting workers' health. A reduction in vibration level of 10 dB can be expected by applying compound Nighthart isolators to jack-leg rock drills and pneumatic grinders, and air cushions to baby rivetting hammers. The isolation system can be designed by simulation on a digital computer, using the equivalent electrical circuits for the mechanical impedance of the tool and the human hand, to establish the spring constant of the isolator from the equivalent low-pass filter. It is most important that the vibration-isolating handles possess a stable, balanced, mechanical structure, so that higher harmonics and coupled vibrations may be avoided.

REFERENCES

1. Timoshenko S. Vibration Problems in Engineering 3rd ed. New York: Van Nostrand, 1955.
2. Crede CE. Vibration and Shock Isolation. New York: Wiley, 1951.
3. Soroka WW. Analog Methods in Computation and Simulations. New York: McGraw-Hill, 1954.
4. Miwa T. Design of a vibration isolator for portable vibrating tools. J Acoust Soc Jpn (E) 1980; 1: 201-208.
5. Pestel EC, Leckie FA. Matrix Methods in Elasto-Mechanics. New York: McGraw-Hill, 1963.
6. Desai CS, Abel JF. Introduction to the Finite Element Method. New York: Van Nostrand, 1972.
7. Miwa T, Yonekawa Y, Nara A, Kanada K. Vibration isolators for portable vibrating tools: part 2, a rock-drill of leg-type. Ind Health (Japan) 1979; 17: 103-122.
8. International Organization for Standardization. Principles for the Measurement and the Evaluation of Human Exposure to Vibration Transmitted to the Hand. Draft International Standard ISO/DIS 5349, 1979.
9. Miwa T, Yonekawa Y, Nara A, Kanada K, Baba K. Vibration isolators for portable vibrating tools: part 1, a grinder. Ind Health (Japan) 1979; 17: 85-101.
10. Miwa T, Yonekawa Y, Nara A, Kanada K. Vibration isolators for portable vibrating tools: part 3, a pneumatic baby-rivetting hammer. Ind Health (Japan) 1979; 17: 131-139.

DISCUSSION

M. Morin: What was the force applied by the hands to the handles during the measurement of attenuation? The force I am referring to is that pushing the tool into the work piece.

Author's Response: The static force applied to the handle was about 100 N.

A. Behar: How much weight is added to the tools by the isolation systems using Nighthart isolators?

Miwa: Vibration isolators

Author's Response: The isolator of the jack-leg drill weighed about 1 kg, that of the grinder about 1.5 kg, and that of the baby hammer about 0.4 kg.

Do you have any reaction from users on the practicality and operation of pneumatic tools with these isolation systems?

Author's Response: The handle of the jack-leg rock drill has been sold by Furukawa Co. and Toyo Ind. Co. in Japan. A users' questionnaire has been evaluated and the responses were favourable. The other isolation systems were only produced in our laboratory. Before being available commercially, various improvements have to be made, especially reduction of their weight.

An Investigation of Chipping Hammer Vibration

E. I. Auerbach

ABSTRACT: Methods for reducing the vibration of chipping hammers have been studied. Vibration measurements were performed with a shock accelerometer rigidly attached to the handle and with a transducer mount hand-held against the chisel, when the chipper was working on iron and operating with no load. Vibration reduction by dynamic absorbers, compliant isolators and internal damping has proved to be ineffective at low frequencies. These frequencies include the peak vibration at the tool impact rate. It is concluded that an active isolation system involving redesign of the chipper to reduce the recoil forces is required.

RESUME: Les méthodes visant à réduire les vibrations engendrées par les marteaux piqueurs ont été étudiées. Les mesures des vibrations ont été réalisées à l'aide d'un accéléromètre solidement fixé à la poignée de l'instrument et avec une monture de transducteur tenue à la main contre la lame, alors que le marteau travaillait sur du fer et fonctionnait sans charge. La réduction des vibrations par des absorbeurs dynamiques, des isolateurs élastiques et un amortissement interne s'est avéré inefficace aux basses fréquences. Ces dernières comprennent la vibration de crête à la fréquence d'impact de l'outil. L'auteur conclut qu'un système actif d'isolation comprenant une modification du marteau piqueur pour réduire les forces de recul, est nécessaire.

INTRODUCTION

Percussive tools, such as chipping hammers, have been major sources of hand-arm vibration since their invention almost a century ago. Efforts to reduce the vibration of these useful tools began soon afterwards, and many patents have been issued over the years for percussive tool vibration isolation systems. Few have been incorporated in the standard product. The chipping hammer of today is almost unchanged from the design of fifty years ago.

The major difficulty with reducing the vibration of the tool has to do with the duty cycles and applications of chipping hammers. The transmissibility of a one-degree-of-freedom mass-spring system is given by (1):

$$T = \frac{(1+\delta^2)^{\frac{1}{2}}}{\{[1-(\omega/\omega_o)^2]^2+\delta^2\}^{\frac{1}{2}}} \qquad (1)$$

where T is the transmissibility, δ the damping factor, ω the forcing angular frequency, and ω_o the natural angular frequency (= $\sqrt{K/M}$, where K is the spring stiffness and M the mass). If $0 < (\omega/\omega_o)^2 < 1$, then $T > 1$ and no isolation is present. If $(\omega/\omega_o)^2 = 1$,

then $T = (1+\delta^2)^2/\delta^2$: for most cases $\delta << 1$ so that $T >> 1$ and amplification or resonance occurs. If $(\omega/\omega_o)^2 = 2$, then $T = 1$ and for $(\omega/\omega_o)^2 > 2$, T is less than unity and isolation begins. Thus, the natural frequency of the isolation system must be such that the lowest frequency of interest is at least $\sqrt{2}$ times higher, and this can usually be achieved only by the use of compliant (soft) isolators or by increasing the mass of the system. Added mass reduces vibration effectively, but a hand-held tool should be as light as possible for operator comfort, safety, and productivity. Soft isolators between the handle and the working end of the chisel reduce vibration but also reduce worker "feel" and control of the operation. This creates chisel bounce, poor finish, and low productivity. In addition, practical isolators cannot be made soft enough to attenuate low frequency vibration because of the low mass of the chipping hammer. Dynamic absorbers that increase the effective mass also tend to be ineffective, due to the large number of harmonics generated by the percussive cycle.

The measurement of chipping hammer vibration has also proved difficult. The impulses caused by the recoil and impact appear to excite the natural frequency of general purpose accelerometers, leading to

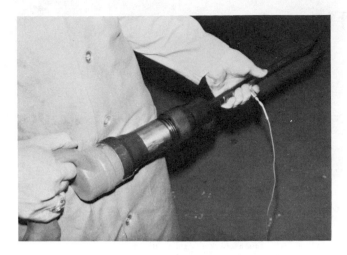

Fig. 1 Accelerometer attached to a sheet metal mount shown held against the chisel.

so-called DC-shifts and, ultimately, to transducer destruction. In consequence, general purpose accelerometers mounted on low-pass mechanical filters, or shock accelerometers with high natural frequencies, directly attached to vibrating surfaces are preferred for such measurements.

In this paper, measurements of chipping hammer vibration are reported. Some of the reasons why attempts to reduce the vibration of these tools have failed are discussed.

I VIBRATION MEASUREMENTS

There are very few accelerometers available that have sufficient sensitivity and resolution at low frequencies combined with durability at high amplitudes and frequencies. One shock accelerometer that seems to meet these criteria is the Endevco 2225, with a charge sensitivity of 0.71 pC/G and natural frequency of 80 kHz. Back-to-back comparison tests of a Bruel & Kjaer (B&K) 4366 general purpose accelerometer, mounted on a B&K UA 0559 mechanical filter, and the Endevco 2225 (2), on a 2.5 cm stroke chipper, yielded results within 1 m/s^2 of each other from 8 to 1000 Hz. Accordingly, the present study of chipper vibration was conducted using two Endevco transducers and charge amplifiers (Kistler, 503), and a Hewlett Packard 3582A dual-channel, real-time analyzer.

Tests were conducted on chippers working on iron and running free. The accelerometers were mounted directly on the handle and to a fixture for the measurement of chisel vibration, which is shown in Fig. 1. The extremely high impact forces on the chisel will destroy even the most hardy transducer if it were rigidly attached to the chisel. Thus the mount, which is

Table 1. Natural Frequencies of Chipper Components.

Component	Frequency (Hz)
Chipper Barrel (5.1 cm Stroke)	6000
Chipper Handle	750
	5125
Standard Chisel (30 cm)	2750
	4960
Internally Damped Chisel (30 cm)	1325
	3320

hand-held against the chisel, provides a means for measuring the vibration entering the hand from the chisel without subjecting the accelerometer to intense vibration at high frequencies.

II RESULTS AND DISCUSSION

Vibration in the frequency range of from 8 to 1000 Hz may affect the hand-arm system. Impulsive natural frequency tests on chipper components, as shown in Table 1, indicate that only the handle fundamental mode lies within this range. This demonstrates that adding damping to the system, including the chisel, is unlikely to reduce vibration, since damping is only effective near resonance.

Measurement of the vibration of standard and internally damped chisels confirmed that damping did not reduce their vibration over the frequency range of interest, as shown in Table 2 and in Fig. 2. Note that

Table 2. Narrow Band Peak Accelerations of Chisels (Radial Direction, Filter Bandwidth 6 Hz).

Tool & Operation	Frequency (Hz)	Narrow-Band Acceleration (m/s^2)
Standard 40.6 cm	40	212
(16 in)	84	236
Paper Stripping	124	182
Chisel	712	135
Running Free	756	139
	796	136
Internally Damped	44	261
40.6 cm (16 in)	88	225
Paper Stripping	120	246
Chisel	160	237
Running Free	204	254
Standard 25 cm	48	83.2
(10 in) Chisel	96	90.7
on Cast Iron	144	78.4
	196	68.1
Internally Damped	44	80
25 cm (10 in)	84	88.5
Chisel on Cast Iron		

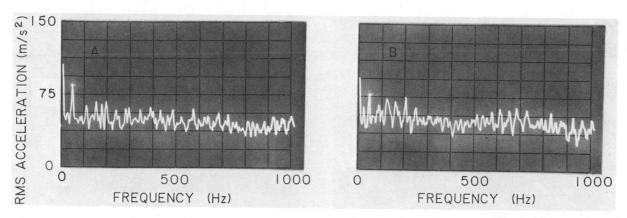

Fig. 2 Narrow band acceleration spectra (6 Hz bandwidth) of A, standard chisel; and B, internally damped chisel.

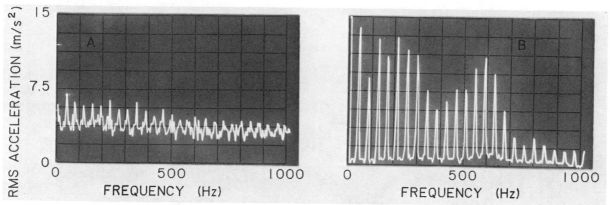

Fig. 3 Narrow band acceleration spectra when tool is A, chipping on iron (4 Hz band-width); and B, free running (6 Hz bandwidth: average of 16 samples).

Table 3. Narrow-Band Peak Accelerations of Chipper Handle (Axial Direction).

Tool & Operation	Frequency (Hz)	Narrow-Band Acceleration (m/s²)
Standard Chipper on Cast Iron (2.5 cm Stroke)	40	14.1
	80	11.1
	128	7.4
	168	7.4
	208	11.6
Chipper with Isolated Handle Running Free (2.5 cm Stroke)	40	44.1
	84	17.6
	128	9.5
Chipper with Isolated Handle on Cast Iron	36	14
	76	7.8
	112	6.9
	148	3.9
	188	2.4

the vibratory level is considerably higher when the chisel is free running rather than working on iron. This may be due to the impact of the chisel flange against the retainer and the lack of energy transfer to a work piece.

As expected, the handle vibration is considerably less than that of the chisel, both when working on iron and running free, as can be seen from Table 3 and Fig. 3. Again, the vibration when running free was greater than when working on iron and the level was highest at the firing frequency. In conventional applications such as metal removal, the chipper is rarely operated running free. However, the chipping hammer is being used more and more as a light demolition tool and this application in-volves free running for as much as 50% of the operating time. Free running or "play off" is hard on the tool and on the oper-ator. Generally, the operator does not hold or guide the chisel, so that most of the vibration is absorbed by the hand and arm holding the handle.

To demonstrate the effect of vibration isolation, a rubber section was added to the handle of the chipper, as shown in Fig. 4. As in previous measurements, accelerometers were attached to the handle and held to the barrel of the chipper. Figure 5 shows a comparison of barrel and handle vibration, and the coherence of these

Auerbach: Chipping hammer vibration

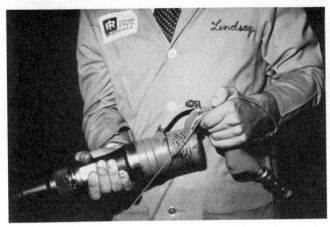

Fig. 4   Photograph showing rubber isolator between the handle and barrel of the chipping hammer.

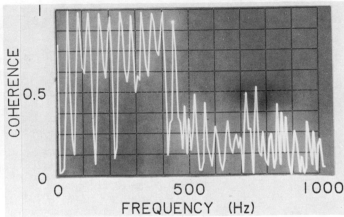

Fig. 6   Coherence between handle and barrel vibration.

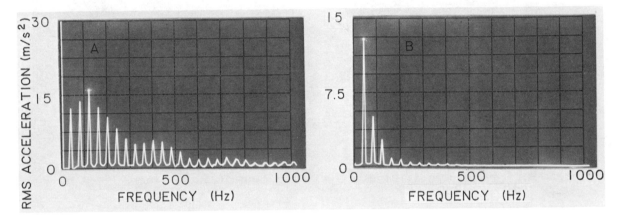

Fig. 5   Narrow band acceleration spectra (8 Hz bandwidth) of A, chipping hammer barrel; and B, isolated handle.

two motions is shown in Fig. 6. These results indicate that the isolator does not attenuate vibration at the fundamental firing frequency (see Table 3). However, higher harmonics are attenuated and the coherence plot indicates that the isolator is very effective above 400 Hz. Most of the standards proposed for assessing hand-arm vibration exposure weight low frequencies (3), so that it is imperative that low frequency vibration be attenuated. This isolator does not reduce the lowest frequency vibration and is not, therefore, an adequate solution to the problem.

We have developed an effective active vibration reduction system for a pavement breaker (see Fig. 7). The recoil forces caused by piston acceleration are cancelled by the motion of a mass in the opposite direction. This type of system could be incorporated in a chipper and timed to the firing frequency. Any higher frequency vibration could then be reduced by passive isolation.

Other chipper designs reduce the vibration when the tool is free running by allowing the air behind the piston to exhaust when the chisel moves past a port. However, the air is exhausted through the front end of the tool, which lets chips and dust blow back at the operator. This design has merit if the exhaust air is deflected away from the work piece and the operator.

The intense vibration of the chisel is presently only isolated from the hand by means of a rubber sleeve, which does not attenuate vibration at the firing frequency. In addition, some chipping is done with short (10 cm) chisels that are shorter than the sleeve. There does not seem to be any viable alternative to the sleeve handgrip at the present time.

III   SUMMARY AND CONCLUSIONS

This study has determined some of the reasons why previous attempts to reduce the

315

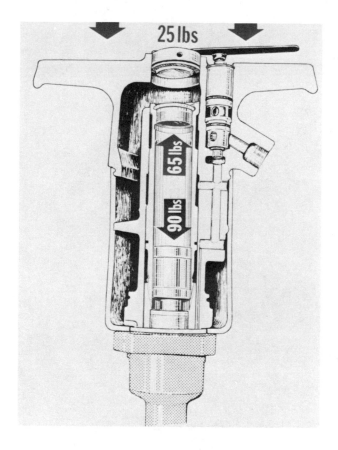

Fig. 7 Sketch showing the operating
principle of the SB-8 road breaker.

vibration of chipping hammers have failed.
It also leads to the conclusion that passive isolation systems are ineffective at
low frequencies and that an active vibration
reduction system is needed. Some design
features that could be incorporated in a
low vibration chipper have been discussed.
     The chipping hammer is an old tool by
power tool standards. Instead of being
phased out to make way for newer tools, the
popularity of the chipping hammer is actually
increasing. New applications for it seem to

be found every year. Since the tool appears
to be here to stay, the design requires
further refinement and improvement for low
noise and vibration, and high efficiency, to
meet the needs of a modern world.

REFERENCES

1.   Snowdon JC. Vibration and Shock in Damped
     Mechanical Systems. New York: Wiley, 1968.
2.   European Committee of Manufacturers of
     Compressors, Vacuum Pumps and Pneumatic Tools.
     Vibrations in Pneumatic Hand Tools: Investi-
     gations on Hand-Held Percussive Tools. (Copies
     available from British Compressed Air Society,
     8 Leicester Street, London WC2H 7BL, England.)
3.   International Organization for Standardization.
     Principles for the Measurement and the Evalu-
     ation of Human Exposure to Vibration Trans-
     mitted to the Hand. Draft International
     Standard ISO/DIS 5349, 1979.

DISCUSSION

     D.E. O'Connor: Am I to understand that your
accelerometer was welded to a plate which was then
held in the hand and pressed against the chisel?
     Author's Response: Yes.

     Then the accelerometer was effectively coupled
to the chisel through some form of low-pass mechanical filter.

     D.E. Wasserman: It is my understanding that
several years ago your company introduced a low
vibration road breaker (model SB-8), and that this
model was subsequently taken out of production
because of lack of sales. It seems that the tool
was not accepted by workers, because the vibration
levels were so low they believed it could not perform satisfactorily, despite the fact that it did.
Is this information correct?
     Author's Response: Yes.

     Then this experience demonstrates that even
when "vibration free" tools can be produced, an
educational process is needed to convince workers to
use them.

Rock-Drill Vibration and White Fingers in Miners

L. A. Rodgers, D. Eglin and W. F. D. Hart

ABSTRACT: The prevalence and degree of severity of vibration-induced white finger (VWF) was established among the miners of the British Steel Corporation's haematite iron-ore mines. Rock-drill vibration from a variety of drilling activities was measured extensively, to establish vibration exposure patterns, to correlate vibration exposures with epidemiological and clinical data, and to set design objectives for anti-vibration devices. Several methods of reducing vibration have been studied. Drilling tests have demonstrated that one reduction method resulted in a 17 dB reduction in the Z axis vibration and a 9 dB reduction in the X axis vibration. The reduction in vibration exposures by the use of gloves that incorporate vibration damping material has also been investigated.

RESUME: La prévalence et le degré de gravité des doigts blancs dûs aux vibrations (VWF) ont été déterminés parmi les mineurs travaillant dans les mines d'hématite de la British Steel Corporation. La vibration des marteaux perforateurs lors d'opérations de perforation diverses ont fait l'objet de mesures complètes pour déterminer les types d'expositions aux vibrations, pour corréler les expositions aux vibrations et les données épidémiologiques et cliniques, et pour établir des objectifs pour les dispositifs anti-vibrations. Plusieurs méthodes de réduction des vibrations ont été étudiées. Des essais de perforation ont révélé qu'une des méthodes réalisait une réduction de 17 dB des vibrations dans l'axe Z et une réduction de 9 dB des vibrations dans l'axe X. La réduction des expositions aux vibrations par l'emploi de gants contenant un matériau amortissant les vibrations a également été étudiée.

INTRODUCTION

In 1976, a comprehensive epidemiological and clinical study of vibration-induced white finger (VWF) was carried out, involving 115 men in four British Steel Corporation (BSC) fluorspar mines in the Northern Pennines (1). In 42 miners who had been exposed to the vibration of pneumatic rotary-percussive rock-drills, the prevalence of VWF was 50%, ranging from 19 to 93% in the individual mines. The results of this investigation led to growing concern for other BSC miners, as well as for the large number of people using other vibratory tools, such as chipping hammers, grinders and swagers.

Accordingly, the European Coal and Steel Community (ECSC) was approached by the BSC for financial assistance to investigate VWF in iron-ore miners at Beckermet in Cumbria. An engineering study of anti-vibration modifications to the drills, and an appraisal of the potential for vibration reduction by gloves were incorporated into

the study, preliminary results of which are reported here.

I STUDY OF DRILL VIBRATION AND MINERS' EXPOSURE PATTERNS

1.1 Working Procedure in Mines

A drill and air-leg unit in use at Beckermet are shown in Fig. 1. Each drill (Holman) used in the iron-ore mines weighs from 23 to 31 kg; the telescopic air-leg (jack-leg) adds another 19 to 23 kg. The hammer action is generated by a reciprocating piston, impacting at 35 to 40 Hz on the drill-rod which simultaneously rotates at a frequency of 6 Hz. There are two controls - a throttle on the drill back-end, which controls the hammering rate, and a valve on the air-leg, which controls the thrust into the rock and also supports the weight of the drill. Typically, the operator will control the air-leg with one hand. With the other hand, he may have to exert a

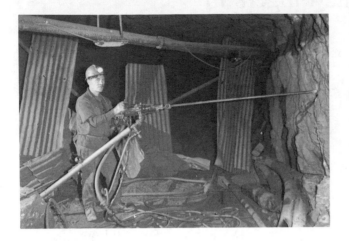 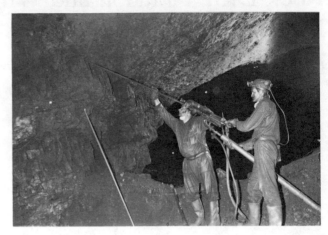

Fig. 1 A rock drill with air-leg in use, employing a 1.8 m drill rod.

Fig. 2 Drilling with a 2.4 m drill rod, prior to using 3.1 m and 3.7 m drill rods in the same hole.

downward force on the drill handle to balance the forces of the drill weight and air-leg thrust. The throttle will be full on, except when starting to drill the hole.

Although running methods vary considerably with the shape, size, and type of ore deposit, a form of bord and pillar working, which is allied to sub-level caving is generally employed. When working in an advancing heading, extensive drilling is required; when robbing back, drilling requirements are more limited. Day to day work will often follow a consistent pattern. If, for example, the company is advancing a typical 2.4 × 3 m heading, the loose rock from the previous day's blasting will be removed by autoloaders (EIMCO 12B or Atlas Copco T2GH) to rail tubs (0.45 m^3 or approximately one tonne loose ore), or to chutes leading to hoppers at the main rail haulage levels. In a typical heading, up to 26 shot holes will be drilled with the 1.6 m drill rods, which are standardized at Beckermet. Drill rods up to 4.8 m in length may be used in other types of operations, as shown in Fig. 2. At the end of the shift, the charges are placed and detonated.

The miners work in pairs, historically known as companies, and all companies are given equal opportunities to work in both advancing and retreating work. Drilling may occupy about 2.5 hours, including the time spent in moving the drill, coping with mishaps and with any natural breaks. Drilling is often shared by the teams, so that the actual time any one man may spend drilling is unlikely to exceed 2 hours for this type of operation. The drills have been observed to produce sound levels of 106 to 110 dBA and the autoloaders 103 to 106 dBA. (Ear muffs are now commonly in use.) Cold water from the workings and from the drill usually washes over the miners' hands and

leads to substantial cooling of the digits. The air temperatures in the mines vary from 12 to 18°C, with a mean of 16.9°C. The mean relative humidity is 94%, varying from 87 to 100%. Air movements may affect the local environment.

1.2 Vibration Measurement

A previous study of rock-drill vibration in the fluorspar mines included only limited vibration measurements (1). The vibration survey at Beckermet was undertaken to provide detailed information on the miners' exposure patterns and vibration "doses", to correlate these with medical data, and to investigate the relationships between vibration and work practices or other operating parameters, such as rock hardness or model of drill.

The measurement system consisted of a mechanical filter (Bruel and Kjaer (B&K) Type UA0559) and piezoelectric accelerometer (B&K Type 4369) mounted on the handle using a hose clip. An oscilloscope (Telequipment Type D32) was used to monitor continuously both the input signal to the tape recorder (B&K Type 7003) and the recorded signal, to evaluate distortion. By using selected low-pass filters in the preamplifier (B&K Type 2635), two series of recordings were made: the first, over the frequency range of 0 to 1000 or 3000 Hz; and the second, over the frequency range of 0 to 100 Hz, to enhance the signal-to-noise ratio of any critical, low frequency components, such as the drill hammering frequency. A B&K accelerometer calibrator Type 4291 was used to calibrate the system. For rapid analysis of the recordings, a microcomputer system (Apple II) was interfaced with a real-time, one-third octave band analyser (B&K Type

Rodgers et al.: VWF in miners

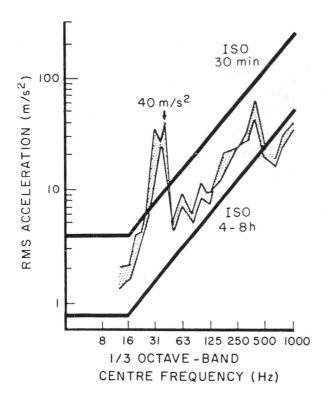

Fig. 3 Vibration measured in the Z axis during the drilling of four holes in hard ore, using 1.6 m drill rods and drilling angles of 45° above to 10° below horizontal. The ISO exposure guidelines for 4 to 8 h and for 30 min are also shown.

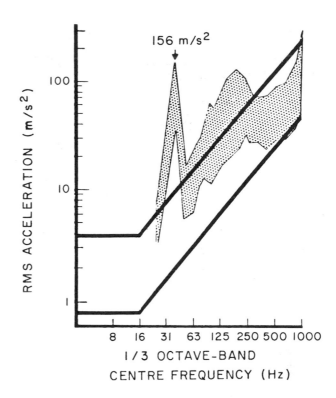

Fig. 4 Vibration measured in the Z axis during the drilling of eight holes in hard ore, using 1.6 and 2.4 m drill rods and drilling angles of 20° above to 20° below horizontal. The ISO exposure guidelines for 4 to 8 h and for 30 min are also shown.

3347), with centre frequencies from 12.5 to 20 kHz. Because it is unable to perform the long time period, true integrations possible with digital analysers, a more representative time averaging was effected by digitizing one-third octave-band analyses of consecutive 20 second determinations of the rms acceleration, and transferring them to the computer, for further processing and conversion to engineering units. The mean value of an appropriate number of samples, for example 10 or 15 depending upon the signal available, was then computed.

1.3 Results and Discussion

The measured rms accelerations, in one-third octave-band spectra, were evaluated in terms of the damage-risk guidelines proposed by the International Organization for Standardization (2). Other guidelines were considered by BSC specialists (3), but were not used as they provided less detailed and authoritative guidance.
Figures 3 and 4 present two series of results illustrating the range of vibration in the Z axis (as defined in Ref. 2) during

the drilling of four holes. The upper exposure guidelines (30 minutes exposure) and the lower exposure guidelines (four to eight hours exposure) are indicated in each diagram. The data shown in Fig. 3 were obtained by drilling in hard siliceous ore with a 1.6 m drill rod and drilling angles varying between 45° above and 10° below horizontal. It is worthwhile noting that the vibration values are similar despite different drilling angles. During this recording, with a company advancing a 2.4 × 3 m heading, eleven holes were monitored, each requiring three minutes to bore. The resulting exposure duration for the shift was eighty minutes for a 26 hole round. The data shown in Fig. 4, which are less typical, were obtained by drilling in soft, friable ore with 1.5 and 2.4 m drill rods at angles of 20° above and 20° below the horizontal. The very large acceleration of 156 m/s² at the hammering frequency was tentatively attributed to a mechanical fault in the drill. In general, throughout the survey, the recommended exposure limit in the 31 Hz third octave band for one to two hours exposure (6 m/s²) was exceeded by a factor of 6 to 9 in the Z axis, and

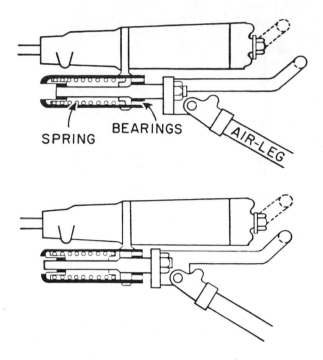

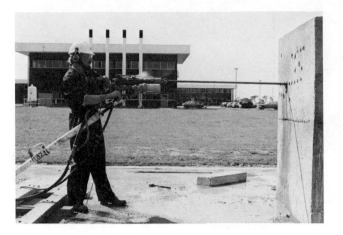

Fig. 6 Performance testing of helical spring anti-vibration handle.

Fig. 5 Cross-sectional sketch of first anti-vibration handle using a helical spring: uncompressed state, upper diagram; during operation, lower diagram (spring compressed by pressure from the air-leg).

by 3 to 4 in the two mutually perpendicular axes.

The amplitude and spectral distribution of drill vibration were monitored in a total of over sixty holes bored by five mining companies in a wide variety of drilling operations. Although considerable differences were found, there was no apparent correlation with the working practices or type of ore body. Based on this evidence, no significant differences would be anticipated in vibration dose. It is clear, however, that individual differences will result from the skill of the miner, the mechanical condition of the drill (particularly the air-leg valve), the type of operation (use of long drill rods at elevated angles require prolonged hand contact), and the grip force (4).

II MEDICAL AND CLINICAL EVALUATION

The medical data are currently being analysed. Only the objectives of the survey and the test methods are described here.

Five test methods were used in the study. First, a questionnaire was administered, to enable estimates to be made of: a) exposure duration before the onset of symptoms; b) exposure duration after the

onset of symptoms; c) the extent to which the fingers were affected by episodes of ischemia; d) frequency of complaints indicating neurological damage, such as numbness or paresthesia; and e) frequency of symptoms suggesting carpal tunnel syndrome. Second, neurological function was examined by esthesiometer, which assessed two point discrimination. Third, the sensitivity to light touch and pin pricks were examined. Fourth, the skin temperature of the fingertips was measured by a thermocouple. Fifth, the prevalence of carpal tunnel syndrome was investigated by applying pressure around the wrists (20 mm Hg above the measured diastolic pressure). One specific objective of the tests was to determine whether a more objective measure of VWF severity could be deduced from a segmental analysis of the hand, identifying those phalanges affected by numbness or ischemia.

Forty-five workers at the mine were found to have been exposed to the vibration from rock-drills. Only eight of the men, whose exposures varied from 3 to 31 years, had no complaints about attacks of white finger. Of the remaining 37 who did complain, exposure varied from 4 to 42 years. The onset of symptoms of white finger was reported as early as one year after starting use of the drills, but onset varied from 1 to 32 years. As had been expected, it proved difficult to date the onset of symptoms with accuracy in this retrospective survey.

III VIBRATION REDUCTION OF ROCK-DRILLS

To comply with the ISO guidelines (2), a 20 dB reduction in drill vibration would be required in the Z direction, and 10 dB in the X and Y directions. Other requirements of anti-vibration (A/V) devices were

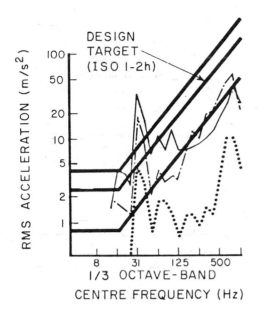

Fig. 7 Vibration measured in the Z direction on the drill body (continuous curve) and on the spring handle (dash-dot curve) during drilling tests of the anti-vibration handle, and, after modification, performance from vibration exciter tests (dotted curve). The ISO exposure guidelines adopted as the design targets are also shown.

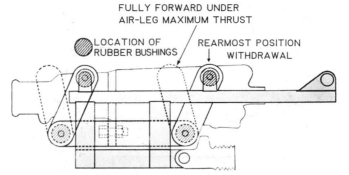

Fig. 8 Cross-sectional sketch of second anti-vibration handle, using rubber bushings in torsion. The link-arms between top and bottom rubber bushings are shown in the relaxed position; dotted outline shows position under maximum air-leg thrust.

established in discussions with the miners, and included their inherent safety, their strength and durability to equal those of the drill and air-leg, their minimal weight, and their effect on drill handling characteristics. It was suggested that handle flexibility should not, under maximum force exerted by the operators, cause a deflection greater than 6 mm, in order that the operator could maintain control of the drill. In retrospect, and considering the work of other researchers (5), this may have been too restrictive.

Early tests on simple replacement handles incorporating rubber in compression or shear confirmed that meeting the stipulation for a relatively firm handle would require an unacceptably high mass to be incorporated in the vibration-isolated part of the device. By adopting the design shown in Fig. 5, the existing mass of the air-leg, to which the repositioned handle is now attached, can be utilized to benefit the degree of isolation. In this design, the air-leg acts via two pistons against two helical steel springs which are, in effect, attached to the front cylinder washer of the drill. The device is shown under test in Fig. 6, when drilling into a large concrete block cast in the ground of the laboratories.

The results from the initial drilling tests, presented in Fig. 7, were

disappointing with only a 6 dB reduction in hammering frequency. However, frictional effects between the plunger and bearings were identified (using a vibration exciter) as the main cause of poor performance. The lower curve in Fig. 7 illustrates the attenuation achieved using the vibration-exciter and subsequently during drilling, after frictional effects had been minimized. Unfortunately, in achieving robustness, the A/V device was massive. A second version using aluminium alloys has been manufactured: further weight reductions could be achieved by using rubber/air springs rather than helical steel springs.

Another design approach, using eight rubber bushings in torsion, is shown in Figs. 8 and 9. The lower bushings, connected to the drill by the cylinder washer, are also, in turn, attached to a framework comprising a tubular handle and support arms to the air-leg connection. For strength and lightness, the device is fashioned from spring steel and high-strength alloy tube. Although it has yet to be tested, the device could probably be further lightened by further simplifying the design.

IV GLOVES AS PERSONAL PROTECTION

Prior to the ECSC's consideration of this research proposal, the use of gloves as a means of reducing vibration exposures had received little attention. However, the question of "anti-vibration" gloves had often been raised by the mines' management. It was known that both the grip force and the hand-arm posture affect the hand's dynamic response. It was also known that there is a dynamic coupling between the hand and any damping material interposed between the hand and a vibrating source (6).

Rodgers et al.: VWF in miners

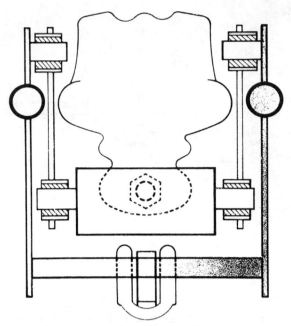

Fig. 9 Front elevation of second
anti-vibration handle, showing the
frame assembly and the attachment to
the drill front cylinder washer.

It was therefore necessary to determine the
transmissibility of gloves while the gloved
hand was vibrated.

  The glove testing apparatus used in
our investigation is shown schematically
in Fig. 10. The apparatus consisted of a
hollow, tubular grip bar rigidly attached
to a vibration exciter. The grip bar incorporated a miniature accelerometer to
measure vibration input to the glove material and a strain gauge to measure grip
force. Vibration at the hand-material
interface was registered by an accelerometer mounted on a small alloy plate between
the glove and the hand. During tests,
subjects held the grip bar as shown in
Fig. 11, with a predetermined grip force
monitored by the strain gauge, while the
bar was subjected to sinusoidal vibration
swept over the frequency range from 20 to
1000 Hz at a constant acceleration amplitude of 10 m/s^2. For each material evaluated, eight subjects underwent two tests
to determine the acceleration amplitude at
the grip bar (nominally constant), and at
the material-hand interface. Signals from
the accelerometer were fed to the one-
third octave real-time analyser and microcomputer, which processed the data to
provide the attenuation of the materials
tested.

  As expected, the performance of a
material was found to vary widely from
person to person. Figure 12 shows a
typical spread of results, and the mean for
one of the polyurethane foam materials.
All demonstrated similar tendencies - effectively zero attenuation below 100 Hz,

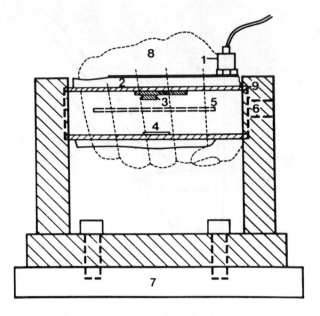

Fig. 10 Instrumented grip bar for glove
material testing. Key: 1, accelerometer
and mounting plate; 2, damping material
under test; 3, miniature accelerometer
and mounting plate; 4, strain gauge;
5, slot in grip bar; 6, lead out for accelerometer and strain gauge; 7, vibrator
platform; 8, hand; and 9, slotted cylindrical grip bar.

followed by two resonant peaks, and an
increasing degree of attenuation above 400-
500 Hz. Gloves have been developed in other
studies to reduce the resonances reported
here (7, and Pechar J, personal communication), and to provide gradually increasing
protection at frequencies above 200 Hz,
resulting in reductions of 6 dB or more at
1000 Hz. It therefore appears that anti-
vibration gloves cannot attenuate the low-
frequency components from the rock-drills'
percussive action. They do, however, play
a direct and valuable role in keeping the
hands warm.

V SUMMARY AND CONCLUSIONS

  An extensive series of hand-arm vibration measurements on rock-drills in the
British Steel Corporation iron-ore mines at
Beckermet in Cumbria have been performed.
Vibration levels at the drill handles were
found to exceed the ISO guidelines by up to
20 dB in the Z axis and 10 dB in the X and
Y axes. Two anti-vibration modifications
to rock drills were developed and drilling
tests on one version have demonstrated 17
and 9 dB reductions in the Z and X axes,
respectively. We are confident that practical modifications to the drills will
reduce the vibration to acceptable levels.
  An examination of the vibration attenuating properties of damping materials

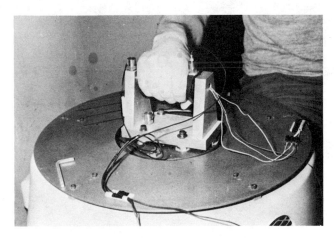

Fig. 11 Subject holding instrumented grip bar for glove material testing.

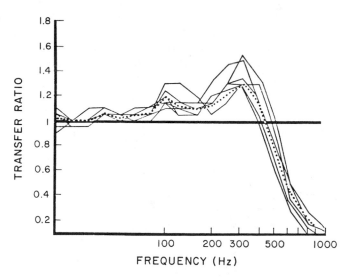

Fig. 12 Glove testing results: Values of attenuation for one material, six subjects, two tests per subject. Mean value is also shown as a dotted line.

suitable for inclusion in gloves has confirmed that no appreciable attenuation of the critical vibration component, the hammering frequency of the drills (35 to 40 Hz), is feasible, although significant attenuation may be possible at higher frequencies.

The statistical analyses of the medical data are not yet complete. Detailed results of both medical and engineering investigations will be published elsewhere.

ACKNOWLEDGEMENTS

This work received financial assistance from the European Coal and Steel Community. The authors also wish to thank Derriton Electronics Ltd. for the invaluable and extended loan of a vibration controller.

REFERENCES

1. Chatterjee DD, Petrie A, Taylor W. Prevalence of vibration induced white finger in fluorspar mines in Weardale. Br J Ind Med 1978; 35: 208-218.
2. International Organization for Standardization. Principles for the Measurement and Evaluation of Human Exposure to Vibration Transmitted to the Hand. Draft International Standard ISO/DIS 5349, 1979.
3. British Standards Institution. Draft for development: Guide to the Evaluation of Exposure of the Human Hand-Arm System to Vibration. London: British Standards Institution, 1975 (publication no. DD43).
4. Reynolds DD. Hand-arm vibration: a review of three years' research. In: Wasserman DE, Taylor W, Curry MG, eds. Proc of the Int Occup Hand-Arm Vibration Conf Cincinnati, OH: Dept of Health and Human Services, 1977. (NIOSH publication no. 77-170): 99-128.
5. Miwa T, Yonekawa Y, Nara A, Kanada K. Vibration isolators for portable vibrating tools, part 2: a rock-drill of leg-type. Ind Health (Japan) 1979; 17: 103-130.
6. MacFarlane CR. The Vibration Attenuating Properties of Gloves. Southampton: Inst of Sound and Vibration Research, Univ of Southampton, 1979 (Report to Health and Safety Executive, London). (unpublished).
7. Miwa T, Yonekawa Y and Kanada K. Vibration isolators for portable vibrating tools, part 4: vibration isolation gloves. Ind Health (Japan) 1979; 17: 141.

DISCUSSION

A.J. Brammer: Could the authors please provide the average latent interval with standard deviation for the population and/or the latent intervals reported by the 37 individual workers?

Authors' Response: Of the 37 miners who exhibited signs of VWF, the latent interval was 13.1 years with a standard deviation of 7.5 years, and a normal distribution.

Objective Test for the Vibration Syndrome and Reduction of Vibration During Fettling

K. Sivayoganathan, N. K. Akinmayowa and E. N. Corlett

ABSTRACT: Two studies are reported in this paper. The Renfrew depth esthesiometer has been modified to improve the precision of this sensory clinical test for vibration-induced white finger (VWF), by controlling finger pressure. Results from three groups of subjects showed that the esthesiometer could differentiate between the group of industrial workers with Stage 2 or 3 VWF in Taylor and Pelmear's classification (N=16), a control group of industrial workers of similar age without VWF (N=10), and a group of students (N=25). In the second study, it was shown that most vibration during pedestal grinding occurs when restoring the cutting ability of the grinding wheel ("dressing"). An improved dressing procedure has been developed, which reduces the vibration level both during dressing and when grinding the work piece. The procedure also leads to reduced exposure time.

RESUME: Deux études sont mentionnées dans la présente communication. L'esthésiomètre en profondeur de Renfrew a été modifié pour améliorer la précision de cet essai clinique de détection des doigts blancs dûs aux vibrations (VWF), en réglant la pression exercée par les doigts. Les résultats obtenus pour trois groupes de sujets montrent que l'esthésiomètre pouvait distinguer entre le groupe des travailleurs industriels arrivés aux stades 2 et 3 des doigts blancs selon la classification de Taylor et Pelmear (N=16), un groupe témoin de travailleurs industriels d'âge comparable mais sans doigts blancs (N=10) et un groupe d'étudiants (N=25). Dans la deuxième étude, il fut démontré que la plupart des vibrations accompagnant le meulage à la machine se produisent lorsqu'on rhabille la meule. Une méthode de rhabillage améliorée a été mise au point; elle réduit le niveau de vibration au cours du rhabillage et au cours du meulage de la pièce à travailler. Cette méthode entraîne aussi une réduction du temps d'exposition.

INTRODUCTION

Two studies are reported in this paper. The first is concerned with the search for an objective, clinical test for vibration-induced white finger, or VWF (1, 2), and the second with the reduction of vibration exposure during pedestal grinding.

Of seven clinical tests for VWF studied by Taylor and Pelmear (3), the ridge test using the Renfrew depth sense esthesiometer gave statistically the greatest difference between vibration-exposed and non-exposed populations (4). In part I of this paper, the development and testing of an improved esthesiometer, which provides a controlled and sensitive measure of depth sense, is described (5).

In pedestal grinding, the parts to be ground are held or supported and pushed against the grinding wheel with one or both hands. The cutting agent is usually a large diameter (up to 900 mm), rotating abrasive wheel supported on a pedestal and frame. The process is commonly performed on components produced by casting or forging, to remove unwanted metal, usually in preparation for further processing. There are two basic operations: "dressing" and grinding. The former is used periodically to restore the cutting ability of the abrasive wheel, and involves holding a tool (the "dresser") against the wheel. It has been shown that more vibration is produced during dressing than during the grinding of components (6,7), and for this reason an improved method of dressing the wheel has been developed. This is discussed in part II of the paper.

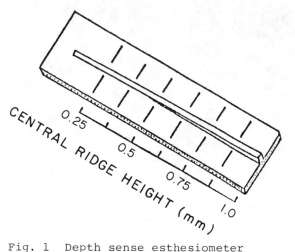

Fig. 1 Depth sense esthesiometer
proposed by Renfrew (Ref. 4).

I AN IMPROVED DEPTH-SENSE ESTHESIOMETER

1.1 Apparatus and Method

The Renfrew esthesiometer (see Fig. 1)
has been modified to enable psycho-physical
test procedures to be adopted, in order to
improve the precision of the depth sense
values obtained.

Sketches of the front and side elevations of the new apparatus are shown in
Fig. 2. A ridge was machined eccentrically

on the periphery of a circular plastic disk
80 mm in diameter, approximately 3 cm wide,
from the surface of the disk to a height of
1 mm. The eccentricity was chosen to
duplicate the dimensions of the Renfrew
esthesiometer. The ridged disk, together
with a 360° protractor, were mounted on a
spindle and concealed in a box. The
position of the ridge, relative to the
disk, can be read in degrees through an
aperture in the side of the box. A larger
aperture on the other side of the box,
level with the periphery of the disk,
allows the subject to insert a finger so
that it can rest on the edge of the plastic
disk. The box was mounted on a channel
between guides and its horizontal movement
was constrained by a light spring.

In use, the pressure of the subject's
finger on the disk pushes the spring-loaded
box towards him. A guide mark indicates
where the subject is required to keep the
box during the test. The subject then
rotates the disk by means of a knurled knob,
using the other hand, until the ridge is
felt to disappear or appear. The subjects
can see neither the ridge nor the protractor
scale during the tests and thus have to rely
solely on detecting the ridge with the
finger.

1.2 Results and Discussion

A total population of 51 subjects was
divided into three groups for the purpose of
evaluating the performance of the esthesiometer. The first group (N=16) consisted
of industrial workers who had been exposed

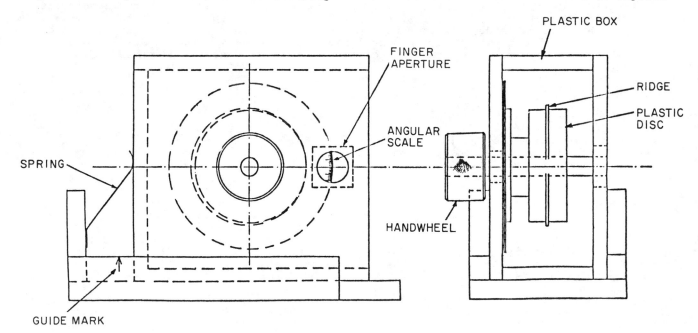

Fig. 2 Sketch of the improved esthesiometer designed to permit better psycho-physical
control of the measurement.

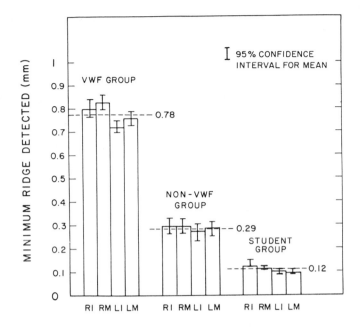

Fig. 3 Mean values and 95% confidence intervals for the sensory thresholds (recognition of the presence of the ridge) of the right and left index fingers (RI, LI) and middle fingers (RM, LM), in three population groups. Data obtained with the new esthesiometer.

to vibration and identified clinically as suffering from Stage 2 or 3 VWF in Taylor and Pelmear's classification (6). The second group (N=10) consisted of industrial workers who had been exposed to vibration but had no signs or symptoms of VWF, and were reasonably matched to group 1 in industrial experience and age (40.7 ± 10.2 and 47.6 ± 12.3 years, respectively). The third group (N=25) consisted of students who had a lower mean age (25.8 ± 1.4 years).

The minimum ridge heights detected by the three groups of subjects are shown in Fig. 3. The data are for the index and middle fingers of each hand and are given in terms of the mean value and 95% confidence interval (vertical bar). It is evident that the industrial group with VWF can be clearly differentiated from the other two groups, with a mean ridge height detected of 0.78 mm, as compared with 0.29 mm for industrial workers not suffering from VWF, and with 0.12 mm for students. In one advanced case of VWF, the subject could not feel the maximum ridge height of 1 mm.

A revised version of the esthesiometer is in preparation with an increased maximum ridge height.

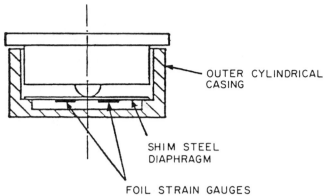

Fig. 4 The transducer used to record grip force. It was sewn into an industrial glove. (Overall diameter approximately 15 mm).

II VIBRATION REDUCTION DURING PEDESTAL GRINDING

2.1 Apparatus

Initial pilot studies in industry confirmed the work of Kitchener (7), that dressing the grinding wheels usually produced the highest vibration levels experienced by operators. Other factors influencing vibration exposure were: the use of modified dressers; the varying sizes of work pieces; differences in the presentation of work or dresser to the wheel; the use of aids to lever components against the grinding wheel; and bumping the grinding wheel with the work piece as a substitute for wheel dressing.

A new dresser was constructed to improve the dressing of the grinding wheel. It used the existing cutters, which were supported by a bracket and were free to move on a guide bar, operated by a lever. The device can be locked into position on the work rest of the pedestal grinder, and the cutter distance from the grinding wheel adjusted to provide various depths of cut. (It is envisaged that in the production version the dresser will swing into position, and be locked to the work rest when needed.)

Vibration measurements were made in three mutually perpendicular directions: horizontally and vertically, in directions radial to the grinding wheel (the latter also being approximately tangential to the wheel at the point of contact during grinding), and lateral, that is parallel to the rotational axis of the wheel (which is horizontal).

The outputs from three accelerometers (Bruel & Kjaer (B&K) 4367) were amplified,

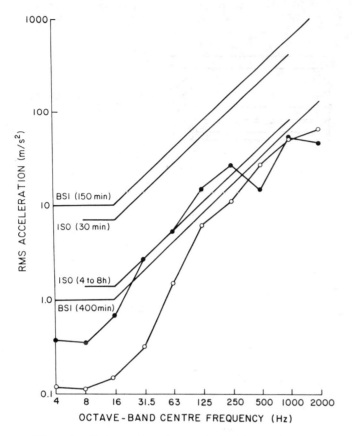

Fig. 5 Octave-band accelerations in the horizontal direction when using a hand-held or stand-mounted dresser (shown by closed and open circles, respectively). Also shown, for comparison, are the vibration limits proposed by the ISO and the British Standards Institution (8,9).

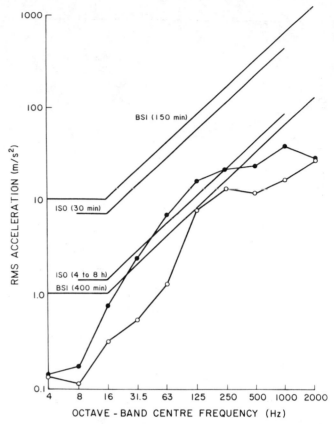

Fig. 6 Octave-band accelerations in the vertical direction when using a hand-held or stand-mounted dresser (shown by closed and open circles, respectively). Also shown, for comparison, are the vibration limits proposed by the ISO and the British Standards Institution (8,9).

low-pass filtered, and then recorded on a multi-channel tape recorder. The signals were observed on an oscilloscope for evidence of overloading prior to recording. The recorded signals were subsequently analysed by an analogue system, consisting of an amplifier (B&K 2606), a band-pass filter (B&K 1614) and a level recorder (B&K 2305), and were also analysed by computer (Digital Equipment Corp. PDP 11/34).

A glove equipped to measure grip force and a force platform were used to identify the forces exerted by the hand and arm during vibration measurements. A small cylindrical load cell containing miniature strain gauges mounted on a diaphragm was attached to a close fitting glove. The centre of the diaphragm was deflected by compression of the cap of the load cell (Fig. 4), as occurred when gripping a component. The force platform measured the horizontal (push) force exerted radial to

the wheel, by means of a hydraulic cylinder resisting the movement of the platform.

2.2 Results and Discussion

Octave-band acceleration spectra in the horizontal, vertical and lateral directions during dressing are shown in Figs. 5 to 7, respectively. Also included in these diagrams are guidelines for vibration exposure proposed by the International Organization for Standardization (ISO/DIS 5349) and the British Standards Institution (DD 43) (8,9).

It can be seen that the vibration of the stand-mounted dresser was generally less than that of a hand-held dresser, and always less than the 400 min daily exposure limit of the British proposal. A significant reduction in vibration occurred in those directions in which the mounted dresser provided some constraint to motion (the

Sivayoganathan et al.: Apparatus

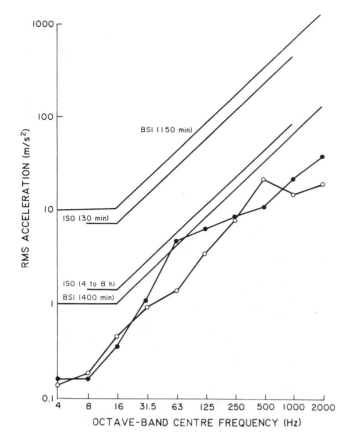

Fig. 7 Octave-band accelerations in the lateral direction when using a hand-held or stand-mounted dresser (shown by closed and open circles, respectively). Also shown, for comparison, are the vibration limits proposed by the ISO and the British Standards Institution (8,9).

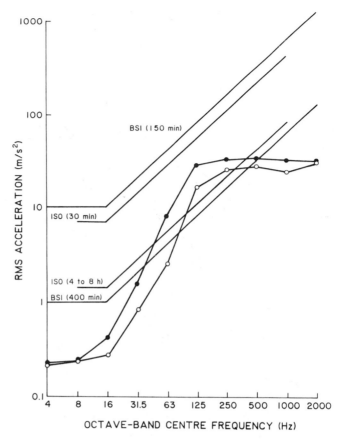

Fig. 8 Octave-band accelerations in the horizontal direction during grinding after using a hand-held or stand-mounted dresser (shown by closed and open circles, respectively). Also shown, for comparison, are the vibration limits proposed by the ISO and the British Standards Institution (8,9).

horizontal and vertical components). Vibration in the lateral direction, which was also the direction in which the dresser moved, showed less improvement, and differed little from the hand-held value. These results, which were obtained in industry, confirmed earlier laboratory measurements that demonstrated there was a reduction in vibration energy during use of the stand-mounted dresser.

Octave-band acceleration spectra, when grinding a component after using the two alternate methods of dressing, showed less improvement (see Figs. 8-10). However, these results from industry were consistent with laboratory measurements, and confirmed that the vibration in each octave band was reduced after using the stand-mounted dresser.

As reported elsewhere, there were considerable improvements in the rate of removing metal when using the more circular

(unlobed) grinding wheel produced by the stand-mounted dresser (10). There was thus also a reduction in vibration exposure time (per component). These factors provide an economic incentive to industry to adopt the more effective dresser design.

III CONCLUSIONS

The results indicate that the apparatus used in a sensory test for VWF can be improved, and that better dressing practices can lead to reductions in vibration exposure during pedestal grinding. It appears that the improved control of wheel dressing may make softer grinding wheels economic, which in turn could result in a further reduction in vibration. This and other aspects of grinding technology require further investigation.

Sivayoganathan et al.: Apparatus

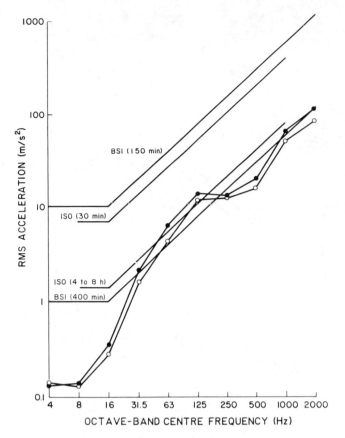

Fig. 9 Octave-band accelerations in the vertical direction during grinding after using a hand-held or stand-mounted dresser (shown by closed and open circles, respectively). Also shown, for comparison, are the vibration limits proposed by the ISO and the British Standards Institution (8,9).

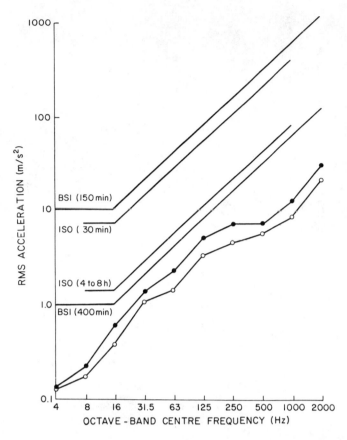

Fig. 10 Octave-band accelerations in the lateral direction during grinding after using a hand-held or stand-mounted dresser (shown by closed and open circles, respectively). Also shown, for comparison, are the vibration limits proposed by the ISO and the British Standards Institution (8,9).

ACKNOWLEDGEMENTS

Financial support for this project was provided by the Health and Safety Executive (UK), the Department of Industry (UK), and Guest, Keen and Nettlefolds Ltd. We are grateful for the advice and co-operation of the management and workers involved in the study. The technical support of Professor N.A. Dudley, the former Head, and of Professor K.B. Haley the present Head of the Dept. of Engineering Production, Univ. of Birmingham, are also acknowledged.

REFERENCES

1. Taylor W. The Vibration Syndrome. London: Academic Press, 1974.

2. Industrial Injuries Advisory Council. Vibration White Finger. London: Her Majesty's Stationery Office, 1954, 1970, 1975 and 1981. (Reports to the Dept of Health and Social Security).

3. Pelmear PL, Taylor W, Pearson JCG. Clinical objective tests for vibration white finger. In: Taylor W, Pelmear PL, eds. Vibration White Finger in Industry. London: Academic Press, 1975: 53-81.

4. Renfrew S. Fingertip sensation. A routine neurological test. Lancet 1969; I: 396, ibid 1970; I: 1011.

5. Corlett EN, Akinmayowa NK, Sivayoganathan K. A new aesthesiometer for investigating vibration white finger (VWF). Ergonomics 1981; 24: 49-54.

6. Taylor W, Pelmear PL. Vibration White Finger in Industry. London: Academic Press, 1975.

7. Kitchener R. The measurement of hand-arm vibration in industry. In: Wasserman DE, Taylor W, Curry MG, eds. Proc of the Int Occup

331

Hand-Arm Vibration Conf. Cincinnati, OH: Dept of Health and Human Services, 1977 (NIOSH publication no. 77-170): 153-159.

8. International Organization for Standardization. Principles for the Measurement and the Evaluation of Human Exposure to Vibration Transmitted to the Hand. Draft International Standard ISO/DIS 5349, 1979.

9. British Standards Institution. Draft for Development: Guide to the Evaluation of Exposure of the Human Hand-Arm System to Vibration. London: British Standards Institution, 1975. (publication no. DD 43).

10. Sivayoganathan K, Corlett EN. The effect of wheel profile in metal removal rate in hand-fettling. Sixth Conf on Production Research. Yugoslavia, 1981. (unpublished).

DISCUSSION

M.R. Noble: What was the proportion of time spent dressing the wheel versus grinding?

Authors' Response: In a four hour sample of workers grinding forgings, each man dressed the wheel about thirty times, taking, on average, about ten seconds. However, the time spent dressing will depend on the wheel, the operator's ability and the material being dressed. Hence a true estimate of the contribution from dressing to the total vibration exposure can be made only in relation to specific circumstances.

What proportion of the total vibration dose was due to dressing?

Authors' Response: From our results, it is not possible to give a definitive answer to this question, primarily because the test pieces were all from the same component, which was cut and reduced in weight, to permit other measurements to be made. Within these limitations, the rms weighted acceleration (weighted according to Ref. 8) observed with hand-held and stand-mounted dressing are given in Table D1.

Table D1. RMS Weighted Accelerations During Dressing, and Grinding a Component (m/s^2).

Vibration Source		Weighted Acceleration (m/s^2)		
		Vertical	Horizontal	Lateral
Hand-held dressing	Dresser	1.57	1.68	0.84
	Component	1.51	2.37	0.72
Mounted dressing	Dresser	0.7	0.82	0.6
	Component	1.24	1.44	0.48

It should be made clear that these results are tentative, since a range of machines, components and operators need to be investigated before representative industrial dose levels can be established.

Sivayoganathan et al.: Apparatus

Resilient Handgrips

C. W. Suggs and J. M. Hanks

ABSTRACT: The vibration reduction of foam rubber and foam plastic handle coverings suitable for power and hand tools has been measured by a lightweight transducer at the hand-handgrip interface. The use of from 1 to 3.6 cm thickness of foam, with compressional stiffness in the range ∿1 to 10 N/cm, reduced the overall acceleration from an electric, reciprocating sabre saw and a gasoline powered chain saw by at least 50%, and from a hammer by 95%. Most of the attenuation occurred at frequencies in excess of 300 to 500 Hz; little or no attenuation was observed at lower frequencies. The results suggest that high frequency vibration can be significantly reduced by resilient handle covers, but that the frequencies commonly associated with the Vibration Syndrome can only be reduced at the handle-tool interface or at the source.

RESUME: La réduction des vibrations que permettent les revêtements en caoutchouc mousse et en mousse de plastique des poignées des outils mécaniques et manuels, a été mesurée par un transducteur léger, à la surface intermédiaire comprise entre la main et la poignée. L'utilisation d'une mousse d'une épaisseur comprise entre 1 et 3,6 cm, d'une résistance à la compression comprise entre ∿1 et 10 N/cm, a réduit l'accélération générale d'une scie à chantourner électrique alternative et d'une tronçonneuse à essence d'au moins 50%, et celle d'un marteau, de 95%. La plus grande partie de l'atténuation se produit à des fréquences supérieures à 300-500 Hz; il n'y a que peu ou pas d'atténuation à des fréquences plus basses. Les résultats suggèrent que les vibrations haute fréquence peuvent être grandement réduites par des revêtements de poignée souples, mais que les fréquences associées couramment au syndrome de vibration ne peuvent être réduites qu'à la surface intermédiaire de la poignée et de l'outil ou à la source.

INTRODUCTION

Hand-held tools powered by internal combustion engines and electric, or compressed air, motors have all been found to produce significant vibration, either from impacts between the tool and work piece, or from the reciprocating nature of the tool or power source (1-3). In many current tool designs, the handle is combined with the main body of the device, so that it cannot be vibration isolated at the tool body-handle interface, as has been achieved with chain saws (4), without a significant amount of redesign. Also, the integration of the handle with the tool housing simplifies design and reduces construction cost in many cases. In consequence, the use of resilient handgrips is an attractive approach to vibration isolation.

The purpose of the work reported here was to determine whether resilient handgrips reduced the vibration reaching the hands of operators of both manual and hand-held power tools. In addition to measuring the overall attenuation, a further objective of the study was to determine what frequencies could be attenuated and what material thickness and stiffness could be used.

I METHODS AND MATERIALS

A rubber foam and a plastic foam material were evaluated as potential handle covers. The stiffness of these two materials was evaluated by compressing 1 cm cubes of each on an Instron stress-strain measuring machine, which resulted in the force-deformation curves shown in Fig. 1. As can be seen from the diagram, neither of the responses was linear, so that estimates of sample stiffness will be dependent on its compression as well as its size. (The sample of the softer material appeared to behave like a slender column undergoing buckling.)

At the compressive forces to be expected on handgrips, the stiffnesses of the 1 cm cubes of foam rubber and plastic were 11.7 N/cm and 1.2 N/cm, respectively.

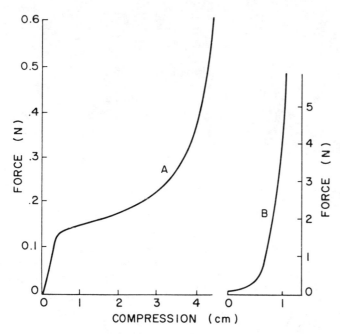

Fig. 1 Load-compression curves for 1 cm cubes of the materials used for handle covers: A, foam plastic; and B, foam rubber.

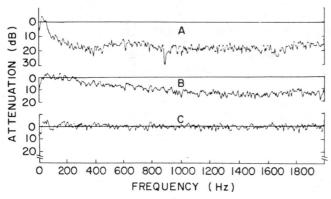

Fig. 2 Attenuation of foam covered handles when hand-held and excited by broad-band vibration: A, handle covered with 3.6 cm thick plastic foam; B, handle covered with 1.15 cm thick rubber foam; and C, bare handle.

A 1.15 cm thick sheet of the foam rubber was judged to be of approximately the right thickness and stiffness to be used as a handle cover for a power tool. The foam plastic was considered to be too soft for the intended application, as the forces required to grip and support most tools would cause it to be almost completely compressed. However, results obtained with 3.6 cm thickness of this material are included for comparison.

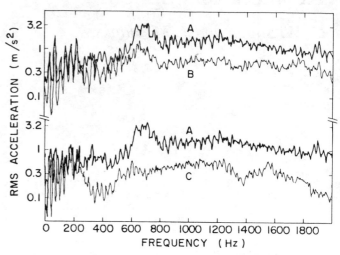

Fig. 3 Handgrip acceleration of a reciprocating sabre saw, with and without foam covering, when used to cut wood: A, bare handle; B, handle covered with 1.15 cm thick foam rubber; and C, handle covered with 7.2 cm thick foam plastic.

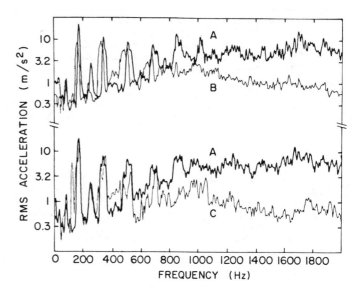

Fig. 4 Handgrip acceleration of a gasoline powered chain saw, with and without foam covering, when used to cut wood. A, bare handle; B, handle covered with 1.15 cm thick foam rubber; and C, handle covered with 3.6 cm foam plastic.

The two foams were next formed into handle covers and their attenuation measured when excited by an electrodynamic shaker. The vibrator was driven at the same acceleration at all frequencies in the range of interest, by the amplified signal from a white noise generator. Two accelerometers (Bruel & Kjaer, type 4344) monitored the

Suggs et al.: Resilient handgrips

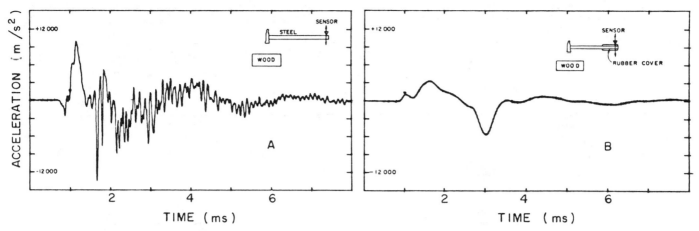

Fig. 5 Vertical component acceleration of the handgrip of a 0.88 kg ball pein hammer striking a wooden block: A, bare handle; and B, handle covered with rubber sleeve.

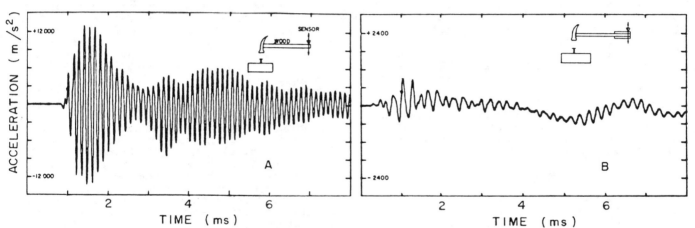

Fig. 6 Vertical component acceleration of the handgrip of a claw hammer striking a 16 penny nail: A, bare handle; and B, handle covered with 1.15 cm thick foam rubber.

vibration; one was attached directly to the handle and one to a thin sheet of metal bent to fit between the handgrip cover and the operator's hand, in accordance with the procedure recommended by the ISO (5). A 400 line real-time frequency analyzer (Nicolet, type 446A) produced spectrograms of the vibration amplitudes. A companion instrument plotted the results in the form shown in some of the diagrams.

In the second experiment, the two materials were used to cover the handle of an electric saw with a blade that reciprocated from 2800 to 3000 times per minute, or at about 50 Hz. A third experiment similarly involved a small gasoline-powered chain saw operating at about 10 000 rpm, or at about 170 Hz. In a fourth experiment, the effect of resilient handgrips on the vibration of hammer handles was investigated.

II RESULTS AND DISCUSSION

The three curves in Fig. 2 show the acceleration of the handle with white noise excitation. Since the acceleration was measured at the hand-handle interface, the values shown are also the acceleration inputs to the hand. Curve C is for the bare handle with no resilient cover and indicates that the acceleration was about 1 m/s^2 over the entire frequency range (100 to 2000 Hz). Curve B gives the acceleration at the hand-resilient cover interface for a 1.15 cm layer of the stiffer foam, when the handgrip was hand-held. Under these conditions, there is no attenuation at frequencies below about 250 Hz, but at higher frequencies the vibration is attenuated from 10 to 15 dB. A 3.6 cm layer of the 1.2 N/cm foam, curve A, provided from 15 to 20 dB of attenuation at frequencies above 200 Hz, with decreasing amounts at frequencies down

Suggs et al.: Resilient handgrips

Table 1. Transmission of Vibration Through Various Types and Thicknesses of Resilient Handle Covers (Expressed as a Percentage of the Overall Acceleration Observed with No Cover).

Source of Vibration	Overall Acceleration with No Cover (m/s^2)	Vibration Transmitted (%) Approximate Stiffness and Thickness of Handle Cover		
		11.7 N/cm 1.2 cm	1.2 N/cm 3.6 cm	1.2 N/cm 7.2 cm
Electric Shaker	18.5	42	21	–
Electric Reciprocating Saw	48.5	50	47	33
Gasoline Chain Saw	100.8	42	36	–
Hammer	14 000	5	–	–

to 50 Hz. The thick layer of softer foam clearly gave better vibration isolation but the resulting handle diameter was too great to grip comfortably. However, it would be possible to construct a small diameter handle to which this resilient material could be attached.

We would expect attenuation to occur at frequencies above $\sqrt{2}$ times the effective natural frequency at the hand-handle interface, with the amount of attenuation dependent on the damping inherent in the material and on the frequency. Neglecting the frequency shift due to damping, the natural frequency of a simple one-degree-of-freedom system is:

$$f_n = \frac{1}{2\pi} \sqrt{(K/m)} \qquad (1)$$

where K is the effective spring constant and m the mass being vibrated. If we neglect the elastic properties of the hand, the spring constant may be approximated by the unit stiffness of the foam material times the area of the hand gripping the handle, which was measured and found to be about 75 cm^2. The mass of the hand coupled to the vibrating handle is expected to decrease with frequency because the hand itself is not rigid and, according to Mishoe (6), decreases from about 0.36 Kg at 40 Hz to 0.004 Kg at 1000 Hz. Substituting an intermediate-frequency hand mass of 0.09 Kg, the stiffness of the foam cube, a foam thickness of 1.15 cm and the palm area into eqn. 1 gives a natural frequency of 147 Hz. Thus, attenuation would be expected at frequencies above about 207 Hz. This is, in fact, about the frequency at which attenuation was found to occur (curve B of Fig. 2).

The handle cover that led to curve A was both softer and thicker. These two factors taken together gave an overall handle cover stiffness about one-thirtieth of the value for the middle curve. We would, therefore, expect attenuation to occur down to frequencies $1/\sqrt{30}$ times 207 Hz, the value found for the stiffer

material, or 37 Hz. Curve A of Fig. 2 indicates that attenuation is actually obtained at frequencies of 50 Hz and above, suggesting that the stiffness has been underestimated for the deflection occurring in this application. The agreement between calculation and measurement is, nevertheless, within about 25%.

In the second experiment, the handle vibration of an electric, reciprocating sabre saw when cutting wood was compared to the vibration on the surface of a resilient handle cover. For a 1.15 cm thick cover of the stiffer foam, the attenuation was approximately 10 dB for frequencies above 500 Hz, (Fig. 3). A 7.2 cm thick cover of the softer foam resulted in an attenuation of from 10 to 20 dB at frequencies of 250 Hz and above. It is evident by comparing Figs. 2 and 3 that less attenuation was obtained at low frequencies when the foams were attached to the saw handle. This was probably due to the need to hold the saw with a firm grip and push it against the work piece, in order to cut the wood. In at least part of the handgrip, the foam cells were completely compressed, so that the actual stiffness would be greater than that obtained from the force-displacement measurements. This could account for the increase in frequency at which attenuation was first observed.

The third experiment was similar to the second, with the foam materials now attached to the handles of a gasoline-powered chain saw. The results are given in Fig. 4 and are similar to the preceding case, with from 10 to 20 dB of attenuation at high frequencies and little, if any, attenuation at frequencies below about 300 to 500 Hz. Once again, the problem appears to be due to the grip force completely compressing the cells of the foam material.

In hammering, as in fact with most impact-delivering hand tools, significant high frequency vibration occurs (see Figs. 5A and 6A). A commercially supplied resilient handgrip reduced the overall acceleration to about 32% of the original value, while a 1.15 cm thick layer of the stiffer foam reduced the overall acceleration to about 5% when driving 16 penny nails, (see Figs. 5B and 6B).

The results of the four experiments are summarized in Table 1, which shows the percentage vibration transmitted to the hand through three different materials. The transmission of vibration (when not frequency weighted) was never more than 50% and in one case was reduced to 5%, as already noted.

DISCLAIMER

The use of trade names in this publication does not imply endorsement by the North Carolina Agricultural Research Service of the products named, nor criticism of similar ones not mentioned.

REFERENCES

1. Abrams CF, Suggs CW. Chain saw vibration isolation and transmission through the human arm. Trans Am Soc Agricultural Engrs 1969; 12: 423-425.
2. Gullander A, Petersson NF. Arbetsbelastning samt buller- och vibrationsexponering vid arbete med handslipmaskiner (Physical strain, noise and vibration from work with hand sanding machines). Stockholm: Arbetarskyddsstyrelsen Arbetsfysiologiska enheten, 1977. (in Swedish).
3. Suggs CW, Hanks JM, Robertson GT. Vibration of power tool handles. In: Brammer AJ, Taylor W, eds. Vibration Effects on the Hand and Arm in Industry. New York: Wiley, 1982.
4. Hansson JE, Klysell L, Krantz S, Ohlsson G, Petersson NF. Impact Power Drills: An Ergonomic and Hygienic Study. Stockholm: National Board of Occup Safety and Health, 1973. (Report 21/725).
5. International Organization for Standardization. Principles for the Measurement and the Evaluation of Human Exposure to Vibration Transmitted to the Hand. Draft International Standard ISO/DIS 5349, 1979.
6. Mishoe JW. Dynamic modeling of the human hand using driving point mechanical impedance technique. North Carolina State Univ., 1974. Ph.D. Thesis. (unpublished).

DISCUSSION

J. Starck: Have you considered measuring the vibration after it enters the hands, as mounting an accelerometer on foam can introduce errors?

Authors' Response: We have considered measuring vibration after it enters the hand, but not in this study. The accelerometer was not mounted on the foam but on a thin metal sheet bent around the foam.

M.J. Griffin: What was the mass of the accelerometer and mount used in the experiment, and what fraction was it of the hand mass used to predict the natural frequency (eqn. 1)?

Authors' Response: The estimated vibrating hand mass used in the calculation was 90 g. The combined mass of the accelerometer and mount was 22 g or about 1/4 of the hand mass.

M.R. Noble: Was any attempt made to control the grip force?

Authors' Response: No, except that subjects were instructed to maintain a reasonable grip.

Can you, then, comment on the possible effects of changes in grip force occasioned by a change in handle diameter, such as results from the addition of foam material?

Authors' Response: As grip force is increased we would expect to see an increase in the intensity of the vibration transmitted to the hand. In general, a decrease in the stiffness of the material between the hand and the handle will attenuate hand vibration.

M.J. Griffin: Table 1 refers to unweighted rms (and peak) accelerations. The results are therefore entirely dependent on the bandwidth of the spectra, and make no allowance for any differential sensitivity to vibration acceleration at different frequencies. What happens to the percentage vibration transmitted (or the attenuation) if the accelerations are frequency-weighted according to the Draft International Standard, ISO/DIS 5349?

Authors' Response: The measurements summarized in Table 1, and associated graphs, were designed to describe the vibration-isolating characteristics of various resilient handle covers rather than the improvement in the operator's working conditions. Therefore it is difficult to answer your question quantitatively. However, since transmission was lowest at higher frequencies where the ISO weighting factor is lowest, the "ISO adjusted" transmission would be higher than listed in Table 1.

LEGAL IMPLICATIONS

Legal Aspects of the Vibration Syndrome in Japan

T. Fukui

ABSTRACT: The status of the Vibration Syndrome under the occupational disease scheme in Japan is described and legal disputes involving vibration "disease" are discussed. The one court case in Japan which has come to judgment is considered in detail, particularly the court's findings on the nature of the Syndrome, the way of assessing severity of the Syndrome, and the level of compensation to be rendered to the victims. Critical views are expressed regarding this court judgment in Japan. Reference is made to the legal approach to this Syndrome in the United Kingdom.

RESUME: On décrit le statut du Syndrome de vibration sous le régime des maladies professionnelles au Japon et on examine les litiges au sujet de cette maladie. On étudie en détail le seul procès, au Japon, qui ait donné lieu à un jugement; une attention particulière est accordée au verdict du tribunal concernant la nature du syndrome, la façon d'en déterminer la gravité et l'importance des compensations à accorder aux victimes. On critique le verdict rendu par ce tribunal japonais et référence est faite à la position juridique du Royaume-Uni au sujet de cette maladie.

INTRODUCTION

Physical disorders caused by vibratory tools such as pneumatic rock-drills and rivet guns have been designated as an occupational disease under Japanese law since 1947 (1). In 1965, the chain saw was officially recognized as one of the tools which caused vibration disease (2). Physical disorders considered within the scope of this occupational disease category included not only vibration-induced white finger (VWF) but other conditions involving nerve and bone damage. As a result, the terms "vibration disease" or "vibration hazard" are generally used instead of VWF when referring to these disorders.

In order to receive benefits, the victim of this disease must be officially certified by the authorities with the help of physicians. The authorities do not check complainants in a strictly scientific and objective manner, and a large number of persons have therefore been certified as suffering from this disease, most of whom are chain saw workers. The total number of chain saw workers certified since 1965 is 3460 Government forestry workers and 3969 private sector forestry workers (as of December, 1978).

Following certification, a worker receives all medical expenses incurred for future treatment of the disease and almost full compensation for subsequent days off work directly attributable to the disease.

Both the union involved and the workers themselves, however, are not satisfied with the present compensatory measures. They have recently filed a number of lawsuits against the employers, the saw manufacturers and the saw importers, claiming additional monetary compensation for their pain and suffering caused by the disease.

To the best of our knowledge, there have been about twelve lawsuits filed with several trial courts, involving a total of 94 chain saw workers employed by the National Government Forestry Agency, 58 chain saw workers employed by private forestry businesses, and 87 miners employed by a private mining company. The defendants in these cases are: a) the State, i.e. the National Forestry Agency (the employer); b) four general sales agents of chain saws imported from West Germany, the United States and Sweden, and one domestic chain saw manufacturer and its sales agent; and c) a mining company (the employer).

The amount claimed by each plaintiff-worker ranges from approximately US $50 000 to US $200 000. The majority of the plaintiffs are claiming more than US $100 000 each.

I COURT JUDGMENT

Thus far, there has been only one court Judgment handed down in the above-mentioned lawsuits (3). The Judgment was in July 1977, and was in favour of the claimants in their suit against the State (Forestry Agency). The Forestry Agency was ordered to pay each of the twelve plaintiffs, who were ex-chain saw operators of the Agency, compensatory damages in amounts ranging from approximately US $25 000 to US $50 000. The Forestry Agency immediately appealed the decision to the appellate court.

1.1 The Court Findings on the Nature of the Syndrome

In the Judgment, the court made several findings (most of which we cannot agree with) concerning the nature and classification of severity of the disease, and the Forestry Agency's duty of care for the workers' safety.

The Judgment stated that the so-called Andreeva Galanina Classification of the disease (named after a Soviet physician) is reliable and is widely accepted in Japan. The court therefore accepted the following classification table, which is strongly influenced by the Soviet classification, for estimating the severity of vibration disease.
a) Level I: Several symptoms are claimed, including a sensation of heaviness in the fingers and hands with intermittent pain and numbness, abnormal dullness or abnormal sensitivity. There may be stiffness of the neck and shoulders, and heaviness in the arms and the waist.
b) Level II: Level I symptoms increase, occur more frequently, and spread to other parts of the body. Fingers and hands may become cold and discolored. Symptoms of vegetative stigmata, such as headaches, dizziness, irritability, sweating and forgetfulness may also occur.
c) Level III: Level II symptoms increase and Raynaud's Phenomenon appears. Symptoms of numbness, pain, or dulling of sensation in the arms intensify. There are changes in the muscles, such as muscle contracture, muscle atrophy, and reduced muscle strength, resulting in reduced movement. There may also be neurasthenia-like symptoms, or a decrease in sexual desire.
d) Level IV: Raynaud's Phenomenon occurs with increasing frequency and in more and more parts of the body. Angiospasms spread from the extremities throughout the body. In the brain, this results in catatonia. Symptoms may appear which resemble those of angina pectoris, Ménière's syndrome, the interbrain syndrome, as well as those resulting from diseases of, or injury to, the spinal cord.

The damage in each individual system, such as the circulatory, autonomous nervous, and muscle-tendon-joint-ligament systems, does not necessarily progress uniformly. The damage in one system may progress to a more severe degree and at a faster rate than in the others.

Under the above classification, most of the twelve plaintiffs (eight were over age sixty) were found to have damage due to vibration, not only of peripheral nerves and blood vessels, but also of muscles and tendons, elbow and shoulder joints. Moreover, subjective complaints such as headache, irritability, sweating, and impotency were also attributed to vibration exposure. Thus all plaintiffs, but one, were classified as victims of level III or IV. Several of them were found to require hospitalization for treatment.

It is questionable whether many of the symptoms involving muscles, nerves, bones, joints, ligaments, and tendons described in the above classification have been proven to be attributable to the vibration of chain saws. We do not find any consensus of opinion among medical practitioners specializing in this field that would permit such findings to stand in a court of law. In my opinion, the court may well have been misled by the very limited information supplied by certain public health doctors who had been acting for the plaintiffs.

1.2 The Court Findings on the Duty of the Forestry Agency

The court stated that the Forestry Agency was liable for the non-performance of its duty concerning the care and safety of workers, for the following reasons:
a) Before introducing the chain saw to the Forestry Agency around the mid 1950's, the Agency had an obligation to investigate its effects on the human body. Vibration "disease" caused by pneumatic tools was already known in Japan at this time. The chain saw should have been introduced only after the Agency had confirmed that the machine was harmless. However, investigations were not undertaken because the vibration of chain saws was thought not to be as intense as that of pneumatic tools.
b) The Forestry Agency made no serious effort to deal with the occurrence of vibration disease in chain saw operators. This was in spite of evidence, as early as 1960, which included complaints by several workers to their supervisors of white fingers, and a questionnaire survey conducted by a research laboratory of the Forestry Agency revealing symptoms of whitening of fingers among the workers.
c) The Forestry Agency tended to restrict the vibration "disease", for which victims could be certified, to Raynaud's Phenomenon, regardless of the fact that vibration

damage was recognized in 1966 by the National Personnel Agency to affect the entire body. Furthermore, certification was delayed because examining physicians were limited to those physicians retained by the Forestry Agency. Because lower level effects were not recognized, and certified patients were directed to continue using vibration tools, the effects of the disease were exacerbated.

d)   As long as vibration disease continued to occur, Forestry Agency was required to discontinue the use of chain saws, or to adjust their use in such a way that the disease would be prevented. The Forestry Agency did take some precautionary measures such as the introduction of anti-vibration saws. However, it was not until April 1969 that the Forestry Agency finally agreed to a time restriction on the use of chain saws (4), which had long been demanded by the Forestry Agency's Workers Union.

Based upon these reasons, the court's Judgment was in favour of the claimants in their suit against the State (Forestry Agency). The court's reasoning and its conclusion seem to be unwarranted, and to raise the standard of legal duty of care far beyond that normally required for an employer in the forestry industry. If these standards were to be enforced, timber production would of necessity be reduced, and the forestry industry might cease to exist.

II   THE BRITISH APPROACH

There is a distinct contrast between the Japanese approach to the Vibration Syndrome described above, and the approach followed in the United Kingdom, one of the few industrialized countries where the Syndrome has not yet been recognized as a Prescribed Disease.

We ascertained that in 1975, the Industrial Injuries Advisory Council of the United Kingdom turned down VWF as a Prescribed or Scheduled Disease (5). In its conclusions, it stated that:
"The object of prescription would, of course, be to compensate those workers who are disabled in any real sense by vibration, particularly those who lose earnings. From the evidence we have received we have concluded that such workers form a very small proportion of the total, affected in some measure by VWF, for the great majority of whom the right assessment would probably be less than 1 percent which the law lays down as the minimum needed to attract benefit. Even if there were a reliable and acceptable way of sifting out the few deserving cases, the trouble and cost could be considerable and might well be regarded as disproportionate to the results. In fact there is no such way."

We have also learned that in one court case between the UK Forestry Commission

and a chain saw operator who developed VWF (Stage 3) through his work with the Commission from 1971 to 1974 (6), the Judgment decreed that the Forestry Commission was not negligent in its exercise of care towards the operator (plaintiff).

The Judgment reached this conclusion on the following grounds:
a)   In 1968, it was brought to the notice of the Forestry Commission that chain saws which they were using were causing VWF.
b)   Immediately thereafter, the Forestry Commission started investigation of anti-vibration saws and such saws were actually put into service within a relatively short period.
c)   Although the Forestry Commission faced difficulties in deciding a safety limit for vibration of the saws at the early stage of the investigation, since relevant and reliable information was not available, the Commission, and in particular its Safety Officer, tried to keep abreast of new information as it became available. They actually utilized the information to establish an up-to-date safety limit.
d)   In the light of further research in the future, it might be shown that the applied safety limit was incorrect. However, having regard to the information which was available during the period from 1971 to 1974, the Forestry Commission, and its Safety Officer, should be considered to have taken all reasonable steps to inform themselves of the up-to-date safety limit for exposure to vibration of the saws, and to have applied it with due care.

From the viewpoint of the Japanese court, it appears that the UK Forestry Commission would be held liable for the VWF of the chain saw operator, on the grounds that: a) the Forestry Commission was too late in noticing the occurrence of VWF among chain saw operators in 1968; and b) the Commission's efforts to establish a safety limit for vibration, and to introduce anti-vibration saws were not sufficient, since they did not succeed in preventing the occurrence of VWF.

III   CONCLUSIONS

It appears that the legal issues relating to vibration disease have not been handled in a proper and reasonable manner in Japan. Both the administration and the court seem to have been misguided about the nature of vibration disease, and both have shown over-reaction to the problem. The standards or criteria to be applied for assessing the severity of the disease and the level of compensation for victims should be re-examined. Closer access to information from abroad, and more frequent communication with information sources will help to reach a reasonable solution to the problem.

REFERENCES

1. Enforcement Ordinance of the Labor Standards Law. Article 35, 1947.
2. Labor Standards Bureau Chief of the Labor Ministry. Directive 595, 1965.
3. Matsumoto et al. v Forestry Agency. Kochi District Court, July 28, 1977.
4. Japan Forestry Agency. Time Restriction - April, 1969: 2 hours per day, 5 days per week, less than 3 days continuous use per week, 40 hours per month, 10 minutes per hour.
5. Industrial Injuries Advisory Council. Vibration Syndrome. London: Her Majesty's Stationery Office, 1975 (cmnd 5965).
6. Murphy v UK Forestry Commission. Court of Session, Edinburgh, Scotland, May 30, 1979.

DISCUSSION

T. Matsumoto: I have been investigating the Vibration Syndrome relating to chain saw operators in Japan. I have two comments to make on this presentation. First, with regard to Japan, it has been claimed that the principal symptoms of the Vibration Syndrome are mainly peripheral functional disturbances. However, it should be pointed out that central function, ennervated through the autonomic nervous system, and the endocrine system may also be involved. Second, chain saws were introduced into the national forest in Japan in 1954. In the sixth year after this introduction, in 1959, the Vibration Syndrome became an occupational hazard. Twelve years before the introduction of chain saws, in 1947, the Ministry of Labor of Japan recognized the Vibration Syndrome as an occupational disease (Rule of Labor Standard Law, No. 35). I think, therefore, that the Forestry Agency introduced the chain saw without considering the effect of vibration and without any safety consideration. They continued introducing machines for the next 15 years. Furthermore, they did not take any counter measures to reduce the signs and symptoms of the Vibration Syndrome in their chain saw operators.

Author's Response: To the first comment, although I am not a medical specialist, I do not think that any consensus among medical specialists in Japan has been reached with regard to the view that the central nervous system as well as the endocrine system could be adversely affected by exposure to vibration. To the second comment, I think that chain saws were first introduced in Japan for trial use around 1954 and were put into industrial use around 1957.

Other than the above, I agree with your chronological statements, with the qualification that in 1947, the Ministry of Labor recognized only the Vibration Syndrome caused by pneumatic tools, such as rock drills and rivet guns, as an occupational disease. This recognition was based on regulations in other countries, and not upon our own research.

It may be true that at the time when the Forestry Agency of Japan first introduced chain saws into its operations, it did not foresee that exposure to chain saw vibration would jeopardize workers' safety by causing VWF. In my view, the Forestry Agency should not be blamed for this as nobody in the world at that time had ever foreseen such danger.

I cannot agree with the last statement that the Forestry Agency did not take any preventive measures against the Vibration Syndrome. In fact, the Forestry Agency:
a) conducted a nationwide questionnaire survey in 1963, and special medical examinations for complainants of VWF among chain saw operators since 1965;
b) since 1965, has started a number of medical as well as engineering research projects requiring many outside specialists;
c) introduced A/V saws and gloves in 1969; and
d) implemented time restrictions for chain saw use in the same year.

In my view, Japan is one of the most sensitive and responsive countries in the world to VWF. Japan has spent a great amount of time and money to prevent VWF. However, much of this has not yet contributed to solving the problem.

Legal Aspects of Vibration White Finger:
Joseph v *Ministry of Defence (Navy)*

T. P. Oliver

ABSTRACT: The means by which a workman can obtain compensation in the United Kingdom are briefly described. A synopsis of the only case concerning vibration white finger that has been heard in the English High Court is given, together with an account of the proceedings in the Court of Appeal. The problems raised and future prospects are discussed.

RESUME: Les moyens par lesquels un travailleur peut obtenir des prestations d'invalidité dans le Royaume-Uni font l'objet d'une courte description. Un résumé du seul cas concernant les doigts blancs dûs aux vibrations qui a été entendu dans une Cour supérieure britannique est donné, ainsi qu'un résumé des événements en Cour d'appel. Les problèmes et les perspectives d'avenir sont abordés.

INTRODUCTION

There are two ways in which an employee can obtain compensation for industrial injury or disease in the United Kingdom. Firstly, he can claim benefit in the form of a disability pension, or a single payment from the Department of Health and Social Security under the Industrial Injuries Provisions of the Social Security Act 1975; and/or secondly, he can sue any party, normally his employer, in court. In this context, precedent, i.e. case law, can be important. Success with a claim for a Prescribed Industrial Disease gives, in many cases of permanent disability, a good opening for proceeding with the second option, with the intention of securing further monetary damages for the malady. Such actions are often paid for by the employee's union.

In the United Kingdom, there are currently 50 conditions listed as Prescribed Diseases together with the various pneumoconioses. Before a disease is prescribed, it must be possible to establish, or presume with reasonable certainty, in the individual case that the disease is attributable to the prescribed occupation. Despite two references to the Industrial Injuries Advisory Council (1,2), the body which advises the Minister, they have been unable to present other than a majority view against prescription in the case of vibration-induced white finger (VWF). Another such reference is now collecting evidence. Thus no employee can directly claim benefit from the State: compensation can only be sought in the courts against a third party.

The case with which this paper is concerned relates to a caulker/riveter employed by the Ministry of Defence (Navy) (MOD(N)), in the naval base at Portsmouth. The introduction of the all-welded ship, as distinct from one in which the plates were held together by rivets, has led to the demise of the riveter in the shipyard world, and his replacement by the caulker. Although some of the more elderly dockyard caulkers started work as riveters (or even rivet boys), most of their working life has been spent as iron caulkers.

The task of the caulker is to remove excess metal, particularly where two metal plates have been welded together. For this purpose he uses an air-driven gun, whose hammer drives a cutting tool. The gun weighs about 10 kg and is held in one hand (which also operates the trigger), with the other hand holding the cutting tool in the gun (there being no locking device), and guiding it. The gun is generally held in the dominant hand. The work is intermittent and it has been estimated that about four hours actual work, i.e. exposure to vibration, is done per day. The vibration characteristics of the tools are in excess of the proposed British Standard (3).

Leather industrial gloves are normally worn by the operators of this type of tool, not only due to the rough nature of the task but also because work is often in the open air and in all weather. They also diminish the discomfort of the cold air exhausted from the tools. These tools are also extremely noisy, giving rise to sound levels in excess of 100 dB(A). Noise-induced hearing loss from the use of such tools in shipyards is a Prescribed Disease.

I THE TRIAL

1.1 The High Court Proceedings

The case was heard before Mr. Justice Watkins VC in the Queen's Bench Division of the High Court in July 1978.

The burden of the Plaintiff's case was that the MOD(N) had been negligent. They were also in breach of their duty of care in that the Plaintiff was disabled by VWF, which the employer ought to have foreseen and about which the employer had knowledge, both at first hand from the bundle of scientific papers to be placed in evidence before the Court, and from their medical advisors who had discussed the disease. The defendants admitted the Plaintiff had VWF from the use of the tools, but denied negligence or breach of duty. Following the opening addresses by Counsel for both sides, Mr. Joseph, the Plaintiff, was called. He told the Court he was found to be suffering from VWF in 1973 when he was aged 59. He had then been employed as a caulker/riveter in the dockyard for a period of 23 years. He alleged he first developed numbness and whiteness of his finger tips in September 1972. By February 1973 all his fingers and his thumbs were affected at work with whiteness, numbness and pain, and he was unable to hold his tools. As a result he "collapsed" at work.

This he reported to his own general practitioner (not the dockyard occupational physician), and it was from his own doctor that the latter first heard of the case. On his return to work he was taken off caulking duties and employed elsewhere, until his retirement some four years later, on medical grounds unconnected with VWF. The second witness called by the Plaintiff was a fellow caulker/riveter and a shop steward of his Union. He stated that he never had white fingers in his 35 years in the trade, but knew other caulkers who had. On cross-examination, he admitted that the men accepted this as part of the penalty of the job, and never made any official complaints to management or the medical authority about the condition.

The third witness was another workman who alleged he had VWF, and who said the condition was widespread in the dockyard at Portsmouth. Two expert witnesses were called by the Plaintiff. The first was an eminent cardiovascular surgeon. The defence had no quarrel with his description of Raynaud's Phenomena and VWF. However, his views on preventive measures, the right type of gloves, compliant handles and

interval medical examination were challenged on cross-examination, on the basis that there was no support in the literature put forward by the Plaintiff, rather the reverse, and that no alternative supporting evidence for his ideas could be produced. The Plaintiff's other expert witness was an engineer, presented as experienced in sound and vibration measurement. In his evidence he gave the Court to understand that vibration measurements had been relatively easy to make since the early 1950s, and that there were several people competent so to do. However, he had to admit the instruments he used to measure the dockyard tools were borrowed from Salford University. Concerning papers in engineering journals on the subject that appeared before the relevant time (i.e., 1972), he stated he believed he had seen none.

Although they had an engineering report of their own, the Defendants called only one witness, a Senior Naval Occupational Physician. He admitted that he and his colleagues were aware of the VWF problem. He recounted his surprise when involved with Taylor and Pelmear in a survey at Rosyth Dockyard (one of the scientific papers used by the Plaintiff) that 46% of the vibrating tool workers had Stage 1 or 2 VWF, and a latent period of the order of 15 years (4). These findings had been discussed with his Naval Occupational Physician colleagues.

Several lines of action had been explored, a fuller survey, accurate measurement of vibration characteristics, and possible recommendations to management. On these matters, the Plaintiff had asked for transcripts of the discussions as recorded at the time, and various internal Ministry correspondence. He explained the ethical dilemma involved in surveys, in what to tell the workforce, and the possible destruction of a man's livelihood in removing him from his trade.

The trial closed with a closing address by Counsel.

1.2 The Judgment

Judgment was reserved and given on 29 September 1978. It covers 26 pages of foolscap typescript and ends (5): "So on the balance of probabilities I am firmly of the view that the Plaintiff cannot succeed upon this basis. Accordingly his claim fails and there must be judgment for the Defendants."

Why did the Plaintiff not succeed? There were several reasons and these are amplified in the following discussion by passages from the Judgment. He was an atypical case in clinical terms - 23 years work with no symptoms, then disabling VWF within five months. "From the first sign of the condition to the final incapacity a remarkably short period of time elapsed. No other comparable case was referred to me by Mr. M. or anyone else. There is no evidence that any other man had deteriorated so rapidly."

The dismissal by the Judge of the evidence 1) by the Plaintiff's expert witness on vibration measurement, and his failure to provide any evidence in the engineering journals, and 2) by his medical consultant in matters relating to the protection of workers by gloves, damping devices, etc. was as follows:

"I thought Mr. S wandered beyond his competence and knowledge and upon those aspects I found him to be an unconvincing and unsatisfactory witness. This comment also applies to some extent to Mr. M when he speculated upon what remedial measures might be provided to lessen the effect of vibration. Neither of them persuaded me that an improved glove or compliant material fitted to the tool would have any noteworthy effect in this respect. It would, in my opinion, require the results of experiments to advance with confidence such propositions. The assertion of Mr. S that there has been since the early 1950s at least a dozen highly competent people dealing with the reduction of the effects of vibration - although I bear in mind the device fitted to chain saws in the late 1960s - I treat with considerable reserve. ...It is only in the last year that Mr. S has seen engineering articles upon this subject appear."

The symptoms up to and including Stage 2 symptoms were trivial:

"The triviality of the illness in question, the rareness of its manifestations in a severe stage, the complete absence of complaint by workmen of suffering and a loss of work caused thereby are but several of the many factors which alone, or in combination, could have the probable effect of excusing an employer from looking for the appearance of some physical harm to his workmen brought about by the use of his tools."

The acceptance of the evidence of the Defence's only witness, "a splendidly honest and frank witness" regarding the following matters:

a) Decisions of priority between the noise hazard and that of vibration.

"He has observed the work of caulking and riveting on many occasions. He was thus impressed by the challenge to a workman's hearing created by these occupations and, as I have said, actively concerned himself with the study of this problem from 1967 onwards, which he regards insofar as I am able to judge, rightly regards, as far more serious than that posed by the condition of Raynaud's Phenomenon."

b) The question of a survey or other means to ascertain the extent of VWF and act upon it.

"I think the survey at Rosyth was partly instigated by Captain O. ... Then it is said that they did not act upon the results of this survey. The Defendants' internal memoranda oppose this assertion."

c) The introduction of interval health screening for these workers.

"However the obligations thus cast upon an employer do not mean that because he is aware that tools of the kind used by his workmen are known by him to cause, for example, Raynaud's Phenomenon, he is by reason of that fact only and automatically in breach of duty to his workmen if he does not by medical examination... ."

d) The difficulty of accurately measuring the vibration.

"Assistance was sought to measure vibrations. There were problems in the way of doing so. Moreover, Dr. Taylor advised the Defendants to await the assistance of the British Standards Institution."

e) The Defendants did not inform the workmen of the nature of Raynaud's Phenomenon.

"It is obvious that the Defendants consciously took a decision not to do this. It seems to have been a judgment formed on medical grounds and for, as I say, a reason of which Captain O approved. The Defendants decided to make measurements of vibrations their first objective. This may have been a wrong though not necessarily a negligent decision."

II THE APPEAL

The case was taken to Appeal in the Supreme Court on the basic grounds that the Judge's decision "was wrong in law and against the weight of the evidence." In the Plaintiff's Appeal, all charges of negligence were dropped and the evidence of their expert engineering witness was not used.

The transcript of the Judgment of Lord Justic Megaw and his two fellow Lord Justices runs to 21 pages and is unanimous. A few quotations will illustrate (6):

"But a fair summary of the evidence appears to us to be that up to and including Stage 2, as defined, the condition is not fairly to be described as serious. It is, rather, a matter of inconvenience, which may prevent or discourage the sufferer from pursuing hobbies which involve exposure of the fingers to cold conditions."

"There is no dispute as to the principle of law to be applied. It is as set out in the passage which was cited by Mr. Justice Watkins from the Judgment of Mr. Justice Swanwick in Stokes v Guest, Keen, and Nettlefolds (Bolts and Nuts) Ltd. (1968). I take this from the Judgement of Mr. Justice Watkins. At page 18 of the Judgment he quotes Mr. Justice Swanwick as follows (7):

'The overall test is still the conduct of the reasonable and prudent employer, taking positive thought for the safety of his workers in the light of what he knows or ought to know ... where there is developing knowledge, he must keep reasonably abreast of it and not be too slow to apply it ... . He must weigh up the risk in terms of the likelihood of injury occurring and the potential consequences if it does; and he must balance against this the probable effectiveness of the precautions that can be taken to meet it and the expense and inconvenience they involve.'

If Mr. M's evidence is to be taken literally, the employees would have to be told (perhaps by a note in their first pay-packet), 'If when you make your periodic visit to the Medical Centre it is discovered that there has been any deterioration in your VWF condition, you will no longer be allowed to work as a caulker, or with vibratory tools'."

The Appeal Court decided that on the facts of the case it had not been shown that the Defendants were in breach of duty towards the Plaintiff, and, following the disclosure of the Rosyth survey, the Defendants acted as reasonable and prudent employers having regard to the degree of the condition thereby disclosed. The appeal was dismissed (with costs).

III DISCUSSION AND CONCLUSIONS

The Rosyth survey featured in the trial has been followed up by Oliver, Pethybridge and Lumley (3). Their study showed 75% of the caulkers in Portsmouth and Devonport Dockyards (i.e., 147 out of 195) had VWF in Stages 1 or 2 but none were found in Stage 3 (Table 1). The exposure to vibration ranged from 1 to 50 years.

Table 1. Dockyard Caulkers by Category of Vibration White Finger (%)

Dockyard	N	0	0_TN	1	2
Devonport	120	21	3	40	36
Portsmouth	75	12	7	42	33

The question of prescription is again before the Industrial Injuries Advisory Council. During the trial described, the Judge remarked "he was not moved by the failure to prescribe the disease". However, the whole question of Prescribed Diseases is under scrutiny and could be dropped in favour of individual proof. The Society of Occupational Medicine, in its evidence on this subject, pointed out the 'two bites at the cherry' situation, which arises with a successful claim under the Prescribed Diseases regulations providing 'prima facie' evidence for a court claim (8).

It appears that an important point of case law may have been established for the future over the question of the medical examination of workers at risk, with a distinction between risk which can be fatal and that which is trivial. However the occupational physician will still be faced with the dilemma of when to say to an employee "enough is enough" and remove him from work with vibrating tools.

The establishment of an acceptable standard of "safe" vibration exposures, the availability of tools that match that standard, and a reliable method of objective measurement of the extent of VWF would be of major assistance in establishing the medical and legal parameters. On the other hand, an unconnected technological advance may remove the problem overnight. Thus the future position as of today lies very much in the hands of the courts, the credibility of the expert witnesses called, and the normality, if that is not a paradox, of the plaintiff's signs and symptoms.

ACKNOWLEDGEMENTS

I acknowledge the permission of the Medical Director General (Naval), Surgeon Vice Admiral Sir John Harrison QHP, to publish this paper, and my indebtedness to Mr. H. Grange of the Treasury Solicitor's Dept. for his help in legal matters.

DISCLAIMER

The views expressed in this paper are those of the author and do not necessarily represent those of the Ministry of Defence.

REFERENCES

1. Industrial Injuries Advisory Council. Raynaud's Phenomenon. London: Her Majesty's Stationery Office, 1954 (cmnd 9347).
2. Industrial Injuries Advisory Council. Vibration Syndrome. London: Her Majesty's Stationery Office, 1975 (cmnd 5965).
3. Oliver TP, Pethybridge RJ, Lumley KPS. Vibration white finger in dockyard workers. Arh Hig rada toksiko 1979; 30: 683-693.
4. Tayler W, Pelmear PL, Pearson JCG. Vibration-induced white finger epidemiology. In: Taylor W, Pelmear PL, eds. Vibration White Finger in Industry. London: Academic Press, 1975: 1-13.
5. Joseph v Ministry of Defence (Navy). Judgment. Royal Courts of Justice, Transcript Sept 29, 1978.
6. Joseph v Ministry of Defence (Navy). Appeal. Royal Courts of Justice, Transcript Feb 29, 1980.
7. Stokes v Guest, Keen, Nettlefolds (Nuts and Bolts). Weekly Law Report 1968; 1776: 1783.
8. Society of Occupational Medicine. Evidence to Industrial Injuries Advisory Council. J Soc Occup Med 1980; 30: 123.

DISCUSSION

M. Morin: Is an individual's susceptibility to VWF considered in cases such as you have described?

Author's Response: The short answer is no. We have no way of identifying susceptible individuals.

J.A. Rigby: With regard to the Musto v Saunders Valve Co. case, one of the judgments against the defendants was that the company physician had not warned the employee of his condition and its associated hazards. Since then, an out-of-court settlement has occurred because a company physician had not warned an employee, and the company's insurer decided that the claim could not be defended. Would you like to comment on the impact of this Judgment on future common law cases?

Author's Response: Perhaps I might refer to the appeal Judgment on this matter in the case I have described. "It is obvious the Defendants took a decision not to do this, ... this may have been a wrong though not necessarily a negligent decision." I suspect in law that a positive decision is a better defence than a decision implied by default.

W. Taylor: In the case of Murphy v UK Forestry Commission (1980), the Judgment was in favour of the Forestry Commission and found that the Defendant was not negligent in that it had: a) investigated the prevalence of VWF in its forests in 1968; and b) kept abreast of advancing knowledge, by carrying out chain saw vibration measurements and by replacing non-A/V chain saws with A/V saws in 1971 to 1972. The VWF impairment was Stage 3.

Author's Response: I think that this case is similar to the situation you have given. In both cases, management did all that was reasonably possible, even if they did not prevent an individual suffering from the Phenomenon.

Canadian Compensation Law and Vibration-Induced White Finger: A Preliminary Description

J. C. Paterson

ABSTRACT: Compensation for vibration-induced white finger (VWF) under Canadian law is reviewed. The historical information available in claims data is indicated with specific reference to British Columbia. The basis upon which the disease is recognized for compensation purposes in British Columbia is described. Reference is made to the status of VWF in the compensation schemes of other provinces. The limitations of the current approaches are noted.

RESUME: La compensation financière pour les doigts blancs dûs aux vibrations prévue par le législateur canadien est examinée. Les renseignements historiques disponibles dans les données relatives aux réclamations sont indiquées dans le contexte particulier de la Colombie-Britannique. Les critères de reconnaissance de la maladie aux fins des prestations d'invalidité en Colombie-Britannique sont décrits. Les auteurs décrivent le statut des doigts blancs dûs aux vibrations dans les programmes de compensation des autres provinces. Les lacunes des approches actuelles sont notées.

INTRODUCTION

Compensation for vibration-induced white finger (VWF) in Canada has not been the subject of extensive published information or analysis. Indeed, the subject of workers' compensation in Canada has seldom been researched and analyzed in the legal literature. In this respect, Canada compares very unfavourably to Europe and the United States. No understanding of compensation for VWF in Canada can be achieved without an awareness of the basic context of workers' compensation and industrial disease law (1).

The central philosophy of workers' compensation in Canada is that it is a compulsory, state-administered, no-fault, mutual insurance scheme which replaces the right of the worker to sue his employer in civil court for work-related diseases or injuries. Compensation is generally paid for wage-loss, medical aid, pensions for permanent disabilities, dependents' pensions in fatal cases and vocational rehabilitation. As an alternative to compensation, the worker can elect to sue a negligent "third party" manufacturer (where the manufacturer is not an employer in the jurisdiction). Alternatively, the agency administering workers' compensation in each province can sue as a "subrogated" party. Such actions are rare, however, partly due to immature Canadian products' liability and status laws.

Workers' compensation schemes are provincial jurisdictions, and were started first in Ontario and Nova Scotia (1915), followed by British Columbia and Manitoba (1917), Alberta (1918), New Brunswick (1919), Saskatchewan (1929), Quebec (1931), Prince Edward Island (1949), Newfoundland (1951), Yukon Territory (1973) and Northwest Territories (1977). The schemes are financed by an assessment (tax) levied on every employer at the point of production. The assessment rates vary according to the historical hazard rating of the industry group to which each employer belongs. The rate levied against an individual employer can be adjusted, if there is a merit or demerit assessment of that employer.

Although compensation statutes and their administration have been oriented to injury and trauma, industrial diseases are also covered under every provincial scheme. However, industrial disease claims constitute only a very small percentage of all claims. One study estimated that only 2% of all fatal claims and 0.8% of all permanent disability awards (excluding hearing loss) were related to industrial disease (2). Most claims are for medical aid (approximately 60%) or wage loss (approximately 40%). Wage loss compensation and pensions are paid where real wage loss occurs (projected wage loss is pensionable in some jurisdictions). There are no awards in any compensation scheme for pain and suffering, or for social or recreational losses. There is no on-going, automatic, administrative search for disease incidence. And no compensation law requires epidemiological work to be conducted.

I CLAIMS DATA

An historical analysis of claims made to any Provincial Workers' Compensation Board (WCB) is difficult. Few have fully utilized computer data storage and retrieval methods. Where they are used, the historical claims file data are not all necessarily available. Statistics are not usually maintained on both claims received and claims paid; generally, only claims paid are registered. In addition, the information available in any computer file is limited by the design of computer coding; generally only the "nature of disease" and the "source of injury" are provided. The pension percentage, length of wage-loss payment, or nature and amount of medical aid or vocational rehabilitation may not be described.

For example, the British Columbia WCB has reliable computer recall established to 1972. However, it is only since June 1980 that all industrial disease claims have been computer coded. The reliability of earlier data cannot be confirmed, and claims filed in each jurisdiction must be used. An example of the current British Columbia WCB computer coding for a chain saw operator who has contracted VWF would be as follows:

Type of Accident: "Contact with vibration"
Source of Injury: "Chain saw"
Part of Body: "Circulatory"
Nature of Injury: "Other-industrial disease"

The National Work Injuries Programme is a programme sponsored by Statistics Canada to provide a reliable, national, and uniform basis of jurisdictional comparison. Unfortunately, not all provinces have been involved in the last decade of preparatory work.

II INDUSTRIAL DISEASE RECOGNITION

The inclusion of a disease in a formal schedule generally carries with it great legal benefit for the worker. In such cases, there is a specific legal presumption as to disease etiology, unless disproved by positive evidence provided by the compensation board or the worker's employer. To quote the British Columbia Workers' Compensation Act, R.S.B.C. 1979, C437 as amended at S.6(3): "...the disease shall be deemed to have been due to the nature of that employment unless the contrary is proved."

Of the provinces which utilize a formal scheduled listing of industrial diseases, seven do not include vibration-induced white finger. These are:
1) Nova Scotia (see Workers' Compensation Act, R.S.N.S. 1967, C.343 as amended to date, Schedule A);
2) Quebec (see Workers' Compensation Act, R.S.Q. 1964, C.159 as amended to date, Schedule D);

3) New Brunswick (see Workmen's Compensation Act, R.S.N.B. 1973, C.W.-13, S.76 as amended to date; Regulation 67-13 as amended to date by N.B. Reg. 76-140; 79-30, paragraph 14);
4) Prince Edward Island (see Workers' Compensation Act, R.S.P.E.I. 1974, C.W.-10, as amended to date, Schedule);
5) Newfoundland (see Workers' Compensation Act, R.S.N. 1970, C.403 as amended to date, Schedule);
6) Alberta (see Workers' Compensation Act, S. Alta. 1973, C.87 as amended to date; General Regulations, Alta. Reg. 362/73 as amended to date, S.14); and
7) Ontario (see Workmen's Compensation Act, R.S.O. 1970, C.505 as amended to date; General Regulation 834, as amended to date, Schedule 3).

The lack of an Industrial Disease Schedule or a scheduled inclusion does not mean a VWF claim cannot be accepted. However, in such cases, the onus is on the worker to establish the medical condition and the work-related etiology. The medical diagnosis and legal adjudicatory criteria are commonly unpublished, and perhaps totally discretionary.

2.1 British Columbia

The British Columbia WCB has not developed comprehensive specific written guidelines covering medical diagnosis, medical treatment, claims adjudication, pension entitlement or vocational rehabilitation. There are unpublished internal memoranda, however, which provide some guidelines for disability pension assessment. For example, a disability is recognized "...in that it has the potential to impair earning capacity". A disability does not constitute "...a pre-disposition which was not caused by the work environment". A functional (physical) impairment is recognized, as, for example, "...there is no doubt that there is such an impairment of the circulatory system". The steps for medical diagnosis and criteria for disability entitlement currently being utilized by the British Columbia WCB are the Laroche modified version of the American Medical Association's (AMA) "Guides to the Evaluation of Permanent Disability" (3,4). Cases are assessed on an individual basis. Use is made of the 'Guidelines for Adjudication' developed for the Ontario WCB by Dr. D. Burton (5).

The British Columbia WCB has formally recognized the following condition as an industrial disease (6):

Description of Disease: "Vascular disturbances of the extremities"
Description of Process/Industry: "where there is prolonged exposure to excessive vibrations at low temperature"

It is not presently clear when this condition was first scheduled, or what initiative or field research prompted its inclusion. There is a reference to at least one earlier study originating within the British Columbia WCB (7). It would, however, be relevant to know what is meant in the schedule by prolonged exposure, excessive vibrations, and low temperature; whether all three criteria need to be established (as an unpublished decision of WCB Commissioners seems to indicate (8)); and whether there are minimum requirements.

Tables 1 and 2 summarize the numbers of wage loss and pension claims for VWF in British Columbia which are presently known to us. A fixed pension award of 4% for total disability has prevailed in British Columbia since 1978 for those cases where there has been no return to the previous or equivalent occupation, and for which there is no evidence of vascular damage from physical, radiologic, or arteriographic examination.

Table 1. British Columbia Wage Loss Claims Data for VWF (Mason K, personal communication).

Year	Wage-Loss Claims First Paid	Employer Class[1] Against Which Claim Charged (No. of Claims)
1972	0	-
1973	2	102(2)
1974	0	-
1975	2	102(1), 906(1)
1976	4	403(2), 706(1), 707(1)
1977	2	102(1), 1302(1)
1978	3	102(1), 411(1), 1401(1)
1979	9	102(7), 104(1), 726(1)
1980	2	102(2)
Total to Date:	24	102(14), 403(2), Misc(8)

[1] 102-"Logging or Reforestation"; 403-"Gravel, Quarrying, etc."; 906-"Fish Canning or Processing"; 706-"Building Construction"; 707-"Metal Manufacturing"; 1302-"B.C. Government"; 411-"Metal Mining"; 1401-"Municipal Construction"; 726-"Construction General"; and 104-"Pulp & Paper Mill".

There are several points to be considered in VWF awards. First, for sawyers with long exposures, the worker is likely to have other physical disabilities from the work such as hearing loss, spinal deterioration, and/or a variety of trauma-induced ailments. Job mobility is adversely affected by factors such as education and age. In addition, private retirement pensions may not be available. Therefore, the worker's job alternatives are limited. Second, the 4% pension is equivalent to

Table 2. Pensions Established for VWF in British Columbia (Mason K, personal communication).[1]

1975	0
1976	1
1977	0
1978	1
1979	2

[1] The four claims averaged a $16 000 pension reserve set aside in the year of the award for future payment. The functional percentage award in each case was not available.

other scheduled awards, including "Loss of One Thumb (either hand) at I.P. Joint", and "Loss of One Index or Middle Finger (either hand) at M.P. Joint" (9). It is questionable whether the loss of digits described above would generally necessitate leaving one's employment, as VWF does with a chain saw operator, faller, miner, or operator of any other type of vibrating tool. It may be that historical social values regarding physical disfigurement are the source of the apparent incongruity.

Only a specified method for evaluating a real or projected loss-of-earnings can adequately address the problem. However, not all Canadian jurisdictions have such a method. Statutory wage ceilings also limit the economic justice to be accorded, even where such a method is used.

The numbers of workers in British Columbia exposed to hand-arm vibration through the use of chain saws has been estimated by the Research Department of the International Woodworkers of America (IWA), the largest industrial union in British Columbia representing most unionized fallers. They estimate that there are approximately 1625 IWA fallers using chain saws, of which 1030 are in the Coast Master Agreement, 500 are in the Coast Independent Agreements, 70 are in the Southern Interior Master Agreement, and 25 are in the Northern Interior Master Agreement (Scott D, personal communication). There are, in addition, unknown numbers of sawyers who are non-unionized in British Columbia. Other users of chain saws include forest industry workers on landing work, bridge construction, and right-of-way clearing. It has been estimated that coastal fallers average from 3.5 to 4.5 hours exposure per day.

A 1979 sawyers' survey by the IWA and Portland State University covered workers in the U.S. Pacific Northwest States (Washington, Oregon, Idaho) and the Canadian western provinces (British Columbia, Alberta, Saskatchewan, Manitoba) (10). Of 156 replies, only 10% of respondents reported no symptoms, such as burning sensation or numbness. Approximately 43% of respondents reported difficulties under cold conditions. Use of gloves, tight grips, warming, and rest periods were reported as defensive techniques. Very few saws are presently used that do not have anti-vibration devices, such as rubber isolators.

These results may be compared with the symptomatic response received by Brubaker et al. (11), indicating that 51% of British Columbia coast sawyers surveyed complained of some form of vibration-induced white finger.

2.2 Alberta

Alberta has no adjudicatory or diagnostic guidelines, but basically follows those of Ontario. The province has no scheduled condition recognized as an industrial disease (i.e. it does not utilize a legal presumption methodology on industrial disease claims). Therefore, each case is considered on its own merits. Advisory Medical Panels may be used at the initial decision-making level. The members are appointed as experts in groups of two or three by the Director of Medical Services. Appeal Medical Panels also exist for medical disputes. Alberta uses a physical (functional) loss method for pension awards. This may now be modified by a Disability Evaluation Committee to a loss-of-earnings methods (Hall WF, personal communication).

2.3 Saskatchewan

Saskatchewan had a formal scheduled listing in its former Schedule II (Workers' Compensation Act, S.S. 1973-74, C.127), since circa 1963, as follows: Description of Disease: vascular disturbances in the upper extremities due to continuous vibration from pneumatic or power drills, riveting machines or hammers; and Description of Process: arising out of, and in the course of, employment.

Saskatchewan no longer maintains an industrial disease schedule (Workers' Compensation Act, 1979, S.S. 1979, C.W.-17.1, S.84(1)(2), proclaimed effective 1 October 1979, remainder of Act proclaimed effective 1 January 1980). Saskatchewan also no longer defines the term "industrial disease" by statute. Formerly, it was defined as "any of the diseases mentioned in Schedule II, and any other disease that by the regulations is declared to be an industrial disease".

The first claims date from the early 1960's, with cases in northern underground miners working in extremely cold and wet conditions. Since that time, working conditions have improved and claims received now number only one to two per year.

Pensions paid prior to 1 January 1980 average 7.5% to 10% of salary. Since 1980 and the new Act, a fixed lump sum of

approximately $1000 is paid (Elliot GF, personal communication).

2.4 Ontario

Interest in this subject was awakened with an "avalanche" of claims from the mining industry in 1977. The claims (allowed) for this condition as of the 30 April 1981 total approximately 580. Functional pensions awarded range from 0% to 13% of salary, with awards of 4% being the average or median (Burton D, personal communication).

III CONCLUSIONS

It may be concluded from the preliminary survey of Canadian workers' compensation practice that:
1. Canadian compensation boards do not have a uniform legal or medical approach to VWF.
2. Some Canadian boards appear to have little or no specific, formalized legal or medical approach whatsoever.
3. Where there is uniformity, Ontario's approach is the model, which places reliance upon the Laroche modified version of the American Medical Association's "Guides to the Evaluation of Permanent Disability" (4).
4. In adjudicating awards, the traditional physical impairment method still predominates, and is not well-suited for dealing with VWF.
5. Compensation for VWF in the form of wage loss and pensions has been variable from province to province.
6. Pension awards have been modest, both in numbers and the percentage disability awarded.
7. It is probable that hundreds more undiagnosed and uncompensated cases exist in Canada, primarily from chain saw use in the forest industry.
8. Canadian workers' compensation law and its administration have been of limited use in the recognition, treatment and prevention of VWF, and in the income and employment needs of workers who suffer from this condition.
9. Legal and administrative decisions outside of medical diagnosis and treatment are being influenced heavily by internal WCB medical staff. This is primarily the result of inadequate legal attention and administrative direction.
10. Statistical computer coding methods require increased uniformity, specificity, and historical coverage across Canada to assist in VWF description and evaluation, and for administrative and policy planning purposes.
11. There does not appear to be any organized effort for epidemiological investigation, or for claims solicitation.

Unless the disease incidence is fully recognized and properly compensated, workers lose social and economic opportunities to which they are entitled. In addition, unless the actual incidence and real costs of VWF are registered fully within the compensation system, a "total loss cost" approach to prevention cannot be expected to perform well. It is through the impact of employer assessment costs and compensation costs that prevention, technological and medical research will be stimulated.

ACKNOWLEDGEMENTS

I wish to express my appreciation to the trade union, medical and WCB correspondents and direct sources listed in this paper. In particular, I would thank Dr. W. Whitehead and Mr. K. Mason of the British Columbia WCB who provided responses on short notice and with unfailing courtesy.

REFERENCES

1. Reasons CE, Ross L, Paterson C. The Assault on the Worker. Occup Health and Safety in Canada, Scarborough Ont: Butterworth, 1981.
2. Ison TG. The dimensions of industrial disease. Kingston Ontario. Queen's University, Industrial Relations Centre, 1978. (Research and Current Issues 35: 1-2).
3. Laroche GP. Traumatic vasospastic disease in chain saw operators. Can Med Assoc J 1976; 115: 1217-1221.
4. American Medical Association. Vascular disease affecting the extremities. AMA Guides to the Evaluation of Permanent Impairment. Chicago: American Medical Association, 1977.
5. Burton D. Vibration-Induced White Finger Disease. Sub nom "Raynaud's Phenomenon," "White Hand Syndrome": Guidelines for Adjudication. Ontario Workman's Compensation Board. Claims Adjudication Branch Procedure Manual. Toronto Ont: Government of Ontario, 1977.
6. British Columbia Workers' Compensation Board. Certain industrial diseases. Decision #333, Reporter Series, 1981; 5: 96-98.
7. McKinnon CR, Kemp WN. Vibration syndrome. Can Med Assoc J 1946; 54: 472-477.
8. British Columbia Workers' Compensation Board. Decision of the WCB Commissioners, Claim #XY78068461, 27 June 1980.
9. British Columbia Workers' Compensation Board. Permanent Disability Evaluation Schedule - "Upper Extremity". Items A(8), A(16), A(19).
10. International Woodworkers of America. Survey of Professional Chain Saw Users. IWA Research Department 1979. (unpublished).
11. Brubaker RL, Bates DV, Mackenzie CJG, Eng PR. The Prevalence of Vibration White Finger Disease Among Fallers in Coastal British Columbia. Vancouver BC: Univ of British Columbia, 1982. (unpublished).

DISCUSSION

T.P. Oliver: In the United Kingdom, compensation payments for Prescribed Diseases are for disability only. If disability is judged to be less than 5%, a lump sum payment is made. If disability is greater than 5%, a weekly pension is awarded, which can be reassessed at a later date. Recovery for loss of earnings must be made in the courts.

Affections Professionnelles Provoquées par les Vibrations Transmises par Certaines Machines-Outils, Outils et Objets—Aspect Médico-Légal

P. Mereau et L. Roure

RESUME: En France les tableaux des Maladies Professionnelles spécifient, d'une part, l'agent ou la cause responsable de la maladie et, d'autre part, les conditions nécessaires et suffisantes pour que l'origine professionnelle soit légalement reconnue. Des arguments d'ordre technique et médical, issus de travaux de recherche effectués au cours de la dernière décennie, ont montré qu'il semblait pour le moins légitime d'en étendre le bénéfice à tous les travaux exposant habituellement aux vibrations transmises aux mains. Ceci fait l'objet du nouveau tableau nº 69 des Maladies Professionnelles. L'éradication du risque repose évidemment sur des améliorations technologiques et la réduction du temps d'exposition. A cet égard, la norme française E 90-402, publiée en 1980, constitue un guide pragmatique pour la mise en oeuvre d'une bonne prévention technique.

ABSTRACT: In France, Occupational Diseases Tables indicate the agent or cause of a disease, and the necessary and sufficient conditions required for its occupational origin to be legally recognized. Technical and medical arguments stemming from research in the last decade have shown that it is at least legitimate to extend benefits to all occupations in which vibration is habitually transmitted to the hands. This is the subject of the new Occupational Diseases Table No. 69. Elimination of risk clearly depends on improved technology and reduced exposure time. In this respect, French Standard E90-402, published in 1980, is a pragmatic guide for the implementation of a sound system of technical prevention.

INTRODUCTION

Les effets pathologiques résultant du maniement habituel de machines vibrantes, telles que marteau-piqueur, meuleuse, tronçonneuse à dents articulées par exemple, ont été décrits par de nombreux auteurs. Toutefois, trop peu d'entre eux ont réussi à établir des relations bi-univoques entre les paramètres qui caractérisent les vibrations, le temps d'exposition des sujets, la nature et la gravité des lésions observées, pour tenter de définir des limites d'exposition s'appuyant sur des données rigoureuses.

L'analyse des spectres vibratoires des marteaux perforateurs, par exemple, permet à cet égard de comprendre pourquoi des syndrômes angio-neurotiques, surtout observés lors de travaux de meulage, polissage, usinage des soies sur machines à rétreindre et d'utilisation de scies à dents articulées, peuvent également être provoqués par l'utilisation d'autres types de machines.

Dans les tableaux nº 35 et nº 48 en vigueur jusqu'au 15 juillet 1980, la liste limitative des travaux cités, ainsi que la durée trop brève du délai de prise en charge, n'autorisaient pas dans tous les cas l'indemnisation de troubles d'origine professionnelle manifeste. Il semblait donc pour le moins légitime d'en étendre le bénéfice à tous les travaux exposant habituellement aux vibrations transmises aux mains, en harmonie avec le tableau homologue du régime agricole. C'est chose acquise depuis le décret nº 80.556 du 15 juillet 1980 révisant et complétant les tableaux de Maladies Professionnelles nº 35 et nº 48, relatifs à la prévention et à la réparation des accidents du travail et des maladies professionnelles.

La présente communication apporte des commentaires d'ordre technique et médical en faveur des dispositions contenues dans le nouveau tableau nº 69. De plus, nous présentons la norme E 90-402 qui comporte des spécifications en vue d'améliorer l'hygiène industrielle et la prévention technique.

I PRINCIPAUX TROUBLES ENGENDRES PAR DES MACHINES VIBRANTES TENUES A LA MAIN

Pour faire face à la difficulté de se baser sur la notion de preuve ou sur les seules constatations médicales, pour certifier qu'une maladie est d'origine professionnelle ou ne l'est pas, le législateur a établi un certain nombre de conditions médicales, techniques et administratives devant être obligatoirement remplies pour qu'une maladie puisse être indemnisée en tant que maladie professionnelle.

Les tableaux des Maladies Professionnelles spécifient, d'une part, l'agent ou la cause responsable de la maladie et, d'autre part, les conditions nécessaires et suffisantes pour que l'origine professionnelle soit légalement reconnue. Ces conditions sont les suivantes: a) lésions ou symptômes pathologiques que doit présenter le sujet, b) le délai de prise en charge, c'est-à-dire le délai maximum entre l'apparition de l'affection et la date à laquelle le travailleur a cessé d'être exposé au risque, c) les travaux susceptibles de provoquer l'affection en cause.

Les troubles et lésions provoqués par le maniement habituel des machines vibrantes sont localisés essentiellement au niveau des membres supérieurs: coudes, poignets, mains et doigts. Toutefois, l'effort généralement important, exigé pour le travail correct de la machine, et le niveau important de la contraction musculaire qui en résulte, facilitent la transmission des vibrations à tout l'organisme (fig. 1). Ils sont très schématiquement de deux ordres: ostéoarticulaires d'une part, angioneurotiques d'autre part.

Comme de coutume en médecine, les symptômes observés ne sont pas spécifiques d'une étiologie déterminée; néanmoins, ils peuvent apparaître associés en syndromes

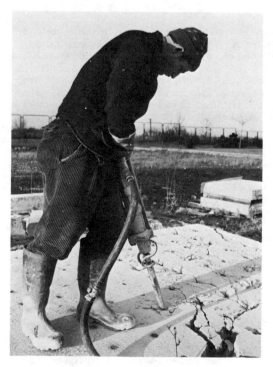

Fig. 1 Ouvrier effectuant un travail au marteau-piqueur. La posture traduit une forte contraction musculaire.

bien caractéristiques ou au contraire réaliser des entités pathologiques mixtes à prédominance de l'une ou l'autre sorte.

1.1 Les troubles ostéoarticulaires

Les plus typiques frappent essentiellement les articulations du coude et du poignet, ainsi que les os du carpe. Ce sont les troubles ostéoarticulaires qui seuls étaient pris en charge au titre des maladies professionnelles indemnisables engendrées par l'emploi habituel des marteaux pneumatiques et engins similaires (tableau nº 35): a) arthrose hyperostosante du coude, et b) lésions du poignet - malacie du semi-lunaire ou maladie de Kienböck, ostéonécrose du scaphoïde carpien ou maladie de Köhler. Le diagnostic de ces affections exigeant un contrôle radiographique.

Les lésions sont en effet objectivables radiologiquement, et l'on observe fréquemment une dissociation étonnante entre les dégâts organiques et la discrétion des signes cliniques et des troubles fonctionnels survenant typiquement au début ou, au contraire, en fin de travail.

1.2 Les troubles angioneurotiques

Ces troubles à composante subjective majeure sont, au contraire des précédents, difficiles à objectiver. Ils voient leur expression localisée essentiellement au niveau de la main.

Leur expression vasculaire se manifeste par des crises à type de doigts morts, dites "syndrome de Raynaud" quand se succèdent, en un laps de temps de l'ordre de quelques minutes à un quart d'heure, les trois phases classiques: "ischémie" des doigts qui apparaissent blancs et insensibles (doigts morts), "cyanose" ou coloration bleue des téguments plus ou moins étendue à toute la main, "récupération" à type de congestion locale douloureuse.

Les troubles nerveux périphériques d'accompagnement altèrent globalement la sensibilité mais surtout sa composante tactile, selon une topographie variable.

Seuls étaient pris en charge, au titre des maladies professionnelles indemnisables, les troubles angioneurotiques limités aux doigts, prédominant à l'index et au médius, s'accompagnant de troubles de la sensibilité provoqués par les travaux de meulage et de polissage avec présentation manuelle de la pièce ou de l'outil, les travaux effectués au moyen de tronçonneuses à chaîne, les travaux sur machine à rétreindre, ainsi que les crampes de la main (tableau nº 48).

II TABLEAU NO 69 DES MALADIES
    PROFESSIONNELLES

En l'état antérieur des tableaux nº 35 et nº 48 du régime général des maladies professionnelles, la liste limitative des travaux cités n'autorisait pas dans tous les cas l'indemnisation de troubles d'origine professionnelle manifeste. Ils ne permettaient pas l'indemnisation de troubles angioneurotiques des extrémités engendrés par la manipulation de marteaux-perforateurs. Or, il apparaît dans ce cas précis que la nature professionnelle de cette maladie invalidante est certaine et que son degré de handicap est fonction de l'ancienneté dans le poste (1 et 2); la confirmation en a été donnée en l'occurrence tant par les épreuves paracliniques mises au point en la circonstance que par l'analyse des spectres vibratoires, qui a permis de comprendre pourquoi les syndromes angioneurotiques peuvent être également engendrés par l'utilisation de marteaux-perforateurs.

De fait, d'autres arguments viennent infirmer une classification des maladies professionelles par trop schématique. Certains auteurs attribuent la survenue d'une pathologie à des phénomènes autres que les vibrations. Amphoux, Gentaz et Sevin avancent l'hypothèse corroborée par les conclusions identiques d'auteurs étrangers (enquête du CEDARR, Centre Viggo-Petersen) et étayée par des arguments cliniques, selon laquelle la maladie de Kienböck pourrait être la forme évoluée d'une fracture méconnue du semi-lunaire (3).

Certains auteurs, tel Christophers (4), vont jusqu'à émettre l'opinion que les vibrations n'ont aucune influence et que seul le froid serait responsable du syndrome de Raynaud. En outre, la distinction classique entre troubles ostéoarticulaires et vasculo-nerveux, en fonction de la fréquence dominante des vibrations d'après le type de machine manié, mérite d'être nuancée.

Ainsi, des études de Mosinger et Col mettent en évidence, à l'aide de techniques d'exploration du système neuro-vasculaire, que ce dernier subit une nette influence sous l'effet des vibrations émises par les marteaux pneumatiques (5).

Dans la perspective de l'établissement d'un nouveau tableau, il est apparu nécessaire d'apporter des éléments nouveaux en cas de maladie constituée. En ce qui concerne la désignation des travaux susceptibles de provoquer la maladie, il a semblé à la fois plus logique et plus légitime d'étendre le bénéfice de la présomption d'origine professionnelle indistinctement à tous les travaux effectués à l'aide de machines-outils tenues à la main figurant au tableau n° 35 qu'au tableau n° 48 du régime général, dans le double souci

Tableau 1. Affections professionnelles provoquées par les vibrations transmises par certaines machines-outils, outils et objets (tableau n° 69 décret du 15 juillet 1980).

Désignation des maladies	Délai de prise en charge	Travaux susceptibles de provoquer ces maladies
Affections ostéoarticulaires: - arthrose hyperostosante du coude, - malacie du semi-lunaire (1) (maladie de Kienböck), - ostéonécrose du scaphoïde carpien (maladie de Köhler). Le diagnostic de ces affections exige un contrôle radiographique.	1 an	Travaux exposant habituellement aux vibrations transmises par: - les machines-outils tenues à la main, notamment les machines percutantes telles que les marteaux piqueurs et les marteaux burineurs, les machines rotopercutantes telles que les marteaux perforateurs, les machines rotatives telles que les meuleuses et les tronçonneuses, les machines alternatives telles que les ponceuses et les scies sauteuses,
Troubles angioneurotiques de la main tels que crampes de la main prédominant à l'index et au médius pouvant s'accompagner de troubles prolongés de la sensibilité.	1 an	- les outils associés à certaines des machines précitées notamment dans les travaux de burinage, - les objets façonnés, notamment dans les travaux de meulage et de polissage et les travaux sur machine à rétreindre.

(1) Malacie ou ramollisement ne doit pas se confondre avec maladie.

Mereau et al.: Affections professionnelles

d'harmonisation avec le tableau homologue du régime agricole et d'équilibrer la protection sociale dont bénéficient les ressortissants des deux régimes. Il était par ailleurs souhaitable d'adopter une classification plus précise qui s'inspire des distinctions introduites selon le mode de transmission des vibrations (corps d'une machine, outil associé, pièce façonnée).

Le délai de prise en charge des troubles angioneurotiques, compte tenu du handicap social persistant, engendré essentiellement par les troubles prolongés de la sensibilité, et susceptible de s'aggraver des mois après cessation de l'exposition au risque, voire de se révéler a posteriori à la faveur d'un changement de climat ou de saison, a été porté à un an à

l'instar des affections ostéoarticulaires. Pour les affections ostéoarticulaires, il est encore difficile de se prononcer en l'absence d'un nombre d'observations suffisant. Toutefois, il est permis de se poser la question à propos d'une observation particuliérement probante d'arthrose des coudes survenue chez un homme ayant travaillé 23 ans au marteau-piqueur, et dont les signes fonctionnels anciens de douleur après effort ne sont devenus invalidants que trois ans après la cessation de l'exposition.

Tout ceci a été pris en compte pour l'élaboration du tableau nº 69 (tableau 1). Il fait l'objet du décret nº 80 556 du 15 juillet 1980 révisant et complétant les tableaux nº 35 et nº 40.

III LES VALEURS LIMITES D'EXPOSITION - LA NORMALISATION

L'éradication du risque repose évidemment sur des améliorations technologiques et la réduction du temps d'exposition. A cet égard, la norme française E 90-402, publiée en 1980, constitue un guide indispensable pour la mise en oeuvre d'une bonne prévention technique.

La norme E 90-402 définit avant tout un domaine d'application (tableau 2) et les méthodes permettant de caractériser l'environnement vibratoire. Elle propose de plus des valeurs en matière de limite provisoire d'exposition (fig. 2). Ces valeurs, dont le principe est admis pour des raisons d'ordre pragmatique, ne sont pas intangibles et devront faire l'objet de révisions périodiques au fur et à mesure de l'amélioration des connaissances.

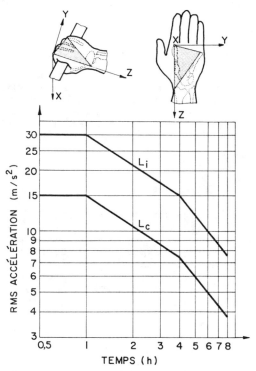

Fig. 2 Valeurs limites de l'accélération équivalente en fonction du temps d'exposition quotidienne (l'accélération équivalente a_{eq} est représentative de la contrainte vibratoire). L_c s'applique à une exposition régulière aux vibrations; L_i s'applique à une exposition intermittente aux vibrations. $a_{eq} = (a_{wx}^2 + a_{wy}^2 + a_{wz}^2)^{\frac{1}{2}}$; a_{wx}, a_{wy}, a_{wz} désignent les valeurs efficaces des accélérations mesurées selon les axes X, Y et Z, puis pondérées au moyen de réseaux produisant l'atténuation suivante: entre 8 Hz et 16 Hz = 0 dB, entre 16 Hz et 1000 Hz = 6 dB/octave.

Tableau 2. Domaine d'application de la norme E 90-402: "guide pour l'évaluation de l'exposition des individus à des vibrations transmises par les mains".

- Vibrations transmises par les mains.

- Vibrations linéaires, périodiques aléatoires et non périodiques dans la gamme de fréquences s'étendant de 8 Hz à 1000 Hz.

  Note: Provisoirement, les excitations répétées du type choc sont prises en considération

- Les limites d'exposition ne concernent que les personnes en bonne santé, c'est à dire aptes à faire fonctionner quotidiennement une machine ou un outil à main vibrant, au cours d'une journée de travail normale.

Mereau et al.: Affections professionnelles

IV CONCLUSION

Le nouveau tableau n⁰ 69 du régime
général des maladies professionnelles abro-
geant et remplaçant les anciens tableaux
n⁰ 35 et n⁰ 48 prend en compte à la fois
des considérations d'ordre médical et des
données techniques récentes.

En effet, en l'état antérieur des
tableaux n⁰ 35 et n⁰ 48, la liste limitative des travaux cités ainsi que la durée
trop brève du délai de prise en charge
n'autorisaient pas dans tous les cas
l'indemnisation de troubles d'origine professionnelle manifeste, qu'il s'agisse de
syndromes angioneurotiques ou d'affections
ostéoarticulaires engendrés indistinctement
par tel ou tel type de machine ou d'outil
vibrant, voire de pièce façonnée tenue à
la main.

BIBLIOGRAPHIE

1. Jayat R, Roure L, Bitsch J. Nature et intensite des vibrations engendrees par les marteaux perforateurs pneumatiques - Troubles angioneurotiques provoques par les vibrations des marteaux perforateurs. lere partie (note documentaire no 1059-87-77).

2. Robert J, Mereau P, Cavelier C, Chameaud J. Enquete effectuee chez 100 mineurs utilisant des marteaux-perforateurs. 2ème partie (note documentaire no 1059-87-77).

3. Amphoux M, Gentaz R, Poli JP, Sevin A. La maladie de Kienböck: un accident du travail? Arch mal prof 1973, 34: 309-319.

4. Christophers AJ. Occupational aspects of Raynaud's disease. Med J Aust 1972; 2: 730-733.

5. Mosinger M, Jullien G, Bourgoin J. Bisschop G. A propos de la pathologie des ouvriers utilisant le marteau-piqueur sur les chantiers du bâtiment et des travaux publics. Arch mal prof 1966; 27: 260-264.

Symbols and Abbreviations

AMP	adenosine-5-phosphate (adenosine monophosphate, muscle adenylic acid)
A/V	anti-vibration (saws, rock drills, etc.)
C	coulomb
°C	degree Celsius
cc	units of swept volumetric capacity of an internal-combustion engine (cm^3)
CNS	central nervous system
cp	centipoise (viscosity)
dB	decibel
dB(A)	A-weighted sound pressure level expressed in dB re 2×10^{-5} Pa
dB(AL)	overall acceleration level expressed in dB re 10^{-5} m/s^2
dB(VL)	overall acceleration level frequency-weighted according to ISO/DIS 5349, 1979, expressed in dB re 10^{-5} m/s^2
DIS	Draft International Standard
div	division (oscilloscope scale, etc.)
ECE/FAO/ILO	Economic Commission for Europe/Food & Agriculture Organization/International Labour Organization
EMG	electromyography
G	acceleration due to gravity
g	gram
GMP	guanosine-5-phosphate (guanosine monophosphate, guanylic acid)
h	hour
HGF	hand grip force
Hz	hertz
IEC	International Electrotechnical Commission
Im	Imaginary part of a complex quantity
in.	inch
I.P.	inter-phalangeal
ISO	International Organization for Standardization
IU	international unit
J	joule
l	litre
ln	logarithm, natural
log	logarithm (to base 10; common logarithm)
m	metre
M	molar
min	minute
M.P.	meta-phalangeal
MVC	maximum voluntary compression force exerted by the hands
N	newton
N	number of subjects
NA	noradrenaline
NIPTS	noise-induced permanent threshold shift
NS	not significant
Pa	pascal
/	per
%	percent
°	phase angle in degrees
p	probability
PT	vibro-tactile threshold of perception
PZT	lead zirconate titanate (transducer material)
r	correlation coefficient
Re	real part of a complex quantity
rms	root mean square

rpm	revolutions per minute
s	second
SD	standard deviation
SEM	standard error of the mean
TOT	Cumulative time exposed to vibration (hours/day × days/year × years)
t-test	Student's t-test
TTS	temporary shift in vibro-tactile threshold of perception
VS	Vibration Syndrome
VWF	Vibration-induced white finger
W	watt
WAS	vector sum of accelerations in three orthogonal directions (usually defined by the coordinate axes of the hand), frequency-weighted according to ISO/DIS 5349, 1979
wk	week
X,Y,Z	coordinate axes of the hand
yr(s)	year(s)

Subject Index

364

see Central nervous system
Axe, handle vibration of, 256

B

Biodynamic models
  dynamic response of the hand-arm:
    see Dynamic response of hand-arm
  four degrees-of-freedom, 121-123, 125-132
    biological implications, 127-128
    comparison with human data, 123, 126-
      127
    dynamic compliance, prediction by, 128
    grip, effect of, 125-126, 129
    physical representation of, 121-122
    theoretical development of, 122, 130-132
    values of parameters for, 125-126
  one degree-of-freedom, 113, 303-304
    comparison with human data, 304
    physical representation of, 304
  three degrees-of-freedom,
    comparison with previous work, 123
    grip, effect of, 124
    values of parameters for, 123-124
  two degrees-of-freedom,
    glove transmissibility, for, 113-114
Blood viscosity
  in the Vibration Syndrome, 67
  whole blood and plasma, 69
Bone changes in VS
  cysts, 5, 180, 184, 186-187
British Standards Institution
  comparison of vibration limits in
    grinding, 328-330, 343, 345

C

Calibration procedure for vibration
    measurement, 229
Callosities
  effect of calluses on permanent vibra-
    tion threshold, 63
  on finger pads and palm, 20
Canadian compensation law and VWF, 349-353
Canadian Standard for chain saw vibration,
    261
Cardiovascular system, effects of vibration
    on blood pressure, 27
  echocardiographic measurements, 26-27
  electrocardiographic findings, 27
Carpal tunnel syndrome
  exclusion in differential diagnosis, 4
  in miners using jack-leg drills, 39-41
Catecholamine, increase in, 29
Caulkers
  compensation for VWF, 343-346
  prevalence of VWF in, 346
Central nervous system and VS
  adaptive response to stressors, 3, 29-30
  autonomic nervous activity, 21, 25, 28, 71
  cardiovascular system, relation with, 25-28
  catecholamine output, 20, 31-37
    excretion of, 274
  cochlear blood flow, 55-58

hypothalmus, excitation of, 29
pathogenesis of VS, 29-30
psychosomatic disorders, 3, 28, 274
regulatory function of, 20-21, 25
role of, 3, 21
stressors, adaptive response to, 3, 29-30
symptoms mediated by 3, 28, 274
  classification of, 5, 340
  compensation for, 339-342
  prevalence of, 273-274
vasoconstriction, influence on, 21, 29-30
    see also: Vasoconstriction and
      Vibration Syndrome
Cessation of exposure, regression of VS with,
    193-195
Chain Saw Manufacturers Association
  vibration test machine, 211-218
Chain saw operators
  blood viscosity levels in, 69
  bone cysts in, 180, 186-187
  compensation for VS, 340-342, 351
  hand grip force in, 45-46
  hearing loss in, 51-58
  latent interval for VWF, 159, 178, 284
  muscle weakness in, 47, 160-161
  nerve disorders in, 181, 273
  noise exposure of, 53
  numbness in, 159-160
  osteoarthritis, osteoporosis in, 180, 186-
    187
  pain in muscles and joints, 272
  prevalence of VS in, 270-274
  prevalence of VWF in, 158-160, 170-171,
    177-178, 263, 270-271
  preventive measures, 170-171: see also
    Prevention of VS
  progression of VS in, 159-162, 269-275
  progression of VWF in, 159-162
    onset, prediction of, 295-296
    prediction of, 285-286
    regression of VWF with use of A/V saws,
      157-167, 169-172, 296-297
    with TOT, 269-276
  tolerable vibration exposures, 297-298:
    see also ISO, and Limits for vibration
    exposure
  vascular disorders in, 16-24, 159, 169-172
    177-185
  vasoconstriction in, 17, 23-24, 163, 270-
    177-185
  vibration exposed to:
    see Chain saw vibration
  vibro-tactile perception, 161-162
  VS in: see also Vibration-induced white
    finger, and Vibration Syndrome
Chain saw vibration
  acceleration data
    A/V saws, 182-184, 199-201, 205-209,
      246-248, 300-301
    comparison with limits, 207, 246-248,
      300-301
    electric, 248, 301
    frequency-weighted component, A/V saws,
      297
    frequency-weighted component, non A/V
      saws, 300
    weighted sum, A/V saws, 204-207, 300-301
    weighted sum, electric saws, 301

369

370

373